EMBODYING INEQUALITY
Epidemiologic Perspectives

Edited by
Nancy Krieger

POLICY, POLITICS, HEALTH AND MEDICINE SERIES
Vicente Navarro, Series Editor

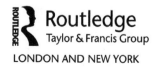

Routledge
Taylor & Francis Group

LONDON AND NEW YORK

First published 2005 by Baywood Publishing Company, Inc.

Published 2017 by Routledge
2 Park Square, Milton Park, Abingdon, Oxfordshire OX14 4RN
711 Third Avenue, New York, NY 10017

First issued in paperback 2016

Routledge is an imprint of the Taylor & Francis Group, an informa business

Library of Congress Catalog Number: 2004045092

Library of Congress Cataloging-in-Publication Data

Embodying inequality : epidemiologic perspectives / edited by Nancy Krieger.
     p. cm. -- (Policy, politics, health and medicine series)
  Includes bibliographical references and index.
  ISBN 0-89503-294-5 (Cloth)
  1. Equality--Health aspects. 2. Diseases--Social aspects. 3. Health--Social aspects. 4. Epidemiology--Social aspects. 5. Social medicine. I. Krieger, Nancy.
II. Series : Policy, politics, health, and medicine series (Unnumbered)

  RA418.E352 2004
  362.1--dc22

                         2004045092

ISBN 13: 978-0-415-78385-9 (pbk)
ISBN 13: 978-0-89503-294-2 (hbk)

Contents

SECTION II
Empirical Investigation: Social Epidemiology at Work

Introduction:
Embodiment, Inequality, and Epidemiology:
What are the Connections?

PURPOSE OF THIS VOLUME: ENHANCING EPIDEMIOLOGIC
ANALYSIS OF SOCIAL INEQUALITIES IN HEALTH

To advance epidemiologic analysis of social inequalities in health, this volume draws from articles published in the *International Journal of Health Services,* which for the past quarter of a century has played a critical role in providing an essential forum for advancing theory, research, and practice, linking social justice and public health (1). Prepared in response to an invitation from Dr. Vicente Navarro, Editor-in-Chief of the *International Journal of Health Services,* this collection considers diverse conceptual, methodologic, and substantive challenges that contemporary social epidemiologists confront when analyzing social disparities in health. The intent is to aid efforts to address these inequities by improving understanding of how population patterns of distributions of disease, disability, and death reflect embodied expressions of social inequality (2–4).

Section I, on "Social Epidemiology: History, Hypotheses, Methods, and Measurement," focuses chiefly on theories and constructs useful for analyzing social inequalities in health involving class, race/ethnicity, gender, sexuality, and disability. Rather than construing these aspects of lived experiences of inequality solely as a matter of personal "identities" and "behaviors," these chapters consider how the political and economic context in which people live enhances—or destroys— their ability to live healthy, dignified lives.

Section II, "Empirical Investigation: Social Epidemiology at Work," moves from considering concepts and critiques to their critical application via concrete analyses of diverse determinants of social inequalities in health. Its chapters explore various aspects of five principal pathways by which people embody social inequality (3, 4), including but not restricted to the psychosocial exposures that are the focus of one prominent strand of contemporary social epidemiologic research (3, 5, 6). These five pathways are:

1. Economic and social deprivation, including lack of access to adequate food, housing, and physical and social recreation;

2. Toxic substances, pathogens and hazardous conditions, at work, in the neighborhood, and more generally;
3. Social trauma, including institutional and interpersonal discrimination and violence, plus additional psychosocial stressors;
4. Targeted marketing of commodities that can harm health, e.g., junk food and psychoactive substances (alcohol, tobacco, and other licit and illicit drugs); and
5. Inadequate or degrading medical care.

Together, these chapters clarify the importance of conceptualizing hypotheses in relation to the political and material as well as psychological conditions in which people live, love, work, fight, play, ail, and die.

Each chapter was selected from prior issues of the *International Journal of Health Services* published between 1990 and 2000 (with the exception of the chapters in the section on history). It is my hope that by bringing together the diverse articles in this volume, critical thinking in social epidemiology will gain yet more critical mass, thereby improving the prospects that this work will contribute significantly to global efforts to secure social equity in health.

SO WHAT ARE THE CONNECTIONS BETWEEN EMBODIMENT, INEQUALITY, AND EPIDEMIOLOGY?

Before jumping into the specific analyses advanced by each chapter in this volume, it is useful first to reflect on their common themes, concerning:

1. Embodiment,
2. Social inequality and injustice, and
3. Social inequalities in health.

The central question being: What are the connections that our human bodies make and manifest every day between injustice, disease, and death, on the one hand, and social justice, human rights, and well-being, on the other (2–4)? Or, stated another way: How do the contours of power and inequity reveal themselves through population distributions of health, body size, disease, disability, and death? And why does it matter?

We humans are mortal, after all. It is no mystery that each of us will die. Yet how we live—and how and when we die, with what degree of suffering—is at once a profoundly social *and* biological question. It is biological because it involves our literal beings and the complex interplay, within our bodies and our embodied minds, of exposure, susceptibility, and resistance across the lifecourse. It is social because current and changing population distributions of the burden of illness, disability, and premature mortality can yield evidence of the range of possibilities of human well-being and delimit the existence and degree of preventable suffering. And it is social *and* biological because, as implied by the concept of "embodiment," what we manifest in our bodies—and how we ail and what therapies we can access—is simultaneously an expression of our experiences in the world and their literal incorporation within us (2–4). While *how* we bring the world into us depends in part on our biological constitution (itself a dynamic interplay between exposure, development, growth, and gene expression), *what* we bring in is historically and socially contingent. Otherwise, there would be no variation in population health across time, place, and social groups.

Or such is the claim of social epidemiology and related fields dedicated to explicating, explicitly, population patterns of health, including social inequalities in health, and their societal determinants (see Box 1) (7–15). The rationale for this work is not to "prove" that injustice is "bad": it is, by definition. Nor is it to suggest that the task of defining, analyzing, or rectifying social disparities in health is uniquely that of epidemiologists or other health professionals. Rather, the purpose of carrying out epidemiologic work pertaining to social disparities in health is threefold. At issue are:

1. *Monitoring:* rigorously documenting current and changing population distributions of—and so disparities in—health, disease, and well-being, to provide a picture of what the problems are within and across diverse societies, over time (9, 16–19);
2. *Etiology:* explaining the observed population patterns in relation to temporally relevant and changing distributions of determinants of and deterrents to the specified outcomes, recognizing that multiple levels and multiple pathways are likely involved (2–6, 8–15); and
3. *Action:* providing evidence relevant to galvanizing public concern about social disparities in health and informing societal efforts, within and across diverse regions and nations, to eliminate these disparities (1–20).

To take on any of these tasks, social epidemiologists necessarily must draw on the theories, concepts, and work of—and often collaborate with—scientists, practitioners, and advocates in myriad disciplines and fields concerned with social justice, human rights, and both ecological and biological integrity. Among the many critical concepts that can be usefully adopted by—but do not originate in—epidemiologic thinking and practice are, in the social realm, inequality, injustice, power, exploitation, oppression, social justice, solidarity, and human rights, and, biologically, those of evolution, growth, development, homeostasis, allostasis, and ecology. By employing a mix of social and biological insights, social epidemiologists can generate quantitative evidence on the population patterning of health, empirically test hypotheses about determinants of these patterns, and provide systematic analysis of the likely strengths and inevitable limitations of these quantitative data and analyses.

To offer but one example of a social epidemiologic theory drawing on social and biological constructs, the theoretical perspective informing this volume is that of ecosocial theory (2–4, 20, 21). This theory explicitly builds on the insights

		Box 1
		An argument for social epidemiology and its use of social and biological reasoning to analyze social inequalities in health (8)
Argument #1	Thesis 1	People are social beings who live in socially constituted societies.
	Thesis 2	People are biological organisms, *Homo sapiens*.
	Deduction	People live in the world simultaneously as social and biological beings.
Argument #2	Thesis 1	Expression of biological traits depends on the conditions under which biological organisms live, including their interactions with other organisms.
	Thesis 2	Disease, disability, death, and health are states of being involving expression of biological traits.
	Deduction	Disease, disability, death, and health are embodied expressions of conditions under which organisms live.
Argument #3	Thesis 1	One component of explaining a phenomenon is HOW it occurs.
	Thesis 2	One component of explaining a phenomenon is WHY it occurs.
	Deduction	Explanations of phenomena that address HOW *and* WHY they occur are more complete than explanations addressing only HOW they occur.
Argument #4	Thesis 1	Epidemiology is the study of population distributions of disease, disability, death, and health and their determinants and deterrents, across time and space.
	Thesis 2	Population patterns of disease, disability, and death reflect population distributions of exposure, susceptibility, and resistance to conditions comprising sufficient causes for (or deterrents to) the specified outcomes and occurring during the etiologically relevant time interval.
	Deduction	Epidemiologic explanations of current and changing patterns of disease, disability, and death must be compatible with temporally relevant and changing distributions of determinants of and deterrents to the specified outcomes.

of related trends of thought pertaining to the social production of disease (9, 14, 15, 22–25), which it complements by weaving in additional insights of evolutionary and developmental biology plus ecology (26–33). In brief, this theory of disease distribution is guided by the question "who and what drives current and changing patterns of social inequalities in health?" Its four core constructs are (2, 3, 21):

1. *"embodiment,"* referring to how we literally embody, that is, biologically incorporate, our lived experience, thereby creating population patterns of health and disease;
2. *"pathways of embodiment,"* referring to how there are often multiple pathways, involving multiple levels, to a given outcome (via diverse physical, chemical, biological, and social exposures);
3. *"cumulative interplay of exposure, susceptibility, and resistance across the lifecourse,"* since all three matter; and
4. *"accountability and agency,"* both for social inequalities in health and for ways they are—or are not—analyzed and addressed.

The "eco" in "ecosocial" thus refers to literal—and not just metaphorical—notions of ecology, recognizing that we simultaneously are but one biological species among many, and one whose labor and ideas literally have transformed the face of this earth. The "social" in turn draws attention to features of the social realm—created by humans, with accountability an option—that shape, if not drive, inequitable population patterns of disease, disability, and death. The goal is to integrate social and biological reasoning to yield new insights into—and new possibilities for addressing—both mechanisms of disease causation and determinants of the population distribution of health.

To see how this kind of thinking is gaining headway in the United States, due largely to the work of many critical analysts of societal determinants of health, consider the model of population health included in the recently released report *Shaping a Vision of Health Statistics for the 21st Century* (24), issued by the U.S. Department of Health and Human Services Data Council, the Centers for Disease Control and Prevention, the National Center for Health Statistics, and the National Committee on Vital and Health Statistics (Figure 1). Importantly, this model explicitly places population health—and its distribution—at the center, literally. Moreover, determinants of this distribution are explicitly framed in terms of "place and time," "context," and "community attributes." Included among the influences on population health explicitly listed are not only the political context, including public policies and laws, but also racism, economics, workplaces and other aspects of the built environment, the "natural" environment, biological characteristics, "collective lifestyles," health services, and public health programs, to name a few. In such a model, the health of a population and its constituent social groups by definition exists in a societal and ecological context and is historically contingent. Thus, at any given moment, the average level and distribution of population health is shaped by the social and physical conditions

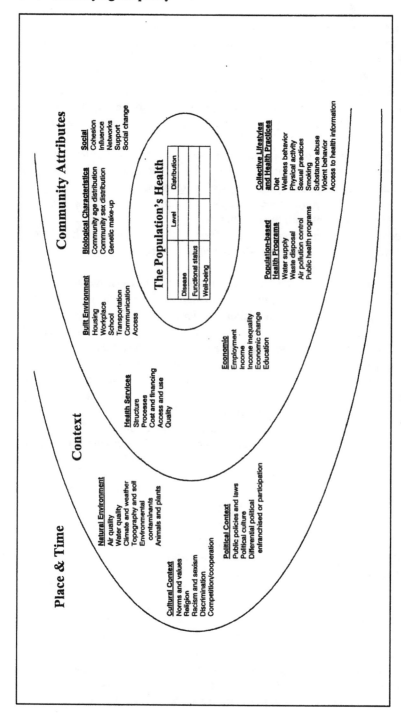

Figure 1. Determinants of population health, as presented in the U.S. federal report "Sharing a vision of health statistics for the 21st century" (2002) (34).

of workplaces, neighborhoods, regional economies and ecologies, and society at large, as they affect social groups across the lifecourse, in successive historical generations.

From this vantage, social epidemiologic perspectives can usefully complement political and social science analyses of social inequities in health, along with those offered by other disciplines in public health and medicine. In particular, epidemiologic analyses can:

a. help draw attention to comparative shapes and secular trends of population distributions of exposures and outcomes, thereby avoiding confusing what is common with what is "normal" or biologically inevitable; and

b. highlight the importance of evaluating postulated links between exposures and outcomes in relation to plausible etiologic periods and biological pathways.

As one example of apt contrasts of population distributions of health, consider epidemiologic evidence, accumulated since the 1950s, showing that while blood pressure typically increases with age in industrialized societies and in urban locales within largely agricultural nations, this increase is not an inevitable expression of human biology (35–38). Why? Because studies have shown no increase of blood pressure with age among adults living in remote rural areas largely outside of the nexus of market economies (36–38).

Consider too how, during the Depression of the 1930s, conservative commentators downplayed its severity by pointing to a lack of increase in the death rate; in his trenchant rebuttal, Edgar Sydenstricker, one of the era's leading social epidemiologists, argued it was ludicrous to focus on mortality (39, 40). Why? Because causes of death rarely operate instantaneously (except for fatal injuries, homicide, or suicide), such that the health impact would first be expected to manifest in changes in morbidity, not mortality. To prove this point, Sydenstricker organized a massive federally-sponsored 10-city study, the first of its kind, on the health impact of the Depression (39, 41). This study not only provided evidence of the Depression's acute effects on morbidity but also provided some of the first large-scale evidence on the contribution of socioeconomic inequality to U.S. health, overall, and to black/white inequalities in health in particular. Still another contribution was to set the basis for the first U.S. National Health Survey, in 1935, forerunner to the current National Health Interview Survey (42).

Nearly three-quarters of a century later, at the time of preparing this volume, debates like those engaging Sydenstricker about the extent and causes of—and solutions to—social disparities in health remain rife within the United States and more globally (1–25, 43, 44). That these arguments continue is no surprise, as contending parties differentially benefiting from and harmed by inequitable distributions of power and property advance their respective positions upholding and opposing the status quo. By generating rigorous evidence that clarifies it is social injustice, not random individual failures or innate inferiority, that produces social inequalities in health, social epidemiologists can make their particular vital contribution to the global discourse animating, and aligned with, efforts to create a more just, caring, and sustainable world.

REFERENCES

1. Navarro, V. Twenty-fifth anniversary: An interview with Vicente Navarro, Editor-in-Chief,. *Int. J. Health Serv.* 25: 1–10, 1995.
2. Krieger, N. Epidemiology and the web of causation: Has anyone seen the spider? *Soc. Sci. Med.* 39: 887–903, 1994.
3. Krieger, N. Theories for social epidemiology in the 21st century: An ecosocial perspective. *Int. J. Epidemiol.* 30: 668–677, 2001.
4. Krieger, N. Embodying inequality: A review of concepts, measures, and methods for studying health consequences of discrimination. *Int. J. Health Serv.* 29: 295–352, 1999.
5. Lynch, J. W., et al. Income inequality and mortality: Importance to health of individual incomes, psychological environment, or material conditions. *Br. Med. J.* 320: 1200–1204, 2000.
6. Elstad, J. I. The psycho-social perspective on social inequalities in health. In *The Sociology of Health Inequalities,* edited by M. Bartley, D. Blane, and G. Davey Smith, pp. 39–58. Blackwell, Oxford, 1998.
7. Krieger, N. A glossary for social epidemiology. *J. Epidemiol. Community Health* 55: 693–700, 2001.
8. Krieger, N. Commentary: Society, biology, and the logic of social epidemiology. *Int. J. Epidemiol.* 30: 44–46, 2001.
9. Shaw, M., et al. *The Widening Gap: Health Inequalities and Policy in Britain.* Policy Press, Bristol, UK, 1999.
10. Berkman, L., and Kawachi, I. (eds.). *Social Epidemiology.* Oxford University Press, Oxford, 2000.
11. Marmot, M., and Wilkinson, R. G. (eds.). *Social Determinants of Health.* Oxford University Press, Oxford, 1999.
12. Evans, T., et al. (eds.). *Challenging Inequities in Health: From Ethics to Action.* Oxford University Press, Oxford, 2001.
13. Leon, D., and Walt, G. (eds.). *Poverty, Inequality, and Health: An International Perspective.* Oxford University Press, Oxford, 2001.
14. Navarro, V. *Crisis, Health, and Medicine: A Social Critique.* Tavistock, New York, 1986.
15. Navarro, V. (ed.) *The Political Economy of Social Inequalities: Consequences for Health and Quality of Life.* Baywood Publishing Co., Amityville, NY, 2002.
16. Krieger, N., Chen, J. T., and Ebel, G. Can we monitor socioeconomic inequalities in health? A survey of U.S. Health Departments' data collection and reporting practices. *Public Health Reports* 112: 481–491, 1997.
17. Krieger, N., et al. Geocoding and monitoring US socioeconomic inequalities in mortality and cancer incidence: Does choice of area-based measure and geographic level matter? *The Public Health Disparities Geocoding Project. Am. J. Epidemiol.* 156: 471–482, 2002.

18. Krieger, N., et al. Race/ethnicity, gender, and monitoring socioeconomic gradients in health: A comparison of area-based socioeconomic measures. *The Public Health Disparities Geocoding Project. Am. J. Public Health,* 93: 1655-1671, 2003.
19. Braveman, P., Starfield, B., and Geiger, H. J. World Health Report 2000: How it removes equity from the agenda for public health monitoring and policy. *Br. Med. J.* 323: 678-681, 2001.
20. Krieger, N., and Gruskin, S. Frameworks matter: Ecosocial and health and human rights perspectives on women and health—The case of tuberculosis. *J. Am. Women's Med. Assoc.* 56: 137-142, 2001.
21. Krieger, N. Ecosocial theory. In *Encyclopedia of Health and Behavior,* edited by N. Anderson. Sage, New York, forthcoming.
22. Navarro, V. U.S. Marxist scholarship in the analysis of health and medicine. *Int. J. Health Serv.* 15: 525-545, 1985.
23. Franco, S., et al. *Debates en Medicina Social [Debates in Social Medicine].* Pan-American Health Organization/Latin American Association of Social Medicine, Quito, Ecuador, 1991.
24. Doyal, L. *The Political Economy of Health.* South End Press, Boston, 1979.
25. Conrad, P., and Kern, R. (eds.). *The Sociology of Health and Illness: Critical Perspectives.* St. Martin's Press, New York, 1981.
26. Mayr, E. *The Growth of Biological Thought: Diversity, Evolution and Inheritance.* Harvard University Press, Cambridge, MA, 1982.
27. Gould, S. J. *The Structure of Evolutionary Theory.* Belknap Press of Harvard University Press, Cambridge, MA, 2002.
28. Sober, E. *Philosophy of Biology,* 2nd ed. Westview Press, Boulder, CO, 2000.
29. Roughgarden, J. *Primer of Ecological Theory.* Prentice Hall, Upper Saddle River, NJ, 1998.
30. Peterson, D. L., and Parker, V. T. (eds.). *Ecological Scale: Theory and Application.* Columbia University Press, New York, 1989.
31. McMichael, A. J. *Human Frontiers, Environments, and Disease: Past Patterns, Uncertain Futures.* Cambridge University Press, Cambridge, UK, 2001.
32. Levins, R., and Lewontin, R. *The Dialectical Biologist.* Harvard University Press, Cambridge, MA, 1985.
33. Kuh, D., and Ben-Shlomo, Y. (eds.). *A Lifecourse Approach to Chronic Disease Epidemiology: Tracing the Origins of Ill-Health from Early to Adult Life.* Oxford University Press, Oxford, UK, 1997.
34. Friedman, D. J., Hunter, E. L., and Parrish, R. G. *Shaping a Vision of Health Statistics for the 21st Century.* Department of Health and Human Services Data Council, Centers for Disease Control and Prevention, National Center for Health Statistics, and National Committee on Vital and Health Statistics, Washington, DC, 2002. www.ncvhs.hhs.gov/hsvision/ (March 2003).
35. Pickering, G. W. *High Blood Pressure,* pp. 216-220. Grune & Stratton, New York, 1955.
36. Carvalho, J. J., et al. Blood pressure in four remote populations in the INTERSALT study. *Hypertension* 14: 238-246, 1989.
37. Eliott, P. High blood pressure in the community. In *Handbook of Hypertension,* edited by C. J. Bulpitt, pp. 1-18. Elsevier, Amsterdam, 2000.

38. Cruickshank, J. K., et al. Sick genes, sick individuals or sick populations with chronic disease? The emergence of diabetes and high blood pressure in African-origin populations. *Int. J. Epidemiol.* 30: 111–117, 2001.

39. Sydenstricker, E. Health and the depression. *Milbank Memorial Fund Quarterly* 12: 273–280, 1934.

40. Sydenstricker, E. *Health and Environment.* McGraw-Hill, New York, 1933.

41. Perrott, G. S. J., and Collins, S. D. Relation of sickness to income and income change in ten surveyed communities. Health and Depression Studies No. 1: Method of study and general results for each locality. *Public Health Rep.* 50: 595–622, 1935.

42. U.S. Department of Health, Education, and Welfare. *Origin and Program of the U.S. National Health Survey.* Health Statistics Series A1, p. 3. May 1958.

43. Navarro, V. A critique of social capital. *Int. J. Health Serv.* 32: 424–432, 2002.

44. Navarro, V., and Shi, L. The political context of social inequalities in health. *Soc. Sci. Med.* 52: 481–491, 2001.

SECTION I

Social Epidemiology: History, Hypotheses, Methods, and Measurement

Preface to Section I

When considering social inequalities in health, the first point, perhaps obvious, is that awareness of class and other social inequalities in health is not exactly new. In fact, descriptions of injurious effects of destitution and hard work on health can be found in documents dating back to the earliest known medical texts.

For example, a document dating back to around 2000 BCE in Egypt, during the time of the prosperous Middle Kingdom, recounted (1, pp. 259–260):

> . . . I have seen the metal worker at this task at the mouth of his furnace. His fingers were like the hide of crocodiles; he stank worse than fish spawn. . . . The stone mason seeks work in every hard stone. When he sits down at dusk, his thighs and his back are broken. . . . The barber shaves till late in the evening. He goes from street to street seeking for men to shave. He strains his arms to fill his belly and works as indefatigably as a bee. . . . The weaver in the workshop is worse off than the women [who must always sit in the house]. He squats with his knees to his belly and does not breathe fresh air. He bribes the doorkeeper with bread that he may see the light. . . .

The Hippocratic treatise, *On Diet,* likely written in the 4th century BCE, likewise observed that only a small minority of the Greek population—its vaunted citizens—had the wherewithal to lead a healthy life (2, p. 240). The vast majority—upwards of 75% of the population—could not (2, 3), including the "metics, freedmen, traders, artisans, farm laborers, and other slaves," described in the treatise as "the mass of people who drink and eat what they happen to get, and who are obliged to work, and to travel by land and sea in order to make a living, who are exposed to unwholesome heat and unwholesome cold, and who otherwise lead an irregular life" and so "who cannot, neglecting all, take care of their health" (2, p. 240).

These kinds of comments, however, were chiefly asides. What these early texts mainly provided was advice on how to live well, directed to those who could afford to live leisured lives precisely because others did the hard labor allowing them this leisure (1–4). Indeed, it would not be for another 2000 years, in the 16th century CE writings of Georg Agricola (1494–1555) and Paracelsus (1493–1541), followed by Bernadino Ramazzini's (1633–1714) celebrated opus, published in 1700, *The Diseases of Workers,* that the question of how work affects health would first attain sustained treatment in European medical texts (4, 5). It likewise would not be until the mid-19th century that the impact of slavery on the health of black Americans would receive serious attention in U.S. medical journals (6–9). Nor would it be until the early 20th century that women's work—whether at home or in the paid labor force—would begin to be legitimately analyzed as a determinant of women's health (10, 11), and not until the late 20th century that the invidious effects of discrimination on the health status of lesbian, gay, bisexual, and transgender populations would be openly considered by leading medical and public health institutions (12, 13). And although serious investigation of socioeconomic inequalities in health can readily be traced to the early 19th century, as discussed below, it has only been in the past decade that this topic has become part of the mainstream U.S. public health agenda.

Which leads to a second point: that class and other forms of inequitable social relationships can shape the very picture people draw of social inequalities in health—and hence what they do (or do not do) to address them. At issue are both description AND explanation. In other words, social inequality can influence: what is seen—or ignored—by whom; how these patterns are—or are not—explained; and what sorts of remedies are—or are not—proposed. One implication is social inequalities in health—however real—can be ignored and rendered invisible if the data to document them are not collected, whether by conscious design or unconscious neglect (16). A second implication is that even if the data are collected, and none dispute the reality of the disparate health status between the groups at issue, there can still be major controversies over WHY these disparities exist and WHO should do WHAT about them.

Consider only centuries of debate in the United States over the poor health of black Americans (6–9). In the 1830s and 1840s, contrary schools of thought asked: is it because blacks are intrinsically inferior to whites?—the majority view—or because they are enslaved and economically impoverished?—as argued by, among others, Dr. James McCune Smith (1811–1865) and Dr. James S. Rock (1825–1866), two of the country's first credentialed African American physicians (6). In contemporary parlance, the questions become: do the causes lie in bad genes?, bad behaviors?, or accumulations of bad living and working conditions born of egregious social policies, past and present (8, 9)? The fundamental tension, then and now, is between individualistic versus contextualized theories, in other words, theories that seek causes of social inequalities in health in innate versus imposed, or individual versus societal, characteristics.

In light of the importance of providing historical context to contemporary social epidemiologic research, the first part of *Section I* focus on "The Historical Roots of Contemporary Social Epidemiology." Chapter 1, by Howard Waitzkin, on "The Social Origins of Illness: A Neglected History," was first published in *International Journal of Health Services* in 1981 (17). Reviving insights about links between social justice and health developed in Europe by Friedrich Engels and Rudolf Virchow in the mid-19th century, and by Salvador Allende in Chile in the 1970s, this chapter usefully delineates how not only health but science is shaped by the politics of its time. Chapter 2, "Measuring Social Inequalities in

Health in the United States: A Historical Review, 1900–1950," by Nancy Krieger and Elizabeth Fee, then considers approaches taken to documenting and analyzing social inequalities in health in the United States in the first half of the 20th century (18). First published in *International Journal of Health Services* in 1996, this chapter was one of several papers prepared for a 1994 workshop on class inequalities in health organized by Nancy Krieger and Nancy Moss under the auspices of the National Institutes of Health (19). Chapter 3, by Richard Crawford, "You are Dangerous to Your Health: The Ideology and Politics of Victim Blaming," first published in *International Journal of Health Services* in 1977, presents a now classic analysis of conservative attempts to obscure the social causation of disease (20). Lambasting apologetics for social inequalities in health in a spirit kindred to that of Engels and Virchow, this chapter remains a timely reminder of the social forces, actors, and frameworks actively deployed to uphold the privilege of a powerful economic minority at the expense of the economic majority.

Taken together, the chapters in this first part of *Secion I* forcefully highlight the fact that issues of class and other social inequalities in health are not new. Instead, conceptual frameworks and the ability to generate empirical evidence to address these issues have existed for over 150 years. Each generation, however, faces the challenges of documenting and advancing knowledge about the determinants of the social inequalities in health that it confronts, recognizing that the causes of disease and death, and their prevalence, change over time.

Acknowledging this challenge, the second set of chapters in *Section I,* grouped under the rubric of "Contemporary Social Epidemiologic Framework and Constructs," elucidate conceptual and methodologic issues germane to analysis of current social inequalities in health involving class, race/ethnicity, gender, sexuality, and disability. Although focused principally on health in the United States and in European countries, these essays raise important ideas with more global relevance.

Thus, Chapter 4, by Nancy Krieger, concerns "Embodying Inequality: A Review of Concepts, Measures, and Methods for Studying Health Consequences of Discrimination," with discrimination considered in relation to race/ethnicity, gender, sexuality, and social class, especially as manifested in the United States (21). First published *International Journal of Health Services* in 1999, plus included in the first textbook on *Social Epidemiology* (22), this chapter constitutes the first systematic review on the ways that discrimination can harm health, both outright and by distorting production of epidemiologic knowledge about determinants of population health. Related, Chapter 5, by David Williams, on "Race/Ethnicity and Socioeconomic Status: Measurement and Methodological Issues," underscores the importance of employing sound, theoretically informed measures to analyze how injurious race and class relations together drive social inequalities in health (23). Prepared for the same 1994 NIH conference as Chapter 2, and first published in *International Journal of Health Services* in 1996, this chapter importantly emphasizes that while racial/ethnic disparities in health cannot be analyzed absent consideration of class, nor can they be reduced to a matter of economics only. Discrimination, migration, and culture also matter.

Further expanding discussion of the health impact of discrimination, via affecting analysis of racial/ethnic disparities in health, Chapter 6, by Carles Muntaner, Craig Nagoshi, and Chamberlain Diala, examines "Racial Ideology and Explanations for Health Inequalities among Middle-Class Whites" (24). One sorry conclusion, given that this chapter was first published in *International Journal of Health Services* in 2001, is that the kind of victim-blaming searingly indicted in Chapter 3 by Crawford regrettably remains alive and well, whereby white university students attributed racial/ethnic inequalities in health chiefly to a mix of innate biology and poor "lifestyle" choices. Importantly, as Muntaner et al. underscore, these kinds of explanations additionally justify class inequalities in health. Why? Because they focus attention on the "bad" health behaviors of the economically disadvantaged rather than on the economic behaviors of those with the power and resources who seek to retain their privilege via economic, labor, and tax policies limiting the economic resources and power of workers and their families, including the working and unemployed poor.

Critical concepts for analyzing economic inequalities in health are then proposed in Chapter 7, by Greg Duncan, on "Income Dynamics and Health," first published in *International Journal of Health Services* in 1996 (25). Also prepared for the 1994 conference on class and health, this chapter usefully highlights the importance of considering not only the impact of fluctuations of income across the lifecourse but also the significance of early life economic circumstances on adult health. The adverse impact of unemployment in health is next considered in Chapter 8 by Samuel E. D. Shortt, in relation to the question "Is Unemployment Pathogenic? A Review of Current Concepts with Lessons for Policy Planners" (26). Augmenting analyses concerned principally with the material effects of economic deprivation, this chapter, first published in *International Journal of Health Services* in 1996, delves into debates regarding psychosocial aspects of the impact of unemployment on health. A central point is that people need to live meaningful lives, replete with meaningful work, above and beyond having access to an income adequate for meeting bodily needs for food, clothing, and shelter. Or, as famously articulated by the textile workers in Lawrence, Massachusetts, in their historic strike at the turn of the 20th century, what is needed are "bread and roses," not just one or the other (27).

Past and present connections between health disparities involving class, race/ethnicity, and gender are then explored in Chapter 9, by Nancy Krieger and Elizabeth Fee, on "Man-Made Medicine and Women's Health: The Biopolitics of Sex/Gender and Race/Ethnicity," first published in *International Journal of Health Services* in 1994 (28). Using an historical perspective to enhance conceptual clarity about distinctions, similarities, and linkages between these different aspects of inequality, the authors argue for alternative approaches to collecting population health data and conducting epidemiologic analyses premised on explicit and conjoint analysis of racial/ethnic, gender, and class inequality. The necessity of employing an historical and theoretically informed approach to understanding health disparities among lesbian and gay populations is likewise evident in Chapter 10, by Kathleen Erwin, on "Interpreting the Evidence: Competing Paradigms and the Emergence of Lesbian and Gay Suicide as a "Social Fact" (29). First published in *International Journal of Health Services* in 1993, this chapter critically compares two interpretations of the same "fact"— higher rates of suicide among lesbians and gays—with one casting this as a sign of innate deviance, the other as an expression of the impact of anti-gay discrimination. Lastly, Chapter 11, by Jae Kennedy and Meredith Minkler, turns attention to "Disability Theory and Public Policy: Implications for Critical Gerontology," and was first published in *International Journal of Health Services* in 1998 (30). Combining critical analyses of aging and disability with a concern for class, racial/ethnic, and gender inequalities in health, the authors urge analysts and policymakers to conduct their work premised on the "moral economy of interdependency over the life course."

Taken together, the different chapters in *Section I* highlight the importance of theoretical clarity, historical perspectives, and explicit analysis of power and politics, for epidemiologic investigation of social inequalities in health. The task of translating these ideas into practice is then addressed in the *Section II*, on "Empirical Investigation: Social Epidemiology at Work."

REFERENCES

1. Sigerest, H. E. *A History of Medicine. Volume I: Primitive and Archaic Medicine.* Oxford University Press, New York 1951 (reissued: 1979).
2. Sigerest, H. E. *A History of Medicine. Volume II: Early Greek, Hindu, and Persian Medicine.* Oxford University Press, New York, 1961 (reissued: 1987).
3. Lloyd, G. E. R. Introduction. In *Hippocratic Writings,* edited by G. E. R. Lloyd, pp. 9–60. Penguin Books, London, 1983.
4. Rosen, G. *A History of Public Health* (1958). Introduction by Elizabeth Fee; Bibliographical essay and new bibliography by Edward T. Morman. Expanded ed. Johns Hopkins University Press, Baltimore, MD, 1993.
5. Porter, D. *Health, Civilization and the State: A History of Public Health from Ancient to Modern Times.* Routledge, London, 1999.
6. Krieger, N. Shades of difference: Theoretical underpinnings of the medical controversy on Black/White differences in the United States, 1830–1870. *Int. J. Health Serv.* 17: 259–278, 1987.
7. Byrd, W. M., and Clayton, L. A. *An American Health Dilemma: The Medical History of African Americans and the Problem of Race.* Routledge, New York, 2000.
8. Krieger, N., et al. Racism, sexism, and social class: Implications for studies of health, disease, and well-being. *Am. J. Prev. Med.* 9(Suppl): 82–122, 1993.
9. Kington, R. S. Racial and ethnic differences in health: Recent trends, current patterns, future directions. In *America Becoming: Racial Trends and Their Consequences,*

Vol. 2, National Research Counsel, edited by N. J. Smelser, W. J. Wilson, and F. Mitchel, pp. 253–310. National Academy Press, Washington, DC, 2001.

10. Doyal, L. *What Makes Women Sick? Gender and the Political Economy of Health.* Rutgers University Press, New Brunswick, NJ, 1995.

11. Messing, K. *One-Eyed Science: Occupational Health and Women Workers.* Foreword by Jeanne Mager Stellman. Temple University Press, Philadelphia, 1998.

12. Solarz, A. L. (ed.). *Lesbian Health: Current Assessment and Direction for the Future.* Committee on Lesbian Health Research Priorities, Neuroscience and Behavioral Health Program and Health Sciences Policy Program, Health Sciences Section, Institute of Medicine. National Academy Press, Washington, DC, 1999.

13. Meyer, I. H. Why lesbian, gay, bisexual, and transgender public health? *Am. J. Public Health* 91: 856–859, 2001.

14. Healthy People 2010. Goal 2: Eliminate health disparities. www.healthypeople.gov/document/html/uih/uih_2.htm#obj (June 2003).

15. Pamuk, E., et al. *Socioeconomic Status and Health Chartbook.* National Center for Health Statistics, Hyattsville, MD, 1998.

16. Krieger, N. The making of public health data: Paradigms, politics, and policy. *J. Public Health Policy* 13: 412–427, 1992.

17. Waitzkin, H. The social origins of illness: A neglected history. *Int. J. Health Serv.* 11: 77–103, 1981.

18. Krieger, N., and Fee, E. Measuring social inequalities in health in the United States: A historical review, 1900–1950. *Int. J. Health Serv.* 26: 391–418, 1996.

19. Krieger, N., and Moss, N. Accounting for the public's health: An introduction to selected papers from a U.S. conference on "Measuring social inequalities in health." *Int. J. Health Serv.* 26: 383–390, 1996.

20. Crawford, R. You are dangerous to your health: The ideology and politics of victim blaming. *Int. J. Health Serv.* 7: 663–680, 1977.

21. Krieger, N. Embodying inequality: A review of concepts, measures, and methods for studying health consequences of discrimination. *Int. J. Health Serv.* 29: 295–352, 1999.

22. Krieger, N. Discrimination and health. In *Social Epidemiology,* edited by L. Berkman and I. Kawachi, pp. 36–75. Oxford University Press, Oxford, 2000.

23. Williams, D. R. Race/ethnicity and socioeconomic status: Measurement and methodological issues. *Int. J. Health Serv.* 26: 483–505, 1996.

24. Muntaner, C., Nagoshi, C., and Diala, C. Racial ideology and explanations for health inequalities among middle-class whites. *Int. J. Health Serv.* 31: 659–668, 2001.

25. Duncan, G. J. Income dynamics and health. *Int. J. Health Serv.* 26: 419–444, 1996.

26. Shortt, S. E. Is unemployment pathogenic? A review of current concepts with lessons for policy planners. *Int. J. Health Serv.* 26: 569–589, 1996.

27. Rowbotham, S. *Women, Resistance & Revolution.* Vintage Books, New York, 1974.

28. Krieger, N., and Fee, E. Man-made medicine and women's health: The biopolitics of sex/gender and race/ethnicity. *Int. J. Health Serv.* 24: 265–283, 1994.

29. Erwin, K. Interpreting the evidence: Competing paradigms and the emergence of lesbian and gay suicide as a "social fact." *Int. J. Health Serv.* 23: 437–453, 1993.

30. Kennedy, J., and Minkler, M. Disability theory and public policy: Implications for critical gerontology. *Int. J. Health Serv.* 28: 757–776, 1998.

PART 1

Historical Roots of Contemporary Social Epidemiology

CHAPTER 1

The Social Origins of Illness:
A Neglected History

Howard Waitzkin

Interest in the social origins of illness, especially disease-generating conditions of the workplace and environment, has grown rapidly. Recent literature often has overlooked the sources of this concern in Marxist thought. Although numerous studies have described occupational and environmental diseases, they generally have not considered the structural contradictions in the capitalist organization of production that foster illness and early death. The social causes of disease also have received little attention in traditional medical sociology.

Three people—Friedrich Engels, Rudolf Virchow, and Salvador Allende— made major early contributions to this field. The historical discontinuities in this perspective are partly explainable by broader forces that affected the work of these individuals. Engels viewed the ill health of the working class as one deprivation among many that demanded revolutionary change. Although Virchow linked his scientific role to political activism, the organization of medical science in Western Europe during the late nineteenth century prevented him from pursuing his commitment to "social medicine." Allende's research in public health receded as he devoted his major energies to the struggle toward socialism in Chile.

In this chapter I try to pick up a thread that has been dropped several times during more than a century. The social origins of illness have been largely forgotten and then rediscovered with each succeeding generation. At our current stage of history, we cannot ignore this problem any longer. Other writers have also concerned themselves with the social etiology of disease. Yet the work of Engels, Virchow, and Allende is important in several respects.

Engels and Virchow provided analyses of the impact of social conditions on health that essentially created the perspective of social medicine. Both men were writing about these issues during the tumultuous years of the 1840s; both took decisive—though quite divergent—personal actions which they saw as leading to the correction of the conditions they described. Allende's work appeared during a

21

later historical period and in a different geopolitical context. While Engels and Virchow documented the impact of early capitalism, Allende focused on capitalist imperialism and underdevelopment. Although little known in North America and Western Europe, Allende's studies in social medicine have exerted a great influence on health planning and strategy in Latin America and elsewhere in the Third World.

The writings of Engels, Virchow, and Allende explicitly or implicitly adopted a Marxist framework to investigate the social origins of illness. While they convey unifying themes that deserve attention, these works also diverge in instructive ways, especially regarding directions of political activism. After critically reviewing the contributions of each man, as well as the personal histories in which their writings emerged, I discuss their similarities and differences.

FRIEDRICH ENGELS

It is difficult to explain Engels's sensitivity to health and illness, since—in contrast to Virchow and Allende—he obtained no formal medical training and did not view public health as a central thrust of his work. Precisely why Engels saw what others missed remains unclear, but some speculations based on his early life are possible.

Engels devoted considerable energy during his late adolescence and early adulthood to the contradictions of his family's religious background. His father and many close relatives were staunch proponents of puritanical Pietism. Engels noted that, in effect, Pietism blamed the poor and the sick for their own suffering. Rather than improving social conditions, Engels concluded, Pietism worsened such problems by giving doctrinal interpretations based on individual responsibility. Engels could not agree that the poor tended to become sick through their own spiritual shortcomings. He also criticized what he saw as a Pietist reluctance to intervene actively in correcting social deprivation (1, pp. 413-432; 2; 3, v. 1, pp. 4-6).

A second experience that heightened Engels's sensitivity was his early journalism, which he undertook at the age of 18. During this period Engels and his family were living in Barmen, an industrial town whose economic base was textile manufacturing (3; 4, v. 1, p. 3; 5, v. 1, pp. 16-17, 183-184; 6). Since several members of Engels's family worked as managers in manufacturing, he had visited local mills and factories many times throughout his youth. In 1839 he began a series of literary activities that included poems, short stories, and newspaper articles. In researching his articles, he observed work processes in factories, interviewed workers, and visited their homes. The result was a sequence of articles called "Letters from the Wupper Valley" (*Briefe aus dem Wuppertal*), which he wrote under a pseudonym (1, 7). These writings gave an impassioned account of workers' sickness and suffering. Engels described the occupational illnesses suffered by weavers, tanners, and other textile workers.

He also claimed that tuberculosis and syphilis spread largely because of difficult working conditions and inadequate housing.

A third influence was Mary Burns, one of the most underrated figures in the history of early socialism. In 1842, shortly after arriving in Manchester to work in his father's factory, Engels met and began living with Burns, an Irish working-class woman. Burns accompanied Engels during his visits and interviews in Manchester. Undoubtedly her presence facilitated Engels's ability to engage in conversations with people who otherwise could not have trusted this manager of a capitalist factory. Burns held radical political views and supported Irish revolutionaries, who frequently stayed in the home that she and Engels shared (3, v. 1, pp. 127-128; 5, v. 2, p. 45; 8, pp. 98-102; 9, p. 477). This was a time of large-scale immigration from Ireland to English manufacturing towns. The major cause of the immigration was the Irish potato famine of 1839 and subsequent years. Engels's relationship with Burns personally exposed him to the hunger and physical degradation that the Irish immigrants faced. Aside from the many complexities of the Engels-Burns connection, it is clear that Burns profoundly affected Engels's perception of working-class life, physical suffering, and radical political action.

In *The Condition of the Working Class in England* (10), Engels's theoretical position was unambiguous. For working-class people, the roots of illness and early death lay in the organization of economic production and in the social environment. British capitalism, Engels argued, forced working-class people to live and work under circumstances that inevitably caused sickness. This situation was not hidden, but was well known to the capitalist class that controlled society.

Engels first considered the effects of environmental toxins. He claimed that the poorly planned housing in working-class districts did not permit adequate ventilation of toxic substances. Workers' apartments surrounded a central courtyard without direct spatial communication to the street. Carbon-containing gases from combustion and human respiration remained sequestered within living quarters. Because disposal systems did not exist for human and animal wastes, these materials decomposed in courtyards, apartments, or the street. Engels described the resulting air and water pollution in minute detail (10, pp. 135-137).

Next Engels discussed infectious diseases caused in large part by poor housing conditions. Tuberculosis, an air-borne infection, was his major focus. He noted that overcrowding and insufficient ventilation contributed to high mortality from tuberculosis in London and other industrial cities. He also considered typhus epidemics. This infection, carried by lice, spread because of bad sanitation and ventilation. In his exposition of typhus, Engels adopted a method he used frequently—the secondary analysis of documents published by the medical profession. Engels doubted the profession's commitment to needed social change. On the other hand, he found extensive data in this literature to justify social change as a means to improve health.

Engels then turned to nutrition and drew connections among social conditions, nutrition, and disease (10, pp. 140-141). He emphasized the expense and chronic shortages of food supplies for urban workers. Lack of proper storage facilities at markets led to contamination and spoilage. Problems of malnutrition were especially difficult for children. Engels discussed scrofula as a disease related to poor nutrition; this view antedated the discovery of bovine tuberculosis as the major cause of scrofula and pasteurization of milk as a preventive measure. He also described the skeletal deformities of rickets as a nutritional problem, long before the medical finding that dietary deficiency of vitamin D caused rickets.

Engels's analysis of alcoholism was an account of the social forces that fostered excessive drinking. In Engels's view, alcoholism was a response to the miseries of working-class life. Lacking other sources of emotional gratification, workers turned to alcohol. Individual workers could not be held responsible for alcohol abuse. Instead, alcoholism ultimately was the responsibility of the capitalist class (10, pp. 141-142):

> Liquor is their [workers'] only source of pleasure. . . . The working-man . . . *must* have something to make work worth his trouble, to make the prospect of the next day endurable. . . . Drunkenness has here ceased to be a vice, for which the vicious can be held responsible. . . . They who have degraded the working man to a mere object have the responsibility to bear.

For Engels, alcoholism was rooted firmly in social structure. The attribution of responsibility to the individual worker was misguided. If the experience of deprived social conditions caused alcoholism, the solution involved basic change in those conditions, rather than treatment programs focusing on the individual.

In this context Engels analyzed the maldistribution of medical personnel. According to Engels (10, pp. 142-143), working-class people contended with the "impossibility of employing skilled physicians in cases of illness." Infirmaries that offered charitable services met only a small portion of people's needs for professional attention. Engels criticized the patent remedies containing opiates that apothecaries provided for childhood illnesses. High rates of infant mortality in working-class districts, Engels claimed, were explainable partly by lack of medical care and partly by the promotion of inappropriate medications.

Engels next undertook an epidemiologic investigation of mortality rates and social class, using demographic statistics compiled by public health officials. He showed that mortality rates were inversely related to social class, not only for entire cities but also within specific geographic districts of cities. He noted that in Manchester the childhood mortality was much greater among working-class children than "children of the higher classes." In addition, Engels commented on the cumulative effects of classes and urbanism on childhood mortality. He gave data that demonstrated higher death rates from epidemics of infectious diseases like smallpox, measles, scarlet fever, and whooping cough among working-class children. For Engels, such features of urban life as crowding, poor housing, inadequate sanitation, and pollution combined with social class position in the etiology of disease and early mortality (10, pp. 144-148).

The social causes of accidents drew Engels's indignation. He linked accidents to the exploitation of workers, lack of suitable child care, and the consequent neglect of children. Because both husband and wife needed to work outside the home in most working-class families, and because no facilities for child care were available when parents were at work, children were subject to falls, drowning, or burns. Engels noted that children's burns were especially frequent during the winter because of unsupervised heating facilities. Industrial accidents were another source of concern, especially the risks that industrial workers faced because of machinery. The most common accidents involved loss of fingers, hands, or arms by contact with unguarded machines. Infection resulting from accidents often led to tetanus.

In other sections of the book, Engels discussed disease entities in particular types of industrial work. He provided early accounts of occupational illnesses that have received intensive study only in recent years.

Many orthopedic disorders, in Engels's view, derived from the physical demands of industrialism. He discussed curvature of the spine, deformities of the lower extremities, flat feet, varicose veins, and leg ulcers as manifestations of work demands that required long periods of time in an upright posture. Engels commented on the health effects of posture, standing, and repetitive movements (10, pp. 190-193):

> All these affections are easily explained by the nature of factory work. . . .
> The operatives . . . must stand the whole time. And one who sits down, say upon a window-ledge or a basket, is fined, and this perpetual upright position, this constant mechanical pressure of the upper portions of the body upon spinal column, hips, and legs, inevitably produces the results mentioned. This standing is not required by the work itself. . . .

The insight that chronic musculoskeletal disorders could result from unchanging posture or small, repetitive motions seems simple enough. Yet this source of illness, which is quite different from a specific accident or exposure to a toxic substance, has entered occupational medicine as a serious topic of concern only in the last two decades.

Engels also singled out the eye disorders suffered by workers in textile and lace manufacturing. This work required constant fine visual concentration, often with poor lighting. Engels discussed such eye diseases as corneal inflammation, myopia, cataracts, and temporary or permanent blindness. After a dry exposition of ocular abnormalities, Engels returned to the passion of his social structural analysis (10, p. 230):

> This is the price at which society purchases for the fine ladies of the bourgeoisie the pleasure of wearing lace; a reasonable price truly! Only a few thousand blind working-men, some consumptive labourers' daughters, a

> sickly generation of the vile multitude bequeathing its debility to its equally
> "vile" children and children's children. . . . Our English bourgeoisie will
> lay the report of the Government Commission aside indifferently, and wives
> and daughters will deck themselves in lace as before.

In passages like this, Engels revealed that his revolutionary commitment grew not only from his view of economic exploitation but also from the experience of physical suffering rooted in class structure. For Engels, the contradictions of class made themselves felt most keenly in symbolic paraphernalia like lace, which the capitalist class enjoyed at the expense of the workers' eyesight.

Engels's observations of occupational and lead poisoning among pottery workers (10, pp. 242-244) are similarly startling, because this disease entity only recently has evoked wide concern in industrial hygiene. He noted that workers absorbed lead largely from the finishing fluid that came into contact with their hands and clothing. The consequences Engels described included severe abdominal pain, constipation, and neurologic complications like epilepsy and partial or complete paralysis. These signs of lead intoxication occurred not only in workers themselves, according to Engels, but also in children who lived near pottery factories. Epidemiologic evidence concerning the community hazards of industrial lead has gained attention in environmental health mainly since 1970, again without recognition of Engels's observations.

His discussions of lung disease were detailed and far reaching. In several instances, Engels described syndromes that medical science did not fully document until well into the twentieth century. His presentation of textile workers' lung disease (10, p. 200) antedated by many years the medical characterization of byssinosis, or "brown lung":

> In many rooms of the cotton and flax-spinning mills, the air is filled with
> fibrous dust, which produces chest affections, especially among workers in
> the carding and combing-rooms. . . . The most common effects of this
> breathing of dust are blood-spitting, hard, noisy breathing, pains in the chest,
> coughs, sleeplessness—in short, all the symptoms of asthma. . . .

Engels offered a parallel description of "grinders's asthma," a respiratory disease caused by inhalation of metal dust particles in the manufacture of knife blades and forks (10, pp. 239-241); he noted the similar pathologic effects of cotton and metal dusts on the lung.

Later in the book, Engels discussed pulmonary disorder among coal miners. He reported that unventilated coal dust caused both acute and chronic pulmonary inflammation that frequently progressed to death. Engels observed that "black spittle"—the syndrome now called coal miners' pneumoconiosis, or black lung—was associated with other gastrointestinal, cardiac, and reproductive complications. By pointing out that this lung disease was preventable, Engels illustrated the contradiction between profit and adequate health conditions in capitalist industry (10, pp. 279-284):

> Every case of this disease ends fatally . . . in all the coal-mines which are properly ventilated this disease is unknown, while it frequently happens that miners who go from well to ill-ventilated mines are seized by it. The profit-greed of mine owners which prevents the use of ventilators is therefore responsible for the fact that this working-men's disease exists at all.

After more than a century, the same structural contradiction impedes the prevention of black lung.

For Engels, the analysis of the social origins of illness was part of a much larger agenda. Like other Marxist scholarship, *The Condition of the Working Class in England* was intended mainly for the purpose of sociopolitical action. Engels quickly focused on additional theoretical and practical concerns. Despite later writings on natural and physical sciences (11, 12), he did not return to the social origins of illness as a major issue in its own right. Yet in a book that aimed toward a broad description of working class life, Engels provided a clear analysis of the causal relationships between social structure and physical illness.

Engels interspersed his remarks about disease with many other perceptions of class oppression. His argument implied that the solution to these health problems required basic social change limited medical interventions would never yield the improvements that were most needed. It is unfortunate that Engels's early work on medical issues has eluded later students and activists. His analysis, however, exerted a major influence, both intellectual and political, on one of the founders of social medicine: Rudolf Virchow.

RUDOLF VIRCHOW

Virchow's life spanned eighty years of nineteenth-century history, more than two thousand publications, numerous major contributions in medical science and anthropology, and parliamentary activity as an elected member of the German Reichstag. His best known work is *Cellular Pathology* (13), which presented the first comprehensive exposition of the cell as the basic unit of physiologic and pathologic processes. Virchow's current reputation rests largely on his research in cellular pathology. Throughout his career, however, he tried to develop a unified explanation of the physical and social forces that cause disease and human suffering. Although Virchow's activism led him in several unproductive directions, his vision of the multifactorial and largely social origins of illness deserves more than the obscurity into which much of his work has fallen.

Although Virchow's complex life is impossible to summarize briefly, some biographical notes give perspective to his contributions. He was born in Schivelbein, a small town in Pomerania. His father, who could not support the family solely by farming, took an extra job as a bureaucrat in the town government and made several unsuccessful attempts to start small businesses. Virchow's mother apparently worked exclusively in the home. Until their death, Virchow maintained an extensive correspondence with his parents which—although carefully edited by his descendants prior to publication—serves as a remarkably honest record of family life and parental reaction to a precocious son (14).

His student years were a time of academic brilliance and humdrum experience. An outstanding record in *gymnasium* led to a full scholarship for medical education at Friedrich-Wilhelms Institut in Berlin. He set himself a Faustian goal for scholarship (14, p. 47): "complete knowledge of nature, from God to earth."[1] After taking his medical degree in 1843, he began an internship and later a position as a clinical pathologist at Berlin's Charité Hospital. There he undertook a multifaceted research project on the cellular basis of pathology, a field that he synthesized during the next two decades. The revolutions of 1848 overtook Virchow and taught him that the microscopic vision, important as it was, could not itself explain—let alone correct—pathologic processes. The events of that year showed that societal problems also caused or fostered pathologic disturbances. Virchow's experience during 1848 engendered the multifactorial view of pathology that pervaded his later publications and teaching. This view often has eluded secondary accounts of Virchow's achievements, which have emphasized cellular observations while downplaying the impact of social forces. The two experiences that were to influence Virchow's thought most deeply were a typhus epidemic in Upper Silesia and the working-class uprising in Berlin.

In late 1847 a typhus epidemic broke out in Upper Silesia, a chronically impoverished area of East Prussia with a large Polish-speaking minority. By the beginning of 1848, thousands were dying and famine complicated the problems. Virchow convinced his superiors to support a pathologically oriented investigation that would lead to recommendations about stopping the epidemic and preventing recurrences. He departed for a brief but intensive field trip to Upper Silesia. Within days of his arrival, the horrors of the epidemic produced a profound emotional impact.

Although he revealed some of these feelings in his formal reports, he reserved most of them for his correspondence with his father. In these letters, Virchow gave a passionate account of suffering. He described the available diet in detail, expressed indignation about the continuing hunger, and began to draw a connection between hunger and disease (14, p. 125): "It is rather certain that hunger and typhus are not produced apart from each other but that the latter has spread so extensively only through hunger." Inadequate housing conditions also predisposed to transmission of the disease. He complained to his father that the epidemic's persistence was the fault of public officials, who did not take aggressive action to correct the social conditions that fostered illness. He also blamed the local medical profession for not attending the poor properly, because of "love of money" and reluctance "to put bills aside" (14, p. 127). Only a "public health service" (*Die Öffentliche Gesundheitspflege*), in which doctors and medical

---

[1] Unless otherwise indicated, I have prepared the translations from the original German or Spanish.

facilities would function under state control, could hope to deal with such problems effectively.

In his publications about the epidemic, Virchow developed a broader theory of multifactorial etiology. He emphasized that a variety of material deprivations interacted with one another to produce disease in the individual and transmission throughout a community (15; 16, v. 1, pp. 128-129, 214-234, 435-464). First, malnutrition predisposed to illness; the government could prevent the impact of malnutrition by distributing foodstuffs to the poor during famine. A second focus of intervention was better housing, since crowding and deprived living conditions encouraged the spread of the epidemic. According to Virchow, adverse climate also contributed to the transmission of disease, but, he claimed, would be a minor factor if adequate food and housing were available. He noted that the typhus epidemic affected the Polish-speaking minority to a larger extent than other groups within Upper Silesia because language differences prevented doctors from communicating with patients. Virchow urged that physicians receive training in local idioms where they practiced.

Virchow noted that the overall material conditions of life created a substratum in which either health or illness flourished. He argued that economic insecurity and political disenfranchisement were, through a complex chain of causality, social problems that generated disease, disability, and early death. Economic stability and active political participation by the poor, in Virchow's view, were necessary for good health. For these reasons, Virchow's policy recommendations included a series of profound economic, political, and social changes such as increased employment, better wages, local autonomy in government, agricultural cooperatives, and a more progressive taxation structure. Virchow's medical solutions, e.g., more clinics or hospitals, were quite limited. Instead, because he saw the origins of ill health in societal problems, the most reasonable approach to epidemics was to change the conditions that permitted them to occur.

Within weeks of his return to Berlin from the grim reality of the typhus epidemic, Virchow plunged into a second experience that was to shape his world view: the 1848 revolution. Virchow's letters to his parents from this period revealed a young man deeply committed to "radical socialism" and to personal participation in revolutionary social change. The correspondence from March 1848 described specific battles of the Berlin uprising and Virchow's own role. He tried to document instances of military brutality against working-class communities. It is clear from these letters that Virchow himself took part in actions on the barricades. Virchow minimized his personal contribution, claiming that it was "relatively unimportant," since he had "only a pistol" (14, p. 137). During the next year direct combat declined, but Virchow pursued a frenetic pace of political activism. In addition to his teaching and scientific publications, Virchow founded and co-edited a weekly newspaper, *Medical Reform* (*Die Medizinische Reform*), written in simple language and directed toward a mass readership—"those who form a medical (trained and practicing) proletariat" (17, p. 99).

He frequently characterized himself as a "socialist" and a member of the "extreme left." In a letter to his mother he described his motivations: "Improving the welfare of the poor, or, to say the same thing, the working class, was not possible under the constitution until now, because the king's will alone was law and the working class had scarcely any means to make their advancement worthwhile." During this period Virchow distinguished between socialism and communism, favoring the former. As he wrote to his father in 1849 (14, p. 197), he believed that communism was "nonsense, if one hoped to achieve it directly." His writings did not clearly distinguish between the two systems, nor did he directly refer to the analysis that Marx and Engels developed during 1848 and subsequent years. His objections to communism seemed to derive from his view that a social system without a state apparatus was a naive goal. On the other hand, he believed that only socialism could create "rational institutions" capable of achieving security for the "masses." Strategically, Virchow was pessimistic about the possibility of a peaceful transition to socialism (14, p. 197):

> This [a socialist system] could happen without violence if men, namely those who have power in hand, would be somewhat rational. Because they are irrational, now as ever, it probably will not come to pass without bloodshed and force.

After 1848 Virchow never again used a pistol or any other instrument of violence in revolutionary struggle. But he also never recanted his early activism, despite many pressures to do so. By 1849 reaction had gained the upper hand in Germany. Virchow decided that continued publication of *Medical Reform* was not worthwhile because, as he put it in the final issue, "the counterrevolution factually has conquered" (17, p. 131). At least temporarily, Virchow retreated from political activity. Meanwhile, his activism during 1848 brought repercussions that threatened the security of his career in academic medicine. In 1849 he wrote his father that both his current teaching position at Charité Hospital in Berlin and a potential professorship at Würzburg were in doubt because of concern about "his radical political tendencies." After nearly a year of uncertainty, the University of Würzburg offered a professorship, which Virchow immediately accepted. Arriving in Bavaria, then a bastion of conservatism, Virchow began a five-year period of intense scholarship and political inaction. His *Cellular Pathology* was a product of the Würzburg years.

Not until 1856, when he returned to Berlin with a chair in pathologic anatomy, did Virchow feel free to renew his public concern for social issues. Throughout his later life Virchow challenged Germany's ruling circles, both inside and outside the medical field. In these activities he consistently chose relatively unthreatening avenues of expression. Shortly after his return to Berlin he began working on sanitation projects, the expansion of medical services for the poor, and other public health efforts. During the next three decades, as an elected member of the

Reichstag, he opposed the conservative policies of Bismarck, who consolidated power in the late 1860s.

Marx, Engels, and others on the left followed Virchow's activities closely and viewed them with a combination of amusement and ambivalence. Engels noted Virchow's parliamentary opposition to Bismarck with approval (18, v. 3, pp. 103, 157). In addition, Engels briefly cited Virchow's pathology as one example of scientific investigation that revealed dialectic processes in nature, although Engels also criticized Virchow for not employing the methodology of dialectics more explicitly (12, pp. 154, 270). Marx apparently tried to influence Virchow's political activities through Ludwig Kugelmann, a gynecologist who was a close friend and adherent of Marx, as well as a professional colleague of Virchow. Kugelmann sought Virchow's attention by presenting him with a description of an unusual case of a uterine polyp the former discovered in his clinical work. Engels replied derisively to Marx's version of this encounter (18, v. 3, p. 383, v. 4, p. 39):

> But the attempt to convert Virchow to communism by means of this polyp resembles an ectopic ["extrauterine"] pregnancy. If V. himself has knowledge and theoretical interest in politics, in respect to economics, then this outstanding bourgeois is much too deeply engaged.

Recent Marxist commentators have criticized Virchow for dropping his radical activism and specifically for ignoring, or even opposing, the practical struggles of European communism during the last part of the nineteenth century. One critic, Boenheim, has gone so far as to claim that Virchow's opposition to Bismarck was more apparent than real ("*Scheinopposition*") (19, pp. 25-27). Although he promoted circumscribed progressive change, in his later life the illustrious professor never took actions that would jeopardize his position in any basic way. He also did not publicly support the theoretical analysis or political work of Marx, Engels, and their followers. In this sense, there is some truth in Boenheim's assertion that Virchow made his peace with the ruling class (19, p. 7; 20-21). Virchow's personal rapprochement with those he had deemed "irrational" in 1848 is not very surprising; nor does it detract from his work on the social origins of illness, which I now shall discuss in somewhat greater detail.

In his analyses of social medicine Virchow acknowledged the impact of many sources, but particularly that of Bacon, Hegel, and materialists like Engels and Arnold Ruge. From Bacon, Virchow derived his commitment to an applied science that would be practically useful. Virchow quoted Bacon's aphorism that "knowledge is power" and claimed: "Knowledge which is unable to support action is not genuine—and how unsure is activity without understanding. This split between science and practice is rather new." After a lengthy critique of the defects of detached science pursued "for its own sake," Virchow concluded (22, pp. 27-29): "It certainly does not detract from the dignity of science to come down off its pedestal—and from the people science gains new strength." From this perspective emerged Virchow's frequent assertion that the most successful science drew its problems largely from concrete social concerns. Science and scientific medicine, according to Virchow, should not be detached from sociopolitical reality. On the contrary, he argued, the scientist must seek to link the findings of research to political work suggested by that research.

Hegel was the main source of Virchow's dialectic approach to both biologic and social problems. On the biologic level, Virchow perceived natural processes as a series of antitheses, such as the humoral-solidistic or vitalistic-mechanistic dualities, that were resolved by syntheses, such as cellular pathology. On the social level, Virchow also viewed historical processes dialectically. For example, in 1847 he anticipated the revolutions of 1848 by claiming that the apparent social tranquility would be "negated" through social conflict in order to reach "a higher synthesis" (23, p. 52). Virchow used a similar dialectic analysis in tracing the process of scientific knowledge. Discoveries, he claimed, emerged from the "kernel of truth" in past observations that scientists initially interpreted erroneously. The dialectic of scientific knowledge therefore required the scientist's awareness of the concrete historical circumstances in which observations and interpretations were made (22, pp. 142-150).

While clearly influenced by Hegel, Virchow rejected Hegelian idealism. Although the dialectic method, in Virchow's view, was applicable to biologic science, it needed grounding in specific material phenomena. Virchow argued for a new "materialism" in medicine that would replace dogma and spiritualism (17, pp. 94-96). In his attempts to construct a dialectical materialist approach in biology, Virchow studied the early work of Engels. He cited with approval Engels's approach in *The Condition of the Working Class in England* and used some of Engels's data to demonstrate the relationships between poverty and illness (16, v. 1, pp. 305, 321-334). During his early years Virchow was influenced to perhaps an even greater degree by Arnold Ruge, who with Marx edited *Die Deutsch-Französischen Jahrbücher*. Virchow referred frequently to Ruge's writings and speeches, especially those on the ambiguities of political authority and on the need to discover "natural laws" of human society (17, pp. 42, 104).

Virchow manifested these orientations—of applied science, dialectics, and materialism—in many ways, but most of all in his analyses of multifactorial etiology and the political role of the medical scientist. In investigating the origins of specific illnesses, Virchow consistently studied a variety of social, political, economic, geographic, climatic, and physiologic factors that interacted with one another in the causation of disease. He emphasized the concrete historical and material circumstances in which disease arose, the contradictory social forces that impeded prevention, and researchers' role in advocating reform. In the analysis of multifactorial etiology, Virchow claimed that the most important causative factors were material conditions of people's everyday lives. This view implied that an effective health care system could not limit itself to treating the pathophysiologic disturbances of individual patients. From Virchow's viewpoint, the responsibilities of the medical scientist frequently extended to direct political action.

Based on the typhus epidemic in Upper Silesia, a cholera epidemic in Berlin, and an outbreak of tuberculosis in Berlin, Virchow worked out a theory of epidemics that emphasized the social circumstances permitting dissemination of illness. He argued that defects of society were a necessary condition for the emergence of epidemics.

Virchow classified certain disease entities as "crowd diseases" or "artificial diseases"; these included typhus, scurvy, tuberculosis, leprosy, cholera, relapsing fever, and some mental disorders. According to this analysis, inadequate social conditions increased the population's susceptibility to climate, infectious agents, and other specific causal factors, none of which alone was sufficient to produce an epidemic (16, v. 1, pp. 121-122):

> Don't crowd diseases point everywhere to deficiencies of society? One may adduce atmospheric or cosmic conditions or similar factors. But never do they alone make epidemics. They produce them only . . . where due to bad social conditions people have lived for some time in abnormal situations.

From this perspective, social change was as important as medical intervention for the prevention and eradication of epidemics, if not more so (23, pp. 125-129): "The improvement of medicine would eventually prolong human life, but improvement of social conditions could achieve this result even more rapidly and successfully." Health workers deluded themselves to think that efforts within the medical sphere alone would ameliorate these problems. The advocacy of social solutions thus became the necessary complement of clinical work.

The defects of society that Virchow emphasized most strongly were the material conditions of social class. He described at length the deprivations that the working class endured and linked disease patterns to these deprivations. For example, he noted that morbidity and mortality rates, and especially infant mortality rates, were much higher in working-class districts of cities than in wealthier areas. As documentation he used the statistics that Engels cited, as well as data he gathered for German cities showing inadequate housing, nutrition, and clothing. Virchow criticized the apathy of government officials for ignoring these root causes of illness. He also attacked the policies of hospitals that required payment from the poor rather than assuming their care as a matter of social responsibility. Virchow expressed his outrage about class conditions most forcefully in his discussion of epidemics like the cholera outbreak in Berlin (17, p. 110):

> Is it not clear that our struggle is a social one, that our job is not to write instructions to upset the consumers of melons and salmon, of cakes and ice cream, in short, the comfortable bourgeoisie, but is to create institutions to protect the poor, who have no soft bread, no good meat, no warm clothing, and no bed, and who through their work cannot subsist on rice soup and camomile tea . . .? May the rich remember during the winter, when they sit in front of

their hot stoves and give Christmas apples to their little ones, that the shiphands who brought the coal and the apples died from cholera. Ah, it is so sad that thousands always must die in misery, so that a few hundred may live well.

For Virchow, the deprivations of working life created a susceptibility to disease. When infectious organisms, climatic changes, famine, or other causal factors emerged, disease arose in individuals and spread rapidly through the community.

Virchow's understanding of the social origins of illness led to the broad scope that he defined for public health and the medical scientist. He envisioned the creation of a "public health service," an integrated system of publicly owned and operated health care facilities, staffed by health workers who were employed by the state. In this system, health care would be defined as a constitutional right of citizenship. Included within this right would be the enjoyment of material conditions of life that contributed to health rather than illness (17, p. 55; 23, pp. 131-138). The activities of public health workers, whom Virchow referred to as "doctors of the poor" (*Armenärzten*), would involve advocacy as well as direct medical care; in this sense, health workers would become the "natural attorneys of the poor." From his observations of the Upper Silesian typhus epidemic, Virchow recommended that doctors learn the local languages and dialects of regions where they practiced. He described with sensitivity the plight of health workers practicing in deprived communities. He claimed that medicine among the poor involved two sets of injustices: those against the poor and those against doctors. Even with the best of motivations, he argued, doctors working among the poor faced continuous overwork and their own impotence to change social conditions fostering illness. For this reason, it was naive to argue for a public health service without also struggling for more basic social change.

Two other principles were central to Virchow's conception of the public health service: prevention and the state's responsibility to assure material security for citizens. Virchow's stress on prevention again derived mostly from his observation of epidemics, which he believed could be prevented by fairly straightforward policies. For example, he found a major cause of the Upper Silesian typhus epidemic in several poor potato harvests preceding the epidemic. Government officials could have prevented malnutrition by redistributing foodstuffs from other parts of the country. Prevention, then, was largely a political problem (17, pp. 108, 127): "Our politics were those of prophylaxis; our opponents preferred those of palliation." It was foolish to think that health workers could accomplish prevention solely by activities within the medical sphere; material security also was essential. The state's responsibilities, Virchow argued, included providing work for "able-bodied" citizens. Only by guaranteed employment could workers obtain the economic security necessary for good health. Likewise, the physically disabled should enjoy the right of public compensation (17, p. 106).

Virchow's vision of the social origins of illness pointed out the enormity of the medical task. To the extent that illness derived from social conditions, the medical scientist must study those conditions as a part of clinical investigation, and the health worker must engage in political action. This is the sense of the connections Virchow frequently drew among medicine, social science, and politics: "Medicine is a social science, and politics is nothing more than medicine in larger scale" (17, p. 117; 22, p. 106). Virchow's analysis of these issues fell from sight largely because of conservative political forces that shaped the course of scientific medicine during the late nineteenth and early twentieth centuries. His contributions set a standard for current attempts to understand, and to change, the social conditions that generate illness and suffering.

SALVADOR ALLENDE

The practice of pathology was an ironic continuity between the lives of Virchow and Allende. Experience in autopsies exposed them to sources of illness and death in problems of social structure. Allende's political career is better known than Virchow's, partly because of the tragedy of its abrupt end. Social medicine, however, was a central concern for them both, and Allende recognized very early that the health problems of the Chilean people derived in large part from the country's economic and political conditions.

Allende came from a professional family. His grandfather, also a physician, had served as director of medical services for the Chilean army. His father, a lawyer, and his mother held liberal political views. Although the family led a comfortable existence, it lacked ties with the financial elite of the country. In fact, several family members who were sympathetic to left-wing politics during the 1920s and 1930s spent short periods of time in prison. While still an adolescent, Allende became deeply interested in politics and the problems of the working class. A shoemaker, Juan Demarchi, introduced him to political theory and was an important influence (24, p. 66).

Allende's medical work further sensitized him to class issues. During medical school and part of his internship he supported himself by working as an assistant in pathologic anatomy. He complained that this work was "very hard and very dull" (24, p. 67). But he later expressed satisfaction that his autopsy experience educated him concerning malnutrition, infectious diseases, and other health problems of the poor. His commitment to popular politics gained clarity as he taught workers at night schools, served as president of the Medical Students' Center, acted as a leader of a student strike that caused his temporary expulsion from the University of Chile, and entered prison briefly because of his opposition to the dictatorship of Carlos Ibañez.

As a medical student Allende studied Marxist theory. In interviews Allende described his own development:

The medical students were traditionally the most advanced. At the time we lived in a humble district, we practically lived with the people, most of us were from the provinces and those of us living in the same hostel used to meet at night for readings of *Das Kapital*, and Lenin, and also Trotsky (24, pp. 63-64).

The first contact [with Marxism] came from our unrest as university students. . . . Above all, the medical student and doctor face head-on very clear social facts. We learned very quickly that the greater the disease, the greater the poverty; the greater the poverty, the greater the disease rate . . . an axiom that inexorably repeats itself. . . . We read the Marxist theorists (25, p. 6).

During the 1930s Allende continued his medical and political work. An organizer of the Chilean Socialist Party, he also helped edit the *Chilean Medical Bulletin* and founded the *Journal of Social Medicine*. Collaborating with José Vizcarra, he wrote his first book, *The Structure of National Health (La Estructuración de Salubridad Nacional)* (26). This volume developed the broad directions of the Chilean National Health Service (*Servicio Nacional de Salud*, SNS), which Allende later helped establish through legislation he proposed during the 1950s as a Senator. In 1938, as a founder of the Popular Front, a coalition of left parties, Allende worked for the election of Pedro Aguirre Cerda, who subsequently appointed Allende as Minister of Health. Shortly after his appointment, Allende completed a major monograph on social medicine, *The Chilean Medico-Social Reality (La Realidad Medico-Social Chilena)* (27). In this book Allende analyzed the connections between illness and the socio-economic reality confronting the Chilean people. It remains a masterpiece of social medicine and deserves a more detailed appraisal. First, however, some notes on Allende's later life are appropriate.

As a Senator and leader of the opposition Socialist Party during the 1940s and 1950s, Allende continued to intertwine medical and political interests. He authored legislation that created the Chilean SNS. Although the SNS suffered from bureaucratic inefficiency, it provided free medical care for about half of Chile's population, additional subsidies for severe illness, prenatal and maternity benefits, and support for provincial hospitals. Allende also kept sight of the relationships between international capitalism and illness in his country his speech to the American Public Health Association in 1941 gave an eloquent analysis of the medical ramifications of imperialism (28).

Allende also maintained a strong interest in medical education. As a faculty member of the medical school of the University of Chile, Allende strove for broader recruitment of medical students from all social classes. In the early 1960s he supported the introduction of the social sciences into the medical curriculum. Moreover, Allende drafted the law that established the Chilean Medical Association (*Colégio Médico de Chile*) during the late 1940s. In its early period,

Allende himself served as the Association's president. Initially the Association adopted a liberal program of modest reforms for the Chilean health system. During the 1950s and 1960s, however, it became increasingly conservative, lobbying for the financial rights of private practitioners and resisting government regulation.

Although Allende did not engage in medical practice after his internship, largely because of the demands of his political work, he did keep his interest in health policy. After losing electoral campaigns as Socialist Party candidate for President in 1958 and 1964, Allende gained a plurality in the 1970 election. In November 1970 he was inaugurated as the first socialist president elected to office in a major country of the Western Hemisphere. During his presidency Allende encouraged a series of reforms in the health system that resembled the legislation he had sponsored as a Senator. At no time did Allende actively seek to nationalize the profession, nor did he attempt to suppress private practice. His proposals generally remained reformist and did not lead to fundamental structural changes in the Chilean health system (29-31).

Allende's understanding of the social origins of illness influenced his political activism, both within and outside the health sector. He worked out his analysis of the relationships among social structure, disease, and suffering most systematically in his classic book, *La Realidad Medico-Social Chilena* (27). *La Realidad* conceptualized illness as a disturbance of the individual that often was fostered by deprived social conditions. This conception implied that social change was the only potentially effective therapeutic approach to many health problems. In its theoretical analysis of disease and its policy proposals, *La Realidad* showed strong similarities to the prior work of both Engels and Virchow. (Although Allende must have been acquainted with these predecessors, direct acknowledgments are not present in currently available writings.) Aside from its substantive content, the organizational format and expository style of *La Realidad* resembled those of Engels's *The Condition of the Working Class in England* and Virchow's monograph on the typhus epidemic in Upper Silesia. After a theoretical introduction on the connections between social structure and illness, Allende presented some geographic and demographic "antecedents" necessary to place specific health problems in context. He devoted the next part of the book to the "living conditions of the working classes." The last sections of the book presented an exhaustive review of health care facilities and services, and a plan for change based on socialist strategy.

The introduction of *La Realidad* developed the position that incremental reforms within the health care system would remain ineffective unless accompanied by broad structural changes in the society. Allende emphasized capitalism and particularly the multinational corporations that extracted profit from Chilean natural resources and inexpensive labor. He claimed that to improve the health care system, a popular government must end capitalist exploitation (27, pp. 6, 8):

> Progress obtained in the output of national production has not yielded a sensible margin of well-being in the popular strata, because international capitalism—economic and financial master of the large centers of production—is interested only in producing to satisfy the demand of the market, and no more. For the capitalist enterprise it is of no concern that there is a population of workers who live in deplorable conditions, who risk being consumed by diseases or who vegetate in obscurity. . . . Therefore, the action of our government is not only the remedial task of transforming the people but moreover of defending against absorption and exploitation by the economic imperialists who encompass the earth. . . . [Without] economic advancement . . . it is impossible to accomplish anything serious from the viewpoints of hygiene or medicine . . . because it is impossible to give health and knowledge to a people who are malnourished, who wear rags, and who work at a level of unmerciful exploitation.

Ill health, in Allende's analysis, was inextricably linked to international capitalism; one could not hope to cure the sick without working toward a socialist economic system.

In his account of working-class life, Allende's analytic tone and statistical tabulations thinly veiled his outrage at the effects of class oppression, underdevelopment, and malnutrition. He focused first on wages, which he viewed as the primary determinant of workers' material condition. Many of his economic observations anticipated later concerns, including wage differentials for men and women, the impact of inflation, and the inadequacy of laws purporting to assure subsistence-level income. He linked his exposition of wages directly to the problem of nutrition and presented comparative data on food availability, earning power, and level of economic development. Not only was the production of milk and other needed foodstuffs less efficient than in more developed countries, but Chilean workers' inferior earning power also made food less accessible. Reviewing the minimum requirement to assure adequate nutrition, he found that the majority of Chilean workers could not obtain the elements of this diet on a regular basis. He argued that high infant mortality, skeletal deformities, tuberculosis, and other infectious diseases all had roots in bad nutrition; improvements depended on better economic conditions for workers.

Allende then turned to clothing, housing, and sanitation facilities. He found that working people in Chile were inadequately clothed, largely because wages were low and the greatest proportion of income went for food and housing. The effects of insufficient clothing, Allende argued, were higher rates of upper respiratory infections, pneumonia, and tuberculosis in Chile than in any economically developed country. In his analysis of housing problems, Allende focused on population density. He noted that Chile had one of the highest rates of inhabitants per residential structure in the world. Overcrowding fostered the spread of infectious diseases and poor hygiene. Again he cited comparative data that showed a correlation between population density and overall mortality. In a style reminiscent of both Engels and Virchow, Allende presented a concrete description of housing conditions. He reviewed the provisions for private initiative in construction, found them unsatisfactory, and outlined the need for major public investment in new housing. Allende then gave data on drinking water and sewerage systems for all provinces of Chile, noting that vast areas of the country lacked these rudimentary facilities.

This view of working-class conditions laid the groundwork for Allende's subsequent analysis of medical problems. When he discussed specific diseases, he looked for their sources in the material environment. He expressed this unifying theme (27, p. 75):

> The individual in society is not an abstract entity; one is born, develops, lives, works, reproduces, falls ill, and dies in strict subjection to the surrounding environment, whose different modalities create diverse modes of reaction, in the face of the etiologic agents of disease. This material environment is determined by wages, nutrition, housing, clothing, culture, and additional concrete and historical factors. . . .

Because disease originated in part from social conditions, health programs could not succeed without changing the illness-generating conditions of society.

The medical problems that Allende considered were maternal and infant mortality, tuberculosis, venereal diseases, other communicable diseases, emotional disturbances, and occupational illnesses. He observed that maternal and infant mortality rates generally were much lower in developed than in underdeveloped countries. After reviewing the major causes of death, he concluded that malnutrition and poor sanitation were major explanations for this excess mortality. In the same section Allende gave one of the first analyses of illegal abortion. He noted that a large proportion of deaths in gynecologic hospitals, about 30 percent, derived from abortions and their complications. Pointing out the high incidence of abortion complications among working-class women, he attributed this problem to economic deprivation. Again, after a dry statistical account of complications, Allende allowed his outrage to surface (27, p. 86):

> There are hundreds of working mothers who, because of anxiety about the inadequacy of their wages, induce abortion in order to prevent a new child from shrinking their already insignificant resources. Hundreds of working mothers lose their lives, impelled by the anxieties of economic reality.

Allende defined tuberculosis as a "social disease" because its incidence differed so greatly among social classes. Writing before the antibiotic era, Allende reached conclusions similar to those of modern epidemiology—that the major decline in tuberculosis followed historical advances in economic development, rather than the therapeutic interventions of medicine. With statistics from the first three decades of the twentieth century, he noted that in economically developed countries tuberculosis had decreased consistently. These trends were clear for essentially all countries of Western Europe and the United States. On the other hand, in economically underdeveloped countries like Chile, little progress had occurred.

In his chapter on venereal diseases, Allende also emphasized socioeconomic problems that favored the spread of syphilis and gonorrhea. For example, he discussed deprivations of working-class life that encouraged prostitution. Citing the prevalence of prostitution in Santiago and other cities, as well as the early recruitment of women from poor families, he argued that social programs to eliminate prostitution must precede significant improvements in venereal diseases.

Other communicable diseases were the topic of Allende's next chapter. He turned his attention first to typhus, the same disease that had shaped Virchow's views about the relations between illness and social structure. Allende began his analysis with a straightforward statement (27, p. 105): "Some [communicable diseases], like typhus, are an index of the state of pauperization of the masses." Like Virchow in Upper Silesia, Allende found a disproportionate incidence of typhus in the working class of Chile. He showed that dysentery and typhoid fever arose and spread because of inadequate drinking water and sanitation facilities in densely populated residential areas. Similar problems fostered other infections, such as diphtheria, whooping cough, scarlet fever, measles, and trachoma. Allende's exposition of social factors in the etiology of infectious diseases antedated many emphases of modern epidemiology. His arguments transcended the search for specific etiologic agents and treatments—the dominant perspective of Western medicine at the time Allende was writing.

Addiction was another topic that Allende discussed passionately. He maintained a concern with addiction throughout his career; one priority of his health policies as President of Chile was a large-scale alcoholism program. In *La Realidad,* Allende analyzed the social and psychological problems that motivated the use of addicting drugs. Allende's analysis (27, p. 119) of the causes of alcoholism was quite similar to Engels's:

> We see that one's wages, appreciably less than subsistence, are not enough to supply needed clothing, that one must inhabit inadequate housing, . . . [and that] one's food is not sufficient to produce the minimum of necessary caloric energy. . . . The worker reaches the conclusion that going to the tavern and intoxicating oneself is the apparent solution to all these problems. In the tavern one finds a lighted and heated place, and friends for distraction, making one forget the misery at home. In short, for the Chilean worker . . . alcohol is not a stimulant but an anesthetic. . . .

Rooted in social misery, alcoholism exerted a profound effect on health. Allende documented this impact for a variety of illnesses, including gastrointestinal diseases, cirrhosis, delirium tremens, sexual dysfunction, birth defects, and tuberculosis. He also traced some of the more subtle societal outcomes of alcoholism;

for example, he offered an early account of the role of alcohol in deaths from accidents.

Allende's brief account of occupational diseases revealed the modesty of his approach when he felt that available data were insufficient to make sweeping conclusions. He recognized that the occupational causes of death and disability were among the most important that the country faced at the time. Indeed, the diseases of work revealed direct links between illness and social structure. Allende noted, however, that knowledge about occupational diseases remained at a rudimentary level. He reviewed such problems as industrial accidents and silicosis. But, reflecting the same dearth of information with which activists must contend forty years later, the most that Allende could advocate was "systematic study and planning of this aspect of our social pathology" (27, p. 124).

In the following chapters of his book, Allende undertook a comprehensive analysis of the Chilean health system. Although these sections did not pertain directly to the social origins of illness, some features of the discussion were noteworthy. Allende's exhaustive catalogue of available medical facilities, programs, laws, regulations, administrative agencies, and personnel set a standard for health care planning. His argument, often overlooked by planners, was that abstract policy making remained meaningless without detailed knowledge of resources that were already available. Another unifying theme involved the lack of overall coordination necessary to achieve a responsive health system. Although many potentially useful facilities and programs existed throughout Chile, he noted, they remained fragmented and disorganized (27, p. 186). For this reason, Allende's political goal was a comprehensive health system that not only provided new services but also reorganized existing ones.

Allende concluded these sections with a critique of the capitalist exploitation of illness by the pharmaceutical industry. In perhaps the earliest analysis of its type, Allende compared the prices of brand-name drugs with their generic equivalents (27, pp. 189-190):

> Thus, for example, we find for a drug with important action on infectious diseases, sulfanilamide, these different names and prices: Prontosil $26.95, Gombardol $20.80, Septazina $21.60, Aseptil $18.00, Intersil $13.00, Acetilina $6.65. All these products, which in the eyes of the public appear with different names, correspond, in reality, to the same medication which is sold in a similar container and which contains 20 tablets of 0.50 grams of sulfanilamide.

Beyond the issue of drug names, Allende also anticipated a later theme by severely criticizing pharmaceutical advertising (27, p. 191): "Another problem in relation to the pharmaceutical specialties is . . . the excessive and charlatan propaganda attributing qualities and curative powers which are far from their real ones." Throughout his career Allende maintained his concern with exploitation by multinational drug companies. As President, he helped develop a national generic drug formulary and proposed nationalization of the pharmaceutical industry that remained dominated by North American firms.

Allende's concluding section set forth the policy positions and plan for political action of the Ministry of Health within the Popular Front government. These passages comprised an extraordinary overview of the social origins of illness and the social structural remedies that were necessary. Allende refused to discuss specific health problems apart from macro-level political and economic issues. He introduced his policy proposals with a chapter entitled "Considerations Regarding Human Capital." Analyzing the detrimental economic impact of ill health among workers, he argued that a healthy population was a worthy goal in its own right, but also for the sake of national development. The country's productivity suffered because of workers' illness and early death. Yet improving the health of workers was impossible without fundamental structural changes in the society. These changes would include "an equitable distribution of the product of labor," state regulation of "production, distribution, and price of articles of food and clothing," a national housing program, and special attention to occupational health problems. The links between medicine and broader social reality were inescapable: "All this means that the solution of the medical-social problems of the country would require precisely the solution of the economic problems that affect the proletarian classes" (27, p. 198). Allende's basic insight was that health policy must transcend the health sector alone.

But he was not content to state this principle in abstract terms. Instead, he proposed general social policies that he viewed as preconditions for an effective health system. First of all, he suggested reforms in the structure of wages, which if enacted would have led to a full-scale redistribution of wealth. Regarding nutrition, he developed a plan to improve milk supplies, fishing, and refrigeration, and suggested land reform provisions to enhance agricultural productivity. Recognizing the need for better housing, Allende proposed a concerted national effort in publicly supported construction, as well as rent control in the private sector.

Thus, Allende maintained the analytic perspective he introduced early in the book. Since the major social origins of illness were low wages, malnutrition, and poor housing, the first responsibility of the public health system was to improve these conditions. Allende did not emphasize programs of research or treatment for specific disease entities. Instead, he assumed that the greatest advances in morbidity and mortality would follow fundamental changes in social structure. This orientation also pervaded his final chapter, which outlined the specifics of the proposed "medico-social program." In this program he suggested innovations including the reorganization of the Ministry of Health, planning activities, control of pharmaceutical production and prices, occupational safety and health policies, measures supporting preventive medicine, and sanitation programs. Forty years later, the insight that the social origins of illness demand social solutions is not particularly surprising. Despite lip service paid to this concept, however, health care analysts have contented themselves with a limited reformism, often arguing that more basic structural change, though needed, is beyond their reach as political actors. Like Engels and Virchow before him, Allende saw major origins of illness in the structure of society. This vision implied that medical intervention without political activism would remain ineffectual and, in a deep sense, misguided.

CONVERGENCE, DIVERGENCE

Sensitivity to the social origins of illness emerged from several directions during the mid-nineteenth century and recently has deepened. In this field, however, the lives and works of Engels, Virchow, and Allende were landmarks. Their varying analyses gave historical depth to these problems, which succeeding generations unfortunately have forgotten and later rediscovered. Although the sources of Engels's interest in illness and death caused by early capitalism remained somewhat obscure, the profound observations of *The Condition of the Working Class in England* made it an overlooked classic. Engels maintained an interest in science, which he developed in several later books, but the breadth of his other theoretical concerns and the intensity of his political activism led him away from medical issues as a prime focus. Virchow's early studies of social etiology in medicine merged with his youthful political radicalism. Both these foci faded later, partly because of the reactionary environment of Western European intellectual life, and partly because of Virchow's own reluctance to risk his prominent academic position. Working during a later historical period and in the much different context of imperialism and underdevelopment, Allende studied medicine as he became a leftist political leader. His commitment to changing the social origins of illness persisted throughout his later career. That he often subordinated health policy to broader social policy was consistent with his view that the most difficult medical problems had their roots in deprivations of class structure and capitalist imperialism. While they overlapped in many ways, the pathbreaking works of these individuals also diverged in crucial respects. Their differences perhaps revealed even more than their similarities.

General Themes

Engels, Virchow, and Allende held divergent, though complementary, views of the social etiology of illness. The divergences reflected more general differences in theoretical orientation. For Engels, economic production was primary. Even in his very early work, Engels emphasized the organization and process of production. Disease and early death, in this view, developed directly from exposure to dusts, chemicals, time pressures, bodily posture, visual demands, and related difficulties that workers faced in their jobs. Environmental pollution, bad housing, alcoholism, and malnutrition also contributed to the poor health of working-class people, but on balance these factors mainly reflected or exacerbated the structural contradictions of production itself. The principal contradiction which permitted illness-generating conditions, of course, was that between profit and safety. Engels noted that changes in the organization of work to prevent occupational illness and accidents, by increasing costs, usually would reduce profits. Engels's early analysis of illness and mortality in the working class anticipated his later emphasis on the primacy of economic production in explaining many problematic facets of capitalist society.

Rather than economic production, Virchow focused on inequalities in the distribution and consumption of social resources. Virchow shared Engels's view that the working class suffered disproportionately. In Virchow's analysis, however, the main sources of illness and early death were poverty, unemployment, malnutrition, cultural and educational deficits, political disenfranchisement, linguistic difficulties, inadequate medical facilities and personnel, and similar deficiencies that affected the working class. He believed, for example, that public officials could prevent epidemics by distributing food more efficiently. Disease and mortality, he argued, would improve if a public health service made medical care more available. Virchow did criticize profiteering by businessmen and the high fees of the private medical profession, but he did not emphasize the illness-generating conditions of production itself. Instead, he viewed unequal access to society's products as the principal problem of social medicine.

Allende also concerned himself with the impact of class structure, but chiefly in the context of underdevelopment and imperialism. The deprivations that the working class experienced in countries like Chile reflected the exploitation of the Third World by advanced capitalist nations. Allende attributed low wages, malnutrition, poor housing, and related problems directly to the extraction of wealth by international imperialism. He recognized that production itself could cause illness but, unlike Engels, devoted little attention to occupational illness *per se*. He did document distributional inequalities of goods and services which, as in Virchow's analysis, ravaged the working class. On the other hand, the most crucial social determinant of illness and death, in Allende's view, was national underdevelopment. Economic advancement of the society as a whole was the major precondition for meaningful improvements in medical care and individual health.

Writing in different historical periods and with divergent (though incompletely developed) theoretical stances, Engels, Virchow, and Allende provided complementary explanations of the social causation of illness. The nature of economic production, distributional inequalities, and underdevelopment all have comprised major causative factors, and the perspectives of these three analysts balanced one another. Their contributions also shared the framework of multifactorial causation. These writings conveyed a vision of multiple social structures and processes impinging on the individual. Disease was not the straightforward outcome of an infectious agent or pathophysiologic disturbance. Instead, a variety of problems—including malnutrition, economic insecurity, occupational risks, bad housing, and lack of political power—created an underlying predisposition to 'disease and death. Although these writers differed in the specific factors they emphasized, they each saw illness as deeply embedded in the complexities of social reality. To the extent that broad social conditions affected individual disease, therapeutic intervention that limited itself to the individual level was both naive and futile. Multifactorial etiology implied social change as therapy, and the latter linked medical practice to political practice.

Another commonality in these early works of social medicine was dialectical materialism. Marx and Engels had not yet developed this analytic method fully by the mid-1840s. On the other hand, Engels had counted himself among the "young Hegelians" of the time, criticizing Hegelian idealism while invoking the principle of dialectic change. Engels's exposition of the health problems of the English working class was a model of the materialist approach. His vivid presentation of the conditions that engendered illness was concretely and historically grounded. He counterposed profit and safety as a central contradiction of capitalist production that only revolutionary political action could resolve. Hegelian philosophy also influenced Virchow, who likewise considered himself a materialist and used the rubric of dialectic contradiction to analyze biologic processes. Although his application of dialectics to biology was not always successful, this theoretical orientation guided Virchow's interpretation of multifactorial etiology in medicine. Virchow's materialism led him to oppose spiritualistic explanations of disease early in his career, as well as facile unifactorial explanations based on germ theory later in the nineteenth century. Virchow maintained a rather consistent position that multiple material factors in the physical and social milieu predisposed to pathologic disturbances at the cellular and organismic levels. Allende explicitly adopted the method of dialectical materialism during his medical student years. His analysis of the diverse conditions that fostered morbidity and mortality emphasized wages, food, and housing. In addition, he introduced the dialectic of imperialism and underdevelopment as a basic contradiction affecting the "medico-social reality" of the Third World. This analysis, as Allende stated, led to a conclusion that effective medical care ultimately required class conflict within nations and the struggle against imperialism.

Engels, Virchow, and Allende shared a surprising consensus about an activist role for medical scientists and practitioners. In his study of the English working class, Engels frequently cited the published accounts of health conditions by liberal physicians. Although he criticized the medical profession for avoiding practice in working-class communities, he commended individual doctors who did make this commitment. On the other hand, he saw little hope that health conditions would improve in any important way through interventions of health practitioners, as opposed to general action by the working class. Despite Virchow's later reputation as a paragon of the laboratory scientist, he advocated the scientist's passionate participation in politics. His own involvement became less radical with passing years, but he continued his civic activities almost until his death. In his view, science and social problems could influence each other beneficially. Not only could scientists contribute to solutions, but social problems could suggest areas of worthwhile research. Skeptical of detached or pure investigation, Virchow argued that medical research and practice properly should take place in a public health service that would overcome barriers of geography, ethnicity, and class structure. Like Engels, Allende undertook his research on medical issues as part of a political agenda. While Engels wrote his book partly for its effect as propaganda, Allende intended his classic analysis mainly as a planning document for an elected progressive government. For Allende, the inseparability of medical and social problems demanded a life-long activism that saw health care reform as one phase of the struggle toward a just society.

Taken together, the published work of Engels, Virchow, and Allende provided an understanding of social epidemiology and health policy that anticipated many concerns of analysts and activists currently working in this area. These three writers documented in great depth the social origins of illness. The deprivations of social class received detailed attention as causes of disease and early death. Engels offered an early account of occupational and environmental health issues. Allende's book gave a pathbreaking analysis of the health effects of under-development and imperialism. Both Engels and Allende documented the social correlates of infant and perinatal mortality, as well as the origins of alcoholism and other addictions in social misery. All three writers traced the complex causal relationships among poverty, malnutrition, and infection. Presently, when interest in these topics has burgeoned, an amnesia that overlooks these major contributions hardly seems justified.

Ahistorical approaches to health policy also are unrewarding. Engels's and Virchow's perceptions of maldistributed health care facilities and personnel are no less applicable to the United States and many other countries than they were a century ago. Engels's and Allende's denunciations of the exploitation of illness by pharmaceutical manufacturers, and calls for public ownership of such enterprises, have an equally modern ring. In somewhat different ways, the three analysts advocated a public health service that would provide medical care across class lines, that would correct maldistribution, and that would restrict profits of practitioners and of the firms that produce drugs and medical supplies. The inhibitions that block such policy alternatives, now as previously, derive mainly from the capitalist class and the private medical profession. Those who benefit from the social conditions that foster illness oppose basic changes in these conditions. The historical continuity of these policy dilemmas, sad as it may be, is also instructive.

Political Strategy

The area of policy raises another crucial divergence. Engels, Virchow, and Allende differed in their views of the political strategies needed to achieve the policies they sought. They also held varying visions of the society in which these policies would take effect. Although their explanations of the social origins of illness converged in many respects, the question of how to change illness-generating conditions evoked quite different strategic analyses.

Even in his early work Engels's strategy involved revolution, not reform. His documentation of the occupational and environmental conditions that caused illness and early death did not aim toward limited reform of those problems. Instead, as noted earlier, he intended his data to serve, at least in part, as propaganda. The purpose was to provide a focus for political organizing among the working class. Notably, Engels did not advocate specific changes in the conditions he described. While he detailed, for instance, the defects of housing, sanitation, occupational safety, maldistribution of medical personnel, and promotion of drugs, he did not explicitly seek reforms in any of these areas. The alternatives that he occasionally suggested, such as the cursory outlines of a public health service, were always speculations about how a more effective system might appear in a post-revolutionary society. The many deprivations of working-class life required fundamental change in the entire social order, rather than limited improvements in each separate sphere. Engels's later writings sometime adopted a more flexible stance about reform in the context of capitalism. The companion piece of *The Condition of the Working Class in England,* however, was clearly *The Communist Manifesto*. The strategic implications of Engels's analysis of health problems were congruent with his role as a primary organizer of the First International. From this perspective, reformism in health care made as little sense as other piecemeal tinkering with capitalist society.

Virchow's strategic approach was quite different. Although he participated in the agitation of the late 1840s, and although he doubted that the ruling circles would permit needed changes in response to peaceful challenges alone, he ultimately opted for reform rather than revolution. While the conditions he witnessed in the Upper Silesian typhus epidemic were horrifying, he believed that a series of reforms could correct the problem. The reforms he advocated transcended medicine to include rationalized food distribution, modifications in the educational system, political enfranchisement, and other changes at the level of social structure. He also adopted a broad view of the systematic reforms that were necessary in health care. An adequate health system, for example, demanded a public health service. In this service, health care professionals would work as employees of the state and would act to correct maldistribution across class, geographical, and ethnic lines. As an overall political goal, Virchow favored a constitutional democracy that would reduce the power of the monarchy and nobility. He supported principles of socialism, particularly those features of socialism that involved public ownership and rational organization of health and welfare facilities. However, Virchow argued against communism, mainly, he said, because of its naive view that a just society was feasible without a strong state apparatus. Virchow firmly believed that limited reforms within capitalist society were both appropriate and desirable, and he was optimistic that they would be effective. During his later life, the reformist slant of his strategic thinking became even clearer.

Allende's conceptualization of political strategy was more complex and differentiated than that of Engels or Virchow. In *La Realidad Medico-Social Chilena,* he stated unambiguously that the health problems of the Chilean working class were inherent in the class structure of society, in the deprivations of underdevelopment, and in the exploitative international relations of capitalist imperialism. Without basic modification of these structural problems, he argued, limited medical reform would prove futile. In Allende's view, revolutionary social change was necessary. But his revolutionary strategy remained that of the peaceful road. Throughout his life, Allende believed that progressive forces could achieve a socialist transformation of society through a sequence of peaceful actions within the framework of constitutional democracy. He and his co-workers based this position on a sophisticated reading of prior socialist strategists, examples of other revolutions, and, most of all, a detailed analysis of Chile's concrete historical and material reality. From this viewpoint, the most important health-related reforms transcended medicine. Allende called for basic improvements in housing, nutrition, employment, and other concrete manifestations of class oppression. Such reforms were the preconditions for reduced morbidity and mortality; without them, changes in health care services could not succeed. On the other hand, structural reforms in the medical system, including a public health service and a nationalized pharmaceutical and equipment industry, were desirable goals en route to a socialist society.

Allende did not accurately anticipate the violent fury of national and international groups about to be dispossessed on the peaceful road to socialism. The balance between reform and revolutionary alternatives remains a crucial and incompletely resolved problem in strategic planning. Chile's tragedy does not detract from the importance of Allende's strategic thinking, in the health sector as in other areas of social life.

CONCLUSION

The social origins of illness are not mysterious. Yet, 135 years after Engels's analysis first appeared, these problems have received remarkably little attention in research or political practice. Industrial hygiene has tended to accept as given the structures of the capitalist system; until recently, activities in occupational health and safety have focused on interventions that would assure an efficient and profitable labor force. On the other hand, medical sociology generally has adopted, or modified only slightly, the medical model of etiology. In this model, social conditions may increase susceptibility or exacerbate disease, but they are not primary causes like microbial agents or disturbances of normal physiology. Since investigation has not clarified the social structural causes of illness, political strategy—both within and outside medicine—seldom has addressed the roots of disease in society.

The social pathologies that distressed Engels, Virchow, and Allende remain with us (32-33). Inequalities of class, exploitation of workers, and conditions of capitalist production cause disease now as previously. Likewise, the constraints of profit and lack of societal responsibility for personal economic security still inhibit even incremental reforms. Stimulated in part by the deepening crisis of world capitalism, current and future research promises to clarify the links between social structure and disease, as well as the contradictions between profit and health. An understanding of these roots of illness also reveals the scope of reconstruction that is necessary for meaningful solutions.

Acknowledgments—Hans-Ulrich Deppe, Eberhard Göpel, David Himmelstein, Tela Long, Vicente Navarro, and Barbara Waterman provided extremely useful criticism and support, although they may disagree with some of this chapter's conclusions.

REFERENCES

1. Engels, F. Briefe aus dem Wuppertal. In *Werke,* by K. Marx and F. Engels, v. 1, pp. 413-432. Dietz Verlag, Berlin, 1961.
2. Kupisch, K. *Von Pietismus zum Kommunismus: Zur Jugendentwicklung von Friedrich Engels.* Lettner-Verlag, Berlin, 1965.
3. Mayer, G. *Friedrich Engels: Eine Biographie.* Kiepenheuer & Witsch, Cologne, 1932.
4. Henderson, W. O. *The Life of Friedrich Engels.* Frank Cass, London, 1976.
5. Ulrich, H. *Der Junge Engels.* VEB Deutscher Verlag der Wissenschaften, Berlin, 1961.
6. Engels, F. *Zwischen 18 und 25: Jugendbriefe von Friedrich Engels.* Dietz Verlag, Berlin, 1965.
7. Machackove, V. *Der Junge Engels und die Literatur.* Dietz Verlag, Berlin, 1961.
8. Marcus, S. *Engels, Manchester, and the Working Class.* Vintage, New York, 1974.
9. Lafargue, P. Personliche Erinnerungen an Friedrich Engels. In *Erinnerungen an Marx und Engels,* p. 477. Dietz Verlag, Berlin, 1965.
10. Engels, F. *The Conditions of the Working Class in England.* Progress Publishers, Moscow, 1973.
11. Engels, F. *Herr Eugen Dühring's Revolution in Science (Anti-Dühring).* International, New York, 1878.
12. Engels, F. *Dialectics of Nature.* International, New York, 1940.
13. Virchow, R. *Cellular Pathology.* DeWitt, New York, 1860.
14. Virchow, R. *Briefe an Seine Eltern.* Engelmann, Leipzig, 1907.
15. Virchow, R. *Ueber den Hungertyphus und einige verwandte Krankheitsformen.* Hirschwald, Berlin, 1868.
16. Virchow, R. *Gesammelte Abhandlungen aus dem Gebiet der Öffentlichen Medicin und der Seuchenlehre.* Hirschwald, Berlin, 1879.
17. Virchow, R. *Werk und Wirkung.* Rütten & Loening, Berlin, 1957.
18. Marx, K., and Engels, F. *Gesamtausgabe.* Marx-Engels-Verlag, Berlin, 1931.

19. Boenheim, F. Einleitung. In *Werk und Wirkung*, by R. Virchow, pp. 7-31. Rütten & Loening, Berlin, 1957.
20. Deppe, H.-U. Rudolf Virchow Kampf um die Preussische Verfassung. *Blatter für deutsche und internationale Politik* 13: 961-974, 1968.
21. Deppe, H.-U., and Regus, M. *Seminar: Medizin, Gesellschaft, Geschichte*. Suhrkamp Verlag, Frankfort am Main, 1975.
22. Virchow, R. *Disease, Life and Man*. Translated by L. J. Rather. Stanford University Press, Stanford, 1958.
23. Ackerknecht, E. H. *Rudolf Virchow: Doctor, Statesman, Anthropologist*. University of Wisconsin Press, Madison, 1953.
24. Debray, R. *The Chilean Revolution: Conversations with Allende*. Vintage, New York, 1971.
25. North American Congress on Latin America. *New Chile*. Waller Press, Berkeley, 1972.
26. Allende, S., and Vizcarra, J. *La Estructuración de la Salubridad Nacional*. Santiago, 1935.
27. Allende, S. *La Realidad Medico-Social Chilena*. Ministerio de Salubridad, Prevision y Asistencia Social, Santiago, 1939.
28. Chile Departamento de Planificación. *Biografía del Presidente Allende*. Departamento de Impresos, Santiago, 1972.
29. Waitzkin, H., and Modell, H. Medicine, socialism, and totalitarianism: Lessons from Chile. *N. Engl. J. Med.* 291: 171-177, 1974.
30. Modell, H., and Waitzkin, H. Medicine and socialism in Chile. *Berkeley Journal of Sociology* 19: 1-35, 1974.
31. Modell, H., and Waitzkin, H. Socialism and health care in Chile. *Monthly Review* 27: 29-40, May 1975.
32. Waitzkin, H. A Marxist view of medical care. *Ann. Intern. Med.* 89: 264-278, 1978.
33. Waitzkin, H., and Waterman, B. *The Exploitation of Illness in Capitalist Society*. Bobbs-Merrill, Indianapolis, 1974.

CHAPTER 2

Measuring Social Inequalities in Health in the United States: A Historical Review, 1900–1950

Nancy Krieger and Elizabeth Fee

Social inequalities in health have long been documented in the United States. From the successive smallpox epidemics of the early 1600s, which killed many settlers but decimated the American Indian population (1–3), and the first colonial bills of mortality, which separately tabulated deaths among whites and "negroes" (4), up to the most recent federal publications on the *Health Status of the Disadvantaged* (5) and the *Health Status of Minorities and Low-Income Groups* (6), U.S. records of births, deaths, and disease have revealed disturbing disparities. Since the start of the modern public health movement in the mid-1800s, and as exemplified by John Griscom's groundbreaking 1845 report on *The Sanitary Conditions of the Laboring Population of New York with Suggestions for Its Improvement* (7; see also 8, pp. 213–217), U.S. public health reformers and public health professionals have prepared reports to document the magnitude of social inequalities in health and to provide benchmarks for evaluating progress in addressing these problems.

Surprisingly, however, U.S. vital statistics—unlike those in Great Britain and several other European countries (9)—have not routinely reported birth and death rates stratified by socioeconomic measures. Instead, they have been tabulated principally by age, sex, and race (6, 10, 11). The same holds true for many other forms of routinely reported public health data, spanning the gamut from notifiable communicable diseases to cancer registries. Even in cases where socioeconomic information is included, the data are often stratified separately by socioeconomic position, by race/ethnicity, and by gender, rather than cross-tabulated.

These conventions would, at first blush, suggest that the relationship between socioeconomic conditions and the public's health has not been accorded serious attention by U.S. public health agencies and public health professionals. The usual explanation is that government officials in the past have liked to assume that the United States is a "classless" society and that the concept of "social class" is not relevant to the health of the U.S. population (10–14). It may therefore be a surprise to discover that, during the first third of this century, questions of socioeconomic inequalities in morbidity and mortality ranked high on the agenda of federal and other public health agencies, and routine reporting of U.S. vital statistics and health survey data by socioeconomic measures was nearly institutionalized. This history has largely been lost.

To recapture this history, we focus our chapter on the period from 1900 to 1950 and examine how public health researchers, both within and outside federal health agencies, conceptualized and analyzed socioeconomic inequalities in health. We first consider the early work of the Bureau of the Census in standardizing and reporting U.S. vital statistics, and the investigations of researchers within the U.S. Public Health Service who were involved in numerous specialized studies of socioeconomic factors in health. We then discuss the contributions of other groups within the larger public health movement, such as the U.S. Children's Bureau and the National Tuberculosis Association, which were also interested in socioeconomic inequalities in health but found that their needs for relevant data were not being met by U.S. vital statistics or by the Public Health Service. By considering the activities of these different agencies, as framed by the sociopolitical context of their times, we recover a rich history that can inform current debates over how to collect and evaluate data relating socioeconomic conditions to health and disease.

STANDARDIZING U.S. VITAL STATISTICS: EARLY WORK OF THE BUREAU OF THE CENSUS

At the start of the 20th century, vital statistics in the United States were just beginning to be organized on a national basis. In 1842, Massachusetts became the first state to mandate state-wide registration of vital statistics (8, p. 217; 15). Other states gradually followed suit, but, since each was responsible for collecting its own data, the quality varied considerably. In 1880, the U.S. government created a "Federal Registration Area for Deaths" that included two states, the District of Columbia, and several cities whose vital statistics were considered to be reasonably complete; during the next two decades, this region expanded to include another seven states, mainly in the industrial east and the agrarian mid-west (16, p. 44; 17). To improve the accuracy and compatibility of the states' data, in 1900 the Bureau introduced the first standardized birth and death certificates (18). It could, however, do no more than recommend their adoption, since states' rights were as carefully guarded in the collection of health data as in many other areas (19). In 1902, when the Bureau of the Census was established as a permanent federal agency, it was given statutory authority for developing registration areas for births and deaths and began to publish annual reports on mortality rates in the Federal Registration Area (16–18). In 1915, the Bureau established a federal Birth Registration Area, containing 15 states, and began publishing annual reports on birth rates; as of 1933, the Death and Birth Registration Areas encompassed the entire nation (17, pp. 96–99). The Bureau continued to be responsible for U.S. birth and death certificates and for U.S. national vital statistics until 1946, when responsibility was transferred to the Public Health Service (16, 18).

The first government report based on the standard certificates of 1900 presented birth and death rates by age, sex, nativity, and color (20). Color—later transmuted to "race" and erroneously considered a relatively simple and unambiguous biological characteristic—has continued to be a central category for vital statistics classification from 1900 to the present (6, 14, 16, 21, 22). By contrast, the measurement of class has always been deemed difficult and complicated. At the turn of the century, the Bureau of the Census was interested in gathering data on the relationship of health to occupation, spurred by social and political concerns about the effects of rapid industrialization on the health and fertility of the laboring population (23, p. 2). In 1900, the Bureau included questions on "occupation" in the first standardized death and birth certificates, referring, respectively, to the occupation of the decedent and to that of the infant's mother and father (18, pp. 18, 21); data on the mother's occupation were intended to measure the effects of maternal employment on infant mortality (24, pp. 98–99). In 1910, questions on "business and industry" were added to the standardized death certificate (18, p. 21). The Bureau did not, however, publish reports based on these occupational data because they considered them too inaccurate to justify publication (25).

In Britain, in the same period, the collection and analysis of vital statistics and health data by occupation and social class was considerably more advanced. Census records and vital statistics had, since 1837, been centrally collected in the General Registry Office, with compulsory reporting mandated by the Registration of Births and Deaths Act of 1874; the centralized collection of data in the British system greatly facilitated the tabulation of national vital statistics on birth and mortality rates (26–29; 30, p. 71). The Registrar-General's Decennial Supplements prepared by Farr, Ogle, and others combined vital and census statistics to reveal striking differences in mortality rates between male workers in diverse occupations. The life tables likewise showed dramatic differences in life expectancy between those living in healthy, upper-class residential districts and those in unhealthy working-class slums (26; 29, p. 399; 31, pp. 123–153). Throughout the 19th century, such statistics were used by Royal Commissions and groups of reformers to delineate the miserable health conditions of the industrial working classes and to guide public policy (31, pp. 11, 52; 32).

This approach, of analyzing health statistics by occupation and social class, would continue to frame British discussions of national health in the 20th century (30, pp. 286–301; 33, p. x). It was institutionalized in the Registrar-General's system of social classes created in 1911 by the Superintendent of Statistics, T. H. C. Stevenson, and first officially employed in government reports on fertility and infant mortality (34–38). This system divided the population into five broad occupational classes: I. Professional; II. Intermediate; III. Skilled; IV. Partly skilled; and V. Unskilled; and, in addition, it defined three special occupational groups: textile workers, miners, and agricultural workers. Later reports on female mortality classified married women, whether in the paid labor force or not, by the occupational class of their husbands, whereas single women, like single and married men, were classified according to their own occupation (39, 40). With relatively minor changes, this system of classification has been retained to the present (33, p. 40).

THE PUBLIC HEALTH SERVICE:
EARLY STUDIES ON INCOME AND HEALTH

In the United States, by contrast, no single agency was responsible for public health research and vital statistics. The Public Health Service was formally created in 1912 by expanding the Marine Hospital Service; as a completely separate agency from the Bureau of the Census, it had no direct authority over vital statistics. The Public Health Service was assigned the duties of preventing the transmission of communicable diseases across state lines, supervising the health of streams and waterways, gathering data on reportable diseases, conducting research, and assisting the states' public health efforts (41–43).

Within a few years of its establishment, the Public Health Service was to sponsor work that would have enormous influence on scientific and public understanding of socioeconomic inequalities in health. Following the enaction in 1911 of workmen's compensation laws in the United States and national health insurance in Britain, the agency became interested in the links between health, work, and health insurance. Workmen's compensation insurance required a knowledge of the risks of various forms of work in different industries; national health insurance, if enacted, would require knowledge of the relative risks and costs of illness in different sectors of the population. Spurring on this work were several highly publicized workplace disasters, such as the 1911 fire at the Triangle Shirt Waist Factory in New York City, in which 146 women garment workers plunged ten floors to their deaths because the factory had no fire escapes (44), and increasingly militant strikes, such as that of the textile workers in Lawrence, Massachusetts, in 1912, which brought national attention to the plight of underpaid workers (45, pp. 315–349).

In 1916, two Public Health Service officers, Benjamin S. Warren, who held the rank of Surgeon, and Edgar Sydenstricker, the Public Health Service's first statistician, published a study on the health of garment workers in relation to their economic status (46) and, at the request of the Surgeon General, prepared a comprehensive report on "Health Insurance: Its Relation to the Public Health" (47). These two works, complemented by Sydenstricker's subsequent studies, clearly established poverty as the main axis of analysis of socioeconomic differences in health in the United States—at least as far as the Public Health Service was concerned—by contrast to the British Registrar-General's emphasis on occupational mortality and social class.

In the first of these publications, on the health of garment workers, Warren and Sydenstricker explained that although those familiar with conditions among low-paid wage earners believed that low wages harmed the health of the workers and their families, there was "a general lack of statistical data indicating these effects" (46, p. 1299). In a careful study of the health of 3,000 white male and female married garment workers and their families in New York City in 1914, Warren and Sydenstricker performed physical examinations, screened for tuberculosis, measured hemoglobin levels, and gathered data on nutritional status, average weekly and annual earnings, and employment status. Classifying individuals according to the annual earnings of the head of household, they found marked differences in health between the poorest families, with incomes under $500, and those with annual incomes over $700. Child mortality, for example, was 21 percent in the poorest families but 12 percent among the somewhat better-off families. Warren and Sydenstricker concluded that "the greatest number of poorly nourished, anemic, tuberculous workers in an extremely seasonal industry were in that group composed of the lowest paid and the least regularly employed" (46, p. 1305). They were clearly impressed that, even among a relatively poor paid group of workers with the same occupation, small variations in economic level had great implications for their health and the health of their families.

In their subsequent report on the relationship of health to health insurance, Warren and Sydenstricker argued that the United States must follow the lead of several European countries and prepare for the introduction of national health insurance. This, they said, could have very beneficial effects on public health: if employers were to share the costs of their workers' illnesses, they would undoubtedly take more interest in disease prevention. First, however, the government needed to understand the extent of employers' responsibility for disease causation. This required data both on people's occupations and on families' economic levels. Summarizing the admittedly limited literature, Warren and Sydenstricker differentiated between occupational diseases resulting from workplace conditions and the broader health problems stemming from inadequate wages and/or irregularity of employment and caused by such intermediate factors as poor diets, bad housing, and blighted neighborhoods. As in their study on garment workers, they argued that poverty was the main cause of illness. Employers who refused to pay a living wage were thus culpable for diseases of poverty (47, pp. 36–37). Discussing the extent of public and private responsibility for ill-health, Warren and Sydenstricker suggested policies to reduce sickness and impoverishment, and outlined proposals for health insurance and sick benefit plans.

Perhaps Sydenstricker's most important formative experience in health research was his next project, working with Joseph Goldberger and G. A. Wheeler to unravel the etiology of pellagra among impoverished millworkers in the southern United States (48). Sydenstricker brought to this study his dual expertise in economics and statistics, and he gained from it a firm conviction of the centrality of income to health. Prior research in both Europe and the United States had strongly suggested that pellagra was a disease of poverty, associated with rural occupations, but considerable controversy still existed on whether it was a dietary or an infectious disease (49, 50). In this context, one central question Goldberger, Wheeler, and Sydenstricker faced was why, among a group of similarly employed and relatively poor white millworkers, some individuals and their families were stricken by pellagra whereas others were spared. Hypothesizing that pellagra was related to diet, the researchers studied seven cotton-mill towns in 1916 and carefully recorded—during a 15-day period preceding the seasonal peak incidence of pellagra in the early summer—the amount and type of food purchased by each family and consumed by each family member. Through this detailed work, they were able to show that annual family income, the conventional demarcation of economic level, failed to provide a sufficiently sensitive measure of the food available to each individual within the family. A family with one child, for example, would have more to eat than another family at the same income level but with five children. Their work also showed that when resources were short, women tended to give the best food to the adult men and skimp on their own diets. These patterns of actual food consumption had not been previously recorded in epidemiologic research.

To solve the problems posed by the pellagra study, Sydenstricker decided he needed a new and more accurate economic scale. He believed that any measure of economic well-being in relation to health must ultimately be derived from family income: "Whether or not nutritious diet, sanitary housing, adequate clothing, proper facilities for the care of children, opportunity for wholesome recreation, and sanitary neighborhood conditions can be enjoyed is determined mainly by the family's financial status" (51, p. 2830). Because the pellagra study had shown that family income alone was not a sufficient index, Sydenstricker and King developed two new economic scales of the income required to maintain all members of the family (51). These were based on Atwater's scale of the different amounts of food required by infants and toddlers, boys and girls, and adult women and men (52). Sydenstricker's novel contribution was to express these requirements as fractions of a single numerical economic unit, based on the food consumption of an adult male, which he termed the "fammain," short for "food expense for adult male maintenance." This number was higher for adults than children and, for persons aged 12 and older, higher for males than females. An adult male (over 16 years old) was assigned a value of 1.0; an adult female, 0.8;

among adolescents 12 through 16 years old, values for boys were 0.1 unit higher than those for girls (for boys, set at 0.9 for ages 15 to 16, at 0.8 for ages 13 to 14, and at 0.7 for age 12); below age 12, boys and girls were assigned the same value (0.6 for ages 10 to 11, 0.5 for ages 6 to 9, 0.4 for ages 2 to 5, and 0.3 for those under 2 years old).

Using a similar approach, Sydenstricker also developed a more general measure, the "ammain," or "total expense for adult male maintenance," which took into account the costs of food, clothing, tobacco, soft drinks, entertainment, etc. (51). In either case, the total family income divided by the required number of "fammains" or "ammains" yielded Sydenstricker's desired universal measure. Arguing that this index should become the standard for public health research, he wrote: "results derived by the use of these scales would . . . be decidedly superior to those obtained by classifying families on the basis of net income for the family as a whole, without considering its size or composition, or even by figuring the net per capita income for each family" (51, p. 2846). He demonstrated this assertion by successfully using the fammain scale in the pellagra study and, together with Goldberger and Wheeler, decisively proving that the disease was caused by nutritional deficiency (48).

Sydenstricker's work set the standard for research conducted by the Public Health Service. After completing the work on pellagra, he designed the first longitudinal study of ill-health among an urban population, which was carried out in Hagerstown, Maryland, between December 1921 and March 1924 (53). Decrying the use of mortality data as an index of health, he advocated collecting data on morbidity, since regions with low death rates might nonetheless have high rates of debilitating illness—as was the case in areas with high prevalences of pellagra, malaria, and hookworm disease. Aiming to give "glimpses of what the sanitarian has long wanted to see—a picture of the public-health situation as a whole, drawn in proper perspective and painted in true colors" (53, p. 280), Sydenstricker and his staff collected baseline data on the health status and economic conditions of over 7,200 members of white families, and continued to visit each family every six to eight weeks for 28 months to record all new cases of illness. They restricted the study to white families because they did not want to confuse economic and "racial" differences in health (54, p. 417). This project generated vast quantities of novel and useful data about health in relationship to family and community conditions (albeit only among whites) and became a landmark in public health research (55, 56).

In 1926, when Selwyn D. Collins, Associate Statistician of the Public Health Service, published, at the request of the Surgeon General, a monograph on "Economic Status and Health" (57), he drew heavily on Sydenstricker's work, including the pellagra and Hagerstown studies. Reflecting his mentor's profound influence, he noted that "Few field studies of morbidity have been undertaken in recent years that have not attempted in some way to evaluate the effect of economic status on the disease being investigated" (57, p. 1). Citing "rough" estimates of economic status, such as "the amount or class of insurance carried, the section of the city in which the family resides, and the occupation of the person or of the household head," he asserted that "any method based on income" was, of course, "superior to the other methods" (57, p. 4). In this light, he reviewed European data on mortality and morbidity rates by social class and the limited U.S. data on infant mortality by economic level. He concluded that these studies showed the rich generally were healthier and lived longer than the poor and that these advantages could not wholly be attributed to differences in age, race, or occupation.

Two years later, Rollo H. Britten, Associate Statistician in the Office of Industrial Hygiene in the Public Health Service, summarized the British government's report on occupational mortality among men for 1921–1923 (58). This was only the second decennial report to classify occupations according to the Registrar-General's system of social classes. Britten reviewed the British data in some detail, noting that most U.S. public health professionals did not have access to the original report and that the United States lacked comparable data. He suggested that the British could usefully gather mortality data by occupation because British workers rarely changed their jobs; by implication, job mobility in the United States made occupational mortality statistics unreliable. From the perspective of industrial hygiene, Britten's point had some validity; job changes meant that the occupational data on death certificates were not necessarily useful for etiologic studies concerned with occupational exposures. But Britten confused the effects of specific job changes with the less common phenomenon of social class mobility; he was wrong to imply that job mobility made it impossible to calculate U.S. mortality rates by social class.

The architect of the Registrar-General's system of classification by social class, T. H. C. Stevenson, was aware of these U.S. arguments in favor of income data, but remained unconvinced that such data were superior for understanding socio-economic differences in health status. Replying to his American critics, in 1928 he wrote (59, pp. 208–209):

> To some extent comparisons of vital statistics . . . have recently been compiled in the U.S.A., and possibly elsewhere, with distinction of family income. . . . So far as this method can be applied it is, of course, ideal for estimation of the effects of wealth as such. . . . But its drawback is that it may fail altogether as an index to culture, probably the more important influence. The power of culture to exert a favourable influence upon mortality, even in the complete absence of wealth, is well illustrated by the case of the clergy. The income test, if it could be applied, would certainly place them well down the list, yet their mortality is remarkably low. . . . Such a record as this, consistently repeated in each succeeding report, seems to make it quite clear that the lower mortality of the wealthier classes depends less upon wealth itself than upon the culture, extending to matters of hygiene, generally on the whole associated with it. . . . But culture is more

easily estimated, as between occupations, than wealth, so the occupational basis of social grading has a wholesome tendency to emphasize it . . . when one speaks of the more or less comfortable classes one is thinking largely of the more or less cultured classes.

Stevenson's comments articulate the difference between a conventional British understanding of social class, based on generally shared ideas of culture, status, and consciousness, and popular views in the United States which were much more likely to emphasize income as the true measure of social differentiation. To Stevenson, a proper understanding of the full spectrum of health and disease could not be reached simply by focusing on income; consideration of the social as well as the economic milieu was essential.

LINKING SOCIOECONOMIC DATA AND VITAL STATISTICS: CONTRIBUTIONS OF THE BROADER PUBLIC HEALTH MOVEMENT

Other groups within the broader U.S. public health movement had their own reasons for wanting U.S. vital statistics to be stratified by socioeconomic level. W. E. B. Du Bois, for example, in his 1906 review, *The Health and Physique of the Negro American* (60), inveighed against the common belief that a presumed biological inferiority explained the poorer health of the black population compared with the white population. Instead, suggested Du Bois, the differences could be explained on other grounds (60, p. 89);

If the population were divided as to social and economic condition the matter of race would be almost entirely eliminated. . . . In England . . . the poor have a [death] rate twice as high as the rich. . . . In Chicago the death rate among whites of the stock yards district is higher than the Negroes of that city.

Even within the Public Health Service, some argued that reporting vital statistics by race masked the differentiation of health status by economic level. John W. Trask, an Assistant Surgeon General, observed in 1916 that the mortality rate of the colored population of the United States was higher than that of U.S. whites but lower than that of the white population of Hungary, Roumania, Spain, and Austria (61). Reminding his readers of the lower incomes of black households, he raised an important question: "It may be that if in the average community deaths could be classified according to economic status, that is, according to the family or household income, a difference in the mortality rates would be obtained approximately as great as that resulting from a white and colored classification" (61, pp. 258–259). This question would have to remain unanswered as long as data were collected only by race and not by economic level—and as long as the Public Health Service limited its investigations of income and health to white populations, did not engage in studies of mortality, and did not consider the adverse health effects of racial discrimination either within or across economic strata.

Another federal agency, the U.S. Children's Bureau, was interested in vital statistics reported by economic level as well as by race. Created in 1912 as an agency of the Department of Labor, the Children's Bureau was quite separate from, and a good deal more radical than, the Public Health Service (24, pp. 176–185; 62, 63). Its dedicated researchers, most of them women, conducted the first prospective studies of infant mortality in a general urban population (64, 65). In the words of Julia C. Lathrop, the first Chief of the Children's Bureau and the first woman to be in charge of a federal agency (66, p. 270):

> So far as the Bureau was aware, the method employed was new. Instead of basing the inquiry on the children who died, the criterion was really the children born in a given calendar year. The surroundings of each child were traced through his first year of life, or such shorter period as he survived, by women agents of the Bureau who called upon each mother and obtained information through direct personal interviews.

For this project, the Children's Bureau selected eight cities, chosen for their social and industrial conditions, including their ethnic and racial composition (65, p. 28). The researchers examined variations in infant mortality rates by maternal employment; parents' race, nativity, and occupation; and family economic level (measured by the father's earnings). According to Lathrop (66, p. 271):

> Great pains were taken to make the income figures as accurate as possible. . . . Hence, in one of the earliest studies a test was made of the accuracy of the mother's answers to the income questions by comparing them with the facts about the father's earnings collected from as many sources as possible; payrolls were consulted and employers and the fathers themselves were interviewed.

Other socioeconomic data gathered in the field concerned each family's monthly rent, whether their home had a bathtub and/or a private indoor or outdoor latrine, the extent of overcrowding, whether the family kept lodgers or boarders to increase their income, and what type of health care was available during the course of pregnancy and at the birth itself.

Similar care was taken in the analysis and interpretation of the survey results. One quickly apparent finding was that the lowest income groups suffered the highest infant mortality rates: the rate for families with an annual income of less than $550 was 151.4 deaths per 1000 births, but was 64.3 for those with an income above $1250 (65, p. 15; 66). To disentangle the various possible causes of the high infant mortality rates among the poor, the Bureau evaluated the contribution of maternal nationality, race, age, and employment; birth order and interval since preceding birth; and breast-feeding and artificial feeding (in relation to each month of the infant's life) (65, pp. 59–74). After painstaking statistical analyses, the Bureau researchers decided that the correlation between economic level and infant mortality was "independent of type of feeding, of race and nationality, and of the factors involved in frequency of births" and instead reflected the "economic pressure due to low father's earnings" in conjunction with such "intermediate factors" as housing congestion, mother's employment, and kinds of health care available (65, p. 151).

To begin to break the link between economic level and infant mortality, the Children's Bureau called for "the free provision of adequate prenatal and confinement care for mothers and of medical supervision over infants through municipal health centers or clinics," instruction of all girls and women in "the normal hygiene of maternity and infancy," and "community responsibility for decent housing and sanitation" (66, p. 274). Explicitly challenging the prevailing notion that ignorance, rather than poverty, was the chief cause of infant mortality, Lathrop forcefully argued that "a decent income, self-respectingly earned by the father is the beginning of wisdom . . . and the strongest safeguard against a high infant mortality rate" (66, p. 274). To secure data needed for public policy, the Children's Bureau urged the collection of national vital statistics by economic level and was instrumental in getting the federal Birth Registration Area established in 1915 (62, pp. 15–16).

The desire for accurate data on socioeconomic differences in mortality was further revealed by an unusual study published in 1924 by Charles V. Chapin, a leading U.S. public health official (67). Because no contemporary data on income and adult U.S. mortality were available, he laboriously matched 60-year-old death records to the tax information contained in the 1865 census (whose records were no longer confidential) and retabulated the causes of death according to current conventions. Finding that the age-adjusted death rate of those wealthy enough to pay taxes was less than one-half that of poorer, non-tax-paying citizens (10.8 versus 24.8 deaths per 1000 people), Chapin concluded: "When we have definitely determined the incidence of different causes of death on the two classes, we will be prepared for what should be of great value, namely, a study of the habits of life and of the environment which make for the longevity of the well-to-do" (67, p. 651).

The National Tuberculosis Association, one of the United States' oldest and most influential voluntary health organizations, was similarly interested in—and frustrated by the absence of—occupational and socioeconomic mortality data for the adult population in the United States (68, 69). The Association needed this information to help target tuberculosis control programs in industrial settings, beyond their first obvious efforts in the dusty trades. Although appreciative of the information provided by studies of occupational mortality based on the records of large insurance companies, such as those conducted by Louis I. Dublin of the Metropolitan Life Insurance Company (70, 71), the Association recognized that its work was hampered by the absence of data on the health status of the much larger portion of the workforce that lacked insurance. Moreover, the English data, however useful, were limited by the relatively small size of the British population: the United States possessed four times as many workers as Britain, and thus more stable rates could, in principle, be calculated for a much larger number of industries. In the late 1920s, the Association therefore designed a project to furnish "for the first time in the United States death rates by occupation based on United States Census figures" (72). According to Kendall Emerson, the Managing Director of the Association, a comprehensive study on the subject would be valuable "not only for the data on tuberculosis it might reveal, but also for its contribution to the knowledge of heart disease, pneumonia, diabetes, and many other diseases." Such information would be relevant not only to the public health and medical professions but also to "workmen's compensation boards, insurance companies, and to industrial hygiene activities in general" (72).

The project was, from the beginning, aggressively nurtured by Jessamine S. Whitney, the chief statistician of the National Tuberculosis Association (68, pp. 144, 203, 230). Trained as a social worker, Whitney had previously worked as a special agent in the Bureau of Labor in Woman and Child Labor Investigation, under the aegis of the Bureau of the Census (73). In 1913, pursuing her interest in economic matters and social welfare, she became involved with the Children's Bureau's infant mortality studies and directed their project in New Bedford, Massachusetts (74). Thus, by the time Whitney joined the National Tuberculosis Association in 1919, she had accumulated considerable experience investigating the relationship between people's occupations, income, and well-being.

Whitney undertook the National Tuberculosis Association's project with considerable resolve, explaining that "At that time the outlook for sound death rates seemed not very optimistic, but it was thought that only by making a beginning could any results be obtained" (75, p. 11). As a first step, she and a research assistant checked the adequacy of occupational returns of 27,500 death certificates filed during 1927 in urban and rural Ohio and certain industrial cities of New England. Informed by their preliminary results, they next conducted a comprehensive educational campaign in 1929, intended to improve the quality of occupational data, in which they visited 21 state registrars of vital statistics in their home offices and met with seven more state registrars at national or sectional health conferences. Subsequently, at the request of the state registrars of New York, Wisconsin, Illinois, and Alabama, they tested the adequacy of these states' occupational returns and prepared constructive memoranda with suggestions for improvements. When the National Tuberculosis Association contacted William Mott Steuart, the Director of the Census, for permission to work with the 1930 census data, Whitney and her staff had already checked 53,342 death certificates for the adequacy of their occupational information and thus could clearly demonstrate the feasibility of their proposed project.

The Bureau of the Census readily gave permission, and the project became a joint endeavor of the Census Bureau and the National Tuberculosis Association (75); the Public Health Service was not involved. In early 1930, the Bureau of the Census published a pamphlet, the *Pocket Reference of Information on Occupations* (25), and distributed more than 50,000 copies to state and city registrars of vital statistics and undertakers. As noted by Whitney, this pamphlet outlined "the need and importance of death rates by occupation" and gave "simple yet definite instructions" (25; 75, p. 12). To ensure that occupational information on the death certificates would be compatible with that obtained in the 1930 census, the Bureau of the Census incorporated additional and more specific inquiries regarding occupation into the 1930 revision of the death certificate (25). The new questions included the date at which the deceased had last worked at his or her stated occupation, the total number of years spent at that occupation, and whether the disease or injury responsible for death was "related to occupation." Comparable questions on the parents' occupations were added to the 1930 revision of the birth certificate, which for the first time asked about the duration and last date of employment for the mother's and father's stated occupations (18, pp. 18–22; 25).

In addition to desiring data on mortality rates for particular occupations, Whitney was interested in calculating rates for groups of occupations sharing a similar "social-economic" position (75, pp. 12–14). She argued that mortality rates for a given occupation could be affected by two distinct factors: the specific hazards associated with that occupation and the standard of living it afforded. To distinguish between the two, it would be necessary to compare mortality rates among occupations at the same socioeconomic level. Noting that "The question of dividing occupations int a few large economic groups has always been a ticklish one in America" (75, p. 13), Whitney sought the help of the leading expert on occupational classification in the United States, Alba M. Edwards of the Bureau of the Census, who, since at least 1915, had been interested in combining occupational information in death certificates and census records to produce occupational mortality rates (23, p. 2).

Edwards had joined the Bureau of the Census in 1909, and in 1910 was appointed Special Agent in charge of Occupational Statistics, a position he held until his retirement in 1943 (76, 77). In 1911, he published his first foray into classifying socioeconomic groups (78), a system that he revised in 1917 (79) and updated in 1933 (80). His approach divided the United States workforce into two major blocks of "mental" and "manual" workers, each of which was further subdivided—by professional role and status in the case of mental workers, and by level of skill in the case of manual workers. Spurring his work was a contentious national debate around the massive number of Eastern and Southern European immigrants then entering the United States (28, 77, 78). According to widely accepted eugenicist doctrines, the new immigrants were, on account of their "reduced" intelligence, filling the lower ranks of labor and, because of their high fertility rates, were diluting the country's "superior" native stock (81–83). Labor unions also feared that the relatively untrained and unorganized immigrants were threatening the wage rates and living standards of more highly skilled American workers. Attempting to discover which positions the immigrants were actually filling, Edwards realized that the conventional distribution between skilled and unskilled labor was no longer adequate: with increasing mechanization, many previously skilled jobs had become less skilled and yet could not legitimately be grouped with unskilled labor. The creation of the "semi-skilled" category was Edwards' exceptional contribution to the debate and, using this category, he was able to show that the immigrants had not, after all, exclusively entered the ranks of the unskilled; a large proportion were employed as semi-skilled workers (78).

By the time Whitney contacted Edwards to help with her study on occupational mortality, his classification scheme divided the United States workforce into six major socioeconomic groups: 1. Professional Persons; 2. Proprietors, Managers, and Officials; 3. Clerks and Kindred Workers; 4. Skilled Workers and Foremen; 5. Semiskilled Workers; and 6. Unskilled Workers (80). Whitney altered this grouping in only one respect, by creating a single new category of "agricultural workers," which included both farmers (previously included as "proprietors," whether they were owners or tenants) and farm laborers (previously included in "unskilled workers"). She had found in her field studies that farmers and farm laborers both tended to be reported as "farmers" on death certificates, thereby artificially inflating the death rate of farmers and reducing that of unskilled laborers (75, p. 14).

Ultimately, all coding of occupations for Whitney's study—of both the death certificates and the census records—was done under Edwards' direction (75, pp. 14–15). The final study population included all men 15 to 64 years old residing in 10 of the 48 states included in the Federal Registration Area in 1930. These states were selected because their "data were sufficiently accurate to warrant undertaking a compilation of occupational mortality statistics"; together, they contained 39 percent of all gainfully employed men in the United States (75, p. 12). The study population was restricted to men under age 65 because of the difficulty of knowing how to classify retired people; although not stated explicitly, the same logic was apparently used to justify the exclusion of women. Moreover, to avoid spurious variations caused by small numbers, the analysis was restricted to occupations with at least 500 deaths.

Whitney's final report presented data on crude and age-adjusted mortality rates for the seven main social-economic groups, 53 separate occupations, and 17 different causes of death. Results were provided for men in three different age groups (15–24, 25–44, and 45–64 years old) and for all ages combined, but were not separately reported by either race or nativity. Whitney found that the age-adjusted mortality rate among the total population (based on approximately 14 million men and 122,000 deaths) was 8.7 deaths per 1000 men (75, p. 18). Four of the social classes experienced death rates below this level: for professional men, the rate was 7.0; for proprietors, managers, and officials, 7.4; for clerks and kindred workers, 7.4; and for agricultural workers, 6.2. By contrast, for skilled workers and foremen, the rate was 8.1; for semi-skilled workers, 9.9; and for unskilled workers, 13.1 per 1000. These data showed that the overall mortality rate provided little insight into the real distribution of death rates in the population. The two-fold difference between the highest and lowest rates also gave grounds for optimism that public health campaigns could reduce the excessively high death rates.

Whitney's analyses went beyond these fundamental points. Because of her concern about the two ways in which occupation could be related to mortality—by specific hazards and by standard of living—she sought to examine variations in occupational death rates within the seven broad social-economic groups. Her results implied that both pathways were important (75, p. 32). In the case of tuberculosis, for example, the overall age-adjusted death rate was 87.5 deaths per 100,000 men. Among professional men, this rate was only 26.2 (ranging from a low of 18.3 for lawyers and judges to a high of 30.7 for technical engineers); it was 43.2 among proprietors, managers, and officials (ranging from 19.3 for bankers, brokers, and money-lenders to 81.2 for restaurant employees); 65.8 among clerks and kindred workers (ranging from 28.4 for real estate agents to 97.9 for clerks); 46.5 among agricultural workers; 72.1 among skilled workers and foremen (ranging from 34.6 for foremen and overseers in manufacturing to 143.3 for molders, founders, and casters of metal); 102.1 among semi-skilled workers (ranging from 83.8 for bakers to 108.6 for guards); and 184.9 among unskilled workers (ranging from 91.9 for laborers not working in factories or building construction to 227.3 for laborers employed in those industries). These data suggest that, contrary to the views of Sydenstricker and other Public Health Service researchers, understanding patterns of mortality required attention to both occupation and standard of living; either one alone was not sufficient.

Highlighting the study's key findings, Kendall Emerson, who was now also Executive Secretary of the American Public Health Association (68, p. 227), optimistically declared that the results would serve to "whet the appetite of those to whom such figures have value, so that when the next Federal Census is taken, provision may be made for a general study of this sort covering a larger area and giving data in greater detail" (72). Suggesting that the study had caught the attention of researchers in the Public Health Service, Rollo Britten—still active in industrial hygiene—described its results at length in the September 1934 issue of *Public Health Reports* (84), in an article appearing only three months after the publication of Whitney's findings. Emerson's enthusiasm was also bolstered by the increasingly close ties his organization enjoyed with the Roosevelt administration; in 1933, for example, Harry Hopkins, then executive director of the New York City Tuberculosis Association, had been appointed as director of the new Federal Emergency Relief Administration by President Roosevelt (68, p. 227). As it turned out, however, Emerson's optimism was misplaced.

FROM THE DEPRESSION TO THE COLD WAR: RETRENCHMENT OF SOCIOECONOMIC ANALYSES OF MORTALITY, HEALTH, AND DISEASE

One of the many ways the Great Depression influenced public health research in the United States was to focus attention on economic inequalities in disease rather than on mortality. As argued by two of Sydenstricker's associates at the Public Health Service, George St. John Perrott (then a consultant) and Selwyn D. Collins (by then promoted to Senior Statistician) (85, pp. 595–596):

> The ordinary barometers of health—death rates and reports of communicable diseases—do not indicate that harmful effects of the depression upon the health of the population as a whole have taken place. The comfortable conclusion is drawn by many that the physical well-being of the American people not only has not suffered but, in view of the continued low death rate, may have been benefitted by the economic catastrophe. Such a conclusion, based on mortality statistics alone, is open to question. Even in the worst depression the families of the unemployed are a minority, and the trend of mortality in the total population does not necessarily reflect the trend in these severely affected households.
>
> The assumption that *mortality* in the general population is an accurate index of *sickness* in the families of the unemployed is still less tenable. Recent morbidity studies have shown that the important causes of death are *not* the most frequent causes of illness. The number of illnesses severe enough to be remembered and recorded . . . is 75 to 100 times the number of deaths. . . . The desirability of checking up on *all* illnesses before drawing conclusions from data based only on the *fatal* cases seems apparent. . . . Among the now well-recognized indexes of ill health are records of sickness. When properly obtained and analyzed, they reveal some of the reactions of human beings to immediate environmental factors in a far more sensitive degree than the gross death rate. . . . Since no national system for the complete registration of sickness exists, special records must be collected, a difficulty not without its advantages, since it permits information to be obtained for such groups and in such detail as may be desired.

The Public Health Service therefore launched a massive ten-city study on the effects of the Depression upon illness in 12,000 white families, divided into three economic groups—those whose income remained relatively high between 1929 and 1933, those who had lived comfortably in 1929 but were impoverished in 1933, and those who had lived in a condition of poverty in 1929 and 1933 (85–87). As in several previous Public Health Service studies, "colored sections were excluded to avoid the question of racial differences in employment, income, and sickness" (85, p. 597). One of the more notable findings was that, among the three economic groups examined, the disabling illness rate was highest among the "new" poor.

Directing even more resources into national studies of disease prevalence, in 1935 the Public Health Service began a still more ambitious project, the first U.S. National Health Survey (88). This house-to-house canvass covered 2.5 million people, both white and "colored," living in 83 cities, and followed their health during a one-year period. The study was designed to focus chiefly on sickness and, to a lesser extent, mortality, in their "relation to income and other social and economic circumstances" (88, p. 3). The survey provided data for a huge number of publications on such topics as the rates of disabling and chronic illness, occupational morbidity, accidents, impaired hearing, blindness, fertility and family composition, school attendance, housing quality, unemployment, and access to medical care and public health programs (89). Despite extensive collection of socioeconomic data, however, most studies relied upon income as their only measure of social and economic position, and the few that used occupational data (90–92) did not use classification schema comparable to those employed by Edwards and Whitney. Even so, these reports collectively showed, to an unprecedented degree, the importance of socioeconomic factors to health.

In addition to its large studies on white or predominantly white populations, during the Depression the Public Health Service published two special studies on the "Health of the Negro." The first of these, conducted by Dorothy F. Holland and George St. J. Perrott, compared the prevalence of disabling illness among black families living in Central Harlem in 1933 with that of low-income white families living in the Lower East Side (93). Finding the "same inverse relation between the disabling illness rate and economic status" among both groups, the authors concluded that "such factors as standard of living and occupation" must be taken into account when analyzing racial differences in morbidity and mortality (93, p. 15). The second study, prepared by the same authors, was based on data from four of the cities covered in the 1935–1936 National Health Survey (94). Finding a much higher prevalence of disabling illness and poverty among black families than white families, and a high rate of illness among both white and black families on relief, the authors concluded that "Low economic status, rather than inherent racial characteristics . . . appears to account in large measure for the higher disability rate observed among Negroes" (94, p. 34). Following the publication of these two studies, in 1937, another Public Health Service researcher, Clark Tibbitts, then Chairman of the Health Inventory Operating Council (which supervised the conduct of the National Health Survey), prepared a review article on "The Socio-Economic Background of Negro Health Status" (54). After surveying much of the work of Sydenstricker, Perrott, and others, Tibbitts ventured "It seems safe to state the hypothesis that environmental conditions are important in determining Negro health status" (54, p. 428).

Also in 1937, Selwyn D. Collins, now Principal Statistician in charge of Statistical Investigations of the Public Health Service, together with Tibbitts, published, under the auspices of the Social Science Research Council, a large monograph, *Research Memorandum on Social Aspects of Health in the Depression*

(95). Summarizing the growing body of research on health in the Depression, this work also made policy recommendations. Beyond this, it institutionalized the contributions of Edgar Sydenstricker, who had died in 1936, shortly after having written much of the legislation that became the Social Security Act of 1935 (96). Starting with a lengthy quotation from Sydenstricker's comprehensive synthesis, *Health and Environment* (97), Collins and Tibbitts elaborated a history that recounted step-by-step each of Sydenstricker's major studies and the research tradition carried forward by the Public Health Service researchers whom he had influenced.

Following Sydenstricker, Collins and Tibbitts emphasized morbidity over mortality, surveys over vital statistics, and income over occupation. They nonetheless acknowledged that mortality data "are about the only figures that are available in detailed causes for specific age and sex groups over a long period of years, and they cannot be neglected" (95, p. 11). This is where one might perhaps have expected a call for national vital statistics stratified by some socioeconomic measure. Collins and Tibbitts did suggest that it would be useful to have studies of infant mortality and maternal mortality using the occupational information available on birth certificates; at the same time, they tended to dismiss the value of occupational data for the study of adult mortality and doubted the feasibility of obtaining accurate income data in census records. Conceding the usefulness of occupational mortality data in England, they reiterated the standard argument that U.S. workers enjoyed too much occupational mobility for such data to be meaningful in the United States. They cited, but without apparent enthusiasm, Jessamine Whitney's study and, showing that they had not read her work carefully, went on to propose a study to check the accuracy of occupations as recorded on the death certificates: "A study of this kind for 1930 would be an excellent preliminary step to a study of mortality statistics by occupation as based on the 1940 census" (95, p. 31). In fact, Whitney and the National Tuberculosis Association had already gone beyond this suggestion; in addition to checking the accuracy of death certificates before they undertook their study, they had arranged for the 1930 certificates and census data to be coded uniformly.

The outbreak of World War II rendered moot many of the research and policy recommendations proposed by Collins and Tibbitts. It also greatly diminished interest in studies on the health effects of the Depression. By the time the first results of the National Health Survey began to be published in 1938, national attention had shifted to other, more urgent matters. The course of public health and other population-based research would be further transformed during the war years by two related developments: the construction of the first large electronic digital computers and the creation of new methods for conducting and analyzing probability samples. Building on new sampling strategies developed in the mid-1930s to meet the demands for data generated by New Deal programs, in 1943 the Bureau of the Census demonstrated the feasibility of using probability sampling in a new nationally representative survey of the labor force (98). Three years later, the Bureau ordered its first digital computer, thereby entering the emerging world of electronic data processing (99). The new technology and new methods, perhaps not surprisingly, further eclipsed more traditional work in the area of vital statistics.

In the wake of the war, the Public Health Service and other federal agencies were reorganized. Reflecting these changes, authority over vital statistics was transferred in 1946 from the Bureau of the Census to the Public Health Service (16, p. 44). After this transfer, the collection of numerators and denominators for calculation of birth and death rates no longer would be under the purview of one agency. This meant that efforts such as those of Whitney and Edwards to include the same questions in the standard certificates and the decennial census would now be far more difficult. Work on improving morbidity statistics simultaneously received a new boost with the establishment of the National Committee on Vital and Health Statistics in 1949. Embracing the idea of probability sampling, the Committee decided its first priority was to obtain adequate national morbidity statistics, since the only available data—from the 1935–1936 survey—were nearly 15 years old. Their efforts led to the creation of a new National Health Survey in 1958, the forerunner of the current National Health Interview Survey (100).

These technical and organizational changes were important but, in the aftermath of World War II, the larger context framing the course of health research—and the collection of data—was set by the Cold War. The work of Whitney and the National Tuberculosis Association had been conducted during the peak progressive years of the 1930s. Already by 1938, the political climate was changing. A more conservative Congress had been elected, and the New Deal reform period was essentially over (45, pp. 398–434; 101–104). By 1943, when Edwards retired from the Bureau of the Census, the agency was already rejecting his initiatives. A major report on vital statistics prepared for the Bureau by Forrest E. Linder and Robert D. Grove clearly stated that the fundamental categories by which U.S. vital statistics should be tabulated were "geographic area, cause of death, age, race, sex, nativity, and month of death"; by contrast, "special studies" could deal with "other factors," such as "occupation of decedent, duration of disease, extent of hospitalization, type of attendant at death, and date and time of death" (17, p. 9). They thus casually disregarded 30 years of effort to develop socioeconomic measures for routine use in gathering and tabulating vital statistics. Enshrining the triad of "age, race, and sex" as essential characteristics, they relegated socioeconomic conditions to a lesser level, no more important to understanding the health of the population than the date and time at which people expired.

The onset of the Cold War, coupled with the passing away of a generation of progressive public health reformers, affected not only the federal government but also organizations such as the National Tuberculosis Association. In 1941, Jessamine Whitney died at the age of 61. Already writing her out of the record in

1937, Tibbitts, in his article on "The Socio-Economic Background of Negro Health Status" (54) mentioned her 1930 study of occupational mortality, but instead of citing her original report, listed the summary article published by Britten in *Public Health Records* (84) and referred to Whitney's investigation as "Britten's analysis of mortality rates by class and cause of death" (54, p. 426). By 1948, even other researchers concerned about socioeconomic variation in mortality from tuberculosis were attributing Whitney's work to Britten and the Public Health Service (105). Further erasing her contribution, in 1942, Herman E. Hilleboe, a member of the Association's Committee on Medical Research and of the federal government's War Emergency Committee, proposed that the Association and the Public Health Service collaborate in studies on the epidemiology of tuberculosis (68, pp. 289–290). Disregarding Whitney's work, he called for baseline data to be assembled on age-specific death rates by sex, race, and geographical distribution; socioeconomic differentials received no mention (106). A few years later, the Association conducted an evaluation of its own work and, criticizing the attention directed to "neglected groups" in the 1930s, issued a final report explicitly stating that the Association was "unwise" to have focused attention on minority groups and should no longer undertake special programs for industrial workers (68, pp. 280–281).

One telling indication of the chilling effect of the Cold War on public health was a major address on "Poverty and Disease" delivered in 1948 by C.-E. A. Winslow (107), then editor of the *American Journal of Public Health* and one of the most eminent figures in the U.S. public health establishment. In this address, commemorating the 100th anniversary of the passage of the world's first Public Health Act in Great Britain in 1848, Winslow felt compelled to defend a liberal public health agenda, New Deal policies, and concern about the relationship between poverty and health. His central argument was that none of these amounted to Communism and that he was as hostile to Communism as he was to Fascism. Praising the work of public health institutions for "having controlled with marvelous success those factors in morbidity and mortality which are susceptible to direct control by specific sanitary and immunological and epidemiological and nutritional procedures," he nonetheless cited Sydenstricker's work, that of the Children's Bureau, and the 1935–1936 National Health Survey, to argue that the United States was "faced with a residuum of sickness and death which is not amenable to such specific controls and in which poverty remains the outstanding causative factor" (107, pp. 174–175). Vividly describing the grossly unequal distribution of income and wealth within the United States, Winslow declared that "The disease of poverty affects a proportion not far from one-third of our population and it bears acutely on the more than one-sixth of the population below the $1000 level. Surely this is a problem deserving the very serious consideration of the health administrator" (107, p. 177).

To address this problem, Winslow proposed two solutions. One was to embark upon truly comprehensive regional planning, integrating programs for economic development, jobs, housing, health, and education, as exemplified by the unprecedented success of the Tennessee Valley Authority's initiatives, and "accomplished, not by bureaucratic dictation, but by coöperative leadership working through locally constituted authorities" (107, p. 178). The other was to equalize, in some measure, the extreme differences in family income. The two examples he offered were the construction of low-income housing and the establishment of a program for the compulsory sickness insurance, as President Truman was then proposing. Winslow lamented, however, that (107, p. 181):

> public discussion on these matters is not conducted on the plane of reason and experience, but on the plane of emotion and ideology. Even in an A.P.H.A. audience I strongly suspect that there are those who are now saying to themselves, 'Why, this fellow is a Socialist! Or a Communist! He probably has a party member's card in his pocket!'

Disavowing Communism, Winslow fervently defended democratic values. He then challenged those in the United States who were demanding "absolute conformity with the social program of one group which happens for the moment to be in power" and who garnered power by calling "everyone who differs a Communist and everyone who has ever been associated with any organization in which there was ever a Communist member a fellow-traveler." "Such an attitude," Winslow asserted, "enthrones emotion above reason, by discovering Un-American Art and Un-American Music and Un-American Science" (107, pp. 183–184).

Winslow's conclusion was both heartfelt and determined. Affirming that the public health movement had won many battles in the past century and that he himself had "fought in the ranks of the health army for nearly half of those hundred years," he declared (107, p. 184):

> We must now determine that men shall not be physically and emotionally crippled by malnutrition, by slum-dwelling, by lack of medical care, by social insecurity. If there are better ways than public housing, and sickness insurance, and social security, let us find them. If not, let us move forward on the lines which I have tried to outline above.

If someone with Winslow's impeccable record felt compelled to devote the bulk of his address on poverty and disease to the task of warding off accusations of being an un-American Communist, it is no surprise that only a handful of public health researchers and administrators would, in the Cold War era, be so foolhardy—or so brave—as to focus on social inequalities in health.

LOOKING BACKWARD, LOOKING FORWARD

In the 1930s, U.S. public health professionals had nearly succeeded in institutionalizing the collection and reporting of socioeconomic data in the nation's vital statistics and in national health surveys. Building on the earlier Progressive era, whose spirit was embodied in the pioneering studies of Edgar Sydenstricker and of the U.S. Children's Bureau, the 1930s was a period in which creative and committed researchers attempted to grapple with the theoretical and practical issues involved in relating people's health status and mortality rates to their standard of living, their workplace and neighborhood conditions, and overall trends in the U.S. economy. It was also a time in which investigators first seriously evaluated the contribution of socioeconomic conditions to racial/ethnic inequalities in health. This remarkable era was cut short by the onset of World War II, its legacy nearly erased by the Cold War.

The extraordinary work of the 1930s was not without its contradictions. Had Sydenstricker and his colleagues in the Public Health Service been more interested in mortality data, more interested in understanding racial/ethnic inequalities in health, and less dismissive of social class analyses based on occupational data, they might have been more eager to work with state registrars of vital statistics, and perhaps more resources would then have been devoted to ensuring the routine reporting of U.S. vital statistics stratified by socioeconomic level. Similarly, had researchers like Edwards and his counterpart in England, T. H. C. Stevenson, been more interested in the economic and health status of women, perhaps they would have taken on—rather than sidestepped—the difficult question of how best to categorize women by social class, thereby providing a more adequate way to describe socioeconomic trends in women's mortality.

Although the Cold War stymied work on social inequalities in health within the United States, the abiding fact of their existence has continued to inspire efforts to document and address these disparities. In recent years, we have seen greater recognition given to the health issues of people of color, of women, of the elderly, and, to a lesser degree, of the poor. For the most part, those involved in these recent efforts have not been aware of the insights and interests of those whose work we have summarized here. By recovering this rich history, we may be better able to build on these earlier attempts to measure socioeconomic differences in health. This history also contains a warning: to avoid becoming entangled in the older debates about the relative importance of mortality versus morbidity data, vital statistics versus health surveys, income versus occupation, and social class versus race/ethnicity. Each of these matters, vitally. For each type of data, we will need the best socioeconomic measures possible if we are to achieve the "glimpses" that Sydenstricker and others of this generation so deeply desired—of "the public-health situation as a whole, drawn in proper perspective and painted in true colors" (53, p. 280).

Ensuring the routine collection and reporting of U.S. health data stratified by appropriate measures of social class and race/ethnicity, in conjunction with gender and age, will, we believe, establish new possibilities and priorities for eradicating social inequalities in health. This work will require not only originality and precision, but also persistence, political acumen, and political will. Sydenstricker, Whitney, and Winslow would have expected no less.

REFERENCES

1. Thornton, R. *American Indian Holocaust and Survival: A Population History Since 1492*, pp. 65–72, 78–81. University of Oklahoma Press, Norman, 1987.
2. Winslow, C.-E. A. The colonial era and the first years of the republic (1607–1799): The pestilence that walketh in darkness. In *The History of American Epidemiology*, edited by F. H. Top, pp. 11–51. C. V. Mosby, St. Louis, 1952.
3. Duffy, J. *Epidemics in Colonial America*, pp. 16–112. Louisiana State University Press, Baton Rouge, 1953.
4. Cohen, P. C. *A Calculating People: The Spread of Numeracy in Early America*, pp. 86–89. University of Chicago Press, Chicago, 1982.
5. U.S. Department of Health and Human Services. *Health Status of the Disadvantaged*. DHHS Pub. No. (HRSA) HRS-P-DV 90-1. U.S. Government Printing Office, Washington, D.C., 1990.
6. U.S. Department of Health and Human Services. *Health Status of Minorities and Low-Income Groups: Third Edition*. U.S. Government Printing Office, Washington, D.C., 1991.
7. Griscom, J. C. *The Sanitary Condition of the Laboring Population of New York with Suggestions for its Improvement*. Harper, New York, 1845.
8. Rosen, G. *A History of Public Health*. Johns Hopkins University Press, Baltimore, Md., 1993 [1958].
9. Fox, J. (ed.). *Health Inequalities in European Countries*. Gower, Aldershot, 1989.
10. Krieger, N., and Fee, E. Social class: The missing link in U.S. health data. *Int. J. Health Serv.* 24: 25–44, 1994.
11. Navarro, V. Race *or* class versus race *and* class: Mortality differentials in the United States. *Lancet* ii: 1238–1240, 1990.
12. Navarro, V. *Crisis, Health, and Medicine: A Social Critique*. Tavistock, New York, 1986.
13. Terris, M. The lifestyle approach to prevention (editorial). *J. Public Health Policy* 1: 5–9, 1980.
14. Krieger, N., et al. Racism, sexism, and social class: Implications for studies of health, disease, and well-being. *Am. J. Prev. Med.* 9(Suppl. 2): 82–122, 1993.
15. Gutman, R. Birth and death registration in Massachusetts: II. The inauguration of a modern system, 1800–1849. *Milbank Mem. Fund Q.* 36: 373–402, 1958.
16. U.S. Bureau of the Census. *Historical Statistics of the United States, Colonial Times to 1970, Bicentennial Edition, Part 2*. U.S. Government Printing Office, Washington, D.C., 1975.
17. Linder, F. E., and Grove, R. D. *Vital Statistics Rates in the United States 1900–1940*. U.S. Government Printing Office, Washington, D.C., 1943.

18. Tolson, G. C., et al. The 1989 revision of the U.S. standard certificates and reports. *Vital and Health Statistics*, Ser., 4, No. 28. DHHS Pub. No. (PHS) 91-1465. National Center for Health Statistics, 1991.

19. Willcox, W. F. *Introduction to the Vital Statistics of the United States, 1900 through 1930*, p. 13. U.S. Government Printing Office, Washington, D.C., 1933.

20. Bureau of the Census. *Special Reports: Mortality Statistics, 1900 to 1904*. U.S. Government Printing Office, Washington, D.C., 1906.

21. Petersen, W. Politics and the measurement of ethnicity. In *The Politics of Numbers*, edited by W. Alonso and P. Starr, pp. 187–233. Russell Sage Foundation, New York, 1987.

22. Hahn, R. A., and Stroup, D. F. Race and ethnicity in public health surveillance: Criteria for the scientific use of social categories. *Public Health Rep.* 109: 7–15, 1994.

23. U.S. Bureau of the Census (Edwards, A. M.). *Index to Occupations, Alphabetical and Classified*. U.S. Government Printing Office, Washington, D.C., 1915.

24. Meckel, R. A. *Save the Babies: American Public Health Reform and the Prevention of Infant Mortality 1850–1929*. Johns Hopkins University Press, Baltimore, Md., 1990.

25. U.S. Bureau of the Census. *Pocket Reference of Information on Occupations*. U.S. Government Printing Office, Washington, D.C., 1930.

26. Leete, R., and Fox, J. Registrar General's social classes: Origins and uses. *Popul. Trends* 8: 1–7, 1977.

27. Szreter, S. R. S. The G.R.O. and the public health movement, 1837–1914. *Soc. Hist. Med.* 4: 435–463, 1991.

28. Szreter, S. R. S. The official representation of social classes in Britain, the United States, and France: The professional model and 'les cadres'. *Soc. Comp. Study Soc. Hist.* 35: 285–317, 1993.

29. Library of The New York Academy of Medicine. *Vital Statistics: A Memorial Volume of Selections from the Report and Writings of William Farr*. Scarecrow Press, Metuchen, N.J., 1975.

30. Newsholme, A. *The Elements of Vital Statistics in their Bearing on Social and Public Health Problems*. George Allen & Unwin, London, 1923.

31. Eyler, J. M. *Victorian Social Medicine: The Ideas and Methods of William Farr*. Johns Hopkins University Press, Baltimore, Md., 1979.

32. Engels, F. *The Condition of the Working Class in England*, edited and translated by W. O. Henderson and W. H. Chaloner, pp. 109–125. Stanford University Press, Stanford, Calif., 1958 [1844].

33. Townsend, P., Davidson, N., and Whitehead, M. *Inequalities in Health: The Black Report and The Health Divide*. Penguin Books, London, 1990.

34. *Seventy-Fourth Annual Report of the Registrar-General of Births, Deaths, and Marriages in England and Wales (1911)*. His Majesty's Stationery Office, London, 1913.

35. *Supplement to the Seventy-Fifth Annual Report of the Registrar General, Part IV, Mortality of Men in Certain Occupations in the Three Years 1910–1912*. His Majesty's Stationery Office, London, 1923.

36. Stevenson, T. H. C. The social distribution of mortality from different causes in England and Wales, 1910–1912. *Biometrika* 15: 382–388, 1923.

37. Szreter, S. R. S. The genesis of the Registrar General's social classification of occupations. *Br. J. Sociol.* 35: 522–546, 1984.
38. Heath, A. The sociology of social class. In *Biosocial Aspects of Social Class*, edited by G. C. N. Mascie-Taylor, pp. 1–23. Oxford University Press, Oxford, 1990.
39. McFarlane, A. Official statistics and women's health. In *Women's Health Counts*, edited by H. Roberts, pp. 18–62. Routledge, London, 1990.
40. Dale, A., Gilbert, G. N., and Arber, S. Integrating women into class theory. *Sociology* 19: 384–409, 1985.
41. Williams, R. C. *The United States Public Health Service, 1798–1950.* U.S. Public Health Service, Washington, D.C., 1951.
42. Schmeckebier, L. F. *The Public Health Service, its History, Activities, and Organizations.* Johns Hopkins University Press, Baltimore, Md., 1923.
43. Mullan, F. *Plagues and Politics: The Story of the United States Public Health Service.* Basic Books, New York, 1989.
44. State of New York. *Second Report of the Factory Investigating Committee, 1913, Volume I, Transmitted to the Legislature January 15, 1913.* J. B. Lyon, Albany, 1913.
45. Zinn, H. *A People's History of the United States.* Harper-Colophon, New York, 1980.
46. Warren, B. S., and Sydenstricker, E. Health of garment workers in relation to their economic status. *Public Health Rep.* 31: 1298–1305, 1916.
47. Warren, B. S., and Sydenstricker, E. Health insurance: Its relation to the public health. *Public Health Bull.* 76, March 1916.
48. Goldberger, J., Wheeler, G. A., and Sydenstricker, E. A study of the relation of family income and other economic factors to pellagra incidence in seven cotton-mill villages of South Carolina in 1916. *Public Health Rep.* 35: 2673–2714, 1920.
49. Etheridge, B. *The Butterfly Caste: A Social History of Pellagra in the South.* Greenwood, Westport, Conn., 1972.
50. Terris, M. (ed.). *Goldberger on Pellagra.* Louisiana State University Press, Baton Rouge, 1964.
51. Sydenstricker, E., and King, W. I. A method for classifying families according to incomes in studies of disease prevalence. *Public Health Rep.* 35: 2829–2846, 1920.
52. Guggenheim, K. Y. *Basic Issues of the History of Nutrition,* pp. 87–88. Akademia University Press, Jerusalem, 1990.
53. Sydenstricker, E. The incidence of illness in a general population group: General results of a morbidity study from December 1, 1921, through March 31, 1924, in Hagerstown, Md. *Public Health Rep.* 40: 279–291, 1925.
54. Tibbitts, C. The socio-economic background of Negro health status. *J. Negro Educ.* 6: 413–428, 1937.
55. Turner, V. B. *Hagerstown Health Studies: An Annotated Bibliography.* U.S. Public Health Service Pub. No. 148. Federal Security Agency, U.S. Public Health Service, Washington, D.C., 1952.
56. Lawrence, P. S., and Tibbitts, C. Recent long-term morbidity studies in Hagerstown, Md. *Am. J. Public Health* 41(Suppl. 2): 101–107, 1951.
57. Collins, S. D. Economic status and health: A review and study of the relevant morbidity and mortality data. *Public Health Bull.* 165, 1927.
58. Britten, R. H. Occupational mortality among males in England and Wales, 1921–1923: A summary of the report of the Registrar General. *Public Health Rep.* 43: 1565–1616, 1928.

59. Stevenson, T. H. C. The vital statistics of wealth and poverty. *J. R. Stat. Soc.* 91: 207–220, 1928.

60. Du Bois, W. E. B. (ed.). *The Health and Physique of the Negro American.* Atlanta University Press, Atlanta, Ga., 1906.

61. Trask, J. W. The significance of the mortality rates of the colored population of the United States. *Am. J. Public Health* 6: 254–260, 1916.

62. Tobey, J. A. *The Children's Bureau: Its History, Activities and Organization.* The Johns Hopkins University Press, Baltimore, Md., 1925.

63. Ladd-Taylor, M. *Mother-work: Women, Child Welfare, and the State, 1890–1930.* University of Illinois Press, Urbana, 1994.

64. Woodbury, R. M. *Causal Factors in Infant Mortality.* U.S. Children's Bureau Pub. No. 142. U.S. Children's Bureau, Washington, D.C., 1925.

65. Woodbury, R. M. *Infant Mortality and Its Causes.* Williams & Wilkins, Baltimore, Md., 1926.

66. Lathrop, J. C. Income and infant mortality. *Am. J. Public Health* 9: 270–274, 1919.

67. Chapin, C. V. Deaths among taxpayers and non-taxpayers of income tax, Providence, 1865. *Am. J. Public Health* 13: 647–651, 1924.

68. Shryock, R. H. *National Tuberculosis Association, 1904–1954: A Study of the Voluntary Health Movement in the United States.* National Tuberculosis Association, New York, 1957.

69. Brandt, L. The social aspects of tuberculosis based on a study of statistics. In *A Handbook on the Prevention of Tuberculosis,* pp. 36–38. The Committee on the Prevention of Tuberculosis, Charity Organization Society of the City of New York, New York, 1903.

70. Dublin, L. I. *Mortality Statistics of Insured Wage-Earners and Their Families; Experience of the Metropolitan Life Insurance Company, Industrial Department, 1911 to 1916, in the United States and Canada.* Metropolitan Life Insurance Company, New York, 1919.

71. Dublin, L. I., and Vane, R. J. Jr. *Causes of Death by Occupation: Occupational Mortality Experience of the Metropolitan Life Insurance Company, 1922–1924.* Bureau of Labor Stat. Bull., No. 507. U.S. Government Printing Office, Washington, D.C., 1927.

72. Emerson, K. Preface. In *Death Rates by Occupation Based on Data of the U.S. Census Bureau 1930,* edited by J. S. Whitney. National Tuberculosis Association, New York, 1934.

73. Leonard, J. W. (ed.). *Woman's Who's Who of America: A Biographical Dictionary of Contemporary Women of the United States and Canada, 1914–1915,* p. 879. American Commonwealth Company, New York, 1914.

74. U.S. Children's Bureau (Whitney, J. S., and Woodbury, R. M.). *Infant Mortality: Results of a Field Study in New Bedford, Mass., Based on Births in One Year.* Children's Bureau Pub. No. 68. U.S. Government Printing Office, Washington, D.C., 1920.

75. Whitney, J. S. (ed.). *Death Rates by Occupation Based on Data of the U.S. Census Bureau 1930.* National Tuberculosis Association, New York, 1934.

76. *Who Was Who in America,* Vol. 1969–1973, p. 209. Marquis Who's Who, Chicago, 1973.

77. Conk (Anderson), M. Occupational classification in the United States census: 1870–1940. *J. Interdisc. Hist.* 9: 111–130, 1978.
78. Edwards, A. M. Classification of occupations. *J. Am. Stat. Assoc.* 12: 618–646, 1911.
79. Edwards, A. M. Social-economic groups of the United States. *J. Am. Stat. Assoc.* 15: 643–661, 1917.
80. Edwards, A. M. A social-economic grouping of the gainful workers of the United States. *J. Am. Stat. Assoc.* 28: 377–387, 1933.
81. Chase, A. *The Legacy of Malthus: The Social Costs of the New Scientific Racism.* Knopf, New York, 1976.
82. Kevles, D. J. *In the Name of Eugenics: Genetics and the Uses of Human Heredity.* Knopf, New York, 1985.
83. Ludmerer, K. M. *Genetics and American Society: A Historical Appraisal.* Johns Hopkins University Press, Baltimore, Md., 1972.
84. Britten, R. H. Mortality rates by occupational class in the United States. *Public Health Rep.* 49: 1101–1111, 1934.
85. Perrott, G. S. J., and Collins, S. D. Relation of sickness to income and income change in ten surveyed communities. Health and Depression Studies No. 1: Method of study and general results for each locality. *Public Health Rep.* 50: 595–622, 1935.
86. Sydenstricker, E. Health and the Depression. *Milbank Mem. Fund Q.* 12: 273–280, 1934.
87. Perrott, G. S. J., and Sydenstricker, E. Causal and selective factors in illness. *Am. J. Sociol.* 40: 804–812, 1935.
88. U.S. Public Health Service. *Illness and Medical Care among 2,500,000 Persons in 83 cities, with Special Reference to Socio-Economic Factors.* Federal Security Agency, U.S. Public Health Service, Washington, D.C., 1945.
89. U.S. Public Health Service, Division of Public Health Methods. *The National Health Survey, 1935–1936.* Federal Security Agency, U.S. Public Health Service, Washington, D.C., 1951.
90. Hailman, D. E. *The Prevalence of Disabling Illness Among Male and Female Workers and Housewives.* Public Health Bull., No. 260. U.S. Government Printing Office, Washington, D.C., 1941.
91. Kiser, C. V. *Group Differences in Urban Fertility: A Study Derived from the National Health Survey.* Williams & Wilkins, Baltimore, Md., 1942.
92. Goddard, J. G. Comparison of occupational class and physicians' estimate of economic status. *Public Health Rep.* 54: 2159–2165, 1939.
93. Holland, D. F., and Perrott, G. S. J. Health of the Negro. Part I. Disabling illness among Negroes and low-income white families in New York City—A report of a sickness survey in the spring of 1933. *Milbank Mem. Fund Q.* 16: 5–15, 1938.
94. Holland, D. F., and Perrott, G. S. J. Health of the Negro. Part II. A preliminary report on a study of disabling illness in a representative sample of the Negro and white population of four cities canvassed in the National Health Survey, 1935–1936. *Milbank Mem. Fund Q.* 16: 16–38, 1938.
95. Collins, S. D., and Tibbitts, C. *Research Memorandum on Social Aspects of Health in the Depression.* Social Science Research Council Bull. 36. Social Sciences Research Council, New York, 1937.

96. Wiehl, D. Edgar Sydenstricker: A memorial. In *The Challenge of Facts: Selected Public Health Papers of Edgar Sydenstricker*, edited by R. V. Kasius, pp. 3–20. Prodist, New York, 1974.

97. Sydenstricker, E. *Health and Environment*. McGraw-Hill, New York, 1933.

98. Stephan, F. F. History of the uses of modern sampling procedures. *J. Am. Stat. Assoc.* 43: 12–39, 1948.

99. Anderson, M. *The American Census: A Social History*, pp. 194–199. Yale University Press, New Haven, Conn., 1988.

100. Department of Health, Education, and Welfare. *Origin and Program of the U.S. National Health Survey, a Description of the Developments Leading to the Enaction of the National Health Survey Act, and a Statement of the Policies and Initial Program of the Survey*. Washington, D.C., 1958.

101. Gaddis, J. L. *The United States and the Origins of the Cold War, 1941–1947*. Columbia University Press, New York, 1972.

102. Wolfe, A. *The Rise and Fall of the Soviet Threat: Domestic Sources of the Cold War Consensus*. Institute of Policy Studies, Washington, D.C., 1984.

103. Yergin, D. *Shattered Peace: The Origins of the Cold War and the National Security State*. Houghton Mifflin, Boston, 1977.

104. Oshinsky, D. M. *A Conspiracy So Immense: The World of Joe McCarthy*. The Free Press, New York, 1983.

105. Terris, M. Relation of economic status to tuberculosis mortality by age and sex. *Am. J. Public Health* 38: 1061–1070, 1948.

106. U.S. Public Health Service. *Tuberculosis in the United States: Graphic Presentation*, Vols. 1–4. National Tuberculosis Association, New York, 1943–1946.

107. Winslow, C.-E. A. Poverty and disease. *Am. J. Public Health* 38: 173–184, 1948.

CHAPTER 3

You Are Dangerous to Your Health:
The Ideology and Politics of Victim Blaming

Robert Crawford

"All the proposals for National Health Insurance embrace, without qualification, the no-fault principle. They therefore choose to ignore, or to treat as irrelevant, the importance of personal responsibility for the state of one's health. As a result, they pass up an opportunity to build both positive and negative inducements into the insurance payment plan, by measures such as refusing or reducing benefits for chronic respiratory disease care to persons who continue to smoke."

Leon Kass (1, p. 41)

"The idea of individual responsibility has been submerged in individual rights—rights or demands to be guaranteed by beneficent Big Brother and delivered by public and private institutions. . . . One man's or woman's freedom in health is now another man's shackle in taxes and insurance premiums.

"But now the cost of individual irresponsibility in health has become prohibitive. The choice is in fact, over the long range, individual responsibility or social failure."

John Knowles, President, Rockefeller Foundation (2, pp. 2, 3)

"For once we cannot blame the environment as much as we have to blame ourselves. The problem now is the inability of man to take care of himself."

Ernst Wynder, M.D. (2, p. 5)

"We must stop throwing an array of technological processes and systems at life-style problems and stop equating more health services with better health. . . . People must have the capability and the will to take greater responsibility for their own health."

Walter McNerney, President, Blue Cross Association (2, pp. 4, 5)

Although these statements may not appear to reflect class positions, in fact, insofar as they conceal the nature of the current health crisis—the growing contradiction between the social production of disease and the burden of a costly and ineffective medical system—and propose solutions most likely to reproduce existing class relations, they represent a class strategy. In other words, these statements take on the character of an ideology. This is not to suggest that these statements should be viewed in instrumentalist terms. Instead, what must be understood is how ideology functions to reinforce political objectives, even though it is perhaps not initially articulated for that purpose, or is perhaps articulated by people not having a direct stake in the larger political interests which might benefit. Ideology reflects an underlying social structure and emerges from the contradictions present in that structure. A clear understanding of why the victim blaming ideology is gaining so much popularity at this particular historical point can only be achieved by examining those contradictions.

THE CHALLENGE TO MEDICINE

During the last twenty years and especially the last decade we have witnessed a remarkable expansion in the health sector. Health expenditures in the United States were 4.1 percent of the gross national product in 1950, 5.2 percent in 1960, 7.1 percent in 1970, and 8.1 percent in 1976. Estimates are that they will exceed 10 percent of the GNP by the early 1980s. Other growth indicators, including employment, the extent of corporate investment, physical infrastructure, and numbers of people obtaining services, have been steadily climbing. Health sector expansion has been powered by a growth coalition able to win the extension of employee health benefits, the socialization of costs for the aged and many of the poor, and the direct subsidization of medical research and provider and training institutions. Medicine has come to capture the imagination and hope of the American public, some observers claiming that the hospital has become the archetype institution of American life.

In the last few years, however, the hegemony of medicine has been challenged. First, the women's and self-help movements have undercut professional authority and raised the issue of overmedicalization. Of more immediate interest for this discussion has been the profusion of monographs, conferences, and policy statements shifting debate from a concern with issues of equality of access to the irrelevancy or limits of medicine for maintaining health. Impressive evidence on the relative ineffectiveness of medicine in reducing mortality and morbidity is being added to the academic literature by McKeown (3, 4), Cochrane (5), Powles (6), and others, and is being popularized in the United States by Illich (7), Fuchs (8), and Carlson (9). Illich has had a particularly profound effect in writing *Medical Nemesis* and lecturing widely on his views.

More concrete recommendations for a reorientation from medical care to health promotion by the Canadian Minister of National Health and Welfare,

Marc Lalonde (10), have generated considerable interest. In the United States, Anne Somers (11) seems to have sparked a new interest in health education as an alternative to continued expansion of the medical system. Medicine, in short, confronts a number of critiques ranging from what has been called "therapeutic nihilism" (12) to more modest proposals for therapeutic constraint. Together they constitute the most serious challenge to medicine since the pre-Flexnerian period.

The victim blaming ideology as applied to health is emerging alongside the limits of medicine argument. Indeed, that argument is its first premise. Basing itself on the irrefutable and increasingly obvious fact that medicine has been oversold, the new ideology argues that individuals, if they take appropriate actions, if they, in other words, adopt life-styles which avoid unhealthy behavior, may prevent most diseases. "Living a long life is essentially a do-it-yourself proposition," as it was put by one pundit. Policy, it is argued, must be redirected away from the extension of social programs which characterized the 1960s toward a health promotion strategy which calls upon the individual to become more responsible for his or her own health rather than to rely on ineffective medical services.

While the emergence of the new victim blaming ideology seems to have been facilitated by the attack on medicine, it is the conjuncture and contradictions contained in three political phenomena which best explain its emergence and the political functions it has acquired. First, I will briefly discuss each of these phenomena, and then describe how the ideology is a response which functions to resolve the resulting tensions to the favor of dominant economic and political interests.

THE NATURE OF THE CRISIS

The Crisis of Costs

Foremost is the current crisis of costs, a crisis which is transforming the entire political landscape in the health sector. The cost crisis has several dimensions, most of which have been repeated so often that they are all too familiar. High medical costs have always been a problem. What makes health sector inflation so critical in the 1970s is not only its spectacular rate but its concurrence with wider economic and fiscal crises. High medical costs have become a direct threat to the corporate sector, adding significantly to the costs of production through increases in health benefit settlements with labor, aggravating inflation, and diverting private and governmental resources. President Carter recently announced that the average American worker is now devoting one month's worth of his yearly salary just to pay for medical care costs (13).

The costs of production for corporations in unionized sectors have been rapidly escalating, in large part due to increasing costs of benefit settlements. The Council on Wage and Price Stability reports that in the auto, rubber, and steel industries, gross average hourly earnings between 1965 and 1974 increased 83, 59, and 85 percent, respectively, but that in the same industries, negotiated employee benefits jumped 240, 150, and 160 percent for the same period. Overall, between 1966 and 1972, total employer payments for insurance and health benefits increased 100 percent while wages increased only 47 percent (14, p. 94).

General Motors claims it spent more money with Blue Cross and Blue Shield in 1975 than it did with U.S. Steel, its principal supplier of metal. Standard Oil of Indiana announced in 1976 that employee health costs for the corporation had tripled over the past seven years (15). In 1976, Chrysler estimates it paid $1500 per employee for medical benefits or a total of $205 million in the United States (16, p. 656). "Unlike most other labor costs that can and do vary with the level of production," the corporation complains, "medical costs continue to rise in good times as well as in bad" (16, p. 660).

The implications for consumer costs are obvious. GM added $175 to the price of every car and truck in passing on its employee medical benefit costs. In a period in which consumption and investment are stalled, and foreign competition adds an additional barrier to raising prices, figures such as those given above are startling. Corporate and union leaders are expressing in every possible forum their concern over the impact of rising medical costs upon prices, wages, and profits.

Mounting fiscal pressures on both federal and local governments are also worrying political and economic leaders. As the Council on Wage and Price Stability reports (14, p. 94),

> The portion of the Federal budget expended for health has increased from 8.9 percent in 1969 to 11.3 percent in 1975 and is projected to be 11.7 percent in 1977. Only national defense, interest on the national debt, and income security programs now consume a larger share.

The fiscal crisis at the local level is dramatically forcing the issue. Steps are being taken daily to cut back public programs and otherwise to attempt to control the escalating costs. The cost problem has hurt almost every major economic interest group in the country, resulting in a fundamental coalitional shift from support for expansion to "get tough" cost control measures. Large corporate interests and government officials are at the center of the coalition. Substantial political pressures are being mobilized to cut the direct costs to corporations and to cut the indirect costs of social programs generally (17). Just as the politics of expansion dominated the last period in health politics, the politics of cost control will dominate the next (18, 19). The terms of agreement in the new coalition as well as its fragility are still to be tested, but it is clear that expansionary forces are facing their most serious challenge to date.

Politicization of the Social Production of Disease

The second phenomenon underlying the emergence of the ideology of individual responsibility, occurring simultaneously with the cost crisis, is a rapid politicization of the social production of disease. Widely reported scientific and popular critiques of environmental health dangers and occupational health and safety hazards have resulted in a growing awareness, concern, and polarization over these issues. First, there is now almost universal agreement in the scientific community that most cancers are environmentally caused, anywhere from 70-90 percent by most estimates. Many researchers call cancer a disease of epidemic proportions. Samuel Epstein, a noted cancer expert, estimates "that in 1975, 665,000 new cancer cases were diagnosed and that there were 365,000 cancer deaths. Thus, cancer deaths in 1975 alone were approximately five times higher than the total U.S. military deaths in the Viet Nam and Korean war years combined." He claims that "more than 53 million people in the U.S. (over a quarter of the population) will develop some form of cancer in their lifetimes, and approximately 20 percent will die of it" (20, p. 1).

The American people have been inundated in just the last few years with a constant flow of environmental warnings and disasters: air pollution, contamination of drinking supplies, ozone watches in which "vulnerable" people are advised to sharply reduce their activities and to stay indoors, food additive carcinogens, the PCB disaster in Michigan, the asbestos disaster in Minnesota, and the kepone disaster in Virginia, vinyl chlorides, pesticides, the controversy over nuclear power plants, and more. The Environmental Protection Agency, the Occupational Safety and Health Administration, and the Food and Drug Administration have been among the most embattled government agencies in recent years. While there is considerable debate over threshold limit values, the validity of animal research applications to humans, and specific policy decisions by the above agencies, awareness is growing that the public is being exposed to a multitude of environmental and workplace carcinogens. Although many people still cling to the "it won't happen to me" response, the fear of cancer is becoming more widespread. A recent Gallup Poll found that cancer is by far the disease most feared by Americans, almost three times its nearest competitor (21).

From within industry, an occupational health and safety movement is gaining momentum. The UMW, OCAW, USW, and UAW are among the most active unions in developing programs and confronting corporate management on health and safety issues. Occupational health and safety has also sparked some radical challenges to established union leadership (22). Industry has reacted to these events by warning of unemployment, inflation, and economic stagnation if government regulations are expanded, and by presenting industry-sponsored research to alleviate fears. In addition, massive advertising campaigns herald the environmental efforts of public-spirited corporations. The "manufacturers of illness" confront what they fear will be a serious threat to corporate autonomy: the forging of labor, environmental, consumer, and populist groups into a new public health movement, The example of political constraints on the growth of the nuclear power industry is not lost on other industries.

Medical Care as a Right

Third, in the present period people's expectations of medicine have been lifted to their highest point, and the idea that medical care is a right is widely accepted. Belief in medicine is the result of many factors: years of conditioning by the medical profession; a research and philanthropy establishment deeply committed to the medical model; a few spectacular medical successes; a general, society-wide glorification of science and technology; and the medicalization of society, the cultural roots of which extend far beyond professional imperialism (7, 23, 24). Further, in a period in which people feel vulnerable to epidemic-proportion diseases, and powerless to do much about it, the tendency is to rely on medicine all the more. Dependency grows, even as anxiety increases over the inability of medicine to find a cure for the new diseases. The great promise of the twentieth century will not easily be dispelled. The hope of deliverance is perhaps more pervasive than ever. Finally, the idea that access to medical services is an essential component of personal and family security has long been a politicized matter. It has emerged from a long history of union and popular struggles negotiated in labor contracts and promoted through legislation. The campaign for national health insurance goes back several decades, was a primary political force in the adoption of Medicare and Medicaid, and in the last six or seven years has gained a new vitality.

In summary, on the one hand, America is a society ridden with anxiety about disease and yet infatuated with the claims of scientific medicine, in which access to medical care is believed to be a basic right. On the other hand, the cost of medical services and the fiscal crisis are making services more difficult to obtain and are forcing a retreat from public programs. At a time when people seem to want medicine most, its continuing availability and expansion threaten powerful economic and political interests. Further, much to the concern of industry, medicine is clearly inadequate in dealing with the contemporary social production of disease, and is therefore increasingly unable to perform its traditional role of resolving societal tensions which emerge when people identify the social causes of their individual pathologies. In the face of these trends, it is fascinating and revealing that we are witnessing the proliferation of messages about our own personal responsibility for health and an attack on individual life-styles and at-risk behaviors.

THE POLITICS OF RETRENCHMENT

Cost control advocates face two major political obstacles: (a) popular expectations for easy access to medical services and political pressures for protection and extension of entitlements; and (b) the entrenched political positions of the providers and medical-corporate interests. On the one hand, the ideology of individual responsibility for health serves to reorder expectations and to justify a retreat from the language of rights and the policies of entitlements. It may also induce attitudes consistent with a voluntary reduction of help-seeking behavior. On the other hand, it is aimed at convincing legislators, other political and economic leaders, and both academic and media commentators on health policy of the necessity for utilization reduction and other cost control measures. In the campaign to marshall sufficient power to overcome the medical special interests, the ideology, joined with the limits of medicine argument, adds to the persuasive resources of the cost control advocates.

In victim blaming statements, both direct policy proposals and indirect policy implications are abundant, as for example in the following set of remarks. With an implied attack on social programs, Fuchs writes (8, p. 27):

> Some future historian. in reviewing mid-twentieth century social reform literature, may note a "resolute refusal" to admit that individuals have any responsibility for their own stress.

Robert Whalen, Commissioner of the New York Department of Health, more explicitly makes the tie with high medical costs (25):

> Unless we assume such individual and moral responsibility for our own health, we will soon learn what a cruel and expensive hoax we have worked upon ourselves through our belief that more money spent on health care is the way to better health.

And John Knowles is worried as well about some of the political consequences (2, pp. 28-29):

> The only thing we've heard about national health insurance from everybody is that it won't solve the problems. It will inflate expectations and demands and cause more frustrations.

Both Knowles and Kass attack the notion of rights. "The idea of individual responsibility has been submerged in individual rights—rights or demands to be guaranteed by beneficent Big Brother and delivered by public and private institutions," Knowles warns (2, p. 2). Kass writes (1, p. 39):

> But if health is what we say it is, it is an unlikely subject of a right in either sense. Health is a state of being, not something that can be given, and only in indirect ways something that can be taken away or undermined by other human beings. It no more makes sense to claim a right to health than a right to wisdom or courage. These excellences of soul and of body require natural gift, attention, effort and discipline on the part of each person who desires them. To make my health someone else's duty is not only unfair, it is to impose a duty impossible to fulfill. Though I am not particularly attracted by the language of rights and duties in regard to health, I would lean much more in the direction, once traditional, of saying that health is a *duty,* that one has an obligation to preserve one's own good health. The theory of a right to health flies in the face

> of good sense, serves to undermine personal and in addition, places obligation where it cannot help but be unfulfillable.

While these comments do not challenge the right to medical care directly, Kass does speak of "the already ambiguous and dubious right to health care" and the implications of the above remarks for the argument of rights in general are evident. His attitudes toward national health insurance are similar to Illich's image of equalizing access to torts and can be further inferred from the lead-off quotation for this chapter.

Several other commentators have called for "economic sanctions." A guest editorial appeared last year in the *New York Times* introducing the idea of "Your Fault Insurance." The writer asks, "How should 215 million Americans be persuaded to take care of themselves?" His answer is "a reward/punishment system based on individual choices," in this case through a taxation scheme (26). Economic sanctions which are used to reinforce access barriers may be justified under the rubric of "lack of motivation," "unsuitability for treatment," or "inability to profit from therapy" (27). Why waste money, after all, on people whose life-style contravenes good therapeutic results, or, as one commentator put it, on a "system which taxes the virtuous to send the improvident to the hospital?" (quoted in 1, p. 42). In the new system, the pariahs of the medical world and larger numbers of people in general could be diagnosed as having life-style problems, referred to a health counselor or social worker, and sent home. At the very least, the victim blaming ideology will help justify shifting the burden of costs back to users. If you are responsible for your illness, you should be responsible for your bill as well.

The common themes apparent in all these and similar statements emphasize the need to reduce expectations and utilization of ineffective and costly medical services, the necessity instead for individual responsibility, and the requirement for either education or economic sanctions to enlighten and reinforce one's sense of responsibility.

Similar ideologies of individual responsibility have always been popular among providers and academics trying to justify inequality in the utilization of medical services. During the period of rapid health sector expansion, higher morbidity and mortality rates for the poor and minorities were explained by emphasizing life-style habits, especially their health and utilization behavior. These culture of poverty explanations emphasized delay in seeking medical help, resistance, and reliance on unprofessional folk healers or advisors. As Riessman summarizes (28, p. 42):

> According to these researchers, the poor have undergone multiple negative experiences with organizational systems, leading to avoidance behavior, lack of trust, and hence a disinclination to seek care and follow medical regimens except in dire need.

Structural barriers, such as provider resistance or unavailability of services, were rarely mentioned. Neither was lack of money often discussed except in the context of explanations for patient-dumping practices or in lobbying for government reimbursement. Now, in a period of fiscal crisis and cost control, the same higher morbidity rates and demands for more access through comprehensive national health insurance are met with a barrage of statements about the limits of medicine and the lack of appropriate health behavior. Several commentators now link overuse by the poor with their faulty health habits, and the latter are linked with ignorance. Again, education is seen as the solution; and again, the role of the providers or the insurance structure, in this case as promoters of utilization, is rarely mentioned. Previously, the poor were blamed for not using medical services enough, for relying too much on their own resources, and for undue suspicion of modern medicine. Now they are blamed for relying too much on admittedly ineffective medical services and not enough on their own resources.

The various measures being adopted to reduce utilization are by now familiar: the closing or reduction in size of public hospitals; the reorganization of public hospitals to operate more like private institutions; Medicaid cuts and freezes; the dramatic failure of Medicare benefits to keep pace with increased costs so that the aged pay more out of pocket for medical services than in 1965, the year before the law became effective; rising insurance premiums, co-payments, and deductibles, along with shrinking benefits and unfavorable health insurance settlements for labor; the reorganization of private hospital services to reduce or close outpatient services and to insure reliability of payment; Health Maintenance Organizations; and the series of regulatory mechanisms designed to reduce unnecessary hospital admissions, stays, and construction.

Most important, by now it is no secret that the prospects for comprehensive national health insurance have receded behind a shield of rhetoric. When President Carter announced his new hospital cost control program in April, the *New York Times* headlined, "Action on Health Insurance May be Deferred for Years." Carter warned that, "with current inflation, the cost of any national health insurance program . . . will double in just five years." White House aides stressed that Carter's "paramount domestic goal" of balancing the budget by 1981 would probably be impossible if national health insurance were enacted. And HEW Secretary Califano argued that the proposed cost control program is a necessary precondition for the time that national health insurance "or some other system" is in place (13).

Such measures cannot be taken without risking the intensification and broadening of disillusionment, especially in a larger political context of retreat from social programs, economic recession, and disaffection from American institutions. At a time when most people still equate their perceived right to health with the right to medical treatment, and at a time when the promise of universal access to effective medical care has been held out in popular and political rhetoric for more than a decade, the need for a new ideology which can replace the mystifying power of medicine is critical. The argument is explicit. Medical benefits do not need to be expanded. What is important is health and not medicine;

and health is not a right. People will not relinquish their expectations unless their belief in medicine as a panacea is broken and the value of access is replaced with a new preoccupation with boot-strapping activities aimed at controlling at-risk behaviors. In a political climate of fiscal, energy, and cost crises, self-sacrifice and self-discipline emerge as dominant themes. In lieu of rights and entitlements, education, economic sanctions, and "more studies of the American family and value system" are proposed. It is an old scenario.

THE POLITICS OF DIVERSION

Social causation of disease has several dimensions. The complexities are only beginning to be explored. The victim blaming ideology, however, inhibits that understanding and substitutes instead an unrealistic behavioral model. It both ignores what is known about human behavior and minimizes the importance of evidence about the environmental assault on health. It instructs people to be individually responsible at a time when they are becoming less capable as individuals of controlling their health environment (29, 30). Although environmental dangers are often recognized, the implication is that little can be done about an ineluctable, modern, technological, and industrial society. Life-style and environmental factors are thrown together to communicate that individuals are the primary agents in shaping or modifying the effects of their environment. Victor Fuchs, for example, while recognizing environmental factors as "also relevant," asserts that "the greatest potential for reducing coronary disease, cancer, and other major killers still lies in altering personal behavior" (8, p. 46). "Emphasizing social responsibility," he philosophizes, "can increase security, but it may be the security of the 'zoo'—purchased at the expense of freedom" (8, p. 26). Or as Whalen writes (25),

> Many of our most difficult contemporary health problems, such as cancer, heart disease and accidental injury, have a built-in behavioral component. . . . *If they are to be solved at all,* we must change our style of living [emphasis added].

Nor should there be "excessive preoccupations," warns Kass, "as when cancer phobia leads to government regulations that unreasonably restrict industrial activity" (1, p. 42). Thus, the practical focus of health efforts should not be on the massive and expensive task of overhauling the environment, which, it is argued, would threaten jobs and economic growth. Instead, the important, i.e., amenable, determinants of health are behavioral, cultural, and psychological.

The diffusion of a psychological world view often reinforces the masking of social causation. Even though the psychiatric model substitutes social for natural explanations, problems still tend to be seen as amenable to change through personal transformation—with or without therapy. And with or without therapy, individuals are ultimately held responsible for their own psychological well-being.

Usually, no one has to blame us for some psychological failure; we blame ourselves. Thus, psychological impairment can be just as effective as moral failing or genetic inferiority in blaming the victim and reinforcing dominant social relations (31). People are alienated, unhappy, dropouts, criminals, angry, and activists, after all, because of maladjustment to one or another psychological norm.

The ideology of individual responsibility for health lends itself to this form of psychological social control. Susceptibility to at-risk behaviors, if not a moral failing, is at least a psychological failing. New evidence relating psychological state to resistance or susceptibility to disease and accidents can and will be used to shift more responsibility to the individual. Industrial psychologists have long been employed with the intention that the best way to reduce plant accidents in lieu of costly production changes is to intervene at the individual level (32). The implication is that people make themselves sick, not only mentally but physically. If job satisfaction is important to health, people should seek more rewarding employment. Cancer is a state of mind.

In another vein, many accounts of the current disease structure in the United States link disease with affluence. The affluent society and the life-styles it has wrought, it is suggested, are the sources of the individual's degeneration and adoption of at-risk behaviors. Halberstam, for example, writes that "most Americans die of excess rather than neglect or poverty" (quoted in 11, p. 22). Knowles' warning about "sloth, gluttony, alcoholic intemperance, reckless driving, sexual frenzy and smoking" and later about "social failure" (2, pp. 2, 3) are reminiscent of a popularized conception of a decaying Rome. Thus, even though some may complain about environmental hazards, people are really suffering from over-indulgence of the good society. It is that over-indulgence which must be checked. Further, by pointing to life-styles, which are usually presented as if they reflect the problems of a homogenized, affluent society, this aspect of the ideology tends to obscure the reality of class and the impact of social inequality on health. It is compatible with the conception that people are free agents. Social structure and constraints recede amidst the abundance.

Of course, several diseases do stem from the life-styles of the more affluent. Discretionary income usually allows for excessive consumption of unhealthy products; and as Eyer (33) argues, everyone suffers in variable and specific ways from the nature of work and the conditioning of life-styles in advanced capitalist society. But are the well-established relationships between low income and high infant mortality, diseases related to poor diet and malnutrition, stress, cancer, mental illness, traumas of various kinds, and other pathologies (34-38) now to be ignored or relegated to a residual factor? While long-term inequality in morbidity and mortality is declining (39), for almost every disease and for every indicator of morbidity incidence increases as income falls (40, pp. 620-621). In some specific cases, the health gap appears to be widening (41, 42). Nonetheless, Somers reassures her readers that contemporary society is tending in the direction of homogeneity (11, p. 77):

> If poverty seems so widespread, it is at least partly because our definition of poverty is so much more generous than in the past—a generosity made possible only by the pervasive affluence and the impressive technological base upon which it rests.

> This point—that the current crisis is the result of progress rather than retrogression or decay—is vitally important not only as a historical fact but as a guide to problem solving in the health field as elsewhere.

Finally, by focusing on the individual instead of the economic system, the ideology performs its classical role of obscuring the class structure of work. The failure to maintain health in the workplace is attributed to some personal flaw. The more than 2.5 million people disabled by occupational accidents and diseases each year and the additional 114,000 killed (43, 44) are not explained by the hazards or pace of work as much as by the lack of sufficient caution by workers, laziness about wearing respirators or the like, psychological maladjustment, and even by the worker's genetic susceptibility. Correspondingly, the overworked, overstressed worker is offered TM, biofeedback, psychological counseling, or some other "holistic" approach to healthy behavior change, leaving intact the structure of incentives and sanctions of employers which reward the retention of health-denying behavior.

Corporate management appears to be increasingly integrating victim blaming themes into personnel policies. Physical and especially psychological health have acquired more importance for management faced with declining productivity and expanding absenteeism. The problem for management becomes more serious with its growing dependence on high-skilled and more expensive labor, and on a more complex, integrated, and predictable production process. If "lifetime job security" becomes a priority demand of labor, employee health will become all the more important. Holding individual workers responsible for their susceptibility to illness, or for an "unproductive" psychological state, reinforces management attempts to control absenteeism and enhance productivity. Job dissatisfaction and job-induced stress (in both their psychological and physical manifestations), principal sources of absenteeism and low productivity, will become identified as life-style problems of the worker. A Conference Board report on Industry Roles in Health Care observes (45, p. 12),

> Psychological stress is coming increasingly into purview of those concerned with occupational health, as a potential hazard sharing the characteristics and complexities of toxic substances—having, that is, its own threshold values, variations in individual susceptibility, and interconnections with other occupational and non-occupational factors.

Workers who are found to be "irresponsible" in maintaining their health or psychological stability, as manifest in attendance records, will face sanctions, dismissals or early retirement, rationalized as stemming from employee health problems. Simultaneously, sick day benefits will be challenged or tied to productivity considerations.

If such practices do become widespread, the facilitating device will likely be health screening. Screening potential and current employees for behavioral, attitudinal, and health purposes has already gained considerable popularity among large corporations. Among the specific advantages cited for health screening are selection "of those judged to present the least risk of unstable attendance, costly illness, poor productivity, or short tenure"; development of a "medical placement code" to match employees to jobs by health specifications; and "protection of the company against future compensation claims" (45, p. 31). In addition, screening holds out the possibility of cost savings from reduced croup insurance rates. In a 1974 survey of over 800 corporations with more than 500 employees each, 71 percent of the companies gave preemployment health screening examinations to some or all new employees, compared with 63 percent ten years ago. General periodic examinations jumped from 39 to 57 percent over the same period (45). New businesses are now selling employee risk evaluations, called by one firm "health hazard appraisals." The American Hospital Association is also developing health appraisal programs for use by employers. Of course, many screening practices, such as psychological testing for appropriate work attitudes, alcoholism, or screening for mental illness records, have long been in use. The availability to employers of computerized information from health insurance companies for purposes of screening has drawn criticism from groups concerned about invasion of privacy. Women have often been asked questions during job interviews about their use of birth control, and women planning to have children continue to face barriers, especially to those jobs requiring employer investment in training.

Programs are now being expanded to screen workers for susceptibility to job hazards. Not only genetic susceptibility but also other at-risk health behaviors, such as smoking, use of alcohol, or improper diet, help legitimize screening programs But while alerting individual workers to their susceptibility, these programs do not address the hazardous conditions which to some degree affect all workers. Thus, all workers may be penalized *to the extent* that such programs function to divert attention from causative conditions. To the degree that the causative agent remains, the more susceptible workers are also penalized in that they must shoulder the burden of the hazardous conditions either by looking for another, perhaps nonexistent job, or, if it is permitted, by taking a risk in remaining. It is worth noting in this regard that some women of childbearing age barred from working in plants using lead are reported to be obtaining sterilizations in order to regain their jobs. *Dollars and Sense* summarizes one labor leader's remarks on industry's tactics (46, p. 15):

> At a recent UAW conference on lead, UAW President Leonard Woodcock summed up industry's response to hazard control as "fix the worker, not the workplace." He voiced particular concern over exclusion of so-called

"sensitive" groups of workers, the use of dangerous chemical agents to artificially lower workers' blood lead levels, the transfer of workers in and out of high lead areas, and the forced use of personal respirators instead of engineering controls to clean the air in the workplace.

Thus, whether or not the individual is personally blamed for some at-risk behavior, excluding the "susceptible" worker from the workplace is like asking "vulnerable" people to reduce activity during an ozone watch: it may be helpful for particular individuals, but under the guise of health promotion, it may also act as a colossal masquerade.

SOME RELATED ISSUES

It is important to recognize and address the issue that a significant portion of socially caused illness is, at some level, associated with individual, at-risk behavior which can be changed to improve health. A deterministic view which argues that individuals have no choice should be avoided. What must be questioned is both the effectiveness and the political uses (as well as the scientific narrowness) of a focus on life-styles and on changing individual behavior without changing the social and economic environment. Just as the Horatio Alger myth was based on the fact that just enough individuals achieve mobility to make believable the possibility, significant health gains are clearly realizable for those who just try hard enough to resist the incredible array of social forces aligned against healthy behavior. McKinlay has convincingly argued that the frequent failure of health education programs designed to change individual behavior is attributable to the failure to address the social context. In reviewing some of the strategies adopted by the "manufacturers of illness" to encourage profitable at-risk behaviors and to shape conducive self-images in American consumers, McKinlay observes that (47, pp. 9-10):

> . . . certain at-risk behaviors have become so inextricably intertwined with our dominant cultural system (perhaps even symbolic of it) that the routine display of such behavior almost signifies membership in this society. . . . To request people to change or alter these behaviors is more or less to request the abandonment of dominant culture.

Certainly, the development of health education programs should be encouraged. Concurrent with expansion of access to primary medical services, health personnel should be trained to work with patients in developing practices which reduce risk factors. Lack of information about the dangers of smoking, high cholesterol intake, or obesity, for example, could be considerably reduced by such efforts. The solid evidence supporting Belloc and Breslow's (48) prescriptions for a healthier and longer life could be made available. Health educators, however, would be engaging in victim blaming if such efforts were allowed to suffice; and only marginal results would be achieved as well.

Unfortunately, at a time when the health education profession needs to develop a new strategy which, as Podell argues, enlarges the focus "to include the political and social context in which the individual's health-related choices are being made" (40, pp. 171-172), the individual-behavior orientation of the field has become more pronounced in response to the developments described in this chapter. The recent Task Force on Health Promotion and Consumer Health Education, sponsored by the National Institutes of Health and the American College of Preventive Medicine, for example, repeatedly emphasized a victim blaming approach in its report. The Task Force made several recommendations overwhelmingly oriented toward the assumption of individual responsibility. The Task Force reasoned (40, p. 88),

> In view of the overriding importance of individual behavior and lifestyle as major factors in the nation's unsatisfactory health status and ever-rising health care bill, CHE [consumer health education], with its emphasis on education and motivation of the individual and better individual use of the delivery system, must now be recognized as a top priority in the national commitment to health promotion.

Some members of the Task Force pressed for a different, more policy-oriented approach for health education. These concerns were acknowledged and even supported in the report, just as social pressures were also acknowledged. The Task Force, nonetheless, made its priorities clear. In response to the appeal for the alternative orientation, the Task Force warned (40, p. 24),

> However, there is also danger in pushing this view too far. Overemphasis on broad policy issues to the neglect of more traditional individual instruction could lead to loss of identity for health education as a profession. . . . [I]f health education is to survive as a profession, rather than just a movement, or a philosophy of life, it must acquire more precise discipline.

These remarks indicate that the Task Force members are keenly aware of the political constraints that impinge on the growth and prosperity of a profession. They should also caution against placing too much faith in health education efforts. While there are dissenting voices in the profession's hierarchy and probably many more among its rank and file, the profession seems bound to conceptions generated and sustained by political expedience. Indeed, a movement is precisely what is needed to free health promotion activities from professional and political control.

Similarly, the National Consumer Health Information and Health Promotion Act of 1976 is concerned almost exclusively with modifying individual health behavior and encouraging "appropriate use of health care." In providing for support of community programs, for example, funding is mandated only for programs which promote "appropriate use" or which "emphasize the prevention or moderation of illness or accidents that appear controllable through individual knowledge and behavior." In another section, the statute provides support for "individual and group self-help programs designed to assist the participant in using his individual capacities to deal with health problems . . ." (49, quoted in 40, pp. 841-842).[1] The ideological themes noted in the Task Force report are now ensconced in law and constitute national policy.

One other policy consideration, following from my earlier remarks linking the victim blaming ideology with the reordering of expectations and the attack on rights and entitlements, needs explication. Those remarks are in no way intended to imply that access to more services, *regardless* of their utility for improved health status, is a progressive position. Medical services as a means to maintain health have been grossly oversold. As Starr comments about irrelevant services, "it makes no sense to add more where there is already too much" (12, p. 55). But universal, comprehensive, and unhindered access to effective and necessary medical services through a national policy which strengthens the public sector, ensures an equal distribution of medical resources, and removes all financial barriers must remain at the center of a progressive health strategy. Comprehensive national health insurance is an important step in that direction. According to Starr, "a critic like Illich argues that because medical care has made no difference in health, we should not be particularly concerned about access. He has the point turned around. We will have to be especially concerned about inequalities if we are to make future investments in medical care effective" (12, p. 52). The argument here is that medical expenditures are presently distorted toward unnecessary and ineffective activities which serve to maximize income for providers and suppliers (50). Political conditions favoring an effective and just reallocation of expenditures are more likely to develop in the context of a publicly accountable system which must allocate services within statutory constraints and a politically determined budget. In such a system, political struggles against special interests, misallocation, or underfunding will obviously continue, as will efforts to achieve effectiveness and responsiveness. The concept and definition of need will move to the center of policy discussions. With all the perils and ideological manipulations that process will entail, it is better that such a debate take place in public than be determined by the private market.

Further, viable programs of cost control must be formulated, first as an alternative to the cut-back strategy, and second as the necessary adjunct to establishing

---

[1] Throughout this paper; it has been implied that self-help groups are the product of a victim blaming conception in that they expect individuals, often through small groups, to extricate themselves from their plight. But even though many self-help groups are diversionary in this respect, others have been part of a larger political movement. The women's self-help movement is an example. It has challenged professional authority over women's lives and has provided personal experiences which were useful for developing more far-reaching conclusions about the politics of health. The demystification and transfer-of-skills strategies have also encouraged some activity of a more political nature. Many of these groups emerged from people's sense of alienation from the medical system and from the strategic ineffectiveness of other movements. An on-going discussion of the politics of self-help can be found in *Social Policy* over the last few years.

effective and relevant services. Technology-intensive and overuse-related sources of inflationary costs are directly related to the problem of ineffectiveness as well as to iatrogenesis. As Marc Lalonde argues for Canada, if "the cost of present services will go down, . . . this will make money available to extend health insurance to more services and to provide needed facilities, such as ambulatory care centres and extended care institutions" (p. 37). Certainly, such an outcome is not assured; but the prospects for obtaining more essential services are enhanced with the reduction of unnecessary ones. Health workers would also be more supportive of cost control measures if they were linked with a development of new jobs for services more attuned to people's needs.

CONCLUSION

The ideology of individual responsibility promotes a concept of wise living which views the individual as essentially independent of his or her surroundings, unconstrained by social events and processes. When such pressures are recognized, it is still the individual who is called upon to resist them. Nevertheless, an alternate political understanding, directed not toward individuals, but toward relations among individuals, will profoundly influence the politics of health in the coming period. The commercial and industrial assault on health is becoming too grave to be ignored. A crisis characterized by an increasing involvement of unions, consumer groups, and environmental activists in confrontation with the "manufacturers of illness" threatens to extend far beyond the normal boundaries of health politics.

This politicization of environmental and occupational health issues suggests an erosion of the power of medicine to function as a diversion from social causation. This may be occurring even though overall utilization of medical services continues to rise and the hope for medical deliverance remains intense. The failure of medicine to contain the new epidemics is a partial explanation for that erosion. The cost crisis also leads to an ideological shift away from medicine. Given people's expectations and political pressures for protection and extension of entitlements, a justification for retrenchment must be offered. Thus, people are told that they rely too much on ineffective medical services, and they must think instead about prevention. However, to the extent that medicine is delegitimized, its traditional social control function of individualizing disease through the biological model, and of providing a "technological fix" as a substitute for social change, is also weakened. As people come to understand the limitations of medicine and technology as a means to better health, there is in-creasing potential for the development of a movement willing to confront dominant interests over the systematic denial of health.

The ideology of individual responsibility poses an alternate social control formulation. It replaces reliance on therapeutic intervention with a behavioral model which only requires good living. Like medicine, the new ideology continues to "atomize both causation and solution to illness" (51), although now that ideological function is performed outside the therapeutic structure.

The success of such an approach, however, is problematic. A deinstitutionalized individualism cannot perform as an effective social control device in a technological age. For this reason it is important not to overemphasize the abandonment of medicine. If cost control and other organizational reforms can be successfully imposed, and the provision of services divorced from popular demands for rights and entitlements, medicine may again become more amenable to dominant interests. The continuing utility of medicine will come not so much from a newly found effectiveness, but from its potent redemptive and other social control qualities. Although medicine is not the only institution capable of performing such critical functions, the therapeutic ideology will remain the "paradigm for modernized domination" (52, p. 8). Through masking political relations by calling them medical (31), and through the technical definition of social problems, medicine provides an institutionalized form of control that the concept of individual responsibility cannot.

Finally, although the victim blaming ideology is linked with the attack on medicine, there is no inherent reason why the celebration of a "reformed" medicine and notions of individual responsibility cannot coexist. Each counterbalances the weakness of the other. Even as the attack on medicine gains popularity, a reintegration may be under way. After all, victim blaming may let medicine off the hook as well.

Acknowledgments—I would like to thank several friends who provided helpful comments and editorial suggestions, mostly on an earlier draft. They include Evan Stark, Susan Reverby, John McKnight, Nancy Hartsock, Sol Levine, Cathy Stepanek, Isaac Balbus, and participants in the East Coast Health Discussion Group. I am especially indebted to Lauren Crawford who provided many hours of her time in discussion and in preparation of this manuscript. Thanks is also extended to Katie Sosner for two long typing days.

REFERENCES

1. Kass, L. Regarding the end of medicine and the pursuit of health. *Public Interest* No. 40: 11-42, Summer 1975.
2. *Conference on Future Directions in Health Care: The Dimensions of Medicine.* Sponsored by Blue Cross Association, The Rockefeller Foundation, and Health Policy Program, University of California, New York, December 1975.
3. McKeown, T. *Medicine in Modern Society.* G. Allen and Unwin, London, 1965.
4. McKeown, T. An historical appraisal of the medical task. In *Medical History and Medical Care: A Symposium of Perspectives,* edited by T. McKeown and G. McLachlan, pp. 29-55. Oxford University Press, London, 1971.
5. Cochrane, A. L. *Effectiveness and Efficiency: Random Reflections on Health Services.* Nuffield Provincial Hospitals Trust, London, 1972.

6. Powles, J. On the limitations of modern medicine. *Sci. Med. Man* 1(1): 1-30, 1973.
7. Illich, I. *Medical Nemesis: The Expropriation of Health.* Pantheon Books, New York, 1975.
8. Fuchs, V. *Who Shall Live? Health, Economics, and Social Choice.* Basic Books, New York, 1974.
9. Carlson, R. *The End of Medicine.* John Wiley & Sons, New York, 1975.
10. Lalonde, M. *A New Perspective on the Health of Canadians: A Working Document.* Information Canada, Ottawa, 1975.
11. Somers, A. *Health Care in Transition: Directions for the Future.* Hospital Research and Educational Trust, Chicago, 1971.
12. Starr, P. The politics of therapeutic nihilism. *Working Papers for a New Society* 4(2): 48-55, 1976.
13. *New York Times,* April 26, 1977.
14. *The Complex Puzzle of Rising Health Costs: Can the Private Sector Fit It Together?* Council on Wage and Price Stability, Washington, D.C., December 1976.
15. *Chicago Sun-Times,* March 16, 1976.
16. Inflation of Health Care Costs, 1976. Hearings before the Subcommittee on Health of the Committee on Labor and Public Welfare, United States Senate, 94th Congress. U.S. Government Printing Office, Washington, D.C., 1976.
17. O'Connor, J. *The Fiscal Crisis of the State.* St. Martin's Press, New York, 1973.
18. Fox, D., and Crawford, R. Health politics in the United States. In *Handbook of Medical Sociology,* edited by H. E. Freeman, S. Levine, and L. Reeder, Ed. 3. Prentice-Hall, Englewood Cliffs, N.J., forthcoming.
19. Kotelchuck, R. Government cost control strategies. *Health/PACBulletin* No. 75, 1-6, March/April 1977.
20. Epstein, S. The political and economic basis of cancer. *Technology Review* 78(8): 1-7, 1976.
21. *Chicago Sun-Times,* February 6, 1977.
22. Berman, D. Why work kills: A brief history of occupational safety and health. *Int. J. Health Serv.* 7(1): 63-87, 1977.
23. Zola, I. Medicine as an institution of social control. *Sociological Review* 20(4): 487-504, 1972.
24. Ehrenreich, B., and Ehrenreich, J. Medicine and social control. *In Welfare in America: Controlling the "Dangerous Classes,"* edited by B. R. Mandell, pp. 138-167. Prentice-Hall, Inc., Englewood Cliffs, N.J., 1975.
25. *New York Times,* April 17, 1977.
26. *New York Times,* October 14, 1976.
27. Ryan, W. *Blaming the Victim.* Vintage Books, New York, 1971.
28. Riessman, C. K. The use of health services by the poor. *Social Policy* 5(1): 41-49, 1974.
29. Special Issue on the Economy, Medicine, and Health, edited by Joseph Eyer. *Int. J. Health Serv.* 7(1): 1-150, 1977.
30. The Social Etiology of Disease (Part 1). *HMO-A Network for Marxist Studies in Health* No. 2, January 1977.
31. Edelman, M. The political language of the helping professions. *Politics and Society* 4(3): 295-310, 1974.
32. *New York Times,* April 3, 1977
33. Eyer, J. Prosperity as a cause of disease. *Int. J. Health Serv.* 7(1): 125-150, 1977.

34. Hurley, R. The health crisis of the poor. In *The Social Organization of Health,* edited by H. P. Dreitzel, pp. 83-122. Macmillan Company, New York, 1971.
35. *Infant Mortality Rates: Socioeconomic Factors,* Series 22, No. 14. U.S. Public Health Service, Washington, D.C., 1972.
36. *Selected Vital and Health Statistics in Poverty and Nonpoverty Areas of 19 Large Cities, United States, 1969-71,* Series 21, No. 26. U.S. Public Health Service, Washington, D.C., 1975.
37. Kitagawa, E., and Hauser, P. *Differential Mortality in the United States: A Study in Socio-economic Epidemiology.* Harvard University Press, Cambridge, 1973.
38. Sherer, H. Hypertension. *HMO-A Network for Marxist Studies in Health* No. 2, January 1977.
39. Antonovsky, A. Social class, life expectancy, and overall mortality. *Milbank Mem. Fund Q.* 45(2, part I): 31-73, 1967.
40. *Preventive Medicine USA.* Prodist, New York, 1976.
41. Jenkins, C. D. Recent evidence supporting psychologic and social risk factors for coronary heart diseases. *N. Engl. J. Med.* 294(18): 987-994, 1976, and 294(19): 1033-1038, 1976.
42. Eyer, J., and Sterling, P. Stress related mortality and social organization. *Review of Radical Political Economy,* forthcoming.
43. Page, J. A., and O'Brien, M. *Bitter Wages.* Grossman Publishers, New York, 1973.
44. Brodeur, P. *Expendable Americans.* Viking Press, New York, 1974.
45. Lusterman, S. *Industry Roles in Health Care.* The Conference Board, Inc., New York, 1974.
46. *Dollars and Sense,* April 1977.
47. McKinlay, J. A Case for Refocussing Upstream—The Political Economy of Illness. Unpublished paper, Boston University, 1974.
48. Belloc, N. B., and Breslow, L. Relationship of physical health status and health practices. *Prev. Med.* 1(3): 409-421, 1972.
49. Public Law 94-317, Title I. 94th Congress, June 23, 1976.
50. Ehrenreich, B., and Ehrenreich, J. *The American Health Empire: Power, Profits, and Politics.* Random House, New York, 1971.
51. Ziem, G. Ideology, the State, and Victim Blaming: A Discussion Paper for the East Coast Health Discussion Group. Unpublished paper, Johns Hopkins University, 1977.
52. McKnight, J. The Medicalization of Politics. Unpublished paper, Northwestern University, undated.

PART 2

Contemporary Social Epidemiologic Framework and Constructs

Embodying Inequality: A Review of Concepts, Measures, and Methods for Studying Health Consequences of Discrimination

Nancy Krieger

Our future survival is predicated upon our ability to relate within equality.
Audre Lorde, 1980 (1, p. 358)

Inequality hurts. Discrimination harms health. These seem like straightforward, even self-evident, statements. They are propositions that epidemiologists can test, just like any other propositions about health that we investigate.

Yet, epidemiologic research explicitly focused on discrimination as a determinant of population health is in its infancy. At issue are both economic consequences of discrimination and accumulated insults arising from everyday and at times violent experiences of being treated as a second-class citizen, at each and every economic level. In asking whether discrimination harms health, this new work builds on a century and a half of research demonstrating that racial/ethnic economic disparities often—but not always—"explain" U.S. racial/ethnic inequalities in health (2–8). And it extends this work to address health consequences of other types of discrimination, based on gender, sexuality, disability, and age (Table 1).

Testing the hypothesis that discrimination harms health requires clear concepts, measures, and methods. This chapter offers a brief review of definitions and patterns of discrimination within the United States, evaluates analytic strategies and instruments researchers have developed to study health effects of different kinds of discrimination, and concludes by delineating diverse pathways by which discrimination can harm health, both outright and by distorting production of epidemiologic knowledge about determinants of population health. Although the examples I employ are primarily U.S.-based and pertain chiefly to racial discrimination and physical health, the broader issues raised should be

101

Table 1

Basic taxonomy of prevalent types of discrimination, United States, 1990s, by type, constituent dominant and subordinate social groups, justifying ideology, material and social basis, and examples of embodiment as inequalities in health

| Type of discrimination | Constituent social groups | | Justifying ideology | Material and social basis | Examples of embodiment as inequalities in health[a] |
	Dominant	Subordinate			
Racial/ethnic	White, Euro-American	People of color: black; Latino/a and Hispanic; American Indian and Alaska Native; Native Hawaiian and Pacific Islander; Asian[b]	Racism	Conquest, slavery, skin color, property	Higher infant mortality rates (per 1,000 births, 1989–1991) Black: 17.1 American Indian: 12.6 Hispanic: 7.6 Asian/Pacific Islander: 6.6 White: 7.4 Age-adjusted mortality rates 1.52 times higher among blacks vs. whites (84, 108)
Gender[c]	Men and boys	Women and girls	Sexism	Property, gender roles, religion	Longer life expectancy of women (6.4 yrs) offset by higher rates of disability and illness, resulting in fewer years of disability-free life (108, 303) Annually, 1 million women (vs. 140,000 men) battered by spouse or partner, and 500,000 women raped or sexually assaulted (usually by a man they know) (332) By age 18, 1 in 3 or 4 girls and 1 in 10 boys sexually abused (333)

Anti-gay/ anti-lesbian	Heterosexual	Lesbian, gay, bisexual, transgender, transsexual	Heterosexism	Gender roles, religion	Elevated rates of smoking, suicide, and substance abuse (61, 163, 300, 308)
Disability	Able-bodied	Disabled	Ableism	Costs of enabling access	Denial of health insurance; inadequate medical care (30, 297)
Age	Non-retired adults	Youth, elderly	Ageism	Family roles, property	Sexual abuse of children (see Gender, above) Among elderly, poorer survival due to less aggressive treatment (31, 64)
Social class	Business owners, executives, professionals	Working class, poor	Class bias	Property, education	Socioeconomic gradient in excess morbidity and mortality, with risk greatest among the poor (7, 84)

[a]References in parentheses.
[b]Each of these groups is extremely heterogeneous; terminology employed is what will be used in the U.S. 2000 census. Examples (far from exhaustive) of subgroups include: Black: African American, Afro-Caribbean, and Black African; Latino/a and Hispanic: Chicano, Mexican American, Cuban, Puerto Rican, Central and South American; American Indian and Alaska Native: nearly 600 federally recognized and unrecognized American Indian tribes, Aleuts, and Eskimos; Native Hawaiian and Pacific Islander: Native Hawaiian, Samoan, Guamanian; Asian: Chinese, Japanese, Filipino, Korean, Laotian, Hmong, Samoan.
[c]Also called "sex discrimination."

relevant to other countries, to other types of discrimination, to mental health, and to overall well-being.

Throughout, the framework I use to conceptualize and operationalize relationships between discrimination, inequality, and health is ecosocial theory (9–11). Taking literally the notion of "embodiment," this theory asks how we literally incorporate biologically—from conception to death—our social experiences and express this embodiment in population patterns of health, disease, and well-being. Bringing the metaphor of the body politic to life—a body "ruled" by a "head" and sustained by laboring "hands," a body that creates, consumes, excretes, reproduces, and evolves—this theory draws attention to why and how societal conditions daily produce population distributions of health. Critical causal components conjointly include (a) societal arrangements of power and property and contingent patterns of production and consumption, and (b) constraints and possibilities of our biology, as shaped by our species' evolutionary history, our ecologic context, and individual trajectories of biological and social development. These factors together structure inequalities in exposure and susceptibility to—and also options for resisting—pathogenic insults and processes across the lifecourse (9, 12). Ecosocial theory thus posits that how we develop, grow, age, ail, and die necessarily reflects a constant interplay, within our bodies, of our intertwined and inseparable social and biological history. Three additional assumptions, relevant to this chapter, are that we, as human beings, desire and are capable of living fully expressed lives replete with dignity and love, that epidemiologists are motivated to reduce human suffering, and that social justice is the foundation of public health.

Before considering how to conceptualize, measure, and quantify health consequences of discrimination, one caveat immediately is in order: the purpose of studying health effects of discrimination is not to prove that oppression is "bad" because it harms health. Unjustly denying people fair treatment, abrogating human rights, and constraining possibilities for living fully expressed, dignified, and loving lives is, by definition, wrong—*regardless* of effects on health. Rather, the rationale for studying health consequences of discrimination is to enable full accounting of what drives population patterns of health, disease, and well-being, so as to produce knowledge useful for guiding policies and actions to reduce social inequalities in health and promote social well-being.

DISCRIMINATION IN THE UNITED STATES: DEFINITIONS AND PATTERNS

Definitions of Discrimination

According to the Oxford English Dictionary, the word "discriminate" derives from the Latin term *discriminare,* which means "to divide, separate, distinguish" (13, p. 746). From this standpoint, "discrimination" simply means "a distinction (made with the mind, or in action)." Yet, when people are involved, as both agents and objects of discrimination, the meaning and act of discrimination takes on a new meaning: "to discriminate against" is "to make an adverse distinction with regard to; to distinguish unfavorably from others" (13, p. 746). In other words, when people discriminate against each other, more than simple distinctions are at issue. Instead, those who discriminate restrict, by judgment and action, the lives of those whom they discriminate against.

The invidious meanings of adverse discrimination become readily apparent in the legal realm, where people have created and enforce laws both to uphold and to challenge discrimination. Legally, discrimination can be of two forms. One is *"de jure,"* meaning mandated by law; the other is *"de facto,"* without legal basis but sanctioned by custom or practice. Examples of *de jure* discrimination include Jim Crow laws, now overturned, that denied African Americans access to facilities and services used by white Americans (14, pp. 57–111) and current laws prohibiting gay and lesbian marriage (15). By contrast, underrepresentation of people of color and white women in clinical trials constitutes a form of *de facto* discrimination (16–18).

Whether *de jure* or *de facto,* discrimination can be perpetrated by a diverse array of actors. These include: the state and its institutions (ranging from law courts to public schools), non-state institutions (e.g., private sector employers, private schools, religious organizations), and individuals. From a legal or human rights perspective, however, it is the state that possesses critical agency and establishes the context—whether permissive or prohibitive—for discriminatory acts: it can enforce, enable, or condone discrimination, or, alternatively, it can outlaw discrimination and seek to redress its effects (Table 2) (19, 20). A powerful example of the latter is the new post-apartheid South African constitution (21). This document mandates, in the most inclusive language of any national constitution in the world, that "The state may not unfairly discriminate directly or indirectly against anyone on one or more grounds, including race, gender, sex, pregnancy, marital status, ethnic or social origin, colour, sexual orientation, age, disability, religion, conscience, belief, culture, language and birth"; discrimination by individuals on these terms is likewise prohibited.

Despite its legal dimensions, however, discrimination is never simply a legal affair. Conceptualized more broadly, it refers to all means of expressing and institutionalizing social relationships of dominance and oppression. At issue are practices of dominant groups to maintain privileges they accrue through subordinating the groups they oppress and ideologies they use to justify these practices, with these ideologies revolving around notions of innate superiority and inferiority, difference, or deviance. Thus, the *Collins Dictionary of Sociology* defines "discrimination" as "the process by which a member, or members, of a socially defined group is, or are, treated differently (especially unfairly) because of his/her/their membership of that group" (22, p. 169). Extending this definition, the *Concise Oxford Dictionary of Sociology* holds that discrimination involves

Table 2

Selected U.S. laws and international human rights instruments prohibiting discrimination[a]

U.S. laws	International human rights instruments
U.S. constitution	Universal Declaration of Human Rights (1948)
13th amendment (banned slavery) (1865)	Discrimination (Employment and Occupation Convention) (1958)
14th amendment (guaranteed due process to all citizens, excepting American Indians) (1866)	Convention against Discrimination (in Education) (1960)
15th amendment (banned voting discrimination based on "race, color, or previous condition of servitude") (1870)	International Convention on the Elimination of All Forms of Racial Discrimination (1965)
19th amendment (banned voting discrimination "on account of sex") (1920)	International Covenant on Civil and Political Rights (1966)
	International Covenant on Economic, Social, and Cultural Rights (1966)
Civil Rights Act (1875) (declared unconstitutional by U.S. Supreme Court in 1883)	Declaration on the Elimination of Discrimination Against Women (1967)
Civil Rights Act (1964)	Declaration on Race and Racial Prejudice (1978)
Voting Rights Act (1965)	Convention on the Elimination of All Forms of Discrimination against Women (1979)
Fair Housing Act (1968)	Convention on the Rights of the Child (1989)
Equal Opportunity Act (1975)	
Americans with Disabilities Act (1990)	

[a]Sources: references 14, pp. 224–238; 18; 19; 297; 334.

not only "socially derived beliefs each [group] holds about the other" but also "patterns of dominance and oppression, viewed as expressions of a struggle for power and privilege" (23, pp. 125–126). In other words, random acts of unfair treatment do not constitute discrimination. Instead, discrimination is a socially structured and sanctioned phenomenon, justified by ideology and expressed in interactions, among and between individuals and institutions, intended to maintain privileges for members of dominant groups at the cost of deprivation for others.

Although sharing a common thread of systemic unfair treatment, discrimination nevertheless can vary in form and type, depending on how it is expressed, by whom, and against whom. As summarized in Table 3, diverse forms identified by social scientists include: *legal, illegal, overt* (or *blatant*), and *covert* (or *subtle*) discrimination, and also *institutional* (or *organizational*), *structural* (or *systemic*), and *interpersonal* (or *individual*) discrimination (24–27). Although usage of these terms varies, *institutional discrimination* typically refers to discriminatory policies or practices carried out by state or non-state institutions, *structural discrimination* refers to the totality of ways in which societies foster discrimination, and *interpersonal discrimination* refers to directly perceived discriminatory interactions between individuals—whether in their institutional roles (e.g., employer/employee) or as public or private individuals (e.g., shopkeeper/shopper). In all cases, perpetrators of discrimination act unfairly toward members of socially defined subordinate groups to reinforce relations of dominance and subordination, thereby bolstering privileges conferred to them as members of a dominant group.

Patterns of Discrimination

A full accounting of discrimination in the United States today is beyond the scope of this chapter. Instead, to provide a reminder of its ubiquity as well as background to considering how it can harm health, I next review, briefly, five notable ways that discrimination can permeate people's lives.

First, as summarized in Table 1, many groups experience discrimination in the United States today. Dominant types of discrimination are based on race/ethnicity, gender, sexuality (including sexual orientation and identity), disability, age, and, although not always recognized as such, social class (15, 25, 28–35). Other types, more pronounced in the past, include discrimination based on religion and nationality (36, 37). These latter types are still highly relevant for American Indians and other indigenous people in the United States, for whom many governmental policies (e.g., restrictions on religious expression, abrogation of treaty rights, removal of children to non-Indian families) have often been genocidal in effect, if not intent (37–40).

Second, as explicitly recognized by the South African constitution, people often can experience multiple forms of discrimination. Whereas white women

Table 3

Conceptualizing discrimination as a determinant of population health

Aspects of discrimination

Type: defined in reference to constituent dominant and subordinate groups, and justifying ideology (see Table 1)

Form: legal or illegal; institutional, structural, interpersonal; direct or indirect; overt or covert

Agency: perpetrated by state or by non-state actors (institutional or individual)

Expression: from verbal to violent; mental, physical, or sexual

Domain: e.g., at home; within family; at school; getting a job; at work; getting housing; getting credit or loans; getting medical care, purchasing other goods and services; by the media; from the police or in the courts; by other public agencies or social services; on the street or in a public setting

Level: individual, institutional, residential neighborhood, political jurisdiction, regional economy

Cumulative exposure to discrimination

Timing: conception; infancy; childhood; adolescence; adulthood

Intensity

Frequency (acute; chronic)

Duration

Pathways of embodying discrimination, involving exposure, susceptibility, and responses to:

Economic and social deprivation: at home, in the neighborhood and other socioeconomic regions

Toxic substances and hazardous conditions (pertaining to physical, chemical, and biological agents): at home, at work, and in the neighborhood

Socially inflicted trauma (mental, physical, or sexual, ranging from verbal to violent): at home, at work, in the neighborhood, in society at large

Targeted marketing of legal and illegal psychoactive and other substances (alcohol, tobacco, other drugs, junk food)

Inadequate health care, by health care facilities and by specific providers (including access to care, diagnosis, treatment)

Responses to discrimination (protective and harmful)

Protective

Active resistance by individuals and communities (involving organizing, law suits, social networks, social support)

Creating safe spaces for self-affirmation (social, cultural, sexual)

Harmful

Internalized oppression and denial

Use of psychoactive substances (legal and illegal)

Effects of discrimination on scientific knowledge

Theoretical frameworks

Specific hypotheses

Data collection

Data interpretation

may be subject, as women, to gender discrimination, women of color—whether black, Latina, Asian or Pacific Islander, or American Indian—may be subject to both gender and racial discrimination. Moreover, this experience of multiple subordination cannot simply be reduced to the "sum" of each type. Recent U.S. scholarship on gendered racism, for example, has begun to examine how, in a context of overall negative stereotypical portrayals of black Americans as lazy and unintelligent (41, 42), black women—as *black women*—are stereotyped, as Patricia Collins has observed, as "mammies, matriarchs, welfare recipients and hot mammas" (43, p. 67), while black men—as *black men*—are stereotyped as criminals and rapists (25, 27, 43, 44). Understanding discrimination experienced by black women and men thus requires considering the salience of both their race/ethnicity and gender.

Third, singly or combined, different types of discrimination can occur in just about every facet of public and private life (Table 3). The full gamut extends from the grinding daily realities of what Philomena Essed has termed "everyday" discrimination (27) to the less common yet terrifying and life-transforming events, such as being victim of a hate crime (45).

In a typical day, experiences with discrimination accordingly can start—depending on type—in the morning, at home, continue with public encounters en route to or while at school or work or even shopping or eating at a restaurant or attending a public event, and extend on through the evening, whether in the news or entertainment or while engaging with family members (1, 14, 15, 25–28, 30, 31, 46–51). Other common but not typically daily scenarios for experiencing discrimination include: applying for a job (24, 51–53), looking for housing (54–56), getting a mortgage or a loan (57–59), buying a car (60), getting health care (61–67), or interacting with the police or public agencies or the legal system (14, 25, 26, 28, 68).

Fourth, while some experiences of discrimination may be interpersonal and obvious, they are also likely to be institutional and invisible. To know, for example, that you have been discriminated against in your salary, or that you have been denied a mortgage, or an apartment, or been steered away from certain neighborhoods when you are looking for a home, requires knowing how the employer, bank, landlord, or real estate agent treats other individuals (29, 46, 69–71). Typically, it is only when people file charges of discrimination in court that evidence of such patterns of inequality can be obtained. Other clues can be obtained by examining social patterning of economic inequality, since acts of discrimination—whether institutional or interpersonal, blatant or covert—usually harm economic as well as social well-being. Table 4 illustrates this point for racial/ethnic discrimination, depicting marked racial/ethnic inequalities in income, wealth, education, and unemployment.

Fifth and finally, attesting to some of the animosity that feeds and justifies discrimination are, to give but one example, numerous surveys of U.S. racial attitudes (14, 41, 42, 72). Despite declines in racial prejudice over time, reported

Table 4

Selected racial/ethnic inequalities in socioeconomic position, United States, mid-1980s to mid-1990s[a]

Outcome	Black	American Indian and Alaska Native	Asian and Pacific Islander	Hispanic	White
Percent below poverty (1990)	29.5%	31.6%	14.1%	25.3%	9.8%
Ratio to whites	3.0	3.2	1.4	2.6	[1.0]
Median household income (1989)	$19,758	$19,897	$36,784	$24,156	$31,435
Ratio to whites	0.6	0.6	1.2	0.8	[1.0]
Median net worth in lowest income quintile (1991)	$1	N.A.	N.A.	$645	$10,257
Ratio to whites	0.0			0.06	[1.0]
Percent unemployed (adults ≥ 16 yrs old) (1990)					
Men	13.7%	16.2%	5.1%	9.8%	5.4%
Ratio to whites	2.6	3.1	1.0	1.9	[1.0]
Women	12.2%	13.4%	5.5%	11.2%	5.0%
Ratio to whites	2.4	2.7	1.1	2.2	[1.0]
Educational attainment (adults ≥ 25 yrs old) (1990)					
Less than high school	37.0%	34.7%	22.4%	50.2%	22.0%
Ratio to whites	1.7	1.6	1.0	2.3	[1.0]
Bachelor's degree or higher	11.4%	8.9%	36.6%	9.2%	21.5%
Ratio to whites	0.5	0.4	1.7	0.4	[1.0]

[a]Source: references 335, p. 34; 336.

levels remain high, even taking into account that (*a*) people underreport negative social attitudes (41); (*b*) dominant groups typically deny discrimination exists, especially, as Essed (29) has noted, if it is no longer legal (e.g., 73, 74); and (*c*) as Jackman (28) has argued, paternalism combined with friendly feelings toward individual members of subordinate groups coupled with denial of any responsibility for institutional discrimination is as much a hallmark of contemporary discrimination as is outright conflict and negative attitudes. Strikingly, then, data from the 1990 General Social Survey reveal that fully 75 percent of white Americans agree that "black and Hispanic people are more likely than whites to prefer living on welfare" and a majority concur that "black and Hispanic people are more likely than whites to be lazy, violence-prone, less intelligent, and less patriotic" (42, 75). These are ugly social facts, with profound implications for not only our body politic but also the very bodies in which we live, love, rejoice, suffer, and die.

MEASURING DISCRIMINATION TO ESTIMATE ITS EFFECTS ON POPULATION HEALTH

How, then, can epidemiologists study discrimination as a determinant of population health? Figure 1 summarizes three approaches to quantify health effects of discrimination: (*a*) indirectly, by inference, at the individual level; (*b*) directly, using measures of self-reported discrimination, at the individual level; and (*c*) in relation to institutional discrimination, at the population level. All three approaches are informative, complementary, and necessary. I review and provide examples for each method, below.

Indirectly Measuring Health Effects of Discrimination, Among Individuals

One of the more common approaches to studying health consequences of discrimination is indirect. Recognizing that discrimination may be difficult to measure, investigators instead compare health outcomes of subordinate and dominant groups (Figure 1a). If distributions of these outcomes differ, then researchers determine whether observed disparities can be explained by "known risk factors." If so, investigators interpret their findings in the light of how discrimination may shape distribution of the relevant "risk factors." If, however, a residual difference persists, even after controlling for these other risk factors, then additional aspects of discrimination may be inferred as a possible explanation for the remaining disparities (assuming no unmeasured confounders).

Exemplifying this indirect method are U.S. studies examining whether socioeconomic factors "explain" black-white inequalities in health status (6–8, 76–86), exposure to occupational and environmental health hazards (87–91), or receipt of medical services (92–97). In their earliest form, starting in the

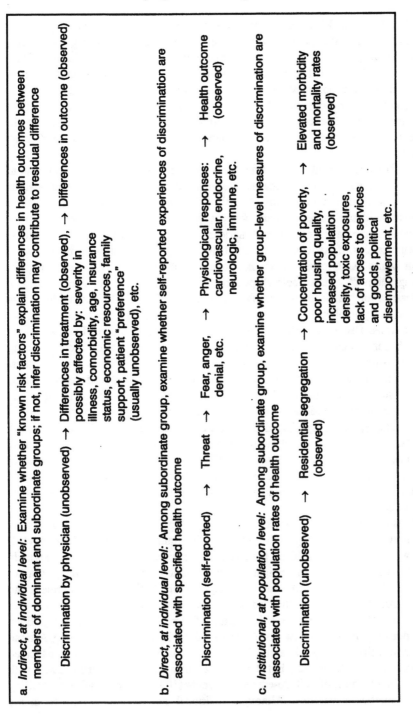

a. *Indirect, at individual level:* Examine whether "known risk factors" explain differences in health outcomes between members of dominant and subordinate groups; if not, infer discrimination may contribute to residual difference

Discrimination by physician (unobserved) → Differences in treatment (observed), → Differences in outcome (observed)
possibly affected by: severity in
illness, comorbidity, age, insurance
status, economic resources, family
support, patient "preference"
(usually unobserved), etc.

b. *Direct, at individual level:* Among subordinate group, examine whether self-reported experiences of discrimination are associated with specified health outcome

Discrimination (self-reported) → Threat → Fear, anger, → Physiological responses: → Health outcome
denial, etc.   cardiovascular, endocrine,   (observed)
neurologic, immune, etc.

c. *Institutional, at population level:* Among subordinate group, examine whether group-level measures of discrimination are associated with population rates of health outcome

Discrimination (unobserved) → Residential segregation → Concentration of poverty, → Elevated morbidity
(observed)   poor housing quality,   and mortality rates
increased population   (observed)
density, toxic exposures,
lack of access to services
and goods, political
disempowerment, etc.

Figure 1. Three main epidemiologic approaches to studying health effects of discrimination.

mid-1800s, these kinds of investigations compared health of enslaved with free blacks and also with poorer and wealthier whites, thereby exposing how slavery and poverty, and not "race" per se, largely explained the poorer health of "the Negro" (5, 98–100). The basic strategy, then and now, is to determine whether "adjusting" for socioeconomic position (along with relevant confounders) eliminates observed racial/ethnic disparities in the specified outcome. If so, economic consequences of racial discrimination are inferred to underlie the observed (unadjusted) disparities; in other words, both racism and class matter (6, 7, 76–81).

If, however, racial/ethnic differences persist, four alternative explanations can be offered. One is that inadequate measurement of socioeconomic position produces residual confounding (6, 101, 102). Consider, for example, a disease whose incidence increases with poverty, with incidence rates identical among African Americans and white Americans at each income level. Under these circumstances, if African Americans below the poverty line were much poorer than white Americans below the poverty line, then analyses adjusting for being "above" versus "below" poverty would fail to explain excess rates of disease among African Americans—even though black-white income disparities in fact fully explained black-white differences in disease incidence. A second hypothesis, discussed in the next section, is that the remaining difference reflects health consequences of unmeasured non-economic aspects of racial discrimination—for example, chronic psychological stress (6, 103). A third explanation, unrelated to discrimination, posits that unexplained differences reflect unmeasured factors that are associated with both race/ethnicity and the specified outcome but are not related to either discrimination or socioeconomic position—for example, culturally shaped patterns of food consumption. Finally, a fourth explanation—often invoked but rarely tested (104, 105)—speculates that innate genetic differences are responsible. Whether and how investigators address these alternative explanations, when interpreting unexplained differences in health status between subordinate and dominant groups, varies considerably across studies.

Illustrating both the importance and the ambiguity of research using indirect methodologies to study health effects of discrimination is research on a well-known public health problem: black-white disparities in risk of low birth weight (106, 107). Numerous investigations have demonstrated that poverty is associated with elevated risk of low birth weight among both African Americans and white Americans and also that "adjusting" for poverty substantially reduces—but does not eliminate—excess risk among African Americans (106, 107). Even so, not only is risk of low birth weight 1.5 to 2 times higher among African American than among white and Hispanic infants born to poor or less educated parents (107; 108, p. 90), but it is also 2 times higher comparing black with white infants born of college-educated parents (109, 110), even after controlling for numerous covariates. Although additional non-economic and economic dimensions of racial discrimination could account for these findings, so too could other unmeasured determinants or confounders. Absent data on these unmeasured factors, discrimination can be at best inferred, not demonstrated, as a determinant of health outcomes. These same caveats apply to the other major strand of research indirectly assessing effects of discrimination and health, which focuses on differentials in diagnosis and treatment of women and men with the same symptoms or diseases (62, 66, 111, 112).

The importance of discrimination in restricting economic resources, coupled with evidence of the profound impact of economic well-being on health (6, 7, 113–116), accordingly suggests that one strategy for reducing ambiguity and improving epidemiologic research is employing appropriate measures of socio-economic position (101, 117–119). Failing to take into account such issues as level of measurement (e.g., individual, household, neighborhood, or region) and time period (e.g., childhood, adult) can introduce bias and produce considerable residual confounding. Using individual-level—instead of household-level—measures of socioeconomic position for women, for example, will rarely be adequate for properly detecting socioeconomic gradients in women's health (116, 120–122). Moreover, as illustrated by a study which found that childhood but not adult measures of socioeconomic position account for adult racial/ethnic disparities in infection by *Helicobacter pylori* (123)—presumably because most infection occurs in childhood—socioeconomic position should be measured at relevant points across the lifespan, in relation to both acute exposures and cumulative disadvantage (12, 117). For guidance on measuring socioeconomic position in epidemiologic studies, overall and with respect to time period and level of management, as well race/ethnicity, gender, and sexual orientation, readers are encouraged to consult the cited references, above.

Lastly, one further indirect approach to measuring health effects of discrim-ination on individuals—albeit relevant only to racial discrimination—addresses associations between skin color and health status. This approach has been employed in 17 U.S. epidemiologic studies focusing on health of African Americans (124–140). Although most of these studies actually were attempting to use skin color as a biological marker for genetic admixture, several also conceptualized skin color as a marker for discrimination. The underlying pre-sumption is that darker skin color increases risk of discrimination above and beyond a powerful "color line" markedly distinguishing people of color from white Americans.

Notably, among these 17 epidemiologic studies, 12 reported associations (all modest) between skin color and the specified outcomes (ranging from blood pressure to all-cause and cause-specific mortality) (124–130, 133, 134, 137, 138, 140). Of these 12, the ten collecting socioeconomic data *all* found that socio-economic position either typically explained or else substantially modified the observed association (124, 126–129, 133, 134, 137, 138, 140). Additionally, the single published U.S. study examining associations between skin color, socioeconomic position, and self-reported experiences of racial discrimination among African Americans documented that while darker skin color was moderately associated with socioeconomic deprivation (among men only), skin color and self-reported experiences of racial discrimination were largely unrelated (141). Other sociologic research similarly has shown that while moderate associations exist between skin color and income among both African Americans and Mexican Americans (chiefly among men), income disparities are far greater comparing African Americans or Mexican Americans with light skin to white Euro-Americans than when comparing African Americans or Mexican Americans with dark versus light skin (142–146). The net implication is that while skin color may serve as a modest indirect marker for aspects of racial discrimination, it is not a direct marker for self-reported experiences of racial discrimination.

Taken together, then, existing research relying upon indirect strategies to measure health effects of discrimination provides precisely this: indirect evidence. These studies do not and cannot explicitly measure direct experiences of discrimination. Nor can they investigate effects related to intensity, duration, or time period of exposure to discrimination. What such studies *can* address, however, are (*a*) health effects of types of discrimination *not readily perceived by individuals* (e.g., treatment decisions of individuals' physicians), and (*b*) whether economic disparities or other factors presumed to be related to discrimination account for observed differences in health between dominant and subordinate groups. For these reasons, studies using indirect approaches to measuring health effects of discrimination can and do provide essential, powerful, and important evidence that discrimination shapes societal distributions of health and disease. To ask and answer the question of how directly perceived discrimination affects health accordingly requires a different set of questions and a different research strategy.

Measuring Self-Reported Experiences of Direct Discrimination and Its Health Effects, Among Individuals

To meet the challenge of explicitly measuring people's direct experiences of discrimination and relating this to their health status, a new generation of public health researchers is devising new methods and approaches. Indicating the novelty of this work, at the time of preparing this chapter I could identify only 20 studies in the public health literature employing instruments to measure self-reported experiences of discrimination (Table 5) (47, 67, 147–164). Of these, 15 focused on racial discrimination (13 on African Americans, two on Hispanics and Mexican Americans), two of which additionally addressed gender discrimination; another solely examined gender discrimination; three investigated discrimination based on sexual orientation; and one concerned discrimination based on disability. I could find no published empirical studies on health effects of self-reported experiences of discrimination based on age.

In Table 5, I summarize measures of discrimination employed in, along with the findings of, these 20 investigations. The most common outcome (ten studies) was mental ill-health, such as depression, psychological distress; the second most common (five studies) was hypertension or blood pressure. Overall, studies consistently reported that higher levels of self-reported experience of discrimination were associated with poorer mental health; associations with somatic health, as discussed below, were more complex.

As indicated by the diversity of questions listed in Table 5, public health research presently lacks a standardized methodology to measure self-reported experiences of direct discrimination. Of particular note is variability in assessing (a) the time period of exposure (ever versus recently), (b) the domain of such exposures (globally or in specific situations), (c) intensity and frequency of exposure (major events or everyday types of discrimination), and (d) the targets of discrimination (respondents only or also members of their family or their group overall). Only eight studies included additional questions asking respondents how much they were upset by and how they responded to experiences of discrimination. Less than half the studies reported psychometric measures regarding validity or reliability of their instruments.

At least two factors underlie proliferation of different measures of self-reported experiences of and responses to discrimination in epidemiologic research. One is the recent emergence of public health research on this topic. Thus, investigators are only now starting to develop, employ, and validate instruments appropriate for large-scale epidemiologic investigations. Methodologic research comparing associations of diverse measures of self-reported discrimination with selected health outcomes, within the same study population, has yet to be conducted. Without such validation research, choice of appropriate measures is likely to remain problematic.

Also contributing to eclectic use of questions about self-reported experiences of discrimination is an overall dearth of empirical studies on this topic, not just in public health but in research more broadly. Often, when epidemiologists decide to measure social phenomena to assess their impact on health, we look to social sciences for guidance. Yet, neither the sociologic nor psychological literature currently offers well-characterized, "ready-to-use," validated instruments appropriate for large-scale empirical studies. Instead, most empirical sociologic studies on discrimination either have focused chiefly on racial attitudes of people who discriminate, rather than experiences of those who have endured discrimination (28, 41), or else, as is also the case in psychological research, they have employed in-depth interviews and qualitative approaches not readily transferable to epidemiologic research (27, 46, 165–170). The net effect is an uncanny silence on empirical estimates of the prevalence (let alone effects) of self-reported

Table 5

Measures of direct discrimination used in or designed for studies with health outcomes[a]

Type of discrimination; study	Study population[b]	Questions asked	Health outcome and association with self-reported experiences of discrimination[c]
Racial/ethnic			
James et al., 1984 (147)	112 African American men in North Carolina	Occupational stressors: race as a hindrance to job success; unfair wages (not paid their worth) *Response format:* yes/no *Psychometric evaluation:* none	Blood pressure ≈↑
Amaro et al., 1987 (148)	303 Hispanic women professionals (national sample)	Ever experienced discrimination at work *Response format:* yes/no *Psychometric evaluation:* none	Psychological distress ↑
Salgado de Snyder, 1987 (149)	140 Mexican immigrant women in Los Angeles	Ever been discriminated against as a Mexican, in the past 3 months (Note: question was one item in an acculturation scale) *Response format:* yes/no; if yes: 4-point Likert scale on extent of related stress, ranging from "not very much" to "very stressful" *Psychometric evaluation:* Cronbach's $\alpha = 0.65$	Depression ≈↑

Study	Population	Measure	Health outcome
Krieger, 1990 (150)	51 black and 50 white women in Oakland, California	Ever discriminated against: at school; getting a job; at work; getting housing; getting medical care; from police or in the courts *Response format:* yes/no *Psychometric evaluation:* none Response to unfair treatment: accept as fact of life or take action; talk to others or keep to self *Response format:* select one of the two specified options *Psychometric evaluation:* none	Hypertension (self-reported) ≈↑
Dressler, 1990 (151)	86 black women and 100 black men in Alabama	Chronic social role stressors: four questions on discrimination at work, regarding pay raises, promotion, job responsibilities, overall pay (Note: questions were items in a scale on chronic stressors) *Response format:* 4-point Likert scale on how often, ranging from "never" to "frequently" *Psychometric evaluation:* none	Blood pressure ∅
Murrell, 1996 (152)	165 African American women in northern California	Perceptions of Racism Scale (337): 20-item self-report inventory, of which 10 questions concern medical, two about lifetime experiences of discrimination *Response format:* 4-point Likert scale ranging from "strongly agree" to "strongly disagree" *Psychometric evaluation:* Cronbach's $\alpha = 0.91$	Stress ↑ Low birth weight ∅

Table 5

(Cont'd.)

Type of discrimination; study	Study population[b]	Questions asked	Health outcome and association with self-reported experiences of discrimination[c]
Krieger and Sidney, 1996 (153)	4,086 black and white women and men in a multicenter study (1,143 black women, 831 black men, 1,106 white women, 1,006 white men)	Discrimination questions: same as in Krieger, 1990, plus one additional situation: ever discriminated against on the street or in a public setting. *Response format:* yes/no. *Psychometric evaluation:* none. Response to unfair treatment: see Krieger, 1990	Blood pressure ≈↑
Jackson et al., 1996 (154)	623 African Americans (national probability sample)	Respondent or family member treated badly because of race (in last 30 days). *Response format:* yes/no. *Psychometric evaluation:* none. Perception of whites' intentions: keep blacks down, better break, don't care. *Response format:* select one of the three specified options. *Psychometric evaluation:* none	Psychological distress Ø; Number of chronic conditions Ø; Disability Ø; Psychological distress ↑; Number of chronic conditions Ø; Disability ≈↓

McNeilly et al., 1996 (47)	165 African American college students and 25 community members in North Carolina (123 women, 67 men)	Perceived Racism Scale (51 items): Frequency domain (items 1–43): frequency of exposure to racist incidents (past year; lifetime) on the job, in academic settings, in public settings (overt and subtle), racist statements *Response format:* for each item, 6-point Likert-like scale, ranging from "almost never" to "several times a day" *Psychometric evaluation:* Cronbach's α = 0.96; test-retest reliability: range = 0.71–0.81 Response domain (items 44–51): emotional responses and behavioral coping responses to perceived racism *Response format:* Emotional responses: 5-point Likert scale for each type of feeling (e.g., angry, sad), ranging from "not at all" to "extremely"; rank importance (from most to least) of four responses to experiencing racism ("think whites have a problem," "think that person being racist has a problem," "feel bad about being black," "feel bad about myself") Behavioral responses: select one or more of 10 options (e.g., "speaking up," "forgetting it," "getting violent," "praying") *Psychometric evaluation:* Cronbach's α = 0.92; test-retest reliability: range = 0.50–0.78	None; designed for use in future public health studies
Broman, 1996 (155)	312 African American adults in Detroit (209 women, 103 men)	See Krieger, 1990 study; rephrased to refer only to discrimination in the past three years	Hypertension (self-reported) Ø Heart disease (self-reported) Ø

Table 5

(Cont'd.)

Type of discrimination; study	Study population[b]	Questions asked	Health outcome and association with self-reported experiences of discrimination[c]
Ladrine and Klonoff, 1996 (156)	149 black students, staff and faculty at a university (location not specified) (83 women, 66 men)	The Schedule of Racist Events: 18-item self-report inventory: frequency of racist events in past year and entire life and appraisal of related stress *Response format:* 6-point Likert scale—frequency: "never" to "almost all the time"; stress: "not at all" to "extremely" *Psychometric evaluation:* Recent discrimination (past year): Cronbach's $\alpha = 0.95$; split-half reliability: 0.93 Lifetime discrimination: Cronbach's $\alpha = 0.95$; split-half reliability: 0.91 Appraisal of stress: Cronbach's $\alpha = 0.92$; split-half reliability: 0.92	Psychiatric distress ↑ Cigarette smoking ↑
Mays and Cochran, 1997 (157)	232 black women and 73 black men (heterosexual) in college, university, and junior college in Los Angeles	Frequency of discrimination: Based on race/ethnicity, gender, or both: in general; personally experienced As perpetrated by three sources (black men, black women, white men): against black person of same gender as respondent; personally experienced As perpetrated by other African Americans against blacks lacking economic resources: in general; personally experienced	Psychological distress ↑

Satisfaction with medical care →

Psychological distress ←

Response format: for each item, 7-point Likert-like scale, ranging from "never" to "fairly often"
Psychometric evaluation: not stated

Degree of upset and relation to perpetrator, for each type of personally experienced discrimination
Response format: 7-point Likert-like scale—upset: ranging from "not at all" to "upset a great deal"; relationship to perpetrator: "mostly by those I know well" to "mostly by complete strangers"
Psychometric evaluation: not stated

Modified Perceptions of Racism Scale (134): reduced to six questions about perception of unfair treatment on basis of race by city officials, restaurant workers, health care providers, school teachers
Response format: 4-point Likert scale, ranging from "strongly disagree" to "strongly agree"
Psychometric evaluation: Cronbach's $\alpha = 0.78$

Respondent or family member treated badly because of race (in last 30 days); for ever-employed persons: own and awareness of others' experiences of racial discrimination at work
Response format: yes/no
Psychometric evaluation: none

Auslander et al., 1997 (158)

55 African American and 103 white children and their mothers or female guardians

Williams and Chung, 1999 (in press) (159)

2,107 African Americans (national probability sample)

Table 5

(Cont'd.)

Type of discrimination; study	Study population[b]	Questions asked	Health outcome and association with self-reported experiences of discrimination[c]
Williams et al., 1997 (160)	586 black and 520 white adults in Detroit	Discrimination—major events; ever unfairly fired or denied promotion, ever unfairly not hired, ever unfairly treated by police; everyday discrimination: sum of ever experiencing nine kinds *Response format:* yes/no *Psychometric evaluation:* Everyday discrimination: Cronbach's α = 0.88	Self-rated ill-health ≈↑ Psychological distress ↑ Psychological well-being ↑ Bed-days →
Gender			
Krieger, 1990 (150)	51 black and 50 white women in Oakland, California	Ever discriminated against at school; getting a job; at work; at home; getting medical care *Response format:* yes/no *Psychometric evaluation:* none Response to unfair treatment: same as Krieger, 1990, for racial discrimination study	Hypertension ≈↑
Ladrine et al., 1995 (161)	294 women students and staff at university; 337 women at an airport (403 white women, 117 Latinas,	Schedule of Sexist Events (1338): 20-item self-report inventory: frequency of sexist events in past year and entire life *Response format:* 6-point Likert scale, ranging from "never" to "almost all the time"	Psychological distress ↑ Premenstrual symptoms ↑

	38 black women, 25 Asian American women, 46 women in other ethnic groups; location of study site not stated	*Psychometric evaluation:* Recent discrimination (past year): Cronbach's α = 0.90; split-half reliability: 0.83 Lifetime discrimination: Cronbach's α = 0.92; split-half reliability: 0.87	
Mays and Cochran, 1997 (157)	232 black women and 73 black men (hetero-sexual) in college, university, and junior college, in Los Angeles	Frequency of discrimination, perpetrator, degree of upset (see entry under "Racial/ethnic," for types of questions, format, psychometric evaluation)	Psychological distress ↑
Sexual orientation Bradford et al., 1994 (162)	1,925 lesbians (national survey; 88% white)	Experiences of discrimination: verbal attack, job loss, physical attack *Response format:* not stated *Psychometric evaluation:* none	Mental distress: high prevalence (compared with U.S. women overall; not analyzed in relation to reported discrimination)
Meyer, 1995 (163)	741 gay men in New York City not diag-nosed with AIDS (89% white)	Prejudice: experienced anti-gay violence, anti-gay discrimination, in past year *Response format:* yes/no *Psychometric evaluation:* none	Psychological distress ↑
		Perceived stigma of being gay: 11-item scale about expectations of rejection and discrimination regarding homosexuality	Psychological distress ↑

Table 5

(Cont'd.)

Type of discrimination; study	Study population[b]	Questions asked	Health outcome and association with self-reported experiences of discrimination[c]
Meyer, 1995 (163) (cont'd.)		*Response format:* 6-point Likert scale, ranging from "strongly agree" to "strongly disagree" *Psychometric evaluation:* Cronbach's α = 0.86	Psychological distress ↑
		Internalized homophobia: 9-item scale about extent to which gay men are uneasy about their homosexuality and seek to avoid homosexual feelings *Response format:* 4-point Likert scale, ranging from "often" to "never" *Psychometric evaluation:* Cronbach's α = 0.79	
Krieger and Sidney, 1997 (164)	204 black and white women and men with at least one same-sex sexual partner in a multicenter study (27 black women, 13 black men, 87 white women, 77 white men)	Ever discriminated against: in family; at home; at school; getting a job; at work; getting medical care; on the street or in a public setting *Response format:* yes/no *Psychometric evaluation:* none Response to unfair treatment: see Krieger, 1990, for racial discrimination study	Blood pressure ≈↑

Disability

| Li and Moore, 1998 (67) | 1,266 U.S. adults with disabilities (Ohio, Michigan, Illinois; 53% women; 78% white, 17% African American; 47% total annual family income < $10,000; 43% multiple disabilities; 23% congenital disabilities) | Perception of discrimination: 4-item scale on beliefs about treatment of disabled regarding friendship, intelligence, treatment in community, being hired for a job. Response format: yes/no. Psychometric evaluation: Cronbach's α = 0.72 | Acceptance of disability → Chronic pain ↑ |

[a]I could find no empirical public health studies on health effects of self-reported age discrimination.

[b]Racial/ethnic categories as designated in each study.

[c] ↑ = positive association (more discrimination associated with higher levels of outcome)

 ↓ = negative association (more discrimination associated with lower levels of outcome)

 ≈↑ = partial positive association (discrimination positively associated with outcome, but not in dose-response relationship)

 ≈↓ = partial negative association (discrimination negatively associated with outcome, but not in dose-response relationship)

 ∅ = no association (between discrimination and outcome)

experiences of discrimination, even as this experience is widely recognized in many other avenues of discourse—law, political science, history, literature, film, other art forms, and the media, to name a few.

Fortunately, epidemiologic principles about considering interplay of exposure and susceptibility in the social context across the lifecourse (9, 12, 171) can nevertheless provide useful guidance for measuring and analyzing self-reported experiences of discrimination and its effects on health. At issue, as in any epidemiologic study, are (a) measurement of exposure, in relation to intensity, frequency, duration, and relevant etiologic period—that is, time between exposure, onset of pathogenic processes, and occurrence of disease; (b) measurement of susceptibility; and (c) effect modification of associations between exposures and outcomes by relevant covariates. In the case of studies of discrimination and health, issues of susceptibility notably include responses to and ways of resisting discrimination, while those involving effect modification require considering how self-reported experiences of discrimination and ways of responding to such experiences may have different meaning or impact depending on a respondent's social position, as related to multiple subordination, degree of social and material deprivation, and historical cohort.

First, regarding measurement of exposure, extant research suggests questions should be direct and address multiple facets of discrimination for *each* type of discrimination being studied. Conversely, studies should avoid global questions about experiences or awareness of discrimination—whether for all types combined or even just for one type of discrimination—since global questions are likely to underestimate exposure and are of little use for guiding interventions and policies to reduce exposure. Recognizing the importance of assessing multiple domains of discrimination, the few large-scale social science surveys investigating self-reported experiences of discrimination—whether racial (28, 172–176), gender (28, 177), or anti-gay discrimination (178–180)—accordingly have asked respondents questions about experiencing distinct types of discrimination or unfair treatment in a variety of policy-relevant situations. Multiple options for questions about responses to discrimination and unfair treatment are likewise advisable, since studies show reactions can span from "careful assessment to withdrawal, resigned acceptance, verbal confrontation, physical confrontation, or legal action" (46, p. 274; see also 181–184).

Studies listed in Table 5 support the recommendation to use specific, rather than global, questions about experiences of discrimination. Thus, rather than ask about experiencing, say, racial discrimination overall, it is likely to be more informative to inquire about experiencing a specific type of discrimination in several different situations, such as at school, at work, on the street. Even better would be asking separately about having experienced racial discrimination in work assignments, promotions, pay, lay-offs, interactions with coworkers, and interactions with supervisors (46, 168). The importance of considering multiple types of discrimination, moreover, is illustrated by one study of anti-gay discrimination which found that while white gay men reported chiefly anti-gay discrimination, white lesbians reported both anti-gay and gender discrimination, and black gay men and lesbians additionally reported racial discrimination (164); another study notably found that lesbian and gay African Americans reported higher rates of depressive distress than would be predicted based on summing risk for their race/ethnicity, gender, and sexual orientation (185).

In addition to specifying domains in which different types of discrimination occur, questions should also address extent of exposure in relation to the presumed etiologic period. Depending on the health outcome(s) under study, both chronic and acute exposures may matter, as will intensity, duration, and frequency of exposure. Thus, in the case of asthma attacks or other outcomes with sudden onsets that can be triggered by adverse events, acute as well as cumulative exposure to discrimination may be relevant. By contrast, in the case of hypertension or other conditions with gradual onset, cumulative exposure, rather than recent or acute exposure, most likely will have greatest etiologic relevance (153). Furthermore, just as "daily hassles" and "major life episodes" often differentially affect health (186), the daily wear-and-tear of everyday discrimination may pose health hazards distinct from those resulting from major episodes of discrimination (such as losing a job) (160). Designing questions about exposure to discrimination accordingly requires careful development of a priori hypotheses about timing and intensity of exposure in relation to the outcome(s) under study.

Additionally, adequate measurement of exposure requires considering whether it is sufficient to ask individuals about only their own experiences of discrimination. Also of concern may be people's fears of experiencing discrimination and their awareness of or fears about discrimination directed against other members of their family or their social group. Notably, recent research on what has been termed "personal/group discrimination discrepancy" documents that people typically report perceiving greater discrimination directed toward their group than toward themselves personally (157, 175, 184, 187, 188). Possible explanations of this phenomenon range from overestimation of group experiences of discrimination to recognition of patterns of discrimination not readily discerned by personal experience (e.g., discriminatory hiring practices, as discussed earlier) to denial of personal experiences of discrimination, positive coping, optimism, and even illusions of invulnerability (46, 174, 175, 187, 189). Fully measuring exposure to discrimination accordingly may entail asking individuals about their lifetime experiences and fears not only for themselves but for their family members and their appraisal of risk for their social group more generally. These estimates of individual and group exposure, moreover, may be influenced by period and cohort effects due to historical changes in legal status, intensity, and domains of discrimination, for example, coming of age before, during, or after the heyday of the U.S. Civil Rights Movement in the 1960s.

Even assuming questions adequately address the breadth of individuals' experiences, awareness, and fears of discrimination, however, data on self-reported experiences of discrimination necessarily—and importantly—are inherently subjective. Issues of validity are thus the same as those with any epidemiologic data on self-reported exposures, particularly those about personal social experiences (186, 190).

In the case of discrimination, at least four factors may contribute to individuals reporting different experiences of discrimination even when subjected to the same "exposure" (e.g., a specific act). The first involves what has been termed "internalized oppression," whereby members of subordinated groups—especially those experiencing greater social and material deprivation—internalize negative views of the dominant culture and accept their subordinate status and related unfair treatment as "deserved" and hence nondiscriminatory (27, 44, 46, 150, 153, 163, 174, 175, 191). The second concerns ways in which members of subordinate groups relate to "positive" traits—if any—attributed to them by dominant groups; for example, some women may interpret men looking them over sexually in public as evidence of their own sexual attractiveness and hence self-worth, whereas other women may perceive such staring as public harassment (28, 50, 192). Third, people consciously or unconsciously may shape answers to be "socially acceptable" (41, 86), and may also vary in whether they find it helpful or distressing to speak about their problems (193). And fourth, individuals may exaggerate experiences of discrimination (system-blame) to avoid blaming themselves for failure (194).

If operative, any of these biases could potentially affect not only estimates of directly perceived discrimination but also its impact on health. It is important to emphasize, however, that existence of these potential biases does not render epidemiologic research on discrimination and health impossible or unfalsifiable. The logical inference, for example, of a study reporting comparable health status (controlling for relevant confounders) among, say, women reporting no, moderate, and high levels of discrimination within each and every specified sociodemographic stratum (e.g., class, race/ethnicity, age, sexual orientation) would be that discrimination is not causally related to the health outcome(s) under study. By contrast, if associations were, in some instances, a dose-response relationship (more discrimination associated with greater risk of poor health) or, in others, a J-shaped curve (since internalized oppression may affect meaning of a "no" reply), the data would offer suggestive evidence of links between self-reported experiences of discrimination and health.

The salience of these kinds of conceptual and methodological issues for studying self-reported experiences of discrimination in relation to health is illustrated by a recent investigation I conducted on racial discrimination and blood pressure (153). Participants were members of the Coronary Artery Risk Development in Young Adults (CARDIA) study, a prospective multi-site community-based investigation established in 1985–1986 that enrolled slightly over 5,000 young black and white women and men, in fairly equal proportions, who were 18 to 27 years old at baseline (195). Questions on racial discrimination included in the Year 7 CARDIA examination are described in Table 5. To analyze data on exposure to discrimination, I set as referent group African Americans reporting moderate racial discrimination, defined as reporting racial discrimination in one or two of seven specified situations. I based this choice on the a priori logic that moderate exposure constitutes a normal experience for people subject to racial discrimination, and I further hypothesized—based on prior research— that this referent group would be at lower risk of elevated blood pressure than African Americans reporting no or extensive discrimination (150).

Key findings for the African American participants were that, first, 80 percent reported having ever experienced racial discrimination (28 percent in one or two, and 52 percent in three or more of seven specified situations); 20 percent, however, reported having never experienced racial discrimination. Second, systolic blood pressure (SBP) was independently associated with both self-reported experiences of racial discrimination and response to unfair treatment. Third, adjusting for relevant confounders, SBP was significantly elevated by 2 to 4 mm Hg among (a) working-class men and women and professional women reporting substantial versus moderate discrimination, and (b) working-class men and women reporting no versus moderate discrimination; conversely, (c) among professional men, blood pressure was over 4 mm Hg lower among those reporting no versus moderate discrimination. Fourth, within economic strata, a net difference of 7 to 10 mm Hg in average SBP existed when comparing extremes of experience involving racial discrimination and responses to unfair treatment. Additional novel analyses, also adjusted for relevant confounders, showed that (a) black-white differences in SBP would be reduced by 33 percent among working-class women and by 56 percent among working-class men if SBP of all black working-class women and men were equal to that of those reporting only moderate discrimination (whose SBP was the same as that of their white working-class counterparts), and (b) no black-white differences in SBP occurred among professional black women and men reporting, respectively, moderate and no discrimination, as compared with their white professional counterparts.

One plausible interpretation of why a response of no versus moderate racial discrimination was associated with *elevated* SBP among working-class African American women and men but *lower* SBP among professional black men is that, as discussed above, the meaning of "no" may be related to social position, in this case, gender and class (153). Thus, for people with relatively more power and resources, a "no" may truly mean "no." By contrast, among more disenfranchised persons, especially those subject to multiple forms of subordination or deprivation, a "no" may reflect internalized oppression. In such cases, a disjuncture between words and somatic evidence may be an instance of the body revealing experiences—translated into pathogenic processes—that people cannot readily articulate with words. In my view, this is the interpretation that makes the most sense, which takes as real the patterns evinced by blood pressure levels in relation to self-reported experiences of racial discrimination. The body can teach us something here, together with our words. Adding plausibility to this interpretation are results of two additional smaller studies, both of which found higher blood pressure among members of groups subjected to discrimination (black women, in one; white gay men, in the other) who said that they had experienced no versus moderate discrimination (150, 164).

Resolving conceptual and methodological questions raised by emerging research on self-reported discrimination and health will require conducting appropriate validation studies. I accordingly describe three complementary research strategies that could potentially be useful, involving smaller, in-depth studies as well as larger surveys.

One approach would be to employ qualitative interviews to assess respondents' perceptions of discrimination and to probe meanings of their answers to survey questions about experiences of discrimination. Along these lines, one small British study found that people who initially stated on the questionnaire that they had not experienced racial discrimination later said, in subsequent in-depth interviews, that they had experienced such discrimination but found it too hard—or too frightening or too pointless—to discuss (169). Were this finding to be replicated, and were discrepancies between survey responses and in-depth answers about experiencing discrimination found to be greatest among those most subject to subordination or deprivation, it would underscore the need for (a) developing more sensitive approaches to eliciting information on people's self-reported experiences of discrimination, and (b) taking into account effect modification, by social position, of observed associations between self-reported experiences of discrimination and health status.

A second strategy could build on new research about people's physiological responses to adverse stimuli pertaining to the type(s) of discrimination being studied. Several recent experimental studies, for example, have shown that blood pressure and heart rate among African Americans increase more quickly upon viewing movie scenes or imagining scenarios involving racist incidents than when viewing non-racist but angry, or neutral, encounters (196–198). These kinds of studies could be extended by also querying study participants about their self-reported experiences of discrimination, and then analyzing associations between their responses to these questions and their experimentally induced physiological responses to witnessing or imagining discrimination.

A third approach, feasible for large-scale surveys, would be to include questions assessing identity formation, political consciousness, stigma, and internalized oppression (163, 199–201). The purpose would be to examine whether these expressions of self- and social-awareness modify associations between health status and self-reported experiences of discrimination. Notably, each of these constructs is distinct from—and cannot be reduced to—"self-esteem" and "self-efficacy." At least among African Americans, research indicates that awareness that discrimination hinders black people from getting a good education or good jobs is *not* associated with self-esteem, and is only modestly associated with self-efficacy—presumably because people derive their self-esteem chiefly from relations with family and peers, and their sense of self-efficacy from how much they are able to influence their immediate conditions, even while understanding that societal discrimination exists (194, 202).

Measuring Population-Level Experiences of Discrimination and Health Effects

Individual-level measures of exposures and responses to direct interpersonal discrimination, however, no matter how refined, can, by their very nature, describe only one of several levels of discrimination that affect people's lives. Also potentially relevant are population-level experiences of discrimination, such as residential segregation, and population-level expressions of empowerment, such as representation in government. A small but growing body of research accordingly has begun to examine whether aspects of discrimination that can be measured only at the population level themselves determine population health. Thus far primarily focused on racial discrimination, studies employing this third strategy have examined associations of African American morbidity and mortality rates with residential segregation, racial/ethnic political clout, and racial attitudes (203–209).

A study on relationships of black residential segregation and political empowerment with infant postneonatal mortality (the death rate of infants 2 to 12 months old) exemplifies this third approach to quantifying health consequences of discrimination (204). Following prior sociological research on residential segregation (58, 210–212), this investigation used an index of dissimilarity to measure degree of residential segregation. This index ranges from 0 to 100 and essentially measures the percentage of African Americans who would have to relocate so that the ratio of blacks to white in every neighborhood would be the same as that for the city as a whole. Black political empowerment (199) in turn was assessed with two measures: (*a*) relative black political power, defined as the ratio of the proportion of black representatives on the city council divided by the proportion of the voting-age population that was black, and (*b*) absolute black political power, defined as the percentage of city council members who were black. This latter measure was conceptualized as reflecting "the level at which African-Americans are empowered to control the political and policy-making apparatus of the city" (204, p. 1084). Analyses showed an increased risk of black neonatal mortality was independently associated with higher levels of segregation and poverty and lower levels of relative (but not absolute) black political power, even when controlling for intra-city allocation of municipal resources (e.g., per capita spending, by neighborhood, on health, police, fires, streets, and sewers). One implication is that community organization, in addition to other community conditions, may affect population health, a finding likewise suggested by recent research on income inequality, community marginalization, and mortality (213–217).

As in the case of studies of self-reported discrimination, however, research on population health in relation to population-level measures of discrimination or empowerment is in its infancy. Potentially promising measures include population-level indicators of social inequality and discrimination created by the United Nations Development Programme (UNDP) (218), none of which have been employed in epidemiologic studies. The UNDP's gender empowerment measure, for example, includes data pertaining to (a) "economic participation," operationalized as the percentage of women and of men in administrative and managerial positions and in professional and technical jobs; (b) "political participation and decision-making power," measured as the percentage of women and of men in parliamentary seats; and (c) "power over economic resources," operationalized as women's and men's proportional share of earned income (based on the proportion of women and men in the economically active workforce and their average wage) (218, p. 108). Similar measures of economic participation and political empowerment could be developed for other subordinate groups, such as the lesbian and gay or disabled populations. Also likely to be informative, though not yet incorporated in epidemiologic studies, are measures of (a) economic segregation of neighborhoods (219, 220), (b) occupational segregation of jobs by gender and race/ethnicity (14, 25, 87, 221), (c) voter registration and voting rates of subordinate and dominant groups, and (d) sociodemographic composition of additional branches of government, such as the judiciary.

A related strategy—also not yet employed in epidemiologic research—would be to examine population health in relation to government ratification and enforcement of diverse human rights instruments, including the existence and enforcement of national laws prohibiting discrimination (e.g., in the United States, the Civil Rights Act and the Americans with Disability Act) (Table 2). For example, the United States has ratified the International Convenant on Civil and Political Rights (1966) and the International Convention on the Elimination of All Forms of Racial Discrimination (1965), but not the Universal Declaration of Human Rights (1948), the International Convenant on Economic, Social and Cultural Rights (1966), the Convention on the Rights of the Child (1989), or the Convention on the Elimination of All Forms of Discrimination against Women (1979) (218, p. 216). Any or all of these human rights instruments could provide important benchmarks for assessing how discrimination related to violation of these internationally stipulated rights affects population health. From a policy perspective, this could be particularly useful, since popular movements and professional organizations can hold governments, and sometimes even non-state actors, accountable for stipulations in these human rights instruments (19, 20,

222). Epidemiologic research, for example, could analyze rates of domestic violence against women in relation to state funding for police training about domestic violence (a type of spending called for by the Convention on the Elimination of All Forms of Discrimination against Women), or racial/ethnic disparities in infant mortality in relation to public expenditures to improve race relations (a type of spending called for by the International Convention on the Elimination of All Forms of Racial Discrimination).

Any studies investigating associations between population-level measures of determinants and outcomes, however, must address two concerns, regarding (a) etiologic period and (b) ecologic fallacy. In the case of etiologic period, at issue—as in the case of studies using individual-level measures of discrimination—are distinctions between acute and cumulative exposures and between outcomes with short and longer latency periods. Thus, from a temporal standpoint, an association of higher levels of residential segregation or negative racial attitudes with, say, concurrent infant mortality rates or childhood morbidity rates or homicide rates would provide more compelling evidence of health effects of segregation or racial attitudes than would its association with all-cause mortality among adults, given the much longer latency period for most causes of death (e.g., cardiovascular disease, cancer). If, however, current levels of segregation reflected past levels and little bias were introduced by residential mobility, then inferences about links between segregation and adult mortality rates could be warranted. Comparable caveats about temporal plausibility have been raised for studies examining current levels of income inequality in relation to adult mortality rates: these associations make sense only if current income inequality is a marker for systematic underinvestment in human resources over time (223).

Second, regarding ecologic fallacy, concern centers on whether causal inferences at the population level are valid at the individual level. As well described in both social science and public health literature, ecologic fallacy chiefly results from confounding introduced through the grouping variable (e.g., census tract, city, state, nation) used to define the group-level dependent and independent variables (224–228). The classic case, reported by W. S. Robinson in 1950 (224), was that although state-level data showed strong associations between high illiteracy rates and the proportion of states' population that was black (Pearson correlation coefficient = 0.946), within these states the relationship between illiteracy and race/ethnicity was much weaker (Pearson correlation coefficient = 0.203).

A subsequent critique of Robinson's analyses demonstrated that grouping by state added an important confounding variable: state level of spending on public education (229). Because southern states—the ones with relatively high proportions of black residents—had a low tax base and spent relatively less on public education, illiteracy in these states was also high among their white residents. Had Robinson taken into account state per capita spending on education, a phenomenon that can only be measured at the group level, not

only would the computed ecologic correlations have been less affected by aggregation bias but the study also would have identified how state funding for
education determines literacy rates. In other words, had Robinson used relevant
population-level data, his study would have avoided what has been termed
"individualistic fallacy": erroneous inferences about explanations of patterns
observed at the individual level because they rely only upon individual-level
data (6, 225, 228).

In addition to highlighting the importance of population-level determinants of
outcomes measured among individuals, the critique of Robinson's study implies
that population-level measures of discrimination could perhaps be meaningfully
combined with individual-level measures to yield even more informative
analyses of health consequences of discrimination (6, 103, 230). Methodologically, this approach entails use of contextual or multilevel analyses, a technique
first developed in the social sciences (228, 231–234). Using such methods, U.S.
epidemiologic studies have begun to show that health profiles of, say, poor
people who live in poor neighborhoods generally are worse than those of equally
poor people who live in more affluent neighborhoods (235–239). Residential
segregation or community political empowerment could likewise conceivably
modify experiences, perceptions, and effects of—as well as responses to—
individually reported experiences of discrimination. The study design of
contextual analysis, however, has yet to be used in epidemiologic research on
health effects of discrimination.

HOW COULD DISCRIMINATION HARM HEALTH?

Prompting development of the kinds of research strategies I have been
describing is the persistent question: why does health status differ among
subordinate and dominant groups? More than methodology, however, is required
to conduct valid and informative analysis of health consequences of discrimination. Equally vital is systematic and explicit consideration of ways that
discrimination can harm health. Theory matters. At issue is comprehending
not only direct health consequences of discrimination that we embody but also
how discrimination can harm our very ability to understand—and provide knowledge useful for effectively intervening upon—the public's health.

Pathways to Embodying Discrimination

From an ecosocial standpoint, one useful concept for understanding links
between discrimination and health is "biological expressions of discrimination,"
to extend a terminology I developed with Sally Zierler to discuss connections
between gender and health. We defined biological expressions of gender
(including gender discrimination) to mean "incorporation of social experiences
of gender into the body and expressed biologically, in ways that may or may not

be associated with biological sex" (10). One example would be how girls' and women's bodybuild and exercise patterns are affected by underfunding of girls' athletic programs (240). By the same logic, biological expressions of racial discrimination (or race relations, more broadly) refer to how people literally embody and biologically express experiences of racial oppression and resistance, from conception to death, thereby producing racial/ethnic disparities in morbidity and mortality across a wide spectrum of outcomes (241). Similar terminology could be used to discuss biological expressions of other types of discrimination, whether based on sexual identity or orientation, age, disability, social class, or other characteristics. For each type of discrimination, a key a priori assumption is that disparate social and economic conditions of subordinate and dominant groups will produce differences in their physiological profiles and health status.

Conversely, constructs such as "gendered expressions of biology" (10) or "racialized expressions of biology" (241) are useful for denoting how social relations of dominance and subordination affect expression of health outcomes linked to biological processes and traits invoked to define membership in subordinate and dominant groups. In the case of biological sex and gender, for example, women's ability to become pregnant has been used to define women's roles and to restrict women's employment in certain male and relatively well-paid occupations, even though other less well-paid and typically female occupations may be equally hazardous—with these gendered roles in turn shaping distributions of pregnancy outcomes (10, 242). Or, in the case of race/ethnicity, examples of racialized components of our biology include skin color, hair type, and facial features, and also such genetic disorders as sickle cell anemia, cystic fibrosis, and Tay-Sachs disease. Rather than being conceptualized as particular aspects of human diversity, with varying distributions among populations—distributions notably shaped by geography, conquest, and laws about who can have children with whom—these traits instead typically are construed, tautologically, as evidence of "racial types" (241). Particular biological characteristics accordingly become imbued with meanings of "race," conjuring up notions of fundamental difference on a whole host of other characteristics, even though within-group differences far exceed those between groups (6, 104, 105, 243–247).

From an ecosocial vantage, specific pathways potentially leading to embodiment of experiences of discrimination—whether perpetrated by institutions or individuals, in public or private domains—are legion, as are plausible health outcomes. This is because discrimination creates and structures exposures to noxious physical, chemical, biological, and psychosocial insults, all of which can affect biological integrity at numerous integrated and interacting levels, simultaneously comprised of genes, cells, tissues, organs, and organ systems. The net effect, as discussed in a growing literature on causal pathways leading to inequalities in health across the lifecourse, is to create, using Eric Brunner's (248) term, a "biology of inequality" (6, 7, 12, 113–116, 213, 248–253).

Conceptually, however, the myriad socially structured trajectories—operative throughout the lifecourse—by which discrimination can affect health can be coalesced into five clusters. As delineated in Table 3, these pathways involve exposure, susceptibility, and responses (both social and biological) to:

1. Economic and social deprivation: at work, at home, in the neighborhood, and other relevant socioeconomic regions.
2. Toxic substances and hazardous conditions (pertaining to physical, chemical, and biological agents): at work, at home, and in the neighborhood.
3. Socially inflicted trauma (mental, physical, or sexual, ranging from verbal to violent): at work, at home, in the neighborhood, and in society at large.
4. Targeted marketing of legal and illegal psychoactive substances (alcohol, tobacco, other drugs) and other commodities (e.g., junk food).
5. Inadequate health care, by health care facilities and by specific providers (including access to care, diagnosis, and treatment).

Also relevant are health consequences of people's varied responses to discrimination. These can range from internalized oppression and use of psychoactive substances to reflective coping, active resistance, and community organizing to end discrimination and promote social justice (6, 11, 27, 46, 159, 181, 254–256).

From a theoretical standpoint, the utility of an ecosocial framework is that it encourages development of specific testable hypotheses by systematically tracing pathways between social experiences and their biological expression. Applying these five pathways to the case of racial discrimination and population distributions of blood pressure among black and white Americans, an ecosocial framework thus guides researchers to explore the following kinds of hypotheses:

Pathway 1: Residential and occupational segregation lead to greater economic deprivation among African Americans and increased likelihood of living in neighborhoods without good supermarkets, thereby reducing access to affordable nutritious diets; risk of hypertension is elevated by nutritional pathways involving high fat, high salt, and low vegetable diets (256–260).

Pathway 2: Residential segregation increases risk of exposure to lead among African Americans via contaminated soil (related to proximity of neighborhoods to freeways) and lead paint (related to decreased resources for removing and replacing lead paint); lead elevates risk of hypertension by damaging renal physiology (91, 261–264).

Pathway 3: Perceiving or anticipating racial discrimination provokes fear and anger; the physiology of fear ("flight-or-fight" response) mobilizes lipids and glucose to increase energy supplies and sensory vigilance and also produces transient elevations in blood pressure; chronic triggering of these physiological pathways leads to sustained hypertension (103, 126, 134, 147, 150, 153, 160, 196, 197, 256, 265–267).

Pathway 4: Targeted marketing of high-alcohol beverages to African American communities increases likelihood of harmful use of alcohol to reduce feelings of distress; excess alcohol consumption elevates risk of high blood pressure (256, 258, 268–270).

Pathway 5: Poorer detection and clinical management of hypertension among African Americans increases risk of uncontrolled hypertension, due to insufficient or inappropriate medical care (256, 258, 271–273).

By specifying these discrete pathways—however entangled in people's real lives—ecosocial theory thus provides a coherent way for integrating social and biological reasoning about discrimination as a determinant of population health. Instead of cataloguing an eclectic list of risk factors or presuming genetic explanations as sufficient or fundamental, ecosocial theory proposes that explanations of population health are incomplete—and their ability to guide healthy public policy crimped—unless they take into account interweaving of social and biological determinants of well-being.

Effects of Discrimination upon Epidemiologic Knowledge

Discussion of how theory directs the generation of hypotheses in turn points to one important additional way discrimination can affect population health: its impact on epidemiologic knowledge and public health practice. At issue are the kinds of questions epidemiologists do and do not ask, the studies we conduct, and ways we analyze and interpret our data and consider their likely flaws.

That scientists' ideas are shaped, in part, by dominant social beliefs of their times is well documented by historians of public health, medicine, and science (274–285). Relevant to epidemiology, during the last 20 years a substantial body of literature has begun to document how scientific knowledge and, more importantly, real people, have been harmed by scientific racism, sexism, and other related ideologies, including eugenics, that justify discrimination in relation to class, age, sexual orientation, and disability (5, 6, 31, 61, 65, 66, 105, 276, 286–299).

At issue are both acts of omission and acts of commission. These range from the virtual invisibility of lesbians and gay men in major public health databases (61, 300) to distortions of etiologic and therapeutic knowledge due to underrepresentation of people of color and women in epidemiologic studies, clinical trials, and even medical textbooks (16–18, 301–303), to the conduct of research premised on the view that innate differences underlie poorer health of subordinate groups, absent consideration of how subordination might affect health. Vividly illustrating detrimental effects of discrimination upon the generation and application of scientific knowledge, to choose but one example, is the pernicious and longstanding legacy of "race" epidemiology; comparable accounts exist for eugenic constructions of class-based differences in health (304, 305), for sexist analyses of women's health (66, 253, 290, 295, 306), and to a lesser extent, for heterosexist research on lesbian and gay health (61, 300, 307–309).

Historically, "race" first attained prominence in U.S. medical research in the early 1700s (5, 289, 310). Appearance of "race" as a category relevant to health followed institutionalization of the "one drop rule" in various slave codes established in the mid-to-late 1600s (37, 310–312). This rule specified that if someone had only "one drop" of African "blood," she or he was deemed "black." Embedded in this allegedly biological and innate definition of "race" was the notion of intrinsic "racial" superiority and inferiority. Based on this belief, leading scientists and physicians conducted studies to document (and occasionally fabricate (313–315)) racial/ethnic differences in every physical feature imaginable, and then used these data both to explain observed racial/ethnic disparities in health and to prove the "black race" was innately inferior to the "white race" and "fit" only for slavery (5, 276, 289, 316–318).

During the mid-1800s, however, the first generation of credentialed U.S. black physicians—along with abolitionists—challenged the very category of "race." Arguing that people had more similarities than differences, they instead conducted studies showing diversity of health outcomes among free and enslaved blacks and similarity of health outcomes among blacks and poor whites (5, 98–100). Based on these studies, they accordingly argued that slavery and economic duress—not innate constitution—were the principal reasons black Americans had worse or different health than white Americans. This alternative viewpoint flourished briefly during and after the Civil War. After the destruction of Reconstruction, however, leading medical and scientific researchers again conducted studies and proffered explanations based on the premise that "race"—not racial subordination—was the root cause of racial inequalities in health (5, 276, 289).

The next serious challenge to biological definitions of "race" emerged in the aftermath of World War II, in part in reaction to Nazi racial science, especially its fusion of eugenics and anti-Semitism to justify both "Aryan" supremacy and the Holocaust (305, 319). In 1951, UNESCO released its first statement on race, rebutting its validity as a biological category; subsequent revisions, amplifying this point, were issued in 1964, 1969, and, most recently, 1997 (320–322). All editions emphasize that although distributions of specific genetic traits may vary across geographic regions, no ensemble of linked characteristics exists that delineates distinct "races." Empirical evidence supporting this view is now so well-established that contemporary population geneticists, other biologists, anthropologists, and social scientists all concur that racial categories reflect social and ideological conventions, not meaningful natural distinctions (22, 103, 243, 247, 322). Or, as stated in the 1997 revision of the UNESCO statement: "Pure races, in the sense of genetically homogeneous populations, do not exist in the human species today, nor is there any evidence that they have ever existed in the past" (322).

Yet, despite this scientific consensus, the 1995 third edition of *Dictionary of Epidemiology* (sponsored by the International Epidemiological Association) continues to define "race" as "persons who are relatively homogeneous with respect to biological inheritance" (323, p. 139). Worse, flouting contemporary scientific knowledge, it baldly asserts that "In a time of political correctness, classifying by race is done cautiously," as if only ideology, and not scientific evidence, were at issue. The net effect of such views has been an overemphasis in epidemiologic research on allegedly genetic explanations of racial/ethnic inequalities in health, and a disregard for how racism, rather than "race," drives these disparities (6, 7, 76, 103–105, 246, 295, 298, 324–331). Tellingly, whereas the keyword "race" identifies 33,921 articles indexed in Medline since 1966, only the 16 studies (0.0005 percent) listed in Table 5 have attempted to study self-reported experiences of racial discrimination in relation to health. Correcting this imbalance requires explicit attention to theories guiding research to explain population patterns of health, disease, and well-being.

INTIMATE CONNECTIONS: EPIDEMIOLOGY AND THE TRUTHS OF OUR BODY AND BODY POLITIC

In summary, epidemiologists can draw on a variety of study designs (Figure 1) and concepts (Table 3) to develop and test epidemiologic hypotheses about health consequences of discrimination. Arguably the most fruitful approaches will systematically address discrimination in relation to (*a*) its varied aspects (type, form, agency, expression, domain, level); (*b*) cumulative exposure (timing, intensity, frequency, duration); (*c*) likely pathways of embodiment; (*d*) likely forms of responses and resistance and their health consequences; and (*e*) effects upon scientific knowledge.

Stated simply, the epidemiology of health consequences of discrimination is, at heart, the investigation of intimate connections between our social and biological existence. It is about how truths of our body and body politic engage and enmesh, thereby producing population patterns of health, disease, and well-being.

To research how discrimination harms health, we accordingly must draw on not only a nuanced understanding of the likely biological pathways of embodying discrimination, from conception to death, but also a finely tuned historical, social, and political sensibility, situating both the people we study and ourselves in the larger context of our times. Out of the epidemiologic commitment to reduce human suffering, we can extend our discipline's scope to elucidate how oppression, exploitation, and degradation of human dignity harms health—and, simultaneously, further knowledge and inspire action illuminating how social justice is the foundation of public health. Embodying equality should be our goal for all.

Acknowledgments — Thanks to Lisa Berkman, David Williams, Sally Zierler, Sofia Gruskin, Hortensia Amaro, Donna Sullivan, and Gillian Steele for their helpful suggestions, and to Hannah Cooper, Melissa Abraham, and Shannon Brome for locating references.

Note — This chapter is adapted from the chapter "Discrimination and Health" in *Social Epidemiology,* edited by L. Berkman and I. Kawachi, published by Oxford University Press, New York, 1999.

REFERENCES

1. Lorde, A. Age, race, class, and sex: Women redefining difference. In *Racism and Sexism: An Integrated Study,* edited by P. S. Rothenberg, pp. 352–359. St. Martin's Press, New York, 1988.
2. Du Bois, W. E. B. (ed.). *The Health and Physique of the Negro American.* Atlanta University Press, Atlanta, 1906.
3. Tibbitts, C. The socio-economic background of Negro health status. *J. Negro Educ.* 6: 413–428, 1937.
4. Holland, D. R., and Perrott, G. S. J. Health of the Negro—Part I: Disabling illness among Negroes and low-income white families in New York City—A report of a sickness survey in the spring of 1933. *Milbank Mem. Fund Q.* 16: 5–15, 1938.
5. Krieger, N. Shades of difference: Theoretical underpinnings of the medical controversy on black-white differences, 1830–1870. *Int. J. Health Serv.* 17: 258–279, 1987.
6. Krieger, N., et al. Racism, sexism, and social class: Implications for studies of health, disease, and well-being. *Am. J. Prev. Med.* 9(Suppl. 2): 82–122, 1993.
7. Williams, D. R., and Collins, C. US socioeconomic and racial differences in health: Patterns and explanations. *Annu. Rev. Sociol.* 21: 349–386, 1995.
8. Lillie-Blanton, M., et al. Racial differences in health: Not just black and white, but shades of gray. *Annu. Rev. Public Health* 17: 441–448, 1996.
9. Krieger, N. Epidemiology and the web of causation: Has anyone seen the spider? *Soc. Sci. Med.* 39: 887–903, 1994.
10. Krieger, N., and Zierler, S. Accounting for health of women. *Curr. Issues Public Health* 1: 251–256, 1995.
11. Zierler, S., and Krieger, N. Reframing women's risk: Social inequalities and HIV infection. *Annu. Rev. Public Health* 18: 401–436, 1997.
12. Kuh, D., and Ben-Shlomo, Y. (eds.). *A Lifecourse Approach to Chronic Disease Epidemiology: Tracing the Origins of Ill-Health from Early to Adult Life.* Oxford University Press, Oxford, England, 1997.
13. *Compact Edition of the Oxford English Dictionary.* Oxford University Press, New York, 1971.
14. Jaynes, G. D., and Williams, R. M. Jr. (eds.). *A Common Destiny: Blacks and American Society.* National Academy Press, Washington, D.C., 1989.
15. Vaid, U. *Virtual Equality: The Mainstreaming of Gay and Lesbian Liberation.* Anchor Books, New York, 1995.

16. Sechzer, J. A., et al. Sex and gender bias in animal research and in clinical studies of cancer, cardiovascular disease, and depression. *Ann. N.Y. Acad. Sci.* 736: 21–48, 1994.
17. Hamilton, J. A. Sex and gender as critical variables in psychotropic drug research. In *Mental Health, Racism, and Sexism,* edited by C. V. Willie et al., pp. 297–349. University of Pittsburgh, Pittsburgh, 1995.
18. King, G. Institutional racism and the medical/health complex: A conceptual analysis. *Ethn. Dis.* 6: 30–46, 1996.
19. Tomasevski, K. *Women and Human Rights.* Zed Books, London, 1993.
20. Amnesty International, Inter-Sectional Women's Network. *A Guide to Understanding the Issues Arising from the Question of Possible AI Action on Abuses by Non-state Actors.* Amnesty International Working Paper. Washington, D.C., 1997.
21. de Vos, P. Appendix I: Introduction to South Africa's 1996 Bill of Rights. *Netherlands Q. J. Hum. Rights* 15: 225–252, 1997.
22. Jary, D., and Jary, J. (eds.). *Collins Dictionary of Sociology,* Ed. 2. HarperCollins, Glasgow, 1995.
23. Marshall, G. (ed.). *The Concise Oxford Dictionary of Sociology.* Oxford University Press, Oxford, England, 1994.
24. Benokratis, N. V., and Feagin, J. R. *Modern Sexism: Blatant, Subtle, and Covert Discrimination.* Prentice Hall, Englewood Cliffs, N.J., 1986.
25. Rothenberg, P. S. *Racism and Sexism: An Integrated Study.* St. Martin's Press, New York, 1988.
26. Feagin, J. R. *Racial and Ethnic Relations,* Ed. 3. Prentice Hall, Englewood Cliffs, N.J., 1989.
27. Essed, P. *Understanding Everyday Racism: An Interdisciplinary Theory.* Sage, London, 1992.
28. Jackman, M. R., *The Velvet Glove: Paternalism and Conflict in Gender, Class, and Race Relations.* University of California Press, Berkeley, 1994.
29. Essed, P. *Diversity: Gender, Color, and Culture.* University of Massachusetts, Amherst, 1996.
30. Fries, K. (ed.). *Staring Back: The Disability Experience from the Inside Out.* Plume, New York, 1997.
31. Minkler, M., and Estes, C. L. (eds.). *Critical Perspectives on Aging: The Political and Moral Economy of Growing Old.* Baywood, Amityville, N.Y., 1991.
32. Sennett, R., and Cobb, J. *The Hidden Injuries of Class.* Alfred A. Knopf, New York, 1972.
33. Jackman, M. R., and Jackman, R. W. *Class Awareness in the United States.* University of California Press, Berkeley, 1983.
34. Mirowsky, J., and Ross, C. E. *Social Causes of Psychological Distress.* Aldine de Gruyter, New York, 1989.
35. Aneshensel, C. S. Social stress: Theory and research. *Annu. Rev. Sociol.* 18: 15–38, 1992.
36. U.S. Equal Employment Opportunity Commission. *Facts About Religious Discrimination.* U.S. Government Printing Office, Washington, D.C., 1992.
37. Zinn, H. *A People's History of the United States 1492–Present.* HarperPerennial, New York, 1995.

38. Thorton, R. *American Indian Holocaust and Survival: A Population History since 1492.* University of Oklahoma Press, Norman, 1987.
39. Brown, D. A. *Bury My Heart at Wounded Knee: An Indian History of the American West.* Henry Holt, New York, 1991 [1970].
40. Nabokov, P. (ed.). *Native American Testimony: A Chronicle of Indian-White Relations from Prophecy to the Present, 1492–1992.* Viking, New York, 1991.
41. Schuman, H., Steehm, C., and Bobo, L. *Racial Attitudes in America: Trends and Interpretations.* Harvard University Press, Cambridge, Mass., 1985.
42. Kinder, D., and Mendelberg, C. Cracks in American apartheid: The political impact of prejudice among desegregated whites. *J. Polit.* 57: 402–424, 1995.
43. Collins, P. H. *Black Feminist Thought: Knowledge, Consciousness, and the Politics of Empowerment.* HarperCollins Academic Press, London, 1990.
44. hooks, b. *Killing Rage: Ending Racism.* Henry Holt, New York, 1995.
45. Pierce, C. M. Stress analogs of racism and sexism: Terrorism, torture, and disaster. In *Mental Health, Racism, and Sexism,* edited by C. V. Willie et al., pp. 277–293. University of Pittsburgh Press, Pittsburgh, 1995.
46. Feagin, J. R., and Sikes, M. P. *Living with Racism: The Black Middle Class Experience.* Beacon Press, Boston, 1994.
47. McNeilly, M. D., et al. The perceived racism scale: A multidimensional assessment of the experience of white racism among African Americans. *Ethn. Dis.* 6: 154–166, 1996.
48. *Allison, D. Two or Three Things I Know for Sure.* Dutton, New York, 1995.
49. Crull, P. Sexual harassment and women's health. In *Double Exposure: Women's Health Hazards on the Job and at Home,* edited by W. Chavkin, pp. 100–120. Monthly Review Press, New York, 1984.
50. Gardner, C. B. *Passing By: Gender and Public Harassment.* University of California Press, Berkeley, 1995.
51. Faderman, L. *Odd Girls and Twilight Lovers: A History of Lesbian Life in Twentieth-Century America.* Penguin, New York, 1991.
52. Turner, M. A., Fix, M., and Struyk, R. J. *Opportunities Denied, Opportunities Diminished: Racial Discrimination in Hiring.* Urban Institute Report 91-9. Urban Institute Press, Washington, D.C., 1991.
53. Riccucci, N. M., and Gossett, C. W. Employment discrimination in state and local government—The lesbian and gay male experience. *Am. Rev. Public Admin.* 26: 175–200, 1996.
54. Turner, M. A. Limits on neighborhood choice: Evidence of racial and ethnic steering in urban housing markets. In *Clear and Convincing Evidence: Measurement of Discrimination in America,* edited by M. Fix and R. Struyk, pp. 118–147. Urban Institutes Press, Washington, D.C., 1993.
55. Rosenbaum, E. Racial/ethnic differences in home ownership and housing quality, 1991. *Soc. Prob.* 43: 403–426, 1996.
56. Bobo, L., and Zubrinsky, C. Attitudes on residential integration: Perceived status differences, mere in-group preference, or racial prejudice? *Soc. Forces* 74: 883–909, 1996.
57. Pol, L. G., Guy, R. F., and Bush, A. J. Discrimination in the home lending market: A macro-perspective. *Soc. Sci. Q.* 63: 716–728, 1982.

58. Massey, D. S., and Denton, N. A. *American Apartheid: Segregation and the Making of the Underclass.* Harvard University Press, Cambridge, Mass., 1993.

59. Oliver, M. L., and Shapiro, T. M. *Black Wealth/White Wealth.* Routledge, New York, 1995.

60. Ayers, I. Fair driving: Gender and race discrimination in retail car negotiations. *Harvard Law Rev.* 104: 817–872, 1991.

61. Stevens, P. E. Lesbian health care research: A review of the literature from 1970 to 1990. *Health Care Women Int.* 13: 91–120, 1992.

62. McKinlay, J. G. Some contributions from the social system to gender inequalities in heart disease. *J. Health and Soc. Behav.* 37: 1–26, 1996.

63. Geiger, H. J. Race and health care—An American dilemma? *N. Engl. J. Med.* 335: 815–816, 1996.

64. Grant, L. D. Effects of ageism on individual and health care providers' responses to healthy aging. *Health Soc. Work* 21: 9–15, 1996.

65. Gamble, V. N. Under the shadow of Tuskegee: African Americans and health care. *Am. J. Public Health* 87: 1773–1778, 1997.

66. Ruzek, S. B., Olesen, V. L., and Clarke, A. E. (eds.). *Women's Health: Complexities and Differences.* Ohio State University Press, Columbus, 1997.

67. Li, L., and Moore, D. Acceptance of disability and its barriers. *J. Soc. Psychol.* 138: 13–25, 1998.

68. Lusane, C. *Pipe Dream Blues: Racism & the War on Drugs.* South End Press, Boston, 1991.

69. Crosby, F. *Relative Deprivation and Working Women.* Oxford University Press, New York, 1982.

70. Fix, M., and Struyk, R. (eds.). *Clear and Convincing Evidence: Measurement of Discrimination in America.* Urban Institute Press, Washington, D.C., 1993.

71. Badgett, M. V. L. The wage effect of sexual orientation discrimination. *Ind. Labor Rel. Rev.* 48: 726–735, 1995.

72. National Conference of Christians and Jews. *Taking America's Pulse: A Summary of the National Conference Survey on Inter-Group Relations.* New York, 1994.

73. Herrnstein, R. J., and Murray, C. *The Bell Curve: Intelligence and Class Structure in American Life.* Free Press, New York, 1994.

74. Thernstrom, S., and Thernstrom, A. *America in Black and White: One Nation, Indivisible.* Simon & Schuster, New York, 1997.

75. Associated Press. Whites retain negative view of minorities, survey finds. *New York Times,* January 10, 1991, p. A15.

76. Lillie-Blanton, M., and LaVeist, T. Race/ethnicity, the social environment, and health. *Soc. Sci. Med.* 43: 83–92, 1996.

77. Syme, S. L., et al. Social class and racial differences in blood pressure. *Am. J. Public Health* 64: 619–620, 1974.

78. Wise, P. H., et al. Racial and socioeconomic disparities in childhood mortality in Boston. *N. Engl. J. Med.* 313: 360–366, 1985.

79. Kessler, R. C., and Neighbors, H. W. A new perspective on the relationships among race, social class, and psychological distress. *J. Health Soc. Behav.* 27: 107–115, 1986.

80. Bassett, M. T., and Krieger, N. Social class and black-white differences in breast cancer survival. *Am. J. Public Health* 76: 1400–1403, 1986.

81. Navarro, V. Race or class versus race and class: Mortality differentials in the United States. *Lancet* 2: 1238–1240, 1990.

82. McCord, C, and Freeman, H. P. Excess mortality in Harlem. *N. Engl. J. Med.* 322: 173–177, 1990.

83. Bacquet, C. R., et al. Socioeconomic factors and cancer incidence among blacks and whites. *J. Natnl. Cancer Inst.* 83: 551–557, 1991.

84. U.S. Department of Health and Human Services. *Health Status of Minorities and Low-Income Groups,* Ed. 3. U.S. Government Printing Office, Washington, D.C., 1991.

85. Geronimus, A. T., et al., Excess mortality among blacks and whites in the United States. *N. Engl. J. Med.* 335: 1552–1558, 1996.

86. Davey Smith, G., et al., Mortality differences between black and white men in the USA: Contribution of income and other risk factors among men screened for the MRFIT. *Lancet* 351: 934–939, 1998.

87. Mullings, L. Minority women, work, and health. In *Double Exposure: Women's Health Hazards on the Job and at Home,* edited by W. Chavkin, pp. 121–138. Monthly Review Press, New York, 1984.

88. Commission for Racial Justice. *Toxic Wastes and Race in the United States: A National Report on the Racial and Socio-Economic Characteristics of Communities with Hazardous Waste Sites.* United Church of Christ, New York, 1987.

89. Brown, P. Race, class, and environmental health: A review and systematization of the literature. *Environ. Res.* 69: 15–30, 1995.

90. Montgomery, L. E., and Carter-Pokras, O. Health status by social class and/or minority status: Implications for environmental equity research. *Toxicol. Ind. Health* 9: 729–773, 1993.

91. Northridge, M. E., and Shepard, P. M. Environmental racism and public health. *Am. J. Public Health* 87: 730–732, 1997.

92. Himmelstein, D. U., et al. Patient transfers: Medical practice as social triage. *Am. J. Public Health* 74: 494–497, 1984.

93. Council on Ethical and Judicial Affairs, American Medical Association. Black-white disparities in health care. *JAMA* 263: 2344–2346, 1990.

94. Giles, W. H., et al. Race and sex differences in rates of invasive cardiac procedures in US hospitals. Data from the National Hospital Discharge Survey. *Arch. Intern. Med.* 155: 318–324, 1995.

95. Ford, E. S., and Cooper, R. S. Racial/ethnic differences in health care utilization of cardiovascular procedures: A review of the evidence. *Health Serv. Res.* 30: 237–252, 1995.

96. Gornick, M. E., et al. Effects of race and income on mortality and use of services among Medicare beneficiaries. *N. Engl. J. Med.* 335: 791–799, 1996.

97. Peterson, E. D., et al. Racial variations in the use of coronary-revascularization procedures: Are the differences real? Do they matter? *N. Engl. J. Med.* 336: 480–486, 1997.

98. Smith, J. M. On the fourteenth query of Thomas Jefferson's notes on Virginia. *The Anglo-African Magazine* 1: 225–238, 1859.

99. Reyburn, R. Remarks concerning some of the diseases prevailing among the freedpeople in the District of Columbia (Bureau of Refugees, Freedman, and Abandoned Lands). *Am. J. Med. Sci.* n.s. 51: 364–369, 1866.

100. Levesque, G. A. Boston's Black Brahmin: Dr. John S. Rock. *Civil War Hist.* 54: 326–346, 1980.

101. Williams, D. R. Race/ethnicity and socioeconomic status: Measurement and methodological issues. *Int. J. Health Serv.* 26: 483–505, 1996.

102. Kaufman, J. S., Cooper, R. S., and McGee, D. L. Socioeconomic status and health in blacks and whites: The problem of residual confounding and the resiliency of race. *Epidemiology* 8: 621–628, 1997.

103. Williams, D. R. Race and health: Basic questions, emerging directions. *Ann. Epidemiol.* 7: 322–333, 1997.

104. Cooper, R. S., and David, R. The biological concept of race and its application to public health and epidemiology. *J. Health Polit. Policy Law* 11: 97–116, 1986.

105. Williams, D. R., Lavizzo-Mourey, R., and Warren, R. C. The concept of race and health status in America. *Public Health Rep.* 109: 26–41, 1994.

106. Institute of Medicine (U.S.), Committee to Study the Prevention of Low Birthweight. *Preventing Low Birthweight.* National Academy Press, Washington, D.C., 1985.

107. Rowley, D. L., et al. Preterm delivery among African-American women: A research strategy. *Am. J. Prev. Med.* 9(Suppl.): 1–6, 1993.

108. National Center for Health Statistics. *Health, United States 1996–97 and Injury Chartbook.* DHHS Pub. No. (PHS) 97-1232. U.S. Department of Health and Human Services, Hyattsville, Md., 1997.

109. Schoendorf, K. C., et al. Mortality among infants of black as compared with white college-educated parents. *N. Engl. J. Med.* 326: 1522–1526, 1992.

110. McGrady, G. A., et al. Preterm delivery and low birth weight among first-born infants of black and white college graduates. *Am. J. Epidemiol.* 136: 266–276, 1992.

111. McFarlane, M. J., Feinstein, A. R, and Wells, C. K. Necropsy evidence of detection bias in the diagnostic pursuit of lung cancer. *Am. J. Epidemiol.* 128: 1016–1026, 1988.

112. Council on Ethical and Judicial Affairs, American Medical Association. Gender disparities in clinical decision making. *JAMA* 266: 559–562, 1991.

113. Doyal, L. *The Political Economy of Health.* South End Press, Boston, 1979.

114. Townsend, P., Davidson, N., and Whitehead, M. *Inequalities in Health: The Black Report and the Health Divide.* Penguin, London, 1990.

115. Evans, R. G., Barer, M. L., and Marmor, T. R. (eds.). *Why Are Some People Healthy and Others Not? The Determinants of Health of Populations.* Aldine de Gruyter, New York, 1994.

116. Amick, B. C. III, et al. (eds.). *Society and Health.* Oxford University Press, New York, 1995.

117. Krieger, N., Williams, D. R., and Moss, N. E. Measuring social class in US public health research: Concepts, methodologies, and guidelines. *Annu. Rev. Public Health* 18: 341–378, 1997.

118. Krieger, N., and Fee, E. Measuring social inequalities in health in the United States: An historical review, 1900–1950. *Int. J. Health Serv.* 26: 391–418, 1996.

119. Liberatos, P., Link, B. G., and Kelsey, J. L. The measurement of social class in epidemiology. *Epidemiol. Rev.* 10: 87–121, 1988.

120. Dale, A., Gilbert, G. N., and Arber, S. Integrating women into class theory. *Sociology* 19: 384–409, 1985.

121. Arber, S. Revealing women's health: Re-analysing the General Household Survey. In *Women's Health Counts,* edited by H. Roberts, pp. 63–92. Routledge, London, 1990.

122. Krieger, N. Women and social class: A methodological study comparing individual, household, and census measures as predictors of black/white differences in reproductive history. *J. Epidemiol. Commun. Health* 45: 35–42, 1991.

123. Malaty, H. M., and Graham, D. Y. Importance of childhood socioeconomic status on the current prevalence of *Helicobacter pylori* infection. *Gut* 35: 742–745, 1994.

124. Boyle, E. Jr., et al. An epidemiologic study of hypertension among racial groups of Charleston County, South Carolina. The Charleston Heart Study, Phase II. In *The Epidemiology of Hypertension,* edited by J. Stamler, R. Stamler, and T. Pullman, pp. 193–203. Grune & Stratton, New York, 1967.

125. Boyle, E. Jr. Biological patterns in hypertension by race, sex, body weight, and skin color. *JAMA* 213: 1637–1643, 1970.

126. Harburg, E., et al. Socio-ecological stress, suppressed hostility, skin color, and black-white male blood pressure: Detroit. *Psychosom. Med.* 35: 276–295, 1973.

127. Keil, J. E., et al. Hypertension: Effects of social class and racial admixture: The results of a cohort study of the black population of Charleston, South Carolina. *Am. J. Public Health* 67: 634–639, 1977.

128. Harburg, E., et al. Skin color, ethnicity and blood pressure. I: Detroit blacks. *Am. J. Public Health* 68: 1177–1183, 1978.

129. Keil, J. E., et al. Skin color and education effects on blood pressure. *Am. J. Public Health* 71: 532–534, 1981.

130. Coresh, J., et al. Left ventricular hypertrophy and skin color among American blacks. *Am. J. Epidemiol.* 134: 129–136, 1991.

131. Nelson, D. A., Kleerekoper, M., and Parfitt, A. M. Bone mass, skin color and body size among black and white women. *Bone Mineral* 4: 257–264, 1988.

132. Garty, M., et al. Skin color, aging, and plasma L-dopa levels. *J. Auton. Nerv. Syst.* 26: 261–263, 1989.

133. Klag, M. J., et al. The association of skin color with blood pressure in US blacks with low socioeconomic status. *JAMA* 265: 599–602, 1991.

134. Dressler, W. W. Social class, skin color, and arterial blood pressure in two societies. *Ethn. Dis.* 1: 60–77, 1991.

135. Keil, J. E., et al. Skin color and mortality. *Am. J. Epidemiol.* 136: 1295–1302, 1992.

136. Nelson, D. A., et al. Skin color and body size as risk factors for osteoporosis. *Osteoporos. Int.* 3: 18–23, 1993.

137. Knapp, R. G., et al. Skin color and cancer mortality among black men in the Charleston Heart Study. *Clin. Genet.* 47: 200–206, 1995.

138. Gleiberman, L., et al. Skin color, measures of socioeconomic status, and blood pressure among blacks in Erie County, NY. *Ann. Hum. Biol.* 22: 69–73, 1995.

139. Schwam, B. L., et al. Association between skin color and intraocular pressure in African Americans. *J. Clin. Epidemiol.* 38: 491–496, 1995.

140. Churchill, J. E., et al. Skin Color, Blood Pressure and Body Mass in Young Adult Blacks: The CARDIA Study. Paper presented at the 11th International Interdisciplinary Conference on Hypertension in Blacks, New Orleans, July 14–17, 1996.

141. Krieger, N., Sidney, S., and Coakley, E. Racial discrimination and skin color in the CARDIA study: Implications for public health research. *Am. J. Public Health* **88**: 1308–1313, 1998.

142. Belethford, J. H., et al. Social class, admixture, and skin color variation in Mexican-Americans and Anglo-Americans living in San Antonio, Texas. *Am. J. Phys. Anthropol.* **61**: 97–102, 1983.

143. Hughes, M., and Hertel, B. R. The significance of color remains: A study of life chances, mate selection, and ethnic consciousness among black Americans. *Soc. Forces* **68**: 1105–1120, 1990.

144. Telles, E. E., and Murguia, E. Phenotypic discrimination and income differences among Mexican Americans. *Soc. Sci. Q.* **71**: 682–696, 1990.

145. Keith, V. M., and Herring, C. Skin tone and stratification in the black community. *Am. J. Sociol.* **97**: 760–778, 1991.

146. Russel, K., Wilson, M., and Hall, R. *The Color Complex: The Politics of Skin Color among African Americans.* Harcourt Brace Jovanovich, New York, 1992.

147. James, S. A., et al. John Henryism and blood pressure differences among black men. II. The role of occupational stressors. *J. Behav. Med.* **7**: 259–275, 1984.

148. Amaro, H., Russo, N. F., and Johnson, J. Family and work predictors of psychological well-being among Hispanic women professionals. *Psychol. Women Q.* **11**: 505–521, 1987.

149. Salgado de Snyder, V. N. Factors associated with acculturative stress and depressive symptomatology among married Mexican immigrant women. *Psychol. Women Q.* **11**: 475–488, 1987.

150. Krieger, N. Racial and gender discrimination: Risk factors for high blood pressure? *Soc. Sci. Med.* **30**: 1273–1281, 1990.

151. Dressler, W. W. Lifestyle, stress, and blood pressure in a southern black community. *Psychosom. Med.* **52**: 182–198, 1990.

152. Murrell, N. L. Stress, self-esteem, and racism: Relationships with low birth weight and preterm delivery in African American women. *J. Natnl. Black Nurses Assoc.* **8**: 45–53, 1996.

153. Krieger, N., and Sidney, S. Racial discrimination and blood pressure: The CARDIA study of young black and white adults. *Am. J. Public Health* **86**: 1370–1378, 1996.

154. Jackson, J. S., et al. Racism and the physical and mental health status of African Americans: A thirteen year national panel study. *Ethn. Dis.* **6**: 132–147, 1996.

155. Broman, C. L. The health consequences of discrimination: A study of African Americans. *Ethn. Dis.* **6**: 148–152, 1996.

156. Ladrine, H., and Klonoff, E. A. The schedule of racist events: A measure of racial discrimination and study of its negative physical and mental health consequences. *J. Black Psychol.* **22**: 144–168, 1996.

157. Mays, V. M., and Cochran, S. D. Racial Discrimination and Health Outcomes in African Americans. Paper presented at the National Center for Health Statistics 1997 Joint Meeting of the Public Health Conference on Records and Statistics and the Data Users Conference, Washington, D.C., July 28–31, 1997.

158. Auslander, W. F., et al. Mothers' satisfaction with medical care: Perceptions of racism, family stress, and medical outcomes in children with diabetes. *Health Soc. Work* **22**: 190–199, 1997.

159. Williams, D. R., and Chung, A.-M. Racism and health. In *Health in Black America,* edited by R. C. Gibston and J. S. Jackson. Sage, Thousand Oaks, Calif., 1999, in press.

160. Williams, D. R., et al. Racial differences in physical and mental health: Socioeconomic status, stress, and discrimination. *J. Health Psychol.* 2: 335–351, 1997.

161. Ladrine, H., et al. Physical and psychiatric correlates of gender discrimination: An application of the schedule of sexist events. *Psychol. Women Q.* 19: 473–492, 1995.

162. Bradford, J., Ryan, C., and Rothblum, E. D. National lesbian health care survey: Implications for mental health care. *J. Consult. Clin. Psychol.* 62: 228–242, 1994.

163. Meyer, I. H. Minority stress and mental health in gay men. *J. Health Soc. Behav.* 36: 38–56, 1995.

164. Krieger, N., and Sidney, S. Prevalence and health implications of anti-gay discrimination: A study of black and white women and men in the CARDIA cohort. *Int. J. Health Serv.* 27: 157–176, 1997.

165. Barbarin, O. A., and Gilbert, R. Institutional racism scale: Assessing self and organizational attributes. In *Institutional Racism and Community Competence,* edited by O. A. Barbarin et al., pp. 147–171. NIMH DHHS Pub. No. (AMD) 81-907. U.S. Government Printing Office, Washington, D.C., 1981.

166. Mays, V. M., Cochran, S. D., and Rhue, S. The impact of perceived discrimination on the intimate relationships of black lesbians. *J. Homosex.* 25: 1–14, 1993.

167. Mays, V. M. Black women, women, stress, and perceived discrimination: The focused support group model as an intervention for stress reduction. *Cult. Diversity Ment. Health* 1: 53–65, 1995.

168. Bobo, L., et al. Work orientation, job discrimination, and ethnicity: A focus group perspective. *Res. Soc. Work* 5: 45–85, 1995.

169. Parker, H., Botha, J. L., and Haslam, C. "Racism" as a variable in health research—Can it be measured? (abstract). *J. Epidemiol. Commun. Health* 48: 522, 1995.

170. Amaro, H. Love, sex, and power. *Am. Psychol.* 50: 437–447, 1995.

171. Krieger, N. Exposure, susceptibility, and breast cancer risk: A hypothesis regarding exogenous carcinogens, breast tissue development, and social gradients, including black/white differences, in breast cancer incidence. *Breast Cancer Res. Treat.* 13: 205–223, 1989.

172. Campbell, A., and Schuman, H. *Racial Attitudes in Fifteen American Cities.* Survey Research Center, Institute for Social Research, University of Michigan, Ann Arbor, 1968.

173. United States, Kerner Commission. *Report of the National Advisory Commission on Civil Disorders.* Bantam Books, New York, 1968.

174. Sigelman, L., and Welch, S. *Black American's Views of Racial Inequality: The Dream Deferred.* Cambridge University Press, Cambridge, England, 1991.

175. Taylor, D. M., Wright, S. C., and Porter, L. E. Dimensions of perceived discrimination: The personal/group discrimination discrepancy. In *The Psychology of Prejudice: The Ontario Symposium,* Vol. 7, edited by M. P. Zanna and J. M. Olson, pp. 233–255. Erlbaum, Hillsdale, N.J., 1994.

176. Mays, V. M., Coleman, L. M., and Jackson, J. S. Perceived race-based discrimination, employment status, and job stress in a national sample of black women: Implications for health outcomes. *J. Occup. Health Psychol.* 1: 319–329, 1996.

177. Women's Bureau. *Working Women Count: A Report to the Nation.* U.S. Department of Labor, Washington, D.C., 1994.

178. Birt, C. M., and Dion, K. L. Relative deprivation theory and responses to discrimination in a gay male and lesbian sample. *Br. J. Soc. Psychol.* 26: 139–145, 1987.

179. Herek, G. M. Documenting prejudice against lesbians and gay men on campus: The Yale Sexual Orientation Survey. *J. Homosex.* 25: 15–30, 1993.

180. Schatz, B., and O'Hanlan, K. *Anti-Gay Discrimination in Medicine: Results of a National Survey of Lesbian, Gay, and Bisexual Physicians.* American Association of Physicians for Human Rights, San Francisco, 1994.

181. Harburg, E., Blakelock, E. H. Jr., and Roeper, P. J. Resentful and reflective coping with arbitrary authority and blood pressure: Detroit. *Psychosom. Med.* 3: 189–202, 1979.

182. Foster, M. D., Matheson, K., and Poole, M. Responding to sexual discrimination: The effects of societal versus self-blame. *J. Soc. Psychol.* 134: 743–754, 1994.

183. Lalonde, R. N., and Cameron, J. E. Behavioral responses to discrimination: A focus on action. In *The Psychology of Prejudice: The Ontario Symposium, Vol. 7,* edited by M. P. Zanna and J. M. Olson, pp. 257–288. Lawrence Erlbaum, Hillsdale, N.J., 1994.

184. Ruggerio, K. M., and Taylor, D. M. Coping with discrimination: How disadvantaged group members perceive the discrimination that confronts them. *J. Pers. Soc. Psychol.* 68: 826–838, 1995.

185. Cochran, S. D., and Mays, V. M. Levels of depression in homosexually active African-American men and women. *Am. J. Psychol.* 151: 524–529, 1994.

186. Cohen, S., Kessler, R. C., and Gordon, L. U. (eds.). *Measuring Stress: A Guide for Health and Social Scientists.* Oxford University Press, New York, 1995.

187. Crosby, F. The denial of personal discrimination. *Am. Behav. Sci.* 27: 371–386, 1984.

188. Taylor, D. M., et al. The personal/group discrepancy: Perceiving my group, but not myself, to be a target of discrimination. *Pers. Soc. Psychol. Bull.* 16: 254–262, 1990.

189. Dion, K. L., and Kawakami, K. Ethnicity and perceived discrimination in Toronto: Another look at the personal/group discrimination discrepancy. *Can. J. Behav. Sci.* 28: 203–213, 1996.

190. Kelsey, J. L., Thompson, W. D., and Evans, A. S. *Methods in Observational Epidemiology,* Ed. 2. Oxford University Press, New York, 1996.

191. Fanon, F. *The Wretched of the Earth,* translated by Constance Farrington. Grove Press, New York, 1965.

192. Gurin, P. Women's gender consciousness. *Public Opinion Q.* 49: 143–163, 1985.

193. Ross, C. E., and Mirowsky, J. Explaining the social patterns of depression: Control and problem solving—or support and talking? *J. Health Soc. Behav.* 30: 206–219, 1989.

194. Neighbors, H. W., et al. Racism and the mental health of African Americans: The role of self and system blame. *Ethn. Dis.* 6: 167–175, 1996.

195. Cutter, G. R., et al. Cardiovascular risk factors in young adults: The CARDIA baseline monograph. *Control. Clin. Trials* 12: 1S–77S, 1991.

196. Armstead, C. A., et al. Relationship of racial stressors to blood pressure responses and anger expression in black college students. *Health Psychol.* 8: 541–556, 1989.

197. Jones, D. R., et al. Affective and physiological responses to racism: The roles of afrocentrism and mode of presentation. *Ethn. Dis.* 6: 109–122, 1996.

198. Morris-Prather, C. E., et al. Gender differences in mood and cardiovascular responses to socially stressful stimuli. *Ethn. Dis.* 6: 123–131, 1996.

199. Bobo, L., and Gilliam, F. D. Race, sociopolitical participation and black empowerment. *Am. Polit. Sci. Rev.* 84: 377–393, 1990.

200. Waters, M. C. Ethnic and racial identities of second-generation black immigrants in New York City. *Int. Migration Rev.* 28: 795–820, 1995.

201. Waters, M. C., and Eschbach, K. Immigration and ethnic and racial inequality in the United States. *Annu. Rev. Sociol.* 21: 419–446, 1995.

202. Hughes, M., and Demo, D. H. Self-perceptions of Black Americans: Self-esteem and personal efficacy. *Am. J. Sociol.* 95: 132–159, 1989.

203. Potter, L. Socioeconomic determinants of white and black males' life expectancy differentials, 1980. *Demography* 28: 303–321, 1991.

204. LaVeist, T. A. The political empowerment and health status of African-Americans: Mapping a new territory. *Am. J. Sociol.* 97: 1080–1095, 1992.

205. LaVeist, T. A. Segregation, poverty, and empowerment: Health consequences for African Americans. *Milbank Q.* 71: 41–64, 1993.

206. Wallace, R., and Wallace, D. US apartheid and the spread of AIDS to the suburbs: A multi-city analysis of the political economy of spatial epidemic thresholds. *Soc. Sci. Med.* 41: 333–345, 1995.

207. Polednak, A. P. *Segregation, Poverty, and Mortality in Urban African Americans.* Oxford University Press, New York, 1997.

208. Collins, C. A. Residential Segregation, Poverty, and Mortality. Paper presented at the National Center for Health Statistics 1997 Joint Meeting of the Public Health Conference on Records and Statistics and the Data Users Conference, Washington, D.C., July 28–31, 1997.

209. Kennedy, B. P., et al. (Dis)respect and black mortality. *Ethn. Dis.* 7: 207–214, 1997.

210. Duncan, O. D., and Duncan, B. A methodological analysis of segregation indexes. *Am. Sociol. Rev.* 20: 210–217, 1955.

211. White, M. J. The measurement of spatial segregation. *Am. J. Sociol.* 88: 1008–1018, 1983.

212. White, M. J. Segregation and diversity measures of population distributions. *Popul. Index* 52: 198–221, 1986.

213. Wilkinson, R. G. *Unhealthy Societies: From Inequality to Well-Being.* Routledge, London, 1996.

214. Kennedy, B. P., Kawachi, I., and Prothrow-Smith, D. Income distribution and mortality: Cross sectional ecological study of the Robin Hood index in the United States. *BMJ* 312: 1004–1007, 1996.

215. Kaplan, G. A., et al. Inequality in income and mortality in the United States: Analysis of mortality and potential pathways. *BMJ* 312: 999–1003, 1996.

216. Kawachi, I., and Kennedy, B. P. Health and social cohesion: Why care about income inequality? *BMJ* 314: 1037–1040, 1997.

217. Wallace, R., and Wallace, D. Community marginalisation and the diffusion of disease and disorder in the United States. *BMJ* 314: 1341–1345, 1997.

218. United Nations Development Programme. *Human Development Report 1996.* Oxford University Press, New York, 1996.
219. Jargowsky, P. A. Take the money and run: Economic segregation in US metropolitan areas. *Am. Sociol. Rev.* 61: 984–998, 1996.
220. Massey, D. S. The age of extremes: Concentrated affluence and poverty in the twenty-first century. *Demography* 33: 395–412, 1996.
221. Dill, B. T., Cannon, L. W., and Vanneman, R. Race and gender in occupational segregation. In *Pay Equity: An Issue of Race, Ethnicity, and Sex,* pp. 9–70. National Committee on Pay Equity, Washington, D.C., 1987.
222. Mann, J. M. Health and human rights. *BMJ* 312: 924–925, 1996.
223. Davey Smith, G. Income inequality and mortality: Why are they related? *BMJ* 312: 987–988, 1996.
224. Robinson, W. S. Ecological correlations and the behavior of individuals. *Am. Sociol. Rev.* 15: 351–357, 1950.
225. Alker, H. R., Jr. A typology of ecological fallacies. In *Social Ecology,* edited by M. Doggan and S. Rokkan, pp. 69–86. MIT Press, Cambridge, Mass., 1969.
226. Susser, M. The logic in ecological: I. The logic of analysis. *Am. J. Public Health* 84: 825–829, 1994.
227. Susser, M. The logic in ecological: II. The logic of design. *Am. J. Public Health* 84: 830–835, 1994.
228. Diez-Roux, A. V. Bringing context back into epidemiology: Variables and fallacies in multilevel analysis. *Am. J. Public Health* 88: 216–222, 1998.
229. Langbein, L. I., and Lichtman, A. J. *Ecological Inference.* Sage University Series on Quantitative Applications in the Social Sciences. Sage, Beverly Hills, Calif., 1978.
230. Hummer, R. A. Black-white differences in health and mortality: A review and conceptual model. *Sociol. Q.* 37: 105–125, 1996.
231. Blalock, H. M. Jr. Contextual-effects models: Theoretic and methodologic issues. *Annu. Rev. Sociol.*. 10: 353–372, 1984.
232. Bryk, A. S., and Raudenbush, S. W. *Hierarchical Linear Models: Applications and Data Analysis Methods.* Sage, Newbury Park, Calif, 1992.
233. DiPriete, T. A., and Forristal, J. D. Multilevel models: Methods and substance. *Annu. Rev. Sociol.* 20: 331–357, 1994.
234. Iverson, G. *Contextual Analysis.* Sage, Newbury Park, Calif., 1991.
235. Haan, M., Kaplan, G. A., and Camacho, T. Poverty and health: Prospective evidence from the Alameda County Study. *Am. J. Epidemiol.* 125: 989–998, 1987.
236. Krieger, N. Overcoming the absence of socioeconomic data in medical records: Validation and application of a census-based methodology. *Am. J. Public Health* 82: 703–710, 1992.
237. Duncan, G., Brooks-Gunn, J., and Klebanov, P. Economic deprivation and early-childhood development. *Child Dev.* 65: 296–318, 1994.
238. O'Campo, P., et al. Violence by male partners against women during the childbearing year: A contextual analysis. *Am. J. Public Health* 85: 1092–1097, 1995.
239. Diez-Roux, A. V., et al. Neighborhood environments and coronary heart disease: A multilevel analysis. *Am. J. Epidemiol.* 146: 48–63, 1997.
240. Lowe, M. Social bodies: The interaction of culture and women's biology. In *Biological Woman—The Convenient Myth,* edited by R. Hubbard, M. S. Henefin, and B. Fried, pp. 91–116. Schenkman, Cambridge, Mass., 1982.

241. Krieger, N. Racial discrimination and health: An epidemiologist's perspective. In *Report of the President's Cancer Panel. The Meaning of Race in Science— Considerations for Cancer Research (April 9, 1997),* pp. A32–A35. National Institutes of Health, National Cancer Institute, Bethesda, Md., 1998.

242. Scott, J. A. Keeping women in their place: Exclusionary politics and reproduction. In *Women's Health Hazards on the job and at Home,* edited by W. Chavkin, pp. 180–195. Monthly Review Press, New York, 1984.

243. King, J. D. *The Biology of Race.* University of California Press, Berkeley, 1981.

244. Gould, S. J. *The Mismeasure of Man.* W. W. Norton, New York, 1981.

245. Lewontin, R. *Human Diversity.* Scientific American Books, New York, 1982.

246. Krieger, N., and Bassett, M. The health of black folk: Disease, class, and ideology in science. *Monthly Rev..* 38: 74–85, 1986.

247. Cavalli-Sforza, L. L., Menozzi, P., and Piazza, A. *The History and Geography of Human Genes.* Princeton University Press, Princeton, N.J., 1996.

248. Brunner, E. Stress and the biology of inequality. *BMJ* 314: 1472–1476, 1997.

249. Breilh, J. *Epidemiologia Economia Medicina y Politica.* Distribuciones Fontamara, Mexico City, 1979.

250. MacIntyre, S. The patterning of health by social position in contemporary Britain: Directions for sociological research. *Soc. Sci. Med.* 23: 393–415, 1986.

251. Laurell, A. C. Social analysis of collective health in Latin America. *Soc. Sci. Med.* 28: 1183–1191, 1989.

252. Geronimus, A. T. The weathering hypothesis and the health of African American women and infants. *Ethn. Dis.* 2: 207–221, 1992.

253. Doyal, L. *What Makes Women Sick? Gender and the Political Economy of Health.* Rutgers University Press, New Brunswick, N.J., 1995.

254. Cooper, R., et al. Improved mortality among U.S. Blacks, 1968–1978: The role of antiracist struggle. *Int. J. Health Serv.* 11: 511–522, 1981.

255. Friedman, S. R., et al. The AIDS epidemic among Blacks and Hispanics. *Milbank Q.* 65: 455–499, 1987.

256. Anderson, N. B., et al. Hypertension in blacks: Psychosocial and biological perspectives. *J. Hypertens.* 7: 161–172, 1989.

257. Troutt, D. D. *The Thin Red Line: How the Poor Still Pay More.* West Coast Regional Office of Consumers Union, Oakland, Calif., 1993.

258. Fray, J. C. S., and Douglas, J. G. (eds.) *Pathophysiology of Hypertension in Blacks.* Oxford University Press, New York, 1993.

259. Khaw, K. T. Sodium and potassium: Blood pressure and stroke. In *Cardiovascular Disease: Risk Factors and Intervention,* edited by N. Poulter, P. Sever, and S. Thom, pp. 145–151. Radcliffe Medical Press, Oxford, England, 1993.

260. Kuh, D., and Davey Smith, G. The life course and adult chronic disease: An historical perspective with particular reference to coronary heart disease. In *A Lifecourse Approach to Chronic Disease Epidemiology: Tracing the Origins of Ill-Health from Early to Adult Life,* edited by D. Kuh and Y. Ben-Shlomo, pp. 15–41. Oxford University Press, Oxford, England, 1997.

261. Sorel, J. E., et al. Black-white differences in blood pressure among participants in NHANES II: The contribution of blood lead. *Epidemiology* 2: 348–352, 1991.

262. Hu, H., et al. The relationship of bone and blood lead to hypertension. The Normative Aging Study. *JAMA* 275: 1171–1176, 1996.

263. Lanphear, B. P., Weitzman, M., and Eberly, S. Racial differences in urban children's environmental exposures to lead. *Am. J. Public Health* 86: 1460–1463, 1996.

264. Brody, D. J., et al. Blood lead levels in the US population. Phase I of the Third National Health and Nutrition Examination Survey (NHANES III, 1988 to 1991). *JAMA* 272: 277–283, 1994.

265. Gentry, W. D. Relationship of anger-coping styles and blood pressure among Black Americans. In *Anger and Hostility in Cardiovascular and Behavioral Disorder,* edited by M. A. Chesney and R. H. Rosenman, pp. 139–147. Hemisphere, Washington, D.C., 1985.

266. Johnson, E. H., and Broman, C. L. The relationship of anger expression to health problems among Black Americans in a national survey. *J. Behav. Med.* 10: 103–116, 1987.

267. McEwen, B. S. Protective and damaging effects of stress mediators. *N. Engl. J. Med.* 338: 171–179, 1998.

268. Beverly, C. C. Alcoholism and the African-American community. In *Health Issues in the Black Community,* edited by R. L. Braithwaite and S. E. Taylor, pp. 79–89. Jossey-Bass, San Francisco, 1992.

269. Taylor, J., and Jackson, B. Factors affecting alcohol consumption in black women, Part II. *Int. J. Addictions* 25: 1415–1427, 1992.

270. Moore, D. J., Williams, J. D., and Qualls, W. J. Target marketing of tobacco and alcohol-related products to ethnic minority groups in the United States. *Ethn. Dis.* 6: 83–98, 1996.

271. Burt, V. L., et al. Prevalence of hypertension in the US adult population. Results from the Third National Health and Nutrition Examination Survey, 1988–1991. *Hypertension* 25: 305–313, 1995.

272. Svetkey, L. P., et al. Effects of gender and ethnic group on blood pressure control in the elderly. *Am. J. Hypertens.* 9: 529–535, 1996.

273. Ahluwalia, J. S., McNagny, S. E., and Rask, K. J. Correlates of controlled hypertension in indigent, inner-city hypertensive patients. *J. Gen. Intern. Med.* 12: 7–14, 1997.

274. Fleck, L. *Genesis and Development of a Scientific Fact.* University of Chicago University Press, Chicago, 1979 [1935].

275. Rosen, G. *A History of Public Health,* Expanded edition. Introduction by E. Fee; bibliographical essay and new bibliography by E. T. Morman. Johns Hopkins University Press, Baltimore, Md., 1993 [1958].

276. Haller, J. S. Jr. *Outcasts from Evolution: Scientific Attitudes of Racial Inferiority, 1859–1900.* University of Illinois Press, Urbana, 1971.

277. Rose, H., and Rose, S. (eds.). *Ideology of/in the Natural Sciences.* Schenkman, Cambridge, Mass., 1979.

278. Fee, E. *Disease and Discovery: A History of the Johns Hopkins School of Hygiene and Public Health, 1916–1936.* Johns Hopkins University Press, Baltimore, Md., 1987.

279. Ziman, J. *Reliable Knowledge: An Exploration of the Grounds for Belief in Science.* Cambridge University Press, Cambridge, England, 1987.

280. Tesh, S. *Hidden Arguments: Political Ideology and Disease Prevention Policy.* Rutgers University Press, New Brunswick, N.J., 1988.

281. Haraway, D. *Primate Visions: Gender, Race, and Nature in the World of Modern Science.* Routledge, New York, 1989.

282. Rosenberg, C. D., and Golden, J. (eds.). *Framing Disease: Studies in Cultural History.* Rutgers University Press, New Brunswick, N.J., 1992.

283. Keller, E. F., and Longino, H. E. (eds.). *Feminism and Science.* Oxford University Press, Oxford, England, 1996.

284. Porter, R. *The Greatest Benefit to Mankind: A Medical History of Humanity.* W. W. Norton, New York, 1998.

285. Krieger, N. The making of public health data: Paradigms, politics, and policy. *J. Public Health Policy* 13: 412–427, 1992.

286. Jones, J. H. *Bad Blood: The Tuskegee Syphilis Experiment.* Free Press, New York, 1981.

287. Brandt, A. M. *No Magic Bullet: A Social History of Venereal Disease in the United States since 1880.* Oxford University Press, New York, 1985.

288. Navarro, V. *Crisis, Health, and Medicine: A Social Critique.* Tavistock, New York, 1986.

289. Gamble, V. N. (ed.). *Germs Have No Color Lines: Blacks and American Medicine, 1900–1940.* Garland, New York, 1989.

290. Hubbard, R. *The Politics of Women's Biology.* Rutgers University Press, New Brunswick, N.J., 1990.

291. Leslie, C. Scientific racism: Reflections on peer review, science, and ideology. *Soc. Sci. Med.* 32: 891–905, 1990.

292. Thomas, S. B., and Quinn, S. C. The Tuskegee Syphilis Study, 1932 to 1972: Implications for HIV education and AIDS risk education programs in the black community. *Am. J. Public Health* 81: 1498–1505, 1991.

293. Harding, S. (ed.). *The "Racial" Economy of Science: Toward a Democratic Future.* Indiana University Press, Bloomington, 1993.

294. Fee, E., and Krieger, N. (eds.). *Women's Health, Politics, and Power: Essays on Sex/Gender, Medicine, and Public Health.* Baywood, Amityville, N.Y., 1994.

295. Krieger, N., and Fee, E. Man-made medicine and women's health: The biopolitics of sex/gender and race/ethnicity. *Int. J. Health Serv.* 24: 265–283, 1994.

296. Epstein, S. *Impure Science: AIDS, Activism, and the Politics of Knowledge.* University of California Press, Berkeley, 1996.

297. Gill, C. J. Cultivating common ground: Women with disabilities. In *Man-Made Medicine: Women's Health, Public Policy, and Reform,* edited by K. L. Moss, pp. 183–193. Duke University Press, Durham, N.C., 1996.

298. Muntaner, C., Nieto, F. J., and O'Campo, P. The Bell Curve: On race, social class, and epidemiological research. *Am. J. Epidemiol.* 144: 531–536, 1996.

299. Moss, K. L. (ed.). *Man-Made Medicine: Women's Health, Public Policy, and Reform.* Duke University Press, Durham, N.C., 1996.

300. Council on Scientific Affairs, American Medical Association. Health care needs of gay men and lesbians in the United States. *JAMA* 275: 1354–1359, 1996.

301. Mendelsohn, K. D., et al. Sex and gender bias in anatomy and physical diagnosis text illustrations. *JAMA* 272: 1267–1270, 1994.

302. Zane, N. W. S., Takeuchi, D. T., and Young, K. N. S. *Confronting Critical Health Issues of Asian and Pacific Islander Americans.* Sage, Thousand Oaks, Calif., 1994.

303. Ruiz, M. T., and Verbrugge, L. M. A two way view of gender bias in medicine. *J. Epidemiol. Commun. Health* 51: 106–109, 1997.

304. Sydenstricker, E. *Health and Environment.* McGraw Hill, New York, 1933.

305. Kevles, D. J. *In the Name of Eugenics: Genetics and the Uses of Human Heredity.* Knopf, New York, 1985.
306. Apple, R. D. (ed.). *Women, Health & Medicine in America: A Historical Handbook.* Rutgers University Press, New Brunswick, N.J., 1992.
307. Weeks, J. *Sex, Politics, and Society: The Regulation of Sexuality Since 1800.* Longman, New York, 1981.
308. Erwin, K. Interpreting the evidence: Competing paradigms and the emergence of lesbian and gay suicide as a "social fact." *Int. J. Health Serv.* 23: 437–453, 1993.
309. Baker, J. A. Is homophobia hazardous to lesbian and gay health? *AFB Practitioners' Forum,* 7: 255–262, 1993.
310. Stanton, W. *The Leopard's Spots: Scientific Attitudes Towards race in America, 1815–1859.* University of Chicago Press, Chicago, 1960.
311. Banton, M. P. *Racial Theories.* Cambridge University Press, Cambridge, England, 1987.
312. Davis, F. *Who is Black?: One Nation's Definition.* Pennsylvania State University Press, University Park, 1991.
313. Jarvis, E. Insanity among the coloured population of the free states. *Am. J. Med. Sci.* 7: 71–83, 1844.
314. Deutsch, A. The first U.S. census of the insane (1840) and its use as pro-slavery propaganda. *Bull. Hist. Med.* 15: 469–482, 1944.
315. Grob, G. Edward Jarvis and the federal census. *Bull. Hist. Med.* 40: 4–27, 1976.
316. Haller, J. S. Jr. The physician versus the Negro: Medical and anthropological concepts of race in the late nineteenth century. *Bull. Hist. Med.* 44: 154–167, 1970.
317. Cartwright, S. A. The diseases and physical peculiarities of the Negro race. *New Orleans Med. Surg. J.* 7: 691–715, 1850.
318. Nott, J. C., and Gliddon, G. (eds.). *Indigenous Races of the Earth; or New Chapters of Ethnological Enquiry.* J. B. Lippincott, Philadelphia, 1857.
319. Proctor, R. *Racial Hygiene: Medicine under the Nazis.* Harvard University Press, Cambridge, Mass., 1988.
320. Montagu, A. *Statement on Race; An Extended Discussion in Plain Language of the UNESCO Statement by Experts on Race Problems.* Schuman, New York, 1951.
321. Kupper, L. (ed.). *Race, Science, and Society.* UNESCO Press, Paris, 1975.
322. Katz, S. The biological anthropology of race. In *Report of the President's Cancer Panel. The Meaning of Race in Science—Considerations for Cancer Research (April 9, 1997),* pp. A32–A35. National Institutes of Health, National Cancer Institute, Bethesda, Md., 1998.
323. Last, J. M. (ed.). *A Dictionary of Epidemiology,* Ed. 3. Oxford University Press, New York, 1995.
324. David, R., and Collins, J. Bad outcomes in black babies: Race or racism? *Ethn. Dis.* 1: 236–244, 1991.
325. Jones, C. P., LaVeist, T. A., and Lillie-Blanton, M. Race in the epidemiologic literature: An examination of the American Journal of Epidemiology, 1921–1990. *Am. J. Epidemiol.* 134: 1079–1084, 1991.
326. Ahmad, W. I. U. (ed.). *"Race" and Health in Contemporary Britain.* Open University Press, Buckingham, U.K., 1993.
327. James, S. A. John Henryism and the health of African-Americans. *Cult. Med. Psychiatry* 18: 163–182, 1994.

328. Smaje, C. The ethnic patterning of health: New directions for theory and research. *Sociol. Health Illness* 18: 139–171, 1996.

329. LaVeist, T. A. Why we should continue to study race . . . but do a better job: An essay on race, racism, and health. *Ethn. Dis.* 6: 21–29, 1996.

330. Freeman, H. P. The meaning of race in science—considerations for cancer research: Concerns of special populations in the National Cancer Program. *Cancer* 82: 219–225, 1988.

331. Report of the President's Cancer Panel. *The Meaning of Race in Science—Considerations for Cancer Research (April 9, 1997).* National Institutes of Health, National Cancer Institute, Bethesda, Md., 1998.

332. Bachman, R., and Saltzman, L. E. *Violence against Women: Estimates from the Redesigned Survey.* NCJ-154348. U.S. Department of Justice, Washington, D.C., 1995.

333. Cosentino, C. E., and Collins, M. Sexual abuse of children: Prevalence, effects, and treatment. *Ann. N.Y. Acad. Sci.* 789: 45–65, 1996.

334. Foner, E. *Reconstruction: America's Unfinished Revolution, 1863–1877.* Harper & Row, New York, 1988.

335. Indian Health Services. *Trends in Indian Health—1996.* U.S. Department of Health and Human Services, Rockville, Md., 1997.

336. U.S. Department of Commerce. *Household Wealth and Asset Ownership: 1991.* Current Population Reports, Ser. P70, No. 34. U.S. Bureau of the Census, Washington, D.C., 1994.

337. Green, N. L. Development of a Perceptions of Racism Scale. *Image J. Nurs. Sch.* 27: 141–146, 1995.

338. Klonoff, E. A., and Landrine, H. The schedule of sexist events: A measure of lifetime and recent sexist discrimination in women's lives. *Psychol. Women Q.* 19: 439–472, 1995.

CHAPTER 5

Race/Ethnicity and Socioeconomic Status:
Measurement and Methodological Issues

David R. Williams

Race has long been a major basis of social stratification in the United States. American society early developed a racial hierarchy in which Indians were below whites and blacks were below everyone else (1). Article One of the U.S. Constitution reflected this ideology when it mandated that population censuses, for purposes of taxation and political representation, should count black slaves as three-fifths of a person and not enumerate Indians who did not pay taxes (2).

The United States has had a long-standing interest in evaluating a broad range of societal outcomes, including health, on the basis of race. Nineteenth century medical researchers developed a large body of research on racial differences in health. These early studies were used to buttress existing ideologies of racial inferiority and justify the economic exploitation of blacks (3). Current efforts to monitor the socioeconomic progress and well-being of groups within the United States continue to collect and report information on racial and ethnic groups. Unlike most industrialized countries, the United States does not routinely report health status variations on the basis of social class, but focuses instead on racial differences (4).

This chapter reviews current measurement and methodological issues in the study of racial differences in health in the United States. A brief overview of the magnitude of racial variations in health is followed by a review of current problems with racial data and a discussion of the critical role of socioeconomic status (SES) in understanding these disparities.

Table 1 provides recent health data by race for two frequently used indicators of health status (5). Statistical Directive No. 15 of the federal government's Office of Management and Budget (OMB) requires federal agencies in the United States

Preparation of this chapter was supported by grant AG-07904 from the National Institute on Aging.

Table 1

Infant mortality rates and age-adjusted death rates for all causes
by race/ethnicity, United States[a]

	Infant deaths per 1000 live births, 1986–88	Deaths for all causes per 100,000 population, 1992	
		Males	Females
All	9.8	656.0	381.2
White	8.2	620.9	359.9
Black	17.9	1,026.9	568.4
Asian and Pacific Islander	7.3	364.1	220.5
Chinese	5.8		
Japanese	6.9		
Filipino	6.9		
Hawaiian and part Hawaiian	11.1		
Other APIA	7.6		
American Indian and Alaskan Native	13.2	579.6	343.1
Hispanic	8.3	506.1	268.6
Mexican American	7.9		
Puerto Rican	11.1		
Cuban	7.3		
Central and South American	7.6		
Other Hispanic	9.0		

[a]Source: reference 5.

to report statistics for four racial groups (American Indian and Alaskan Native, Asian and Pacific Islander, black, and white) and one ethnic category (Hispanic origin) (6). Infant mortality rates and age-adjusted death rates for all causes are presented for these five subgroups of the population (Table 1). These data reveal that blacks have rates of death that are dramatically higher than those of whites. All of the other racial groups have death rates from all causes that are lower than those of whites, and all but the American Indian population have lower rates of infant mortality than whites.

These overall rates obscure the considerable heterogeneity within each of the racial categories. The data on infant deaths provide detail for subgroups of the Hispanic (or Latino) and the Asian and Pacific Islander American (APIA) populations. In contrast to the overall rate of 7.3 per 1000 live births for the APIA category, the infant mortality rates range from 5.8 for Chinese Americans to 11.1 for Hawaiians. Similarly, the rates for Hispanics range from 7.3 for Cubans to

11.1 for Puerto Ricans. Additional data on death rates reveal that for some causes of death, such as tuberculosis, septicemia, cirrhosis of the liver, diabetes, and homicide, Hispanics have death rates that are higher than those of non-Hispanic whites (7, 8). In addition, Hispanics have rates of infectious diseases such as measles, rubella, tetanus, tuberculosis, syphilis, and AIDS that are considerably higher than in the general population. Rates of chronic conditions such as obesity and glucose intolerance are also elevated for Hispanics.

The American Indian (or Native American) population is also characterized by considerable diversity. There are more than 500 federally recognized tribes and entities. The low overall mortality rate for American Indians seen in Table 1 must be considered in the context of higher than average age-specific death rates so that the low rate reflects in part the young age distribution of American Indians (9). Death rates for American Indians also vary considerably from state to state, with rates being higher in states that have a larger concentration of Indians. The Indian Health Service is a federal agency that is responsible for providing medical services to American Indians who live on or near reservations. It estimates that it serves about 60 percent of the American Indian population. The Indian Health Service indicates that age-adjusted mortality rates for Native Americans in its service area are higher than the national average for several causes of death (10). These include tuberculosis (520 percent higher), alcoholism (433 percent higher), diabetes (188 percent higher), accidents (166 percent higher), homicides (71 percent higher), suicides (54 percent higher), and pneumonia and influenza (44 percent higher). Moreover, considerable tribal-specific variation often exists within a specific state. For example, within the state of New Mexico there are large tribal differences in prenatal care, low birth weight, and infant mortality (11).

Although the APIA population in the United States is geographically concentrated, with almost 80 percent of all APIAs residing in only 10 states, the APIA category lumps together persons from 28 Asian countries and 25 Pacific Island cultures (12). Each of these subgroups has its own distinctive history, culture, and language. Not surprisingly, an overall value on a health status indicator for the APIA population hides the considerable heterogeneity that exists for subgroups within that population. For example, the APIA population in California has a death rate due to homicide and legal intervention for 15- to 24-year-olds that is 17 per 100,000, but the rates range from 6 for Chinese Americans and 13 for Japanese Americans, to 54 for Samoans and 73 for the other Pacific Islander category (13). Similarly, although the APIA population has the lowest death rates of any racial group in the United States (Table 1), Native Hawaiians have the highest death rate due to heart disease of any racial group in the United States (14), and the rate of liver cancer for Chinese Americans is four times higher than that of the white population (12). Researchers have also given inadequate attention to the variations within both the black and white populations. The black population is characterized by cultural and ethnic heterogeneity that is predictive of variations in health status (15).

THE QUALITY OF RACIAL DATA

Health researchers routinely use race in an uncritical manner and give scant attention to the underlying problems of measurement that exist for the current racial categories (16–20). These problems importantly affect the quality of even the information presented in Table 1.

Measurement Error: Observer Bias

The numerators for the death rates reported in Table 1 come from death certificates. There are reliability problems with the assessment of race that suggest an acute problem of undercounting racial/ethnic status for Native Americans, APIAs, and Hispanics. A major source of this undercount is the discrepancy between interviewer-observed race and respondent self-report. Between 1957 and 1977 race was determined by interviewer observation in the Health Interview Survey. In 1978, the year in which the measurement of race was changed in that survey, racial information was collected both by interviewer observation and by respondent self-report. Analyses of the discrepancy between these two measurement strategies revealed that 6 percent of persons who reported themselves as black, 29 percent of self-identified Asian Pacific Islanders, 62 percent of self-identified American Indians, and 80 percent of persons who self-identified with an "other" category (70 percent of whom were Hispanic) were classified by the interviewer as white (21).

Respondent self-report is not an option on the death certificate, but it appears that officials who complete these forms make this decision based on their own judgment instead of obtaining the race of the deceased from the next of kin. In a national survey of vital registrars the authors concluded that only 63 percent of medical examiners, 50 percent of coroners, and 47 percent of funeral home directors use the recommended method of relying on family members for racial information (22). They also indicated that funeral home directors view requesting racial information as imposing a burden on the family. Misclassification of Asian Pacific Islanders or American Indians as white would suppress the death rates for these groups. Some evidence suggests that this does, in fact, occur. Sorlie and colleagues (23) compared race ascertained in a personal interview with a knowledgeable adult household member in 12 Current Population Surveys with race recorded on the death certificates as found in the National Death Index for the years 1979–1985. This study found high agreement for whites (99.2 percent) and blacks (98.2 percent) of self-reported racial status with racial status from death certificates. However, 26 percent of self-identified American Indians, 18 percent of Asian Pacific Islanders, and 10 percent of Hispanics were classified into another racial category on the death certificate. Most of these persons were classified as white.

Other studies of the Indian population provide further documentation of this problem. A study in Oklahoma found that 28 percent of Indian infants were misclassified as another race on the death certificate (24). After adjusting for this misclassification the infant mortality rate doubled from the officially reported 5.8 per 1000 to 10.4 per 1000. Similarly, another study found that only 60 percent of cancer patients registered with the Indian Health Service as American Indians were identified as Indians in the cancer surveillance registry (25). This led to an underestimation of cancer incidence rates for Native Americans. The underrecording of Indian race on death certificates is so severe in some places that the Indian Health Service has excluded mortality data from three areas with large concentrations of Indians (California, Oklahoma, and Portland) because of concerns about data quality (22).

Instructively, studies of the ways in which the race variable is used in health research show that researchers do not indicate how race is measured (17, 19). Williams (17) argues that editors of scientific journals can and should play a role in improving the quality of racial data. They can require, for example, that researchers indicate whether race was assessed by self-report, direct observation, proxy report, or extraction from records.

Reliability: Change in Racial Identity

A study of a large national population found that one-third of the U.S. population reported a different racial or ethnic status one year after their initial interview (26). For example, 6 percent of Negroes, 12 percent of Mexicans, 20 percent of Polish, 34 percent of Germans, and 45 percent of persons who said they were English, Scottish, or Welsh reported a racial or ethnic category in 1972 different from that reported in 1971.

The most dramatic evidence of change in self-identification comes from analyses of trends in the Indian population over time. Between 1960 and 1990 there was a six-fold increase in the American Indian population (27). This dramatic growth of the population cannot be explained either by biological growth or by international migration. It appears to reflect a change in self-definition, with more adults of mixed ancestry identifying themselves as American Indian. This shift in self-identification into the American Indian population is more common at younger ages and does not vary by gender (9, 28).

The nature and strength of identification as American Indian appears to be conditioned by the larger social context. The increase of persons reporting American Indian status in recent censuses is twice as high in "non-Indian" states as in states with large Indian populations (28). Persons residing in Indian areas are also more likely to report a single ancestry of American Indian than are persons who reside outside American Indian areas (9). The degree of identification as Indian may not be very strong for many of these "new Indians" (9, 27, 28). Most persons reporting American Indian ancestry did not report American Indian race, with 77 percent of persons who reported American Indian ancestry in the 1980 Census indicating that their race was white (9). American Indian identification for this group may be optional and contextual, depending on the form of the race question, economic incentives for being American Indian in some states, reduced discrimination against American Indians, an increased willingness to self-identify as American Indian, and the increased use of self-enumeration in the census (9).

Given current rates of intermarriage of Indians with persons of other races there is likely to be continued rapid growth in the pool of persons who will be of some Indian ancestry, but for whom this ethnic identification may not be consequential. Fifty-nine percent of all married American Indians in 1990 were married to non-Indians (27). Rates of intermarriage are lowest in the Southwest and highest in the Midwest and inversely associated with age. A recent study found that 47 percent of minor children in two-parent families, where one parent was Indian, were assigned the race of the American Indian parent. Moreover, children assigned Indian race in areas of high intermarriage had an average degree of Indian descent that was lower than that of children assigned Indian race in regions of low intermarriage (27).

Passel and Berman (9) suggest that self-identification as American Indian may capture some distinctiveness in areas with a large Indian population, but may not be as good an indicator of American Indian status in other areas. They also indicate that respondents' ability to identify a specific tribal designation may distinguish persons who have a weak versus a strong American Indian identification.

Multiracial Status

The discussion of establishing the racial status of American Indians raises the more general problem of establishing the race of an individual whose parents are of different races. Birth certificates in the United States have never listed the race of the child but they include the race of both parents. Prior to 1989 the National Center for Health Statistics used a complicated algorithm to determine the race of children whose parents belonged to different races. According to this scheme, if the father was white the child would be given the race of the mother; but if the father was non-white the child would be assigned the race of the father. If one parent was Hawaiian then the child was Hawaiian. Thus, unlike the assignment of race for all other racial groups, a child would be white only if both parents were white. Since 1989, the National Center for Health Statistics no longer reports vital statistics by the race of the child, but reports all birth data by the race of the mother. However, the Indian Health Service continues to consider a child as Indian if either the mother or the father is American Indian, and there is considerable discrepancy in the publication of infant mortality rates by race of child or by race of mother. For example, in 1989 there were 39,478 American Indian births as calculated by race of mother, but 49,267 as calculated by race of the child (22).

The question of how to classify persons whose parents are of different races continues to be a hotly debated issue in the United States, with some groups pushing for changes in the OMB's racial standards that would include a new category of multiracial status for all persons whose parents come from more than one of the four official racial groups. The current trends of interracial marriage suggest that this question will apply to an ever increasing proportion of the population. Twenty-five to 44 percent of Hispanics marry non-Hispanics, and 25 to 50 percent of APIA subgroups marry persons of other races (29). Rates of black–white intermarriage are considerably lower, but they increased from 2 percent in 1970 to 6 percent in 1990. The states of Ohio and Illinois now require that a multiracial category be added to school forms, while Georgia requires it on all written forms used by state agencies.

Researchers have not given systematic attention to the extent to which the health profile of persons of mixed racial parentage differs from that of the standard racial categories. One recent study suggests that this association may be complex and that any attempt to assess multiracial status should include assessment of the race of both parents. Collins and David (30) found that infants born to black mothers and white fathers had a higher rate of low birth weight than those born to white mothers and black fathers.

Definition of Racial Groups

Definitional problems are not limited to multiracial status. The classification of the entire population into racial groups is neither simple nor straightforward. These problems are readily evident for the American Indian population. Indian tribes do not agree on who is American Indian, with some using a strict definition based on degree of Indian ancestry and others requiring identification with Indian culture or participation in tribal affairs. The U.S. government has also had its difficulties in dividing the population into racial groups. The Census Bureau, for example, has routinely changed its racial categories, with no single racial classification scheme having been used in more than two censuses (31). The current assessment of racial status in the United States is indicative of considerable progress but still reflects major problems. Prior to the mid-1970s, most health data in the United States were reported for the white population and the "non-white" or "other than white" population. This latter group included blacks, American Indians, and Asian and Pacific Islanders, but because blacks make up about 90 percent of the group, this category provided a reasonable approximation for the health status of the black population but no information on the smaller minority racial groups (32).

However, in the wake of a growing awareness that other racial populations comprise an increasing proportion of the U.S. population and the publication of the OMB's Racial and Ethnic Standards in 1978, there have been increasing efforts to capture the racial heterogeneity of the U.S. population. For example,

between 1957 and 1977 the Health Interview Survey, a major annual federal
health survey, categorized respondents into white, Negro, or other but in 1978
changed to the five OMB categories. In 1992, the APIA racial category was
expanded to include nine subgroups.

The categories of race and ethnicity are often assessed differently by various
health agencies and researchers. The Centers for Disease Control and Prevention
uses one question to capture OMB's five required racial categories in its national
notifiable diseases surveillance system. However, many health surveys and other
federal data collection systems use one question to assess race and a separate one
to assess Hispanic origin. Similarly, although the standard birth and death certificates were revised in 1989 to include Hispanic identifiers, the wording of the
question varies from state to state and the data on Hispanic ethnicity are not
completely reported in all states (33).

These differences are important because the size of a racial/ethnic population depends on the wording of the question. In the 1980 Census, 26.5 million
Americans self-identified as "black or Negro" but only 21 million indicated
that they were of Afro-American ancestry (16). Similarly, there were 1.5 million
American Indians based on answers to the race question in the 1980 Census,
but 6.8 million based on responses to the ethnic ancestry question (34). In a
study of 7,300 middle-school students in the Miami area, 67 percent of the
sample reported that they were of Hispanic ancestry, but only 56 percent were
Hispanic based on parental report (35). Interestingly, students who were categorized discrepantly (that is, identified as Hispanic by the ancestry definition
but not by parental report) had higher levels of acculturation and depressive
symptoms.

Respondents also vary in their preferred term for self-identification. National
data for the black population reveal that while 18 percent of blacks preferred to be
called African American, 17 percent favored the term black and 60 percent said it
made no difference (36). Younger adults and persons residing in the Northeast
were much more likely to prefer the term African American than were older
adults and persons in other regions of the country.

Thus, there is a continuing need for uniform assessment of race and ethnicity
in state and federal health data collection systems and in the wider research
community. Moreover, there is also a critical need for the inclusion of identifiers
for subgroups of the APIA and Hispanic populations on all surveys and forms.

The implementation of the OMB's Directive 15 frequently violates an important principle of classification, namely, the creation of a set of exhaustive and
mutually exclusive groups. Valid statistical tests are based on the assumption
that the various categories in the classification system are independent samples.
This assumption is not met for the data presented in Table 1. There are black
Hispanics, Asian Hispanics, American Indian Hispanics, and white Hispanics.
Del Pinal (37) has shown that the overlap of race with the Hispanic category
affects the patterns of racial/ethnic differences not only for Hispanics but for the

other racial categories as well. For example, black Hispanics are more similar in labor force participation to blacks than to white Hispanics. Thus, comparing non-Hispanic whites to blacks and Hispanics (instead of comparing differences among whites, blacks, and Hispanics, as Table 1 does) would increase the Hispanic–white difference but reduce the black–white difference.

Census Undercount

Another problem affecting the quality of the mortality data in Table 1 is census undercount. Census data are used to calculate the denominators for mortality rates. They are also used to construct sampling frames and adjust for nonresponse in population-based epidemiologic studies. The use of a denominator that is undercounted inflates the obtained rate in exact proportion to the undercount in the denominator. Thus, all rates of health events that use census data as denominators are overestimated by the same percentage as the population undercount in the denominator.

For the last several decades the U.S. Census Bureau has been evaluating the extent of undercount by means of demographic analysis. This strategy produces estimates of the population based on administrative data and demographic trends. These analyses consistently reveal that, while the overall undercount for the U.S. population is small, it is larger for blacks than for whites, and despite a steady decline in the undercount rate for blacks between 1940 and 1980, there was an upward trend between 1980 and 1990 (38). The undercount rate for the overall population does not importantly distort health data, but the undercount rate varies considerably for some demographic subgroups. In 1990, the overall undercount was 1.8 percent for the U.S. population as a whole and 5.7 percent for the black population. However, it was dramatically higher for black males (8.5 percent) than for black females (3 percent) and varied by age, with a net census undercount of 11 to 13 percent for all of the 10-year age categories of black males between the ages of 25 and 64 (39). Demographic analysis estimates are available only at the national level and it is likely that the omission of black males from households (the major cause of the undercount of blacks) varies by geographic area. Estimates of undercount based on demographic analyses are only as good as the underlying assumptions, and concerns have been raised about the extent to which the demographic analysis methods are becoming less reliable over time (40).

The evaluation of the undercount problem by the Census Bureau has focused heavily on the black and white populations. However, there is reason to believe that census undercount may also be a significant problem for some of the other racial populations. For the 1990 Census, in addition to demographic analysis, the Census Bureau conducted a Post Census Enumeration Survey (PES) in which undercount was estimated on a case-by-case matching of census records with those obtained in the survey of 165,000 households. According to the PES, the undercount rates for Hispanics (5 percent) and reservation Indians (12.2 percent) were even higher than the rate for blacks (4.6 percent) (41), but the extent to which the undercount for these groups is concentrated in particular age and/or gender groups is not known. The PES undercount was 0.7 percent for non-Hispanic whites and 2.4 percent for Asian and Pacific Islanders.

Other Issues

The availability of adequate data, especially morbidity data, for American Indians, Hispanics, and APIAs is still a major problem. Because of the relatively small sizes of some of these population groups and their geographic distribution, standard sampling strategies for national populations do not yield adequate sample sizes to provide reliable estimates for the distribution of disease in these groups or to explore heterogeneity within a given racial group. Surveys focused on a particular geographic area with a high concentration of a racial subgroup as opposed to national surveys are necessary to provide data for these groups. Combining multiple years of data in ongoing surveys is another useful strategy for obtaining health information for small population groups.

Health researchers must also give greater attention to translating study instruments for persons who have limited proficiency in the English language. These persons are more likely to be members of racial minority populations. For example, in 1990, while only 8 percent of the total U.S. population was foreign born, 74 percent of APIAs were foreign born (12). Currently, major federal health surveys, such as the Health Interview Survey, do not routinely translate the questionnaire into other languages. This survey is currently being redesigned to provide for continuous oversampling of blacks and Hispanics. In addition to translating the survey instruments, researchers must also ensure that their new instruments meet the test of conceptual, scale, and norm equivalence (42). Conceptual equivalence refers to similarities in the meanings of the concepts used in the assessment. Scale equivalence is the use of questionnaire items that are familiar to all groups, while norm equivalence ensures that the norms developed for the targeted group are appropriate and not arbitrarily assigned from another group.

UNDERSTANDING RACIAL DIFFERENCES

Traditional explanations for health status differences between the races have focused on biological differences between racial populations. Nineteenth century medical research, for example, attempted to document that blacks were biologically inferior to whites and therefore more susceptible to a host of illnesses (3). Most current research on racial differences has abandoned blatant racist ideology, but much of it still assumes that racial variations in disease are due to underlying differences in biology. The biological approach views racial taxonomies as meaningful classifications of genetic differences between human population groups. It assumes that race is a valid biological category, that the genes determining race also determine the number and types of health problems that an individual will have (43). The available scientific evidence suggests that race is a social and not a biological category. First, the concept of race developed long before modern valid scientific theories of genetics existed. In the context of slavery and imperial colonialism race was a useful construct, not only for classifying human variation but also to provide an apparent scientific rationale for the exploitation of groups that were regarded as inferior (44). Second, the extant racial categories do not represent biological distinctiveness. There is more genetic variation within races than between them. Irrespective of geographic origin or race, all human beings are identical for 75 percent of known genetic factors (45). In addition, some 95 percent of human genetic variation exists within racial groups, with relatively small and isolated populations such as Eskimos and Australian Aborigines contributing most of the between-group variation (46). Our current racial categories are thus more alike than different in terms of biological characteristics and genetics, and there are no specific scientific criteria to unambiguously distinguish different racial groups.

Moreover, single-gene disorders account for only a small part of racial differences in health. Sickle cell anemia, for example, occurs more frequently in African Americans than the rest of the U.S. population. However, it accounts for only 0.3 percent of the total number of excess deaths in the black population and is thus not a major cause of the overall higher rates of disease for African Americans (47). Sickle cell anemia appears to have been a protective biological adaptation to environmental conditions. It is not limited to African Americans but occurs at higher rates in persons who originate in regions of the world where malaria was endemic (48).

Race and SES

Since the discrediting of biological explanations, researchers have been giving increasing attention to the role of social class or socioeconomic status as a determinant of racial differences in health. Race is strongly associated with socioeconomic status and many researchers view race as a proxy for SES. Table 2 presents selected SES characteristics for the five OMB categories (10). The overall patterns for racial/ethnic groups in Table 2 mask the considerable variations that exists within each of the categories. Supplemental data will be used to illustrate this heterogeneity for the Asian American population, but it must be remembered that similar patterns and variation exist for all racial groups.

The data on educational attainment reveal that blacks, Hispanics, and American Indians have considerably lower rates of educational attainment than whites. Rates of high school completion for Asian and Pacific Islanders are comparable to those of whites, with APIAs having even higher levels of college graduation than whites. The higher educational attainment for APIAs is explained in part by

Table 2

Selected economic profiles for the United States, 1990 Census[a]

	White	Black	Asian and Pacific Islander	American Indian and Alaskan Native	Hispanic
Educational attainment (persons 25 yrs and older), percent					
Less than 9th grade	8.9%	13.8%	12.9%	14.2%	30.7%
High-school graduate or higher	77.9	63.1	77.5	65.3	49.8
Bachelor's degree or higher	21.5	11.4	36.6	8.9	9.2
Employment status by sex (persons 16 yrs and older), percent					
Unemployed, males	5.3%	13.7%	5.1%	16.2%	9.8%
Unemployed, females	5.0	12.2	5.5	13.5	11.2
Median household income in 1989	$31,435	$19,758	$36,784	$19,865	$24,156
Below the poverty level by age, percent					
All ages	9.8%	29.5%	14.1%	31.7%	25.3%
Under 5 yrs	13.8	44.0	17.5	43.3	33.4

[a]Source: reference 10.

the selective migration of better educated persons to the United States. However, the overall data on educational attainment for the APIA population obscure the overrepresentation of the population at both ends of the educational distribution. There are low rates of education completion among some subgroups of the Asian population. In a 1993 study, only 26 percent of APIAs from Laos and 38 percent of those from Cambodia had completed high school (12). Asian American men are twice as likely, and Asian American women three times as likely, to have completed only three to four years of elementary education compared with the total population (12).

The unemployment data show a similar pattern, with APIAs and whites having the lowest rates and the rates being considerably higher for American Indians, blacks, and Hispanics, in that order. Unemployment rates for some Asian subgroups are also high. The 1980 unemployment rates were 20 percent for the Hmong, 15 percent for Laotians, 11 percent for Cambodians, and 10 percent for Samoans (42).

The median household income for American Indians ($19,865) is very similar to that of blacks ($19,758) and both are considerably lower than that of the white population ($31,435). The median household income for Hispanics is higher than that of blacks and American Indians but lower than that of whites, while the Asian population has the highest level of median household income in the United States. However, Asian families are larger and have more earners per family than the total population. Thus, the 1990 per capita income of Asians ($13,420) was lower than that of whites ($15,270) (12). The Asian population is also disproportionately located in high-income-earning geographic regions of the country such as the West and New York, where median family income is higher than the national average.

The data on poverty also follow the now familiar pattern. The highest rates of poverty are found for American Indians and blacks—rates that are about three times that for whites. Hispanics have rates that are substantially higher than that of whites, but lower than those of blacks and American Indians. The poverty rates for the APIA category are slightly higher than that of whites. Again, there is considerable variation within the Asian group, with rates of poverty being particularly high among Southeast Asian immigrant groups. One-third of Vietnamese immigrants and over half of Cambodian and Laotian immigrants lived in poverty in 1980 (42).

SES and Racial Differences in Health

Given this strong association between SES and race, it is widely recognized that racial differences must be controlled for SES. Adjusting racial (black–white) disparities in health for SES sometimes eliminates, but always substantially reduces, these differences (20, 49–51). However, a frequent finding is that within each level of SES blacks still have worse health status than whites. Table 3 illustrates this pattern. It presents the association between household income and years of formal education with self-assessed health for blacks and whites (52). Self-assessed health is a robust indicator of health status that is strongly related to overall mortality and other objective measures of health.

Table 3 indicates that irrespective of race, there are large disparities in health by income and education. For example, for persons living in households with a total income of less than $20,000, 16.6 percent of whites and 19 percent of blacks report their health to be poor. The comparable numbers for households with incomes greater than $20,000 are 5.1 and 7.6 percent for whites and blacks, respectively. Thus the differences by income and education are much larger than those by race. At the same time, these data reveal that even when education and income level are held constant blacks have higher levels of ill-health than

Table 3

Average annual percentage of persons reporting to be in fair or poor health
by income and education, for blacks and whites[a]

Education	Income <$20,000		Income >$20,000	
	Whites	Blacks	Whites	Blacks
Less than 12 yrs	33.1%	38.8%	16.1%	20.5%
12 yrs	15.2	17.9	6.8	9.6
More than 12 yrs	9.2	13.2	3.7	5.9
Total	16.6%	19.0%	5.1%	7.6%

[a]Source: reference 52.

whites. This pattern suggests that although most of the racial differences in health are accounted for by SES, race may have an effect on health that is independent of SES.

Other studies have documented a similar pattern. Schoendorf and colleagues (53) found higher rates of infant mortality among college-educated black women than among college-educated whites. Moreover, the black–white gap in infant mortality increases with rising SES (20). In a recent analysis of infant mortality rates during the period 1964–1966, compared with 1987, Singh and Yu (54) found that blacks at all levels of education and income had higher infant mortality rates than whites, with the black–white gap being greater at higher levels of SES. Moreover, the racial disparity across SES levels was greater in 1987 than in the earlier period.

Racism and SES

This pattern of results clearly indicates that, while there is considerable overlap between race and SES, race reflects more than SES and that fully under-standing racial differences in health will require researchers to move beyond the traditional approaches. Several researchers have noted that our fundamental assumptions about what race is will shape the research questions developed to understand racial disparities in health (15, 20, 49, 55). These researchers emphasize that the failure of the traditionally used SES indicators to completely explain racial differences in health reflects the interactive and incremental role of racism as a determinant of health. The construct racism incorporates ideologies of superiority, negative attitudes and beliefs toward racial and ethnic outgroups, and differential treatment of members of these groups by both individuals and societal institutions (51).

Race has been a fundamental organizing principle of society (56). Historically, attitudes and beliefs about racial groups have been translated into policies and societal arrangements that limited the opportunities and life chances of stigmatized groups. Minority populations' disproportionate representation at the lower levels of SES reflects the successful implementation of social processes designed to relegate groups with undesirable physical characteristics such as skin color to positions and roles consistent with the dominant society's evaluation of them.

Racism can affect health by giving rise to racial discrimination at the individual and institutional level. The former is an important but neglected stressor that can lead to adverse changes in health status, while the latter can result in the inequitable distribution of desirable institutional resources including medical ones. However, Williams and associates (15) emphasize that racism is causally prior to SES and exerts its most profound impact by transforming SES such that an equivalent value on a traditional SES measure represents important differences in social and economic circumstances for persons belonging to different racial groups.

Residential racial segregation is one of the primary mechanisms by which racism produces differential socioeconomic outcomes (57). Historically, a web of discrimination orchestrated by banks, federal and local governments, and the housing industry created racially distinct residential zones for blacks (58). This residential segregation effectively concentrated African Americans in the least desirable neighborhoods. There has been a very modest reduction in segregation in recent decades driven largely by the development of new housing in younger metropolitan areas in the south and west (59), but there has been little decline in segregation in the older, larger, metropolitan areas where most blacks live (57).

Racial segregation has pervasive adverse effects on opportunities for education, employment, and socioeconomic mobility. Unless one has the economic resources to purchase alternative schooling, place of residence determines school attendance. Residential segregation thus ensures that blacks do not receive a high-quality education. Even when black and white students attend the same school, blacks are more likely to be placed or "tracked" into low-ability, less academically challenging classrooms that are under the supervision of teachers who have low expectations (58). Under these conditions, it is not surprising that the high-school dropout rate is high for blacks in many urban areas.

Compared with whites, blacks who complete high school have lower levels of skills and knowledge and are less prepared for both higher education and the job market. Thus, high-school completion represents very different realities and opportunities for members of different racial groups. In terms of income, national data reveal that a white male high-school graduate working full-time in the labor force has a median annual income of $26,500 compared with $20,300 and $20,900 for his black and Hispanic counterparts, respectively (60). This pattern of lower income returns for education exists at both high and low levels of education, with blacks and Hispanics, males and females, earning less income than whites.

In addition to being less prepared to enter the labor force, blacks are also more likely to experience discriminatory hiring practices (61). Moreover, employed blacks are more likely to experience job loss. For example, a *Wall Street Journal* study of 35,000 companies that employ more than one-third of the U.S. workforce found that during the economic downturn of 1990–1991, blacks lost a disproportionately high share of the jobs that were cut and received a disproportionately low share of new jobs (62). African Americans had a net job loss of 59,500 jobs, compared with net gains of 71,100 for whites, 55,100 for Asians, and 60,000 for Latinos. Blacks experienced a net loss of jobs even in the traditionally low-paying service and sales sectors. This lack of job security also exists for middle-class blacks (63). College-educated blacks, for example, are about four times more likely to experience unemployment than their white peers (64). In addition, employed blacks are more likely to experience pathogenic occupational conditions. Even after adjustment for job experience and training, blacks are more likely than whites to be exposed to occupational hazards and carcinogens at work (65).

Table 2 noted large racial differences in income, but income disparities understate racial differences in household economic resources. Financial assets or reserves are an important part of household economic resources and may be more strongly tied to social class location than earned income. It is instructive that racial differences in wealth are larger than those for income. While white households have a median net worth of $44,408, the median net worth is $4,604 for black households and $5,345 for Hispanic households (66). Moreover, racial differences in wealth exist at all income levels. For example, for the poorest 20 percent of the U.S. population (where African Americans and Hispanics are overrepresented) white households have a net worth of $10,000 compared with $1 for blacks and $575 for Hispanics. Thus, compared with whites at equivalent levels of income, blacks and Latinos have substantially less economic security and are less able to cushion a shortfall of income. Studies that seek to understand the association between race and SES in affecting health status should devote more attention to assessing wealth.

Residential segregation also leads to the withdrawal of commercial enterprises from black neighborhoods (57). Thus, a disproportionate number of African Americans live in communities bereft of high-quality goods and services. These conditions and racial discrimination combine to ensure that the purchasing power of a given level of income is much greater for whites than for blacks. Studies reveal that compared with whites, African Americans pay higher prices for new cars (67), higher property taxes on homes of similar value (68), and higher costs for food (69) and mortgages (70). These racial differences in purchasing power illustrate the nonequivalence of a given level of income across race in terms of its ability to procure goods and services in society.

Race and SES: A Research Agenda

The preceding discussion highlights the inadequacy of attempting to understand racial differences in health status merely by adjusting for SES. Some have argued that because race is causally prior to SES such statistical adjustment is "overcontrol" (47). Krieger and colleagues (20) provide a helpful critique of this perspective. They conclude that although it is important to recognize the nonindependence of race and SES, adjusting racial disparities for SES is not necessarily an inappropriate analytic strategy. They indicate that such an approach should be complemented by more routine presentation of results stratified by SES within racial groups and by renewed attention to directly assessing the health consequences of neighborhood effects and the noneconomic aspects of discrimination.

In a reanalysis of data from eight epidemiologic surveys, Kessler and Neighbors (71) demonstrated the importance of systematically testing for interactions between race and socioeconomic status. They found that although controlling for SES reduced the association between race and psychological distress to nonsignificance, low-SES blacks had higher rates of distress than low-SES whites. However, the findings have not been uniform. Analyses of data from a large mental health study found that low-SES white males had higher rates of psychiatric disorders than their black peers (72). Among women, low-SES black females had higher levels of substance abuse disorders than their white peers. These findings suggest the importance of examining multiple outcomes and attending to the interactions among race, gender, and class.

A growing body of evidence reveals that experiences of racial discrimination and the internalization of racist ideology by minority group members are adversely linked to physical and mental health (20, 51). However, much work is yet to be done in the conceptualization and measurement of race-related stressors. Research has yet to identify the broad range of racialized experiences that might affect health. It is currently unclear how acute and chronic, major and minor, experiences of racial bias combine with traditional measures of stress, psychosocial resources, and coping patterns to affect health and functioning.

More attention also needs to be given to using multiple measures of SES. Measures of social class at the individual household and neighborhood level each capture exposure to different health risks, and all are necessary as part of a comprehensive assessment of position in the social structure (50). Assessment of neighborhood characteristics must also include more attention to identifying the health effects of segregation. Some recent studies have documented a positive association between segregation and mortality (73, 74). The extent to which various SES indicators may be differently predictive of health status for various racial/ethnic populations should also be addressed. It was recently noted, for example, that the traditional SES indicators tend not to be related to variations in at least some health outcomes for Mexican Americans (51).

Much prior research has viewed SES in a static manner and paid scant attention to changes in SES over the life course. This issue may be especially relevant to the study of racial differences in health. Members of racial/ethnic minority populations are more likely to experience sharp losses in income during adulthood and to have experienced poor economic conditions as a child. An adult's health status is a function not only of current SES but of the SES conditions experienced over the life course (51). There is mounting evidence that the quality of the health and socioeconomic conditions experienced in childhood has profound and lasting effects on health and well-being. Williams and Collins (51) have recently noted that some of the documented associations between early life conditions and adult health status are directly relevant to understanding black–white differences in adult health status. For example, it is well known that black adults have rates of hypertension that are twice that of whites and black infants are twice as likely as their white peers to be low birth weight. Several studies reveal that growth retardation during the fetal period and low birth weight are associated with hypertension in adulthood (75). Thus it is plausible that these early life conditions play a role in racial disparities in high blood pressure.

The comprehensive assessment of social position for minority populations should also include the assessment of alternative indicators of social position. Skin color appears to be one such indicator. Analyses of a national representative sample of African Americans found that darker skin color was inversely related to income, education, and occupational status (76). Moreover, skin color was a stronger predictor of adult occupational status and income than was parental SES. Darker skinned blacks also reported higher levels of racial discrimination.

Dressler (55) has argued that skin color determines exposure to racial bias, access to valued resources, and the intensity of the effort necessary to obtain them. He has used skin color as an objective indicator of SES within the black population in examining the association between status inconsistency and hypertension. He found that darker skin color was an indicator of social status independent of education level. Klag and colleagues (77) also found an interaction between skin color and SES in a sample of blacks. Darker skin color was associated with elevated rates of hypertension for low-SES but not high-SES blacks.

The role of skin color as an indicator of SES may not be unique to the African American population. A national sample of almost 1,000 Mexican Americans found that a measure of phenotype that combined skin color and degree of European appearance was strongly associated with SES (78). Mexican Americans who were dark skinned and Indian in physical appearance were lower on multiple indicators of SES and reported higher levels of discrimination than their peers who were light complexioned and European in appearance. More generally, in virtually all cultures the color black is associated with negative attributes (79), and experimental data suggest that at least in some social situations the color black may be a subtle cue for changes in social perception (80).

The discussion of skin color highlights the importance of paying attention to the unique characteristics of each racial population. African Americans are more likely to be dark in skin color than any other racial group in the United States and this may account in part for the higher levels of segregation (57) and the greater difficulties in social mobility (81) that they have experienced compared with other immigrant groups. Researchers must also give greater attention to the ways in which the unique migration history and mode of incorporation into the United States for each racial/ethnic group interact with SES to affect the distribution of disease. Rates of infant mortality, low birth weight, cancer, high blood pressure, adolescent pregnancy, and psychiatric disorders increase with length of stay in the United States for Hispanics, with foreign-born Hispanics having a better health profile than their U.S.-born counterparts (8). The contribution, if any, of SES to this pattern of disease is unclear (51). However, the ways in which socio-economic status interacts with migration experience, acculturative stress, and health-enhancing cultural resources have yet to receive serious research attention.

Acknowledgment — Thanks to Car Nosel for assistance in preparing the manuscript.

REFERENCES

1. Gould, S. J. American polygeny and craniometry before Darwin: Blacks and Indians as separate, inferior species. In *The Mismeasure of Man*, pp. 30–72. W. W. Norton, New York, 1981.
2. Anderson, M. J. *The American Census: A Social History*. Yale University Press, New Haven, Conn., 1988.
3. Krieger, N. Shades of difference: Theoretical underpinnings of the medical controversy on black/white differences in the United States. *Int. J. Health Serv.* 17: 259–278, 1987.
4. Navarro, V. Race *or* class versus race *and* class: Mortality differentials in the United States. *Lancet* 336: 1238–1240, 1990.
5. National Center for Health Statistics. *Health United States, 1994.* (PHS) 95-1232. U.S. Public Health Service, Hyattsville, Md., 1995.
6. Office of Management and Budget. Statistical Directive No. 15: Race and ethnic standards for federal agencies and administrative reporting. *Federal Register* 43: 19269–19270, May 4, 1978.
7. Sorlie, P. D., et al. Mortality by Hispanic status in the United States. *JAMA* 270: 2464–2468, 1993.
8. Vega, W. A., and Amaro, H. Latino outlook: Good health, uncertain prognosis. *Annu. Rev. Public Health* 15: 39–67, 1994.
9. Passel, J. S., and Berman, P. A. Quality of 1980 census data for American Indians. *Soc. Biol.* 33: 163–182, 1986.
10. National Center for Health Statistics. *Trends in Indian Health—1993*. U.S. Dept. of Health and Human Services, Indian Health Service, Rockville, Md., 1993.
11. Halasan, C., et al. *1990–1991 New Mexico Tribe-specific Vital Statistics*. State of New Mexico, Department of Health, Public Health Division, Bureau of Vital Records and Health Statistics, Sante Fe, 1992.

12. Lin-Fu, J. S. Asian and Pacific Islanders: An overview of demographic characteristics and health care issues. *Asian Am. Pacific Islander J. Health* 1: 20–36, 1993.
13. Suh, D. Cooperative agreements to advance the understanding of the health of Asian and Pacific Islander Americans. In *Proceedings of the 1993 Public Health Conference on Records and Statistics*, pp. 352–356. DHHS Pub. No. (PHS) 94-1214. Centers for Disease Control and Prevention, National Health Center for Health Statistics, Hyattsville, Md., 1993.
14. Chen, M. S. A 1993 status report on the health status of Asian Pacific Islander Americans: Comparisons with *Healthy People 2000* objectives. *Asian Am. Pacific Islander J. Health* 1: 37–55, 1993.
15. Williams, D R., Lavizzo-Mourey, R., and Warren, R. C. The concept of race and health status in America. *Public Health Rep.* 109: 26–41, 1994.
16. Hahn, R. A. The state of federal health statistics on racial and ethnic groups. *JAMA* 267: 268–271, 1992.
17. Williams, D. R. The concept of race in *Health Services Research*: 1966 to 1990. *Health Serv. Res.* 29: 261–274, 1994.
18. LaVeist, T. A. Beyond dummy variables and sample selection: What health services researchers ought to know about race as a variable. *Health Serv. Res.* 29: 1–16, 1994.
19. Jones, C. P., LaVeist, T. A., and Lillie-Blanton, M. Race in the epidemiologic literature: An examination of the *American Journal of Epidemiology*. *Am. J. Epidemiol.* 134: 1079–1084, 1991.
20. Krieger, N., et al. Racism, sexism, and social class: Implications for studies of health. *Am. J. Prev. Med.* 9: 82–122, 1993.
21. Massey, J. T. Comparison of interviewer observed race and respondent reported race in the National Health Interview Survey. In *Proceedings of the American Statistical Association*, pp. 425–428. American Statistical Association, Washington, D.C., 1980.
22. Scott, S., and Suagee, M. *Enhancing Health Statistics for American Indian and Alaskan Native Communities: An Agenda for Action*. Report to the National Center for Health Statistics. American Indican Health Care Association, St. Paul., Minn., 1992.
23. Sorlie, P. D., Rogot, E., and Johnson, N. J. Validity of demographic characteristics on the death certificate. *Epidemiology* 3: 181–184, 1992.
24. Kennedy, R. D., and Deapen, R. E. Differences between Oklahoma and Indian infant mortality and other races. *Public Health Rep.* 106: 97–99, 1991.
25. Frost, F., Taylor, V., and Fries, E. Racial misclassification of Native Americans in a surveillance epidemiology and end results cancer registry. *J. Natl. Cancer Inst.* 84: 957–962, 1992.
26. Johnson, C. E. *Consistency of Reporting Ethnic Origin in the Current Population Survey*. U.S. Department of Commerce Technical Paper No. 31. Bureau of the Census, Washington, D.C., 1974.
27. Eschbach, K. The enduring and vanishing American Indian: American Indian population growth and intermarriage in 1990. *Ethnic Racial Stud.* 18: 89–108, 1995.
28. Harris, D. The 1990 census count of American Indians: What do the numbers really mean? *Soc. Sci. Q.* 75: 580–593, 1994.
29. Rumbaut, R. G. The crucible within: Ethnic identity, self-esteem, and segmented assimilation among children of immigrants. *Int. Migration Rev.* 28: 748–794, 1994.
30. Collins, S., and David, R. J. Race and birthweight in biracial infants. *Am. J. Public Health* 83: 1125–1129, 1993.
31. Martin, E., Demaio, T. J., and Campanelli, P. C. Context effects for census measures of race and Hispanic origin. *Public Opinion Q.* 54: 551–566, 1990.

32. Wilson, R. W., and Danchik, K. M. A Comparison of 'Black' and 'Other Than White' Data from the National Health Interview Survey and Mortality Statistics. Paper presented at the Annual Meeting of the American Statistical Association, Houston, Tex., 1980.
33. U.S. Public Health Task Force on Minority Health Data. *Improving Minority Health Statistics*. Report 715-025. U.S. Government Printing Office, Washington, D.C., 1992.
34. Snipp, M. *American Indians: The First of This Land*. Russell Sage, New York, 1989.
35. Zimmerman, R. S., et al. Who is Hispanic? Definitions and their consequences. *Am. J. Public Health* 84: 1985–1987, 1994.
36. McAneny, L. 'African-American' or 'black'? *Gallup Poll Monthly* 348: 11–12, 1994.
37. Del Pinal, J. H. *Exploring Alternative Race-Ethnic Comparison Groups in Current Population Surveys*. U.S. Bureau of the Census, Curr. Popul. Rep., Ser. P23-182. U.S. Government Printing Office, Washington, D.C., 1992.
38. Robinson, J. G., et al. Estimation of population coverage in the 1990 United States Census based on demographic analysis. *J. Am. Stat. Assoc.* 88: 1047–1057, 1993.
39. National Center for Health Statistics. *Vital Statistics of the United States, 1990. Vol. 11, Mortality, Part A*. U.S. Public Health Service, Washington, D.C., 1994.
40. Notes and Comments: Census undercount and the quality of data for racial and ethnic populations. *Ethnicity Dis.* 4: 98–100, 1994.
41. Hogan, H. The 1990 post-enumeration survey: Operations and results. *J. Am. Stat. Assoc.* 88: 1047–1057, 1993.
42. Takeuchi, D. T., and Young, K. N. J. Overview of Asian and Pacific Islander Americans. In *Confronting Critical Health Issues of Asian and Pacific Islander Americans*, edited by N. W. S. Zane, D. T. Takeuchi, and K. N. J. Young, pp. 3–21. Sage, Thousand Oaks, Calif., 1994.
43. Krieger, N., and Bassett, M. The health of black folk: Disease, class and ideology. *Monthly Rev.* 38: 74–85, 1986.
44. Montague, A. *The Idea of Race*. University of Nebraska Press, Lincoln, 1965.
45. Lewontin, R. *Human Diversity*. Scientific American Books, New York, 1982.
46. Lewontin, R. *The Genetic Basis of Evolutionary Change*. Columbia University Press, New York, 1974.
47. Cooper, R., and David, R. The biological concept of race and its application to public health and epidemiology. *J. Health Polit. Policy Law* 11: 97–116, 1986.
48. Polednak, A. P. *Racial and Ethnic Differences in Disease*. Oxford University Press, New York, 1989.
49. Cooper, R. S. Health and the social status of blacks in the United States. *Ann. Epidemiol.* 3: 137–144, 1993.
50. Krieger, N., and Fee, E. Social class: The missing link in U.S. health data. *Int. J. Health Serv.* 24: 25–44, 1994.
51. Williams, D. R., and Collins, C. U.S. socioeconomic and racial differences in health: Patterns and explanations. *Annu. Rev. Sociol.* 21: 349–386, 1995.
52. Ries, P. Health of black and white Americans, 1985–1987. *Vital Health Stats*, Vol. 10. National Center for Health Statistics, Washington, D.C., 1990.
53. Schoendorf, K. C., et al. Mortality among infants of black as compared with white college-educated parents. *N. Engl. J. Med.* 23: 1522–1526, 1992.
54. Singh, G. K., and Yu, S. M. Infant mortality in the United States: Trends, differentials, and projections, 1950 through 2010. *Am. J. Public Health* 85: 957–964, 1995.
55. Dressler, W. W. Health in the African American community: Accounting for health inequalities. *Med. Anthropol. Q.* 7: 325–245, 1993.

56. Omi, M., and Winant, H. *Racial Formation in the United States: From the 1960's to the 1980's*. Routledge, New York, 1986.

57. Massey, D., and Denton, N. A. *American Apartheid: Segregation and the Making of the Underclass*. Harvard University Press, Cambridge, Mass., 1993.

58. Jaynes, G. D., and Williams, R. M. *A Common Destiny: Blacks and American Society*. National Academy Press, Washington, D.C., 1989.

59. Farley, R., and Frey, W. H. Changes in the segregation of whites from blacks during the 1980s: Small steps toward a more integrated society. *Am. Sociol. Rev.* 59: 23–45, 1994.

60. U.S. Bureau of the Census. *Money Income of Households, Families and Persons in the United States*. Curr. Popul. Rep., Ser. P-60, No. 174. U.S. Government Printing Office, Washington, D.C., 1991.

61. Kirschenman, J., and Neckerman, K. M. "We'd love to hire them, but . . .": The meaning of race for employers. In *The Urban Underclass*, edited by C. Jencks and P. E. Peterson, pp. 203–232. The Brookings Institution, Washington, D.C., 1991.

62. Sharpe, R. In latest recession, only blacks suffered net employment loss. *Wall Street Journal*, September 14, 1993.

63. Collins, S. The making of the black middle class. *Sociol. Prob.* 10: 369–382, 1983.

64. Wilhelm, S. M. Economic demise of blacks in America: A prelude to genocide? *J. Black Stud.* 17: 201–254, 1987.

65. Robinson, J. C. Racial inequality and the probability of occupation-related injury or illness. *Milbank Q.* 63: 567–593, 1984.

66. Eller, T. J. *Household Wealth and Asset Ownership: 1991*. U.S. Bureau of the Census, Curr. Popul. Rep. P70-34. U.S. Government Printing Office, Washington, D.C., 1994.

67. Ayres, I. Fair driving: Gender and race discrimination in retail car negotiations. *Harvard Law Rev.* 104: 817–872, 1991.

68. Schemo, D. Suburban taxes are higher for blacks, analysis shows. *New York Times*, August 17, 1994.

69. Alexis, M., Haines, G. H., and Simon, L. S. *Black Consumer Profiles*. Division of Research, Graduate School of Business Administration, University of Michigan, Ann Arbor, 1980.

70. Pol, L. G., Guy, R. F., and Bush, A. J. Discrimination in the home lending market: A macro perspective. *Soc. Sci. Q.* 63: 716–728, 1982.

71. Kessler, R. C., and Neighbors, H. W. A new perspective on the relationships among race, social class, and psychological distress. *J. Health Soc. Behav.* 27: 107–115, 1986.

72. Williams, D. R., Takeuchi, D., and Adair, R. Socioeconomic status and psychiatric disorder among blacks and whites. *Soc. Forces* 71: 179–194, 1992.

73. LaVeist, T. A. The political empowerment and health status of African-Americans: Mapping a new territory. *Am. J. Sociol.* 97: 1080–1095, 1989.

74. Polednak, A. P. Black-white differences in infant mortality in 38 standard metropolitan statistical areas. *Am. J. Public Health* 81: 1480–1482, 1991.

75. Elo, I. T., and Preston, S. H. Effects of early life conditions on adult mortality: A review. *Popul. Index* 58: 186–212, 1992.

76. Keith, V. M., and Herring, C. Skin tone and stratification in the black community. *Am. J. Sociol.* 97: 760–778, 1991.

77. Klag, M. H., Whelton, P. K., and Coresh, J. The association of skin color with blood pressure in U.S. blacks with low socioeconomic status. *JAMA* 266: 599–602, 1991.

78. Arce, C. H., Murguia, E., and Frisbie, W. P. Phenotype and life chances among Chicanos. *Hispanic J. Behav. Sci.* 9: 19–32, 1987.
79. Franklin, J. H. *Color and Race*. Houghton Mifflin, Boston, 1968.
80. Frank, M. G., and Gilovich, T. The dark side of self- and social perception: Black uniforms and aggression in professional sports. *J. Pers. Soc. Psychol.* 54: 74–85, 1988.
81. Lieberson, S. *A Piece of the Pie: Black and White Immigrants since 1880*. University of California Press, Berkeley, 1980.

CHAPTER 6

Racial Ideology and Explanations for Health Inequalities among Middle-Class Whites

Carles Muntaner, Craig Nagoshi,
and Chamberlain Diala

In a recent article entitled "Race in Epidemiology" (1), Professor Stolley asked why, even when the concept of race has been rejected in genetics and anthropology, it is still used in epidemiology and social science. Recent articles have argued that racial ideology (i.e., racism) is common among educated upper-middle-class whites (2), including health professionals (3–6). In addition, several authors have challenged the common wisdom that using "race" as an implicit or explicit biological category to explain health inequalities is the consequence of white irrationality, an unfortunate legacy of the ideas of a remote past of slavery, or old scientific notions that are difficult to abandon (5). Instead, these critics argue that racial ideology justifies a social structure of economic, political, and cultural stratification that benefits whites in contemporary racial social systems (i.e., where race is a hierarchical social relation rather than a personal attribute) (3, 5–8). In this brief empirical report we provide some evidence in support of this view.

The significance of beliefs about race (i.e., racial ideology) in epidemiology has recently been highlighted (8, 9). Essential components of racial ideology are attributions about racial inequality (10). Whites' attributions for explaining racial inequalities have been quite stable in the United States over the last two decades. According to 1996 National Opinion Research Center surveys, close to one-third of U.S. whites point to discrimination as the main explanation for racial inequalities, while "low inborn ability" is openly selected by 10 percent and "low motivation" remains the *most popular* explanation (52 percent) (11). *More than 60 percent* of U.S. whites thus openly attribute racial inequalities to psychological or biological attributes.

Despite the potential of whites' explanations for racial inequalities in health to affect non-whites through social policies such as welfare reform and affirmative

183

action (12), there has been little research in this area. Several authors have highlighted the potential effect of whites' beliefs about racial inequalities in health on the type of questions asked in epidemiology (2–4) and health services (13). In this sociopsychological study we begin to examine the nature of attributions for racial inequalities in health among white university students, who by definition are likely to be involved in research, policy, and service professions. To test our hypothesis on the self-serving nature of middle-class whites' attributions for racial inequalities in health (e.g., Bonilla-Silva's objective interests; see 7),[1] we investigate the degree to which middle-class whites attribute racial inequalities in health to biological, social, or lifestyle factors. If whites tend to attribute their own better health to biology or lifestyle rather than to social factors, this would confirm our hypothesis. In addition, we examine the relationship between middle-class whites' attributions for racial inequalities, causal explanations for health (e.g., locus of control; see 15) and other attitudes (e.g., modern racism; see 16).

METHODS

Participants

Student participants were recruited through an introductory psychology class at Arizona State University. Psychologists are roughly representative of the attitudes of the U.S. upper middle class (17), while this discipline falls midway between biology and sociology, allowing for an expression of the full array of causal explanations about inequalities in health (18). Students earned research participation credits for completing the questionnaire (described below) during one of several scheduled group testing sessions on campus. There were no significant differences in sociodemographic composition between the participating sample and the rest of the student pool with regard to age, gender, race/ethnicity, and educational background. In all, 335 students (143 men, 192 women) completed the questionnaire, but our analyses are limited to the 256 participants (104 men, 152 women) of Caucasian ancestry (whites), as our goal was to study the attitudes of the dominant race and the number of non-white students was limited. The ethnic breakdown for the 76 non-white participants (three of 79 had missing data for this variable and were excluded) was 9 African-American, 29 Hispanic, 8 American Indian, 21 Asian-American, and 9 other. The mean age of the white subsample was 19.2 years (S.D. = 2.6). Based on the categorical scales described below, median father's and mother's education was college graduate, median father's social class was corporate manager or government administrator, and median mother's social class was small business owner or manager.

---

[1] Bonilla-Silva has fully extended to race the systemic-materialist approach that characterizes modern notions of class (14). For an application of similar notions of race to epidemiology and public health, see 3, 5, 6, and 8.

Measures

The questionnaire (available from the authors upon request) contained the following relevant items.

Social class background (Wright's mediated class location). Father's and mother's educational credentials were measured by seven-point scales ranging from 1 = less than 8th grade to 7 = postgraduate degree. Father's and mother's social class was measured by seven-point scales ranging from 1 = unemployed to 7 = professional (doctor, engineer, teacher, etc.). Participants were asked to rate the most recent occupation for retired parents.

Attributions for racial inequalities scale. This scale was developed to assess the degree to which individuals attributed the causes of inequalities in cardiovascular disease in a particular race to a particular type of explanation: biological, social, or lifestyle. The scale contains four items in each of the three types of causal explanations. Participants were told in the questionnaire, "Epidemiological studies in this country find large differences in the incidence and mortality rates of cardiovascular disease between Caucasians (whites), Asian Americans, African Americans (blacks), and American Indians." They then responded to the instruction, "Please rate the importance of the following causal factors in determining rates of cardiovascular disease in [the assigned group]," using a seven-point scale ranging from 1 = not important to 7 = very important. The questionnaires were collated, such that subjects were randomly assigned to rate one of the four racial/ethnic groups listed above. The *biological* subscale contained the items *genetic factors, family history of heart disease, physiological differences,* and *body type/shape differences.* The *social* subscale contained the items *lack of access to good medical care, socioeconomic factors* (e.g., income), *differences in education,* and *availability of health insurance.* The *lifestyle* subscale contained the items *lifestyle choices, lack of exercise, dietary differences,* and *stresses at work and home.* Alpha reliabilities for the three subscales for the present sample were 0.65, 0.77, and 0.77, respectively.

Health locus of control scale (15). This measure includes subscales for beliefs that control over one's health is *internal* (i.e., under one's control), based on *powerful others,* or based on *chance.* Alpha reliabilities for these three subscales for the present sample were 0.72, 0.73, and 0.56, respectively. Higher scores indicate a greater degree of belief in a given type of causal explanation for one's health (i.e., internal, powerful others, or chance).

Modern racism scale (16). This seven-item scale is intended to measure subtle but persistent racist attitudes against African Americans, higher scores indicating higher levels of racism. Alpha reliability for the present sample was 0.68.

Radicalism-conservatism scale (19). This 30-item scale measures social attitudes, with higher scores representing more "liberal" views. Alpha reliability for the present sample was 0.66.

Data Analysis

We used a mixed-design analysis of variance (ANOVA) to test the null hypothesis of no differences in causal attributions made by whites for racial inequalities in health across the four target race groups. Next, we used Pearson product-moment correlation to assess the strength of associations between beliefs in personal control over health (i.e., health locus of control), modern racism, liberal views, and causal explanations for racial inequalities in health.

RESULTS

Table 1 presents the means and standard deviations for the three health attributions subscales (biological, lifestyle, and social) across the four target racial groups (white, African-American, Asian-American, and American-Indian). A mixed-design analysis of variance yielded significant main effects for target group (F (3,244) = 3.37; $P < .05$), with white targets receiving higher attributions than non-white targets, and for type of attribution (F (2,488) = 106.49; $P < .001$), with lifestyle attributions rated higher than biological attributions, which in turn were rated higher than social attributions. This pattern of results is consistent with whites' use of self-serving attributions for threatening health-related events, with ("controllable") lifestyle attributions being more highly rated by whites for their own racial group. Because whites enjoy better cardiovascular health as a group, higher lifestyle attributions for whites means that whites tend to attribute their better health to their own "healthy behavior" (i.e., lifestyle). Although social attributions for African Americans were lowest, which was consistent with our hypothesis, the interaction between types of health attribution by racial group was not significant (F (6,488) = 1.32; n.s.).

Table 2 presents the correlation of the three health attributions subscales between the three health locus of control subscales, modern racism, and radicalism-conservatism for each of the target racial groups. Consistent with whites' self-serving attributions as interpreted above, internal health locus of control among whites is significantly and positively related to lifestyle attributions, particularly for the white-race group. For the white-race group, in turn, chance-based health locus of control is associated with biological attributions.

With the exception of modern racism's association with Asian-American targets, the modern racism and Comrey's social attitude scales were not related to causal health attributions. Correlations were also run for health attributions versus parental credentials and social class within each target racial group. These yielded a few statistically significant correlations, all of them consistent with our hypothesis: for white targets, father's social class had a correlation of 0.29 ($P < .05$) with biological attributions; for African-American targets, mother's social class had a correlation of –0.30 ($P < .05$) with social attributions.

Table 1

Means and standard deviations of causal attributions for racial inequalities in
cardiovascular health by target race/ethnicity and attribution type
among white college students (n = 256)[a,b]

| Race/ethnicity target group | Type of attribution for racial inequalities in health | | | | | |
| | Biological | | Social | | Lifestyle | |
	Mean	S.D.	Mean	S.D.	Mean	S.D.
White	5.19	0.79	4.39	1.29	5.71	0.90
Asian-American	4.70	1.19	4.25	1.37	5.36	1.18
African-American	4.66	0.99	3.84	1.29	5.15	1.15
American-Indian	4.88	1.29	4.36	1.48	5.25	1.34

Source	SS	df	MS	F	P
Race/ethnicity ethnic group	28.20	30	9.40	3.37	<.05
within cells	681.16	244	2.79		
Attribution type	167.31	20	83.65	106.49	<.001
Race/ethnicity × attribution	6.21	6	1.04	1.32	n.s.
within cells	383.33	488	0.79		

[a]Analyses for the 76 non-Caucasians, of whom 70 had complete data for the attributions ANOVA,
with roughly equal N's across the ethnic group targets: Race/ethnic group condition was nonsignificant
($F(3,66) = 1.04$; n.s.); type of attitude was highly significant ($F(2,132) = 17.44$; $P < .001$) and showing
the same pattern as for whites (biological mean = 4.75 (S.D. = 1.04), social mean = 4.44 (S.D. = 1.20),
lifestyle mean = 5.23 (S.D. = 1.05)). The interaction was nonsignificant ($F(6,132) = 1.33$; n.s.).

[b]SS, sum of squares; MS, mean square.

DISCUSSION

The upper-middle-class whites in our sample attributed racial inequalities in
cardiovascular disease mainly to lifestyle choice, followed by biological attributions. Lifestyle and biological causal explanations are self-serving for middle-
class whites because they enjoy better cardiovascular health as a group. Lifestyle
reflects beliefs in individual responsibility for health (20) as it explains racial
inequalities in health by autonomous choices of (21) (e.g., with regard to diet,
exercise, and smoking). This finding probably reflects the generalization of beliefs
in self-determination among whites (12) and among the middle class in particular
(22) to the explanation of health outcomes. Even in the face of well-documented

Table 2

Correlations of causal attributions for health with other scales by
target race/ethnicity

Attribution type	Health locus of control			Modern racism	Comrey radicalism-conservatism
	Internal	Powerful others	Chance		
White target					
Biological	0.20	−.10	0.25*	0.05	−0.02
Social	0.13	0.08	0.07	0.06	−0.26
Lifestyle	0.31*	−0.04	0.09	0.04	−0.11
Asian-American target					
Biological	−0.01	0.01	0.05	0.01	−0.10
Social	0.14	0.04	0.20	−0.14	−0.07
Lifestyle	0.18	−0.14	−0.10	0.30*	−0.03
African-American target					
Biological	0.03	0.23	0.09	0.09	−0.07
Social	−0.11	0.24	−0.06	0.07	−0.10
Lifestyle	0.21	0.10	0.12	−0.01	−0.08
American-Indian target					
Biological	0.22	−0.05	0.01	0.13	−0.20
Social	0.27*	0.27*	0.07	0.09	−0.13
Lifestyle	0.27*	−0.18	−0.07	0.16	−0.11
N (sample size)	60	63	64	63	56

*$P < .05$

lack of opportunity among most non-whites (23) and the growing rejection of race as a biological variable in the scientific community (2, 3, 4, 8), attributions of racial inequalities in health to social factors lagged behind biology. This result also suggests the presence of a protective self-serving bias among middle-class whites (21). Our interpretation is reinforced by the observed correlation between internal locus of control (i.e., the belief in personal control of one's life) and lifestyle attributions for whites' health. That is, whites' cardiovascular health outcomes are seen as the consequence of lifestyle choices that are under their own personal control, as opposed to, say, a consequence of greater access to better goods and services than non-whites due to a racial system that bars non-whites from those goods and services (5). Modern or "subtle" racism was associated with lifestyle attributions for the cardiovascular health of Asian Americans. This is consistent with the notion that Asian Americans compete in the labor market with middle-class whites and that publicly expressed prejudice against Asian Americans might not currently be as unacceptable as prejudice against African Americans or American Indians (11, 24–28). The lack of relationship between attributions for racial inequalities in health and the (social) conservatism-liberalism dimension is not so surprising. Recent surveys show little differences in racial ideology between self-identified Democrats and Republicans (10), and experiments suggest that the major differences in racial attitudes between self-defined liberals and conservatives are in the *open* expression of racial attitudes (13).

Our study has several limitations in its assessment of middle-class whites' causal explanations for racial inequalities. First, we separated "lifestyle" and "biology" attributions, but we did not measure attributions to "ethnicity," a concept that is currently used as an alternative to "race" in public health (29). Thus, the conflation of biology and culture (lifestyle) underlying "ethnicity" or "race/ethnicity" allows whites to attribute racial position to intrinsic attributes of "non-whites" and simultaneously avoid any social responsibility for the experiences of non-whites (30).

Furthermore, we did not assess attitudes toward capitalism. For example, neoliberal attitudes claiming that employment discrimination will soon disappear under competitive market forces might be associated with attribution of racial inequalities in health to culture or biology. The consequence of such attitudes is that the best solution to racial inequalities is to deepen privatization and markets in every aspect of social life. After almost 150 years of African-American experience in postslavery capitalism, it is clear that racial equality has not been experienced by any single generation of African Americans. Therefore, these utopian procapitalist attitudes might promote what has been called "laissez-faire racism" (31).

Overall our results highlight the causal attributions of personal responsibility for racial inequalities in health that might be used by upper-middle-class whites to explain health data broken down by racial categories (3–5). Because middle-class whites have a large influence in generating public health policy and public opinion about racial inequalities in the United States (32), more research is needed to ascertain the generality of our results in population-based studies. Research is also needed to establish the social origins and possible consequences (12, 21) of the so-called "fundamental attribution error" (i.e., the strong tendency to attribute health outcomes to "free will" rather than social circumstances) for public health research and policies (33).

We agree with the conclusion that the concept of race should be reexamined in epidemiology and social science (3–6). We also agree, against the current wisdom that tends to single out epidemiology as the major culprit in propagating the notion of biological determinism, that social science, too, treats race as an implicitly biological or psychological variable (7, 8). In the light of our results on racial ideology among upper-middle-class whites, as well as additional current literature

(7), the most heuristic research program seems to call for a rejection of biological as well as *pragmatic or empiricist* uses of race that perpetuate the status quo (i.e., racial inequalities) and thwart progress in understanding the effects of racism and its relation to class interests, including the racialization of the U.S. working class (5, 6). Epidemiology and social science should thus study race as a social relation in class societies, with researchers investigating the health effects of racial economic exploitation, racial political oppression, and racial ideology (racism) (5). This would allow epidemiology to catch up not only with the theoretical and empirical standards of contemporary anthropology, but with the egalitarian values of public health as well.

Acknowledgment — The authors would like to acknowledge the comments of Eduardo Bonilla-Silva and Sandra Picot.

REFERENCES

1. Stolley, P. D. Race in epidemiology. *Int. J. Health Serv.* 29: 905–909, 1999.
2. Verba, S. *Elites and the Idea of Equality.* Harvard University Press, Cambridge, Mass., 1987.
3. Muntaner, C., Nieto, F. J., and O'Campo, P. The Bell Curve: On race class, and epidemiologic research. *Am. J. Epidemiol.* 144(6): 531–536, 1996.
4. Muntaner, C., Nieto, F. J., and O'Campo, P. Additional clarification re: The Bell Curve: On race, social class, and epidemiologic research. *Am. J. Epidemiol.* 146(7): 607–608, 1997.
5. Muntaner, C. Social mechanisms, race and social epidemiology. *Am. J. Epidemiol.* 150(2): 121–126, 1999.
6. Muntaner, C., Oates, G., and Lynch, J. The social class determinants of income inequality and social cohesion. *Int. J. Health Serv.* 29(4): 715–732, 1999.
7. Bonilla-Silva, E. Rethinking racism: Towards a structural interpretation. *Am. Sociol. Rev.* 62(3): 465–480, 1997.
8. Krieger, N., et al. Racism, sexism and social class. *Am. J. Prev. Med.* 9(Suppl. 2): 82–122, 1993.
9. Williams, D. R. Race and health: Basic questions, emerging directions. *Ann. Epidemiol.* 45: 1075–1087, 1997.
10. Hurwitz, J., and Peffley, M. *Perception and Prejudice.* Yale University Press, New Haven, 1999.
11. Schuman, H., et al. *Racial Attitudes in America: Trends and Interpretations.* Harvard University Press, Cambridge, Mass., 1997.
12. Gilens, M. *Why Americans Hate Welfare.* University of Chicago Press, Chicago, 1999.
13. Whaley, A. L. Racism in the provision of mental health services: A social-cognitive analysis. *Am. J. Orthopsychiatr.* 68: 47–57, 1998.
14. Navarro, V. *Dangerous to Your Health: Capitalism in Health Care.* Monthly Review Press, New York, 1993.
15. Wallston, K. A., Wallston, B. S., and DeVellis, R. Development of the multi-dimensional health locus of control (MHLC) scales. *Health Educ. Monogr.* 6: 161–170, 1978.

16. McConahay, J. B., Hardee, B. B., and Batts, V. Has racism declined in America? It depends on who is asking and what is asked. *J. Conflict Resol.* 25: 563–579, 1981.

17. Frank, R. H., Meyer, J. W., and Miyahara, D. The individualist polity and the prevalence of professionalized psychology: A cross-national study. *Am. Sociol. Rev.* 60: 360–377, 1995.

18. Eysenck, H. J., and Eysenck, S. *Textbook of Human Psychology.* Oxford University Press, Oxford, 1985.

19. Comrey, A., and Newmeyer, J. Measurement of radicalism-conservatism. *J. Soc. Psychol.* 67: 357–369, 1965.

20. Krieger, N., and Zierler, S. What explains the public's health: A call for epidemiologic theory. *Epidemiology* 7: 107–109, 1996.

21. Knight, E. In their own words. In *Perception and Prejudice,* edited by J. Hurwitz and M. Peffley, pp. 202–232. Yale University Press, New Haven, 1999.

22. Phelan, J., et al. Education, social liberalism, and economic liberalism: Attitudes towards homeless people. *Am. Sociol. Rev.* 60: 126–140, 1996.

23. Conley, D. *Being Black, Living in the Red.* University of California Press, Berkeley, 1999.

24. Devine, P. G., and Elliot, A. J. Are racial attitudes really fading? *Personal. Soc. Psychol. Bull.* 21: 1139–1150, 1995.

25. Gandy, O. H., et al. Race and risk: Factors affecting the framing of histories about inequality, discrimination, and just plain bad luck. *Public Opinion Q.* 61: 158–182, 1997.

26. Sidanius, J. Racial discrimination and job evaluation: The case of university faculty. *Natl. J. Sociol.* 3: 223–256, 1989.

27. Thatchenkery, T. J., and Cheng, C. Seeing beneath the surface to appreciate what "is": A call for balanced inquiry and consciousness raising regarding Asian Americans in organizations. *J. Appl. Behav. Sci.* 33: 397–406, 1997.

28. Krysan, M. Privacy and the expression of white racial attitudes: A comparison across three contexts. *Public Opinion Q.* 62: 506–544, 1998.

29. Crews, D. E., and Bindon, J. R. Ethnicity as a taxonomic tool in biomedical and biosocial research. *Ethnic. Dis.* 1(1): 42–49, 1991.

30. Essed, P. *Understanding Everyday Racism.* Sage, London, 1992.

31. Feagin, J. R. *Racist America.* Routledge, New York, 2000.

32. Sniderman, P. M., Brody, R. A., and Tetlock, P. E. *Reasoning and Choice: Explanations in Political Psychology.* Cambridge University Press, Cambridge, 1991.

33. Muntaner, C., Eaton, W. W., and Diala, C. Social inequalities in mental health: A review of concepts and underlying assumptions. *Health* 4(1): 89–111, 2000.

CHAPTER 7

Income Dynamics and Health

Greg J. Duncan

Socioeconomic status (SES) is a pervasive and persistent correlate of health status (1, 2). A robust inverse association between SES and morbidity and mortality is evident from our earliest records and exists in all countries where the relationship between these factors has been examined (3, 4). More than a threshold pattern in which some minimal level of SES distinguishes the healthy from the unhealthy, the relationship between SES and health is better described as a continuous but nonlinear "gradient," with large improvements in health associated with increments in SES at low levels of SES and smaller improvements in health associated with increments in SES at higher levels of SES.

Links between SES and health are not well understood (2, 5). Do low-SES individuals have worse health and shorter life expectancy because of a gradual process of accumulation of disadvantages in the form of reduced access to health care, polluted or accident-prone home and work environments, worse health behavior (e.g., smoking, drinking, and diet), or more stressful and less-supportive family, neighborhood, and employment situations (6, 7)? Or are many of the health differences the result of shorter-run differences in access to economic resources that could be addressed with tax- and transfer-induced changes in the distribution of income? To what extent are linkages between SES and health the spurious result of shared correlations with genetic differences in health status, in which persistent and typically unobserved frailty leads to both lower SES and worse health?

As one might deduce from the term itself, the concept of socioeconomic status is a somewhat nebulous one in the social sciences (8). Past research has used several different indicators of SES, with the choice usually dictated by the available data. British studies of the linkages between SES and health (e.g., 9, 10)

This research was supported by the National Institute for Child Health and Human Development through its Family and Child Well-being Research Network.

typically rely on an occupation-based measure since that is often provided on vital statistics records. Cross-national comparative studies (e.g., 11) often find that years of schooling is the SES measure most comparable across countries. U.S.-based research has measured SES as occupational categories and characteristics (e.g., 12, 13) and prestige (e.g., 14), education (e.g., 15), household income (e.g., 16), and areal measures such as the poverty rate in an individual's neighborhood (17). The proliferation of various measures of SES has obscured rather than clarified the possible causal linkages between SES and health.

The focus of this chapter is on the economic dimension of SES, in particular a household's total income. Most health research focused on SES has not used an income-based measure; important exceptions based on a variety of data sets have established that household income is a powerful correlate of mortality (12, 16, 18), that the beneficial effect of income on mortality appears larger at lower levels of income than at higher levels, and that the strength of the correlation between income and mortality has, if anything, increased over the last 30 years (19). Although these analyses have yielded valuable insights, they are based on income measured over a single annual accounting period and close in time to the possible death, running the risk that the income-mortality correlation reflects the effect of ill-health on income rather than the reverse. In addition, research using income as a measure of SES has usually been forced to rely on low-quality income data and has often failed to control for other, correlated components of SES.

Important income fluctuations occur at the macro level, as the economy flounders during periods of recession, expands during periods of economic growth, or, as has been the case in the past two decades, is marked by a growing disparity between the incomes of the rich and the poor. Some of these macroeconomic fluctuations are translated into income changes among individual households. Recession-induced layoffs cut into a family's total income, while a growing economy boosts wages, creates jobs, and provides opportunities for overtime work, all of which increase a family's income. This chapter presents a brief review of macro-level developments in the United States, focusing on evidence of a striking increase in inequality in the distribution of household income in the United States over the past 25 years.

The discussion focuses mainly on the dynamic aspects of household income and their possible links to health at the micro level. Most prior studies have been limited by having only minimal measures of SES at a single point in time, and researchers have assumed, at least implicitly, that SES does not change much over time. As with recent occupation-based research that has uncovered linkages between mortality and occupational mobility (12, 13), it is fruitful to explore the health consequences of income-based mobility.

I question the conventional wisdom that views household income, apart from predictable life-cycle fluctuations, as fairly constant across time. In fact, household income is quite volatile, even during periods of macroeconomic stability, with fluctuations linked to family and employment-related events such as divorce, widowhood, marriage, or unemployment. A surprising degree of volatility is evident among the elderly. As a result, conceptions of poverty need to distinguish between transitory and persistent components, as do measures of affluence. More generally, it is important to distinguish between average level, trend, and stability components of income-based SES.

Also crucial is an attempt to distinguish the causal effects of income on health, since a household's income level is the component of SES most amenable to change through redistributive policies such as food stamps or Supplementary Security Income transfer programs. Most studies have not attempted to disentangle the causal role played by income because most data sets with high-quality health measures lack high-quality prospective, longitudinal measurement of income. Those studies that have been based on the necessary data tend to find powerful effects of income on health, even after controlling for differences in extensive sets of other measures of SES. I will review several of these studies and discuss their implications for policy and for future research on the SES-health linkage.

MACROECONOMIC CHANGES IN
THE DISTRIBUTION OF HOUSEHOLD INCOME

"Income dynamics" to most people probably connotes changes in the nation's aggregate income as the economy moves in and out of periods of growth and recession. Business cycles have always been with us and will continue to be. Brenner (20) presents suggestive evidence, based on aggregate data, that economic recessions are associated with increased mortality.

Periods of recession and growth affect household as well as aggregate income, as can be seen by the fluctuations in the household income of prime-age (25-to 54-year-old) U.S. adults depicted in Figures 1 and 2. Figure 1 shows the time path from 1969 to 1991 of inflation-adjusted household incomes separating: (a) the highest-income 10 percent (90th percentile) of the adult population from the rest; (b) the top and bottom half (i.e., median) of the adult population (50th percentile); and (c) the lowest-income 10 percent (10th percentile) of adults from the rest.

Looking first at the experiences of adults in the middle of the income distribution, we can see that income grew little over this period. The median adult had a household income (in 1992 dollars) of about $40,000 in 1969 and about $41,000 22 years later. The median income drops consistently during recession years, which are denoted by rectangles in the figure, and increase somewhat during periods of macroeconomic growth. Business-cycle-induced fluctuations are also evident in the time series of breakpoints at the top and bottom deciles of the income distribution.

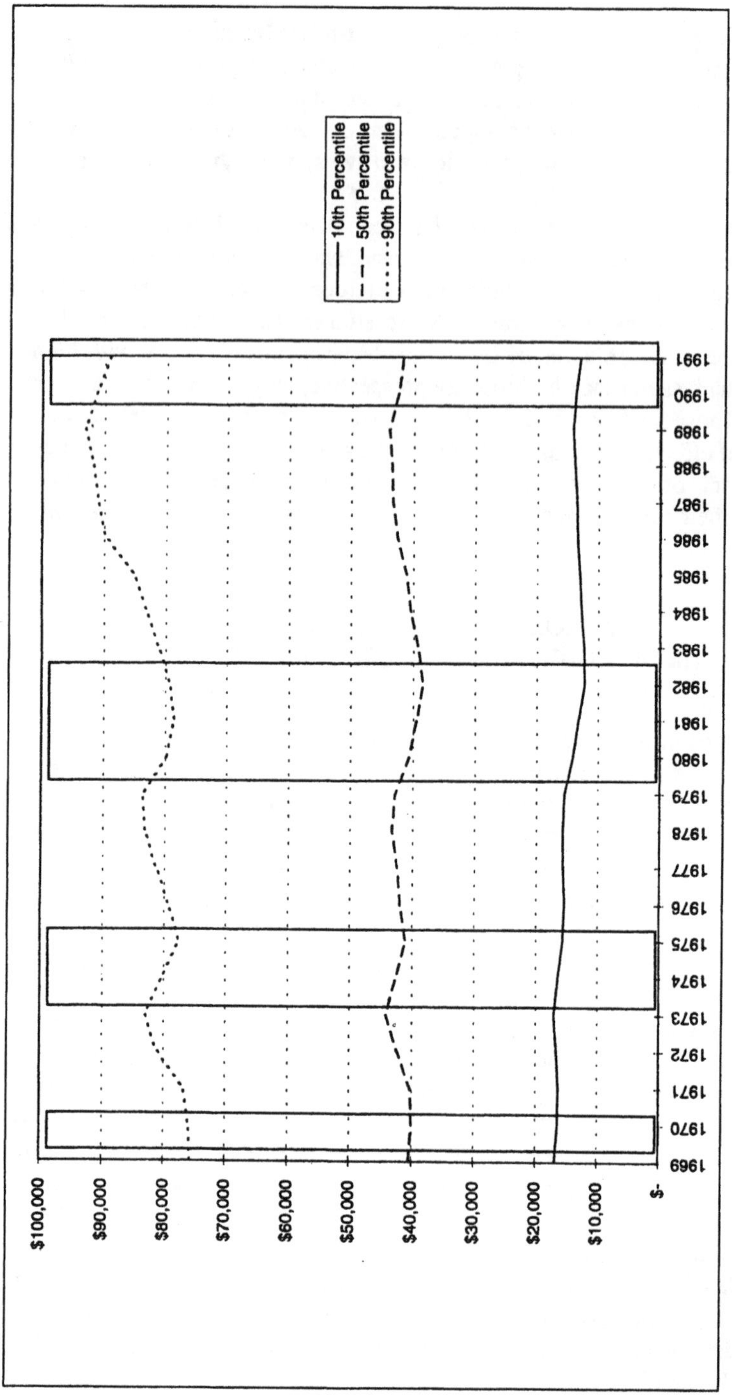

Figure 1. 10th, 50th, and 90th percentile points in household income distribution in 1992 dollars, by year, 25- to 54-year-old adults; all incomes inflated to 1992 price levels using the Consumer Price Index. The rectangles denote periods of recession. Source: Data from U.S. Current Population Reports (32); Current Population Surveys are conducted each year by the Census Bureau and are the primary source of data on poverty and income distribution.

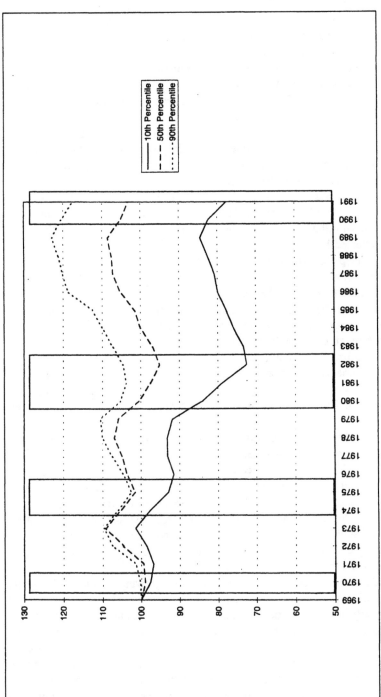

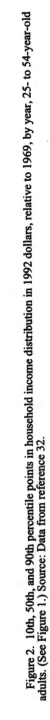

Figure 2. 10th, 50th, and 90th percentile points in household income distribution in 1992 dollars, relative to 1969, by year, 25- to 54-year-old adults. (See Figure 1.) Source: Data from reference 32.

A more revealing, relative, picture of income trends is provided by Figure 2, which takes the data on the three income time series shown in Figure 1 and standardizes them so that the 1969 levels are set equal to 100. Here we see that the proportionate impact of recession tends to be somewhat larger at the bottom of the income distribution than at the top. This was particularly true in the sharp recession in the early 1980s, where the relative drop in the bottom-decile income was more than twice that of the top decile.

But to focus on business-cycle-induced changes in the U.S. income distribution over the past quarter century misses the main point. What is truly new and dramatic at the aggregate level is the enormous growth in the inequality of the distribution of income over the period. Were the extent of income inequality to have remained constant, as was roughly the case between the end of World War II and the end of the 1960s, then the lines depicted in Figure 2 would all be at the same height, with the height determined by the change in income relative to its inflation-adjusted 1969 level.

In fact, the paths are very different: individuals at the top of the income distribution enjoyed modest (about 18 percent) increases in their inflation-adjusted standards of living between 1969 and 1991, while individuals in the lower rungs saw their living standards drop precipitously. The bottom-decile breakpoint was some 22 percent lower in 1991 than 1969.

The picture of growing household income inequality since the mid-1970s has been confirmed in countless studies (e.g., 21). Aggregate data from the National Income Accounts and from wealth surveys (22–24) reinforce this conclusion by showing a growing share of income from capital, a falling share for earnings, and a slightly increasing concentration of wealth among upper-income groups.

Underlying these changes in total household income is a growing inequality in the distribution of earned income, which has occurred not only in the United States but in Western European countries as well (25, 26). Younger and less-educated workers have been especially hard hit. Although the reasons for the growing inequality are still the subject of debate, many researchers point to technological changes in the structure of work that have increased demand for the kinds of skills held by better-educated and more experienced workers and the declining demand for factory-based manual labor typically performed by less-skilled workers.

There are several important implications of this growing inequality for health (27). One results from the nonlinear nature of the association between income and health (28, 29). Most correlational evidence shows that changes in income have a bigger impact on health at low income than at high income levels. In the context of a stagnant macroeconomic environment, growing income inequality causes a drop in the incomes of low-income households and an increase in the incomes of high-income households. If the nonlinear associations between income and health are causal, then growing inequality should worsen the health of individuals in low-income households. Furthermore, in the absence of overall improvement in living standards, growing inequality should cause a decline in the overall health of the population since the decrements in the health of low-income individuals more than offset the improvement in the health of high-income individuals.

Kawachi and associates (27) argue that the effect of income inequality per se on health may be due to people's perception of fairness of their society. Noting evidence that mortality can also increase during periods of rapid economic growth, they suggest that unfulfilled expectations can lead to frustration and stress.

Whatever the reason, evidence from cross-national studies of developed countries confirms that both the level of income and the degree of inequality in its distribution have independent effects on mortality (30, 31).

DYNAMIC ASPECTS
OF HOUSEHOLD-LEVEL INCOME

Income fluctuations can also be observed at the micro level—that is, for individual households across time. Perhaps the most prevalent conception of household-income fluctuations is that they consist of fairly predictable life-cycle changes experienced by individuals as they age. In this view, early adulthood is often seen as a period of relatively low income as career and marital arrangements are being sorted out. Income grows as careers stabilize and, in some cases, blossom and as multiple earners in households increase the household's total income. Pre-retirement years are often the time of maximum household income *per person*, since children have often departed from the parental nest but there is still labor income from one or possibly two adults at the peak of their earning power. Retirement often occasions a drop in both nominal income and work-related expenses. Increasingly generous social security payments have cushioned the income loss brought about by retirement, as have private pensions and other forms of asset income for individuals who acquired these forms of wealth during their working years.

This life-cycle view of income fluctuations conforms closely to (and, indeed, has been developed from) family-income data drawn from representative cross-sections of the population. Life-cycle household income data presented in Table 1 are taken from the Census Bureau's 1992 Current Population Survey and show 1991 median and per-person household income by age of the householder (32, Table 8).

These data show higher levels of household income for older individuals until the late 40s, and then falling levels at older ages. Adjustment for family size pushes the peak income years to the late 50s and increases the relative well-being of households headed by the elderly, most of whom live independently of their children. If we succumb to the temptation to use these cross-sectional data on different families at various life-cycle stages to represent the likely economic path of individuals as they age, then we might view income trajectories as fairly

Table 1

Median household income and average household income per person,
by age of householder, 1991[a]

Age of householder	Median household income, thousands 1991 $	Average household income per household member, thousands 1991 $
15–24	$18.3	$ 9.0
25–29	28.6	12.0
30–34	32.7	12.3
35–39	37.1	13.0
40–44	41.7	14.8
45–49	44.4	16.7
50–54	43.0	18.6
55–59	37.0	18.8
60–64	29.7	17.6
65–69	22.1	15.5
70–74	17.8	14.1
75+	13.9	12.8
All ages	$30.1	$14.4

[a]Source: reference 32, Table 8.

smooth, with major fluctuations occurring infrequently and at discrete points of the life cycle such as early adulthood and retirement.

To what extent does this picture change when longitudinal patterns of income are observed directly? Using data from the Panel Study of Income Dynamics (PSID), Duncan (33) presents various data on the level, trend, and stability of household income by age over the 11-year period between 1969 and 1979. An extension of this analysis by Burkhauser and Duncan (34) shows that the basic patterns changed little between the 1970s and late 1980s. Some of these data are presented in Table 2. Since the longitudinal experiences of men and women are quite different, the household income data are presented separately by sex.

The first column in Table 2 shows that the average level of family income over the 11-year period displays typical life-cycle patterns. As with the data from the Current Population Survey, household incomes are highest for individuals who spent the entire period in their prime earning years and somewhat lower for the initially 46 to 55 year olds, some of whom will have retired during the 11-year period. Most retirements occur among individuals in the next older cohort, who were between the ages of 56 and 65 when the 11-year period began. The average household incomes of this group were substantially

Table 2

Level, trends, and stability of inflation-adjusted and household-size-adjusted household income, 1969–1979, by age and sex[a]

Age in 1969/sex	Avg. level, thousands 1985 $	Avg. level of I:N[b]	Avg. annual growth in I:N	Percent with I:N growing >5% per yr	Percent with I:N falling by >5% per yr	I:N fell by 50% or more at least once	Income loss expected	Poor at least once	Poor for 6 or more yrs
25–45 yrs									
Men	$43.1	4.2	2.9%	35%	6%	18%	9%	13%	2%
Women	40.0	3.9	2.2	32	10	24	6	20	5
46–55 yrs									
Men	38.7	4.7	1.1	22	13	26	12	14	3
Women	32.3	4.4	0.4	21	20	33	24	21	6
56–65 yrs									
Men	29.5	4.3	–3.4	7	38	38	34	17	4
Women	22.1	3.5	–3.1	6	35	39	25	27	9
66–75 yrs									
Men	20.4	3.2	–1.3	6	17	27	42	20	9
Women	16.2	2.6	–1.1	11	16	27	28	35	11

[a]Source: reference 33.
[b]I:N, income-to-needs ratio.

lower than those of individuals in all of the younger cohorts. Incomes of the members of the oldest cohort, all of whom were beyond age 65 when the period began, are the lowest of all.

The gap between the family incomes of men and women increases substantially over the life cycle as a result of the increasing proportion of women without spouses who head their own families. The income gap is below 10 percent in the prime earnings years (e.g., $43,100 versus $40,000 for the 25- to 44-year-olds) and increases to roughly 20 percent for the older cohorts.

Adjustments for family size produce a different life-cycle pattern, especially at older ages. The Census-Bureau-based data in Table 1 were adjusted for family size with a simple division of household income by the number of family members. A more satisfactory method for making family-size adjustments is by dividing family income by the U.S. government's annually calculated poverty thresholds for families with different compositions, producing what has been termed an "income-to-needs" ratio. The poverty threshold for a family of four in 1992 dollars was $14,335. A family of four with a family income of $43,000 would thus have an income-to-needs ratio of 3.0. A family of four with an income of $7,168 would be deemed poor and have an income-to-needs ratio of 0.5.

The emptying nests of parents in the 46- to 55-year age range make them better off in terms of size-adjusted income than the younger cohorts. The economic gap between the sexes is somewhat smaller when one uses the income-to-needs measure, although men in the oldest two age cohorts still enjoy a 15 to 20 percent higher standard of living than women of the same ages.

A unique advantage of panel data is that they make it possible to trace the economic fortunes of the same individuals over substantial portions of their life course. Duncan (33) computed a measure of trend in economic status, defined as the annual average growth rate in size-adjusted family income over the 11-year period 1969–1979. As with the average income figures, the Consumer Price Index was used to deflate each dollar figure, so the calculated growth rate is real rather than nominal. Families with positive real growth rates are those who did better than inflation, and families with negative growth rates are those who did worse. The size of the growth rate is analogous to a compound interest rate. Over an 11-year period, an annual real growth rate of 5 percent will increase a family's real income by over 70 percent; a negative 5 percent rate will cut it almost in half.

The pattern of average growth rates shown in the third column of Table 2 is heavily age-dependent. Prime-age men had the most positive growth; their 2.9 percent average growth rate produced a nearly 40 percent increase in living standards when compounded over the 11-year period. Individuals beginning the period in the pre-retirement, 56- to 65-year-old cohort experienced the most negative changes; the –3.4 percent growth rate for men in this group reduced their standards of living by about one-third over an 11-year period. Average annual changes for women were less positive prior to middle age and less negative afterward when compared with those of their male counterparts.

To what extent do these age-related averages conceal diverse individual experiences? The fourth and fifth columns of Table 2 show the fractions of the sample in various age and sex groups with either very rapid growth (more than 5 percent per year) or sharp declines (falling by more than 5 percent per year) in living standards over the period. Several startling facts emerge, the foremost of which is the prevalence of either large positive or large negative changes in living standards. With the exceptions of 46- to 55-year-old men and post-retirement men and women, at least 40 percent of all groups experienced either large positive or negative changes in income-to-needs. And even among the elderly, for whom economic fortunes are presumed most stable, more than one-quarter experienced either large positive or negative changes. Life-cycle average income figures do indeed obscure a great deal of offsetting change at the individual level.

Large changes in income-to-needs are concentrated among certain age groups. Rapid increases are heavily concentrated in the early adult years, while most of the rapid decreases occur for the retirement cohort. But these groups failed to account for most of the rapid increases and decreases; there are substantial risks of income decline at younger ages and some rapid income increases at older ages.

Duncan's (33) examination of the incidence of adverse economic changes focused on instances in which size-adjusted income fell by 50 percent or more in consecutive years. As reviewed below, this yardstick is similar to that employed by Elder and Liker in their studies of the effects of the Great Depression. They found long-lasting effects of income drops of one-third or more. However, the period over which Duncan measures change is shorter than theirs, his income measure is adjusted for family size, and the cutoff he employs—a 50 percent or greater fall—is somewhat larger.

The incidence of sharp drops in income-to-needs over the life course is shown in the sixth column of Table 2. The overall risk is high: roughly one-third of the population is estimated to have experienced such a drop at least once during the 11-year period. Virtually all of these decreases left the individuals involved with, at best, modest incomes. Some 87 percent of the individuals experiencing these decreases saw their family incomes fall to less than $25,000 (data not shown in Table 2). Not surprisingly, such declines are observed most frequently among the retirement cohort. Again defying the stereotype of economic stability, these data show that more than one-quarter of the elderly experience at least one large drop in their living standards. At younger ages, the risk of income loss is substantially higher for women than men.

Since the PSID asks questions regarding respondents' expectations of future changes in economic status (after a sequence of other questions about household income, PSID respondents were asked "What about the next few years, do you think you will be better off, or worse off, or what?"), it is possible to calculate what fraction of the income drops were preceded by a report that the respondent expected his or her family economic status to decline. The seventh column of Table 2 shows that a majority of all income declines and the vast majority of pre-retirement income declines were unexpected.

Duncan (33) investigated links between the incidence of major income losses and various economic and demographic events such as divorce, death, unemployment, illness, retirement, and disability. Overall, more than half of the income losses can be linked to at least one of the events, with different events being stronger at some points in the life cycle than at others (data not shown in Table 2). Nearly one-quarter of the sharp income-to-needs losses experienced by the 56- to 65-year-old men could be linked to retirement or disability. Divorce or separation could be linked to about one-tenth of the income losses experienced by young adult women, but was much less prominent in the income losses of older women and of men of any age. Widowhood and the moving out of children and other relatives from the home figured most prominently in income losses of older women. Unemployment could be linked to between one-tenth and one-fifth of the income losses of "prime-age" adults and appeared to be considerably more important for these groups than illness-related work losses. Finally, decreases in the market work of wives and, especially, other family members proved surprisingly important for the income-to-needs drops experienced by the pre-retirement cohorts.

In sum, these event-based patterns were consistent with the evidence linking the income losses to expectations: income losses occurring later in life, especially for men near the retirement age of 65, appeared more predictable and linked to the mostly voluntary reductions in work hours by family members. However, income losses occurring during the "prime" working years are not very predictable and, insofar as they can be linked to events, appear to be to a greater extent the result of involuntary rather than voluntary events.

The U.S. government poverty thresholds can also be used to classify years in which an individual's household income falls short of what is judged necessary to cover basic needs. Many descriptions of poverty experiences are possible with the 11-year time period provided by the PSID; perhaps the simplest is a count of the number of years out of the 11 in which an individual lived in a family with total annual income that fell short of the poverty threshold in that year. Such a measure combines information on the level of family resources and the stability of those resources. If poverty were a persistent condition, then the sample would cluster at one of two points—no poverty at all or poverty in all of the 11 years. If much contact with poverty is occasional, then we would expect that the persistently poor would be a small subset of the larger group that had at least some experience with poverty.

The last two columns of Table 2 show what fractions of individuals in the various age-sex groups spent (*a*) at least one of the 11 years below the poverty line and (*b*) more than half of the time (at least six of 11 years) in poverty. The difference in the sizes of these two groups at all stages in the life cycle is striking, indicating the temporary nature of much poverty (35). Depending on the life-cycle stage, between 20 and 35 percent of the women in the sample experienced poverty at least once during the 11-year period. Poverty experiences were most frequent among older women, although they were by no means uncommon for women in their prime years. The risk of poverty was much lower for adult men than women, especially at later life-cycle stages.

Persistent poverty, defined as living in poverty for more than half of the 11-year period, characterized fewer than one-ninth of any of the subgroups. Patterns of persistent poverty over the life course are less differentiated by age, especially for women. An elderly woman's chance of experiencing persistent poverty was roughly that of a 25- to 44-year-old woman and more than five times higher than that of a 25- to 44-year-old man.

LINKS BETWEEN
INCOME DYNAMICS AND HEALTH

The empirical patterns of family income over the life cycle confirm the conventional wisdom that average incomes rise until close to retirement and fall subsequently. But longitudinal data show that it is a mistake to treat this path of average incomes as the typical income course of individuals as they age. Family incomes are quite volatile at nearly every point in the life cycle, making rapid growth or decline in living standards more the rule than the exception. We do not have to look, as Elder and his colleagues have done, to the Great Depression to find frequent instances of economic loss and hardship; the risk of sharp decreases in living standards is still significant at virtually every stage of life. Most of the losses are unexpected. These losses occur despite our system of government and intrafamily transfers that might be expected to reduce or eliminate them.

Among the three dimensions of economic status—level, trend, and stability— the level of average income is surely the most important. Assuming that poverty thresholds are valid indicators of material deprivation, then the poverty incidence and prevalence figures given above show that substantial minorities of individuals are at risk of at least occasional poverty at every stage in the life cycle.

But what about income fluctuations in and of themselves? Few would argue with the propositions that, *ceteris paribus*, higher incomes are better than lower ones, rising incomes are better than falling ones, and stable incomes are better than unstable incomes. But these simple propositions become less clear-cut when one takes into account differences in the conditions that produce income variability. Children leave parental homes and older parents decide not to move in with their adult children, despite economic advantages they would otherwise enjoy, because they value their independence. Although their incomes are lower than before retirement, retired individuals may be better off because they have more leisure time than when they worked, and the predictability of retirement has allowed them time to prepare for its financial and psychological consequences. Despite their unstable incomes, construction workers may be well off because their higher rates of pay compensate them for the instability of their jobs. In short, not all instances of income instability have the same negative implications.

Some have argued that predictable income variability over the life cycle is of little analytic and policy interest (36). Underlying this conclusion are several implicit arguments against concern for predictable fluctuations and against policy interventions aimed at dealing with these fluctuations: (a) steps can be taken to insure against the effects of predictable change, as when the income loss associated with retirement is offset by forced (Social Security, some private pensions) or voluntary savings (Individual Retirement Accounts) to balance consumption between the middle and later years; (b) implementing policies to mitigate the effects of income fluctuations, predictable or otherwise, may discourage productive effort, self-insurance, and the support of family and friends, as when unemployment compensation increases the duration of unemployment (37) or Aid to Families with Dependent Children discourages work (38); and (c) predictability lessens the psychological impact of an adverse economic change (39–40). These propositions suggest that it is crucial to classify income fluctuations according to their predictability and to direct less analytic and policy attention to predictable fluctuations.

It is also important to research the consequences of income level, change, and instability—under what circumstances do they permanently alter the health and development of the individuals involved? We have relatively little evidence on this important question because few data sets combine reliable longitudinal information on family income with well-measured subsequent physiological or psychological outcomes. Much more is known about the consequences of events such as widowhood, unemployment, or divorce that are often associated with income variability, but it is impossible to disentangle the effects of income changes per se from other aspects of the events without measures of both. Such knowledge is crucial for the design of policies to mitigate the adverse effects of income loss. Do, for example, the adverse effects of unemployment on mental health or family stability stem from its more easily remedied *financial* consequences or from the *psychological* consequences of job loss (41, 42)? To what extent are the adverse effects of divorce on children a function of the income losses associated with divorce?

A number of studies have been conducted using data sets that contain (a) prospective, longitudinal measurement of income, (b) measures of other elements of SES, and (c) high-quality measures of health and development. The following is a selective review of these studies, emphasizing the nature of the linkages between dynamic aspects of income and the health outcomes at various stages of life.

Miller and Korenman Study of the Effects of Permanent Income-to-Needs on Children's Nutritional Status

Using data from the National Longitudinal Survey of Youth, Miller and Korenman (43) relate single-year and ten-year average family income to the prevalence of low height-for-weight (stunting) and low weight-for-height (wasting) among children.[1] Their sample is nationally representative of children born to women who were aged 23 to 30 years as of January 1, 1988. Height and weight were assessed in 1988. Data on total family income were gathered in annual interviews conducted with the mothers over the 11-year period from 1978 to 1988. As with the PSID data presented in Table 2, Miller and Korenman adjust family income for family size using the official U.S. poverty threshold, obtaining an income-to-needs ratio that is averaged over their ten-year accounting period.

Of particular interest are comparisons between the effects of income measured in a single year (1988) and over a ten-year period (1978–1987). Table 3 reproduces their key results, which are taken from four logistic regressions that include an extensive set of control variables: age, race, sex, birth order, and number of siblings of the child; marital status, age at first birth, educational attainment, Armed Forces Qualifying Test score, height, and body mass index of the mother; and whether the child was low weight or short length at birth. Income results are expressed as deviations from the omitted category of children living in families with the highest level of income-to-needs (i.e., incomes at least three times the poverty line).

Miller and Korenman find that their single-year measure of size-adjusted family income is never a significant predictor of stunting or wasting, once they adjust for the effects of their extensive set of control variables (regressions 1 and 3 in Table 3). In contrast, almost all categories of their ten-year average income measure are statistically significant at the 5 percent level.[2] Miller and Korenman also reported that with the exception of the effect of mother's education on wasting, none of the other SES-related measures are statistically

---

[1] Miller and Korenman use height-for-weight and weight-for-height standards calculated by the National Center for Health Statistics and the World Health Organization. A child is classified as "stunted" if his or her height is below the tenth percentile for children of the same age and sex, and "wasted" if his or her weight is below the tenth percentile for children of the same age and sex.

[2] Not surprisingly, the effects of income are generally stronger in a version of their models that only controls for age, race, and sex of the child. Respective odds ratios for ten-year average income-to-needs and the stunting outcome are 2.5, 2.5, 2.1, and 1.7. Corresponding odds ratios for the wasting outcome are 2.2, 1.7, 1.5, and 1.5.

Table 3

Effects of single-year and ten-year average household income on
children's stunting and wasting[a]

	Stunting[b]		Wasting[b]	
	O.R.	95% C.I.	O.R.	95% C.I.
1988 income:needs	Regression #1		Regression #3	
<0.5	1.0	0.5–2.0	1.3	0.8–2.3
0.5–1.0	1.0	0.6–1.6	1.4	0.9–2.3
1.0–1.85	1.0	0.6–1.5	1.4	0.9–2.2
1.85–3.0	1.2	0.8–1.8	1.4	0.9–2.0
3.0+ (omitted category)	1.0		1.0	
1978–87 income:needs	Regression #2		Regression #4	
<0.5	1.7	0.9–3.4	2.9	1.4–5.6
0.5–1.0	1.9	1.1–3.2	1.8	1.1–3.1
1.0–1.85	1.7	1.1–2.6	1.6	1.0–2.5
1.85–3.0	1.5	1.0–2.2	1.5	1.1–2.3
3.0+ (omitted category)	1.0		1.0	

[a]Source: reference 43, Tables 2 and 3.
[b]Estimated odds ratios (O.R.) and confidence intervals (C.I.) are taken from logistic regressions that also control for age, race, sex, birth order, and number of siblings of the child; marital status, age at first birth, educational attainment, AFQT score, height, and body mass index of the mother; and whether the child was low weight at birth or short length at birth.

significant predictors of either stunting or wasting once ten-year average income is controlled.

*Duncan, Brooks-Gunn, and Klebanov Study of the
Effects of Transitory and Persistent Poverty
on Age-5 IQ and Behavior Problems*

Duncan, Brooks-Gunn, and Klebanov (44) use data from the Infant Health and Development Program (IHDP) to relate patterns of poverty during the first five years of life to age-5 measures of IQ and behavior problems. The IHDP is an eight-site randomized clinical trial designed to test the efficacy of educational and family-support services and high-quality pediatric follow-up in reducing the incidence of developmental delay in low-birthweight, preterm infants (45). Its measure of cognitive functioning at age 5 is the Wechsler Preschool and Primary Scale of Intelligence (WPPSI) (46). Behavioral functioning is measured by the

Revised Child Behavior Profile (Ages 4 & 5), or Achenbach Behavior Problems indexes (47), a 120-item questionnaire that asks mothers to characterize the behavior of their children over the past six months with respect to two broad factors: internalizing (e.g., too fearful or anxious; unhappy, sad, or depressed) and externalizing (destroys his/her own things; temper tantrums or hot temper) problem behavior. Higher scores on the WPPSI indicate higher IQ; higher scores on the Achenbach Behavior Problems indexes indicate more behavior problems.

In four interviews taken over the child's first five years, the IHDP asked its respondents to provide an estimate of total family income. The duration of poverty was measured by two dummy variables: (a) whether the family was poor some but not all of the time (i.e., whether family income-to-needs was less than 1 in one, two, or three of the four reports); and (b) whether the family was poor all of the time (i.e., family income-to-needs was less than 1 in all four years). Never-poor families are the excluded group in the regressions, so coefficients on the two poverty measures indicate regression-adjusted IQ and behavior problem differences between children growing up in the two kinds of poor families and children raised in never-poor families. Other family-level measures in the IHDP analyses include the birth weight and sex of the child; the completed schooling of the mother, in years; whether the family was headed by the mother; whether the mother was black; and whether the family was in the treatment group.

Table 4 reproduces the main results and shows that after adjustment for other family-level measures, children in persistently poor families have 9.1-point

Table 4

Effects of persistent and transitory family poverty
on age-5 IQ and behavior problems[a,b]

	Age-5 IQ	Age-5 internalizing behavior problem index	Age-5 externalizing behavior problem index
Poor none of the time	Omitted	Omitted	Omitted
Poor some of the time	−4.02 (1.62)	2.44 (1.05)	1.77 (0.97)
Poor all of the time	−9.06 (2.10)	4.02 (1.36)	3.26 (1.25)

[a]Source: reference 44, Tables 4, 5, and 6.
[b]Estimated coefficients and standard errors (in parentheses) are taken from OLS regressions that also control for birth weight and the sex of the child, the completed schooling (in years) of the mother, whether the family was headed by the mother, whether the mother was black, and whether the family was in the treatment group.

(0.52 standard deviation) lower IQs, 4.0-point (0.41 standard deviation) worse scores on the internalizing behavior problem index, and 3.3-point (0.35 standard deviation) worse scores on the externalizing behavior problem index. Occasional poverty is also associated with significantly worse developmental outcomes (for externalizing behavior problems, the relevant coefficient is significant at only the .10 level), although the estimated effect of transitory poverty is not as large as the estimated effect of persistent poverty. An untested alternative interpretation is that they reflect differences in long-run income levels, with transitory fluctuations more likely to push above the poverty line families near the poverty line than families in deep poverty.

Elder, Liker, and Associates Studies of Income Losses During the Great Depression

Some of the most interesting empirical work on the links between income changes and adult outcomes is by Elder and Liker and their colleagues, using longitudinal data collected over several decades as part of the Berkeley Guidance Study from a sample of Berkeley-area married couples with children (48–52). Couples experiencing a drop of 30 percent or more in family income between 1929 and the early 1930s were compared on a range of subsequent outcomes—marital and parent-child relationships and mental health—with couples whose Depression incomes did not fall as much, with some of the outcomes measured several decades later. The researchers found a complex, but ultimately interpretable, pattern of effects that varied with the resources available to the couples at the time of the income loss and with the sex of the individual involved.

For men, the income losses produced uniformly harmful effects on marital and parenting behavior, apparently not so much because of the loss of income per se as because of the stress caused by the loss of status as breadwinner. For women coming from less advantaged families, there were also harmful effects on their marriages, parenting, and subsequent health. For these working-class women, the income loss itself appeared to be the culprit, leaving them with too few resources to perform properly their functions as homemakers.

Interestingly, women from middle-class backgrounds who experienced the income losses did *better* subsequently than otherwise similar women who escaped such adversity. Their resources for coping were apparently adequate and the economic hardship actually made them better able to handle subsequent problems.

McDonough, Duncan, House, and Williams Unpublished Data on Mortality

A final example of research on the associations between components of income and health comes from the nationally representative Panel Study of Income

Dynamics (53). Some 2,776 individuals who were part of the 1968 sample are known to have died between 1969 and 1992, with patterns of mortality by age, race, and sex matching up well with vital statistics sources. Data presented here focus on the possible mortality of individuals age 40 and above.

Although longitudinal data available in the PSID span 22 years, they are treated as if they were a series of 14 independent 10-year panels, the fist spanning calendar years 1967–1976, the second spanning 1968–1977, and so forth, with the last one spanning the decade 1980–1989. Within each 10-year period we used the first five years to measure patterns of household income and the second five years to measure possible mortality. An individual is eligible for inclusion in a given 10-year observation-window sample if he was male, at least 40 years of age in the first of the ten years, alive at least until the interview conducted in the spring of the fifth year, and, over the course of the second five years, either died or was not lost to nonresponse. The first five-year window is used to construct our household income measures, while the second five-year period provides the window over which possible mortality is observed.

Because of the nonindependence of observations across these windows (as well as an initially clustered probability sample), the logistic regression results are estimated using the SUDAAN sampling error program, which relies on Taylor-series approximations to adjust for the clustering of both respondents across time and respondents initially living within the same neighborhood. Data are weighted by the given person's individual weight in the fifth year of the 10-year window. Given the PSID's design and in the absence of nonresponse bias, the weighted sample ought to provide representative national estimates.

The dependent variable in the logistic regressions is whether the individual died during the given five-year period. Observations on annual total family income measured during the first five years are used to form two sets of income variables. The first is five-year average household income, inflated to 1984 dollars and expressed in the intervals $0–10 thousand, $10–15 thousand, $15–20 thousand, $20–35 thousand, $35–50 thousand, and greater than $50 thousand. The second set of income-related variables is based on a count of the number of times over the five-year period that household income fell by 50 percent or more from one year to the next. Dummy variables represent groups for whom income fell 50 percent or more (a) once and (b) two or more times. Individuals for whom income never fell by 50 percent or more constitute the omitted group.

Control variables used in all of the logistic regressions include (a) three dummy variables for age of individual (45–54, 55–64, 65–74, 75+); (b) whether the calendar year of the first year of the window was 1980 or after; (c) race (black versus nonblack); and (d) the average size of the given person's household over the first five years of the window.

Table 5 presents estimated logistic regression coefficients, standard errors, and odds ratios for the two sets of income measures. Average income level is found to have a powerful association with mortality, with individuals in families with

Table 5

Effects of five-year level and stability of household income on
log-odds of male mortality (N = 19,519)[a,b]

	Coefficient (S.E.)	O.R.	Mean (S.D.)
5-year average income level, thousands 1984 $			
<$10	1.11 (0.20)	3.0	0.13 (0.34)
$10–15	0.95 (0.16)	2.6	0.12 (0.32)
$15–20	0.64 (0.17)	1.9	0.12 (0.32)
$20–35	0.37 (0.16)	1.4	0.29 (0.45)
$35–50	0.32 (0.18)	1.4	0.19 (0.39)
>$50 (omitted)		1.0	
No. of times income fell 50% or more			
None (omitted)		1.0	
One	0.24 (0.10)	1.3	0.12 (0.32)
Two or more	0.55 (0.27)	1.7	0.01 (0.12)

[a]Source: unpublished data.
[b]Estimated coefficients and odds ratios (O.R.) are taken from logistic regressions that also control for age, calendar year, race, and average family size. Computations were performed using the SUDAAN sampling error program and take account of the clustered nature of the PSID sample.

incomes under $10,000 having odds ratios three times as high as individuals in families with incomes above $50,000. Mortality risks fall with income but at a decreasing rate. Once income rises above $20,000 the elevated risk of death falls to 1.4—and only at the margin of statistical significance. Thus we cannot be certain in these data that there is any income gradient in the top half of the income distribution.

Income losses are also significant predictors of mortality. Compared with individuals with relatively stable incomes, the relative risk of mortality for individuals who experienced one and two or more sharp income drops was, respectively, 1.3 and 1.7 times as high and statistically significant ($P < .05$ in both cases). It remains to be established whether it is the income fluctuations per se or the events (e.g., unemployment, widowhood) producing them that increase the health risks.

Further analysis showed that the beneficial effects of income level persisted in the presence of controls for more conventional measures of SES, such as completed schooling, as well as for a measure of the initial disability status of the individual (results not shown).

DISCUSSION

This review of recent studies of the linkages between household income and health and development shows very strong associations. What distinguishes most of these studies from their predecessors is that they are able to draw upon high-quality, longitudinal measures of income as well as control for an extensive set of correlated measures of SES and initial health. These results suggest that family income is a powerful (perhaps *the* most powerful) component of SES in its linkage with health. Several of them also suggest that income volatility also matters, although its role is less important than that of income level. The results on income level are consistent with but do not prove that *ceteris paribus* increases in the short-run incomes of low-income families would improve health status.

As argued at the beginning of this chapter, sorting out the causal role of income is crucial from a policy perspective, since family income is the component of SES that is by far the most manipulable through public policy programs. However, the steps between the suggestive associations of the kind found in the existing literature and "smoking gun" causal evidence are many and difficult.

The most convincing evidence that income has a direct, causal impact on health would come from a randomized experimental design. Randomized manipulation of family income was indeed a feature of a series of "negative income tax" experiments undertaken in the 1970s in various sites in the United States (as well as in Canada). Although the primary purpose of these experiments was to gauge the likely effects on work effort of more generous transfer payments to low-income families, some health data were gathered as part of these experiments. Kehrer and Wolin (54) report that mothers in the experimental income groups who had a high risk of adverse pregnancy outcomes had children with birth weights 0.3 to 1.2 pounds higher than those of children of control mothers. These statistically significant improvements came in the absence of any experimental manipulation of health services provided to experimental-group and control-group families. Improved nutrition appears to have been the key intervening factor accounting for the improvements. There seems to be no experimental evidence on the effects of income changes on health at older ages.

In the absence of experimental designs, researchers must resort to data-collection and statistical strategies for estimating causal effects (55, 56). Prospective epidemiological approaches focused on initially healthy individuals are one promising approach, although they must define initial health in terms of observed characteristics and therefore cannot adjust for differences in unobserved frailty.

Longitudinal data on both income and health outcomes provide an opportunity to estimate change models, in which changes in health or developmental outcomes are related to changes in regressors such as income. Suppose, for example, that a health outcome at time t (HEALTH$_t$) is a function of lifetime income up to point t (ΣINCOME$_t$), a "permanent" component of other aspects of SES as measured by completed schooling (SCHOOL), an unobserved permanent degree of frailty (FRAIL), and a random error term (ε_t):

$$\text{HEALTH}_t = \alpha + \beta_1 \, \Sigma\text{INCOME}_t + \beta_2 \, \text{SCHOOL} + \beta_3 \, \text{FRAIL} + \varepsilon_t \qquad (1)$$

Suppose further that this same relationship holds five years later, at $t + 5$:

$$\text{HEALTH}_{t+5} = \alpha + \beta_1 \, \Sigma\text{INCOME}_{t+5} + \beta_2 \, \text{SCHOOL} + \beta_3 \, \text{FRAIL} + \varepsilon_{t+5} \qquad (2)$$

Differencing these two equations eliminates the confounding effects of SCHOOL and FRAIL and gives the following equation relating change in health to the total income between t and $t + 5$:

$$\Delta \, \text{HEALTH}_{t,t+5} = \beta_1 \, \Delta \, \Sigma\text{INCOME}_{t,t+5} + \Delta \, \varepsilon_{t,t+5,} \qquad (3)$$

where $\Delta X_{t,t+5}$ indicates the change in X from year t to year $t + 5$.

In their analysis of the effects of persistent poverty on age-5 IQ and behavior problems, Duncan and colleagues (44) estimate such an equation based on change data between ages 3 and 5 and find highly significant effects of family income between ages 3 and 5 on changes in IQ between ages 3 and 5. Results for the estimated effects of income on changes in behavior problems were in the expected direction but not significant at conventional levels.

Change models estimated on nonexperimental data are not without their problems, since one must still worry about the source of the changes in the righthand-side variables (57). In the context of health change, one needs to make sure that the event causing the income change either did not affect health directly or is somehow controlled in the statistical analysis.

Another model-based approach is to estimate a level equation such as Equation (1) above, but to attempt to remove the spurious correlation between income and health through an instrumental variables procedure. This procedure amounts to replacing the ΣINCOME variable with an instrumental variable for ΣINCOME that is purged of ΣINCOME's spurious correlation with unobserved factors such as FRAIL. The trick for making this work is to find a variable that is highly correlated with ΣINCOME but is not highly correlated with the unobservable component of FRAIL. This task is a difficult one because almost all correlates of ΣINCOME are arguably correlates of unobserved determinants of HEALTH as well.

Change models and instrumental variables procedures such as these may be especially well-suited for research on children's health and development, since, apart from severe child disabilities, changes in family income are almost never caused by changes in children's health. Such independence is more difficult to establish in the case of health of potentially wage-earning adults.

It is also important to move beyond income level and consider income instability as an independent source of health effects. Although the empirical evidence presented herein suggested that income level was the income component by far the most predictive of health outcomes, we also found that income losses had effects on mortality, net of level and other demographic measures. An important extension is to explain why the income losses had the effects they did, starting with an examination of the event underlying the income losses.

The interaction between income level and income fluctuations also leads to the important distinction between transitory and persistent poverty. The finding of differing effects on age-5 IQ and behavior problems of persistent and transitory poverty in the Duncan and associates (44) analysis is suggestive that income changes may matter, although their results are also consistent with an interpretation that income level is all important and is the principal cause of why some children fall into the transitory poverty group while others end up in the persistently poor group. More research is obviously needed on the effects of the various components of income.

Another necessary improvement over the income-dynamics models estimated thus far is the measurement and inclusion of measures of the process by which income (or, for that matter, other components of SES) affects health. The Kehrer and Wolin (54) low-birth-weight study based on experimental data found that nutritional differences associated with higher incomes mattered. Duncan and associates (44) find that roughly one-third of the effect of persistent poverty on children's IQs could be accounted for by differences in home learning environments (e.g., availability of books and educational toys). Neither Miller and Korenman, nor Duncan and colleagues, nor McDonough and colleagues had data on intervening measures such as nutrition and health care access. Augmenting longitudinal data sets with information of this kind as well as data on health behavior, psychosocial characteristics, and important life events such as marital and job instability is clearly a high priority. Ultimate success in understanding how socioeconomic status affects health and development requires the estimation of complete models that account for the many ways in which these effects work.

Acknowledgments — The original empirical work presented in this chapter is part of a joint research project conducted with Peggy McDonough, Jim House, and David Williams, all of whom, along with Johanne Boisjoly, Dorothy Duncan, and Nancy Moss, made helpful comments on the chapter. Pat Berglund provided excellent research assistance.

REFERENCES

1. Bunker, J. P., Gomby, D. S., and Kehrer, B. H. (eds.). *Pathway to Health: The Role of Social Factors*, pp. xv–xxiv. Henry J. Kaiser Foundation, Menlo Park, Calif., 1989.
2. Adler, N., et al. Socioeconomic inequalities in health: No easy solution. *JAMA* 269(24): 3140–3145, 1993.
3. Dutton, D. B., and Levine, S. Socioeconomic status and health: Overview, methodological critique, and reformulation. In *Pathways to Health: The Role of Social Factors*, edited by J. Bunker, D. Gomby, and B. Kehrer, pp. 26–69. Henry J. Kaiser Family Foundation, Menlo Park, Calif., 1989.
4. Williams, D. R. Socioeconomic differences in health: A review and redirection. *Soc. Psychol. Q.* 53: 81–99, 1993.
5. Feinstein, J. S. The relationship between socioeconomic status and health: A review of the literature. *Milbank Q.* 71: 279–322, 1993.
6. Krieger, N., et al. Racism, sexism, and social class: Implications for studies of health, disease and well-being. *Am. J. Prev. Med.* 9(6): 82–122, 1993.
7. House, J., et al. The social stratification of aging and health. *Health Soc. Behav.* 35: 213–234, 1994.
8. Liberatos, P., Link, B., and Kelsey, J. The measurement of social class in epidemiology. *Epidemiol. Rev.* 10: 87–121, 1988.
9. Fox, A. J., Goldbladt, P. O., and Jones, D. R. Social class mortality differentials: Artefact, selection or life circumstances? *J. Epidemiol. Community Health* 39: 1–8, 1985.
10. Marmot, M., et al. Health inequalities among British civil servants: The Whitehall II study. *Lancet* 337: 1387–1393, 1991.
11. Lahelma, E., and Valkonen, T. Health and social inequalities in Finland and elsewhere. *Soc. Sci. Med.* 31(3): 257–265, 1990.
12. Moore, D., and Hayward, M. Occupational careers and mortality of elderly men. *Demography* 27(1): 31–53, 1990.
13. Mare, R. D. Socioeconomic careers and differential mortality among older men in the United States. In *Comparative Studies of Mortality and Morbidity: Old and New Approaches to Measurement and Analysis*, edited by L. Vallin, S. D'Sousa, and A. Palloni. Oxford University Press, London, 1990.
14. Kolter, P., and Wingard, D. The effect of occupational, marital and parental roles on mortality: The Alameda County study. *Am. J. Public Health* 79: 607–612, 1989.
15. Feldman, J. J., et al. National trends in educational differentials in mortality. *Am. J. Epidemiol.* 129: 919–933, 1989.
16. Kitagawa, E. M., and Hauser P. M. *Differential Mortality in the United States: A Study in Socioeconomic Epidemiology.* Harvard University Press, Cambridge, Mass., 1973.
17. Haan, M., Kaplan, G., and Camacho, T. Poverty and health: Prospective evidence from the Alameda County study. *Am. J. Epidemiol.* 125(6): 989–998, 1987.
18. Duleep, H. O. Measuring socioeconomic mortality differentials over time. *Demography* 26: 345–351, 1989.

19. Pappas, G., et al. The increasing disparity in mortality between socioeconomic groups in the United States, 1960 and 1986. *N. Engl. J. Med.* 329: 103–115, 1993.
20. Brenner, M. H. Mortality and the national economy: A review and the experiences of England and Wales, 1936–76. *Lancet* ii: 568–573, 1979.
21. Karoly, L. The trend in inequality among families, individuals, and workers in the United States: A twenty-five year perspective. In *Uneven Tides: Rising Inequality in America*, edited by S. Danziger and P. Gottschalk, pp. 19–98. Russell Sage, New York, 1993.
22. Wolff, E. Trends in aggregate household wealth in the U.S. 1900–1983. *Rev. Income Wealth* 35: 1–30, 1989.
23. Eargle, J. *Household Wealth and Asset Ownership: 1988.* Bureau of the Census, Curr. Popul. Rep., Ser. P-70, No. 22. U.S. Department of Commerce, Washington, D.C., 1991.
24. Kennickell, A., and Woodburn, R. Estimation of Household Net Worth Using Model-Based and Design-Based Weights: Evidence from the 1989 Survey of Consumer Finances. Mimeo. Board of Governors, Federal Reserve System, Washington, D.C., 1992.
25. Danziger, S., and Gottschalk, P. *Uneven Tides: Rising Inequality in America.* Russell Sage, New York, 1993.
26. Levy, F., and Murnane, R. U.S. earnings levels and earnings inequality: A review of recent trends and proposed explanations. *J. Econ. Lit.* 30(3): 1333–1381, 1992.
27. Kawachi, I., et al. Income Inequity and Life Expectancies—Theory, Research and Policy. Mimeo. The Health Institute, New England Medical Center and Harvard School of Public Health, Cambridge, Mass., 1994.
28. Preston, S. The changing relationship between mortality and level of economic development. *Popul. Stud.* 29: 231–248, 1975.
29. Rodgers, S. *Mortality Patterns in National Populations.* Academic Press, London, 1976.
30. Wilkinson, R. G. National mortality rates: The impact of inequality. *Am. J. Public Health* 82: 1082–1084, 1992.
31. LeGrand, J. An international comparison of distribution of ages-at-death. In *Health Inequalities in European Countries*, edited by J. Fox, pp. 75–91. Gower, Aldershot, 1989.
32. U.S. Bureau of the Census. *Money Income of Households, Families and Persons in the United States: 1991.* Curr. Popul. Rep., Ser. P-60, No. 180. U.S. Government Printing Office, Washington, D.C., 1992.
33. Duncan, G. The volatility of family income over the life course. In *Life Span Development and Behavior*, Vol. 9, edited by P. Bates, D. Featherman, and R. Lerner, pp. 317–358. Lawrence Erlbaum Associates, Hillsdale, N.J., 1988.
34. Burkhauser, R., and Duncan, G. Sharing prosperity across the age distribution: A comparison of the United States and Germany in the 1980s. *The Gerontologist* 34: 150–160, 1994.
35. Bane, M. J., and Ellwood, D. T. Slipping in and out of poverty: The dynamics of spells. *J. Hum. Res.* 21: 1–23, 1986.
36. Murray, C. According to Age: Longitudinal Profiles of AFDC Recipients and the Poor by Age Group. Prepared for the Working Seminar on the Family and American Welfare Policy, 1986.
37. Solon, G. Work incentive effects of taxing unemployment benefits. *Econometrica* 53: 295–306, 1985.
38. Moffitt, R. Incentive effects of the U.S. Welfare System: A review. *J. Econ. Lit.* 30(1): 1–61, 1992.

39. Hagestad, G., and Neugarten, B. Age and the life course. In *Handbook of Aging and the Social Sciences*, Ed. 2, edited by R. H. Binstock and E. Shanas, pp. 35–61. Van Nostrand Reinhold, New York, 1985.
40. Antonucci, T. Personal characteristics, social support and social behavior. In *Handbook of Aging and the Social Sciences*, edited by R. H. Binstock and E. Shanas, pp. 94–128. Van Nostrand Reinhold, New York, 1985.
41. Pearlin, L. I., et al. The stress process. *J. Health Soc. Behav.* 22: 337–356, 1981.
42. Turner, J., Kessler, R., and House, J. Factors facilitating adjustment to unemployment: Implications for intervention. *Am. J. Community Psychol.* 19(4): 521–542, 1991.
43. Miller, J., and Korenman, S. Poverty and children's nutritional status in the United States. *Am. J. Epidemiol.* 140(3): 233–243, 1994.
44. Duncan, G., Brooks-Gunn, J., and Klebanov, P. Economic deprivation and early-childhood development. *Child Dev.* 65: 296–318, 1994.
45. The Infant Health and Development Program Staff. Enhancing the outcomes of low birthweight, premature infants: A multisite randomized trial. *JAMA* 263(22): 3035–3042, 1990.
46. Wechsler, D. *Wechsler Preschool and Primary Scale of Intelligence*. The Psychological Corporation, 1967.
47. Achenbach, T. M., and Edelbrock, C. S. Psychopathology of childhood. *Annu. Rev. Psychol.* 35: 227–256, 1984.
48. Elder, G. H. *Children of the Great Depression*. University of Chicago Press, Chicago, 1974.
49. Elder, G. H., and Liker, J. K. Hard times in women's lives: Historical influences across fifty years. *Am. J. Sociol.* 88: 241–269, 1982.
50. Elder, G. H., Liker, J. K., and Cross, C. E. Parent-child behavior in the Great Depression: Life course and intergenerational influences. In *Life-span Development and Behavior*, Vol. 6, edited by P. B. Bates and O. G. Brim, Jr., pp. 109–158. Academic Press, New York, 1984.
51. Elder, G. H., Liker, J. K., and Jaworski, B. J. Hardship in lives: Depression influences in the 1930s to old age in postwar America. In *Life-span Development Psychology: Historical and Generational Effects*, edited by K. A. McCluskey and H. W. Reese. Academic Press, New York, 1984.
52. Liker, J. K., and Elder, G. H. Economic hardship and marital relations in the 1930's. *Am. Sociol. Rev.* 48: 3434–359, 1983.
53. Hill, M. *The Panel Study of Income Dynamics*. Sage, Beverly Hills, 1992.
54. Kehrer, B. H., and Wolin, C. M. Impact of income maintenance on low birth weight: Evidence from the Gary Experiment. *J. Hum. Resources* 14(4): 434–462, 1979.
55. Duleep, H. O. Measuring the effect of income on adult mortality. *J. Hum. Resources* 21: 238–251, 1986.
56. Sickles, R., Taubman, P., and Behrman, J. Black-white mortality inequalities. *J. Econometrics* 50: 183–203, 1991.
57. Heckman, J. J., and Robb, R. Alternative methods for evaluating the impact of interventions. In *Longitudinal Analysis of Labor Market Data*, edited by J. Heckman and B. Singer. Cambridge University Press, New York, 1985.

CHAPTER 8

Is Unemployment Pathogenic?
A Review of Current Concepts with
Lessons for Policy Planners

Samuel E. D. Shortt

At least since the time of Louis René Villermé (1782–1863) and Sir Edwin Chadwick (1800–1890) the connection between chronic poverty and ill-health has been something of an epidemiological truism. But what of more transient deprivation? Does the economic dislocation that accompanies a recession exert an adverse effect on health? More particularly, does unemployment bring with it risk to physical and mental well-being? Answers to this question are of more than academic interest. Many industrialized nations now face a persistent unemployment rate above 10 percent, levels unthinkable in the 1960s. Moreover, the postwar technological revolution has made the very future of work itself a widely debated issue. It is essential, then, that legislators and policy planners have some knowledge of the complex nexus between ill-health and unemployment. It is particularly important that the link between job loss and health status not be viewed as unproblematic, an established certainty that requires no further scrutiny. Unfortunately, in political statements, media commentary, and medical sources, this point is frequently ignored in preference to undocumented generalization about the alleged relationship. Since there are no comprehensive recent surveys of unemployment and health (1), this chapter reviews the existing literature as it applies to developed nations and concludes with general suggestions for future policy formulation.

TIME-SERIES ANALYSIS

Any discussion of contemporary research on the health consequences of unemployment must begin with the controversial but ground-breaking work of M. Harvey Brenner (e.g., 2–6). His studies, national in scope and encompassing time spans of three to four decades, have used aggregate time-series analysis to

219

compare indicators of economic fluctuation to patterns of change in indices of health status. Trends in per capita income, inflation, and particularly unemployment have been compared with age- and sex-specific mortality, cardiovascular mortality, deaths from cirrhosis of the liver, suicide rates, and rates of first admission to mental hospitals. A key concept is that all pathological reactions to unemployment will follow actual job loss at a variable length of time. Acute psychological reactions such as suicide would be expected to occur relatively soon after becoming unemployed, perhaps within a year, while death from physical disorders such as cardiovascular disease would lag by up to half a dozen years to permit adequate progression of the physical pathology.

To Brenner the results are unequivocal: for each of several national experiences ill-health is strongly related to unemployment. In the United States, all age groups demonstrated a significant relationship between unemployment and cardiovascular mortality from 1940 to 1973 in years 2 through 4 after an economic downturn. Mortality from cirrhosis of the liver revealed a significant relationship in the short to medium term for persons over 45 years of age. In general, both suicide rates and first admissions to mental institutions showed similar positive correlations with unemployment (2). In Sweden, from 1950 to 1980, total mortality, mortality due to overall cardiovascular disease, total cerebrovascular disease, total heart disease, and ischemic heart disease were positively related to the unemployment rate at short (2 year) and relatively long (4 to 9 years) lags (5). For the years 1936 to 1976 in England and Wales mortality for all age groups was positively related to unemployment. Suicide revealed an increase within a year of increased job loss, while cardiovascular mortality began to accelerate at 2 to 3 years and continued for 10 to 15 years (3). In several developed nations, then, Brenner's work demonstrated a strong association between unemployment and various forms of ill-health.

How did Brenner account for this relationship? Unemployment, he argued, threatens health in at least three ways. First, it engenders poverty, a state which in turn implies poor nutrition, low housing standards, and, in the United States, impaired access to health care. Second, unemployment creates psychological stress, a documented etiological factor in numerous disorders including cardiovascular disease. Loss of self-esteem, social isolation, and family discord are among the stresses that accompany job loss. Third, unemployment may provoke inappropriate coping techniques such as alcohol abuse, increased tobacco consumption, or illicit drug use, each of which is linked to morbidity (4). Subsequent research has failed to confirm this assertion. While a higher proportion of males who become unemployed smoke compared with males who remain employed, job loss has not been shown to increase either tobacco use or alcohol consumption (7–9).

Despite this plausible line of argument to connect ill-health and unemployment, Brenner is careful to include passing acknowledgment of two constraints on his style of macro analysis. First, while he can clearly demonstrate correlations between unemployment rates and rates for various health indices, these correlations are statements of statistical relationships rather than established causality. Second, aggregate studies can make valid statements only about phenomena at the same macro level but cannot make definitive assertions about behavior at lower levels. Thus, while national unemployment rates may show a positive correlation with morbidity and mortality, it cannot be shown from macro studies that the unemployed are, indeed, those who become sick or die (4). These disclaimers, however, loom small in Brenner's work, perhaps explaining why they are largely ignored by those who debate his methodology.

Brenner's work is certainly not without its critics, the first and most vocal among whom has been Joseph Eyer. While he dismisses some of Brenner's statistical methods, particularly the use of Fourier analysis and the approach to detrending data (10) as "just plain fudge factors" (11, p. 157), in his own work rather similar statistical patterns emerge. The key differences are two-fold. First, Eyer views the peaks in U.S. mortality rates not as a lagged effect of a preceding economic slump, but rather as a relatively immediate effect of a contemporaneous economic boom. Prosperity, in effect, causes death (11). Second, while he accepts the notion that increasing social stress ultimately accounts for much of the increased mortality, this stress does not derive from unemployment but from pathogenic features of capitalist prosperity. For Eyer, "the business cycle is a back-and-forth class struggle between labour and capital over disposition of the economic product" (12, p. 639). Yet actual consumption, inequitably distributed though it is, explains relatively little of the high mortality that he attributes to a typical boom economy. Rather, two aspects of the class struggle itself appear most relevant to fluctuating mortality. First, during recessionary times labor experiences a solidarity forged of conflict with capital which helps to reduce the death rate; similarly, marriages increase at the same point in the economic cycle, also lowering death rates. Second, as recessions recede workers engage in practices such as overwork, employment-seeking migration, or divorce, which tend to accelerate the death rate. Together these solidarity and social disintegration factors "can account for the majority, 72 percent, of the business cycle variation of the death rates" (12, p. 653). Seen in this fashion, the death rate is unlikely to be improved by simply eliminating fluctuation in the economy, as Brenner implied, or instituting ameliorating welfare measures. Instead, Eyer argues, the policy implications of his viewpoint support "the abolition of social hierarchy and the cessation of capital accumulation" (10, p. 143). From this Marxist perspective he concludes that Brenner is little more than an epidemiological apologist for the view of "conventional economists that there is nothing intrinsically pathological about capitalist society when it is working well, in its own terms, 'at full employment' " (10, p. 144).

A number of other critics, none of whom appear to share Eyer's ideological angst, have raised concerns about Brenner's work. Richard Smith, assistant editor of the *British Medical Journal*, succinctly stated a major problem when he observed "the innumerate, which by the standards of Brenner is most of us, can be bewitched by the mathematical magician" (13, p. 1493). It is clear, however, that some statistically sophisticated observers remain unbewitched. Stanislav Kasl (14), for example, notes that Brenner's detrending adjustments distort the basic data and no independent rationale is established for choosing specific lag times. Indeed, Brenner's explanation for choosing lag periods of 0 to 5 years after an economic downturn for various disorders has not been couched in terms calculated to win converts. The methodological rationales, he wrote, "involve considerations of theory, previous empirical research [most of it his own], and measurement issues" (2, p. 595). Spruit dismisses the lag methodology as lacking any theoretical or epidemiological basis (15, p. 1908), while Gravelle and colleagues demonstrate that with a minor and equally plausible statistical manipulation, one obtains results that "do not appear to have any obvious pattern, [and] none of them is significant at the 5% level" (16, p. 678).

Other commentators focus less on statistics than on additional methodological flaws. The raw data used for studies covering a long time course are often of variable quality, while changes such as alterations in diagnostic categories are likely to introduce inconsistencies (17). The choice of a time period to study can, by expanding or reducing its limits, dramatically alter the strength of observed correlations (16). The selection of measures to operationalize concepts of health status and economic conditions has been criticized as highly arbitrary and by no means exhaustive of all relevant variables. Finally, unemployment has not been adequately shown to stand alone and separate in its relationship to ill-health from variables such as income, occupation, education, or housing (16).

On a somewhat more fundamental level, Brenner's critics charge that even were an indisputable correlation established between economic recession and increased morbidity and mortality, it would be impossible to prove causality or the direction in which it flows, that is, from unemployment to ill-health or the converse. As well, while a general pattern may affect large segments of a population, there is no reason to believe any given individual will follow this pattern. Put another way, it is not established that the unemployed are those who die during a recession (18). It matters little that Brenner himself has conceded such methodological limitations. Rather, these concerns reflect a failure on Brenner's part to establish a convincing model from which to explain in precise pathophysiological terms the mechanism by which economic change induces morbidity. That his unidirectional model is at best simplistic is suggested by the complexity and variability of micro-level studies on the health of the unemployed (16). For example, one would assume that if health deteriorates with unemployment in the United States, hospital outpatient department use should increase during recessions, but this has been shown not to occur (19). Despite one supportive paper from Australia (20), researchers in Britain (16), Germany, Denmark, and the Netherlands, using Brenner's approach, have failed to produce similar findings on the issue of mortality and unemployment (15).

It is reasonable to conclude from this review of Brenner's work that his contentions, while plausible, are not proven. This conclusion creates an unfortunate dilemma for policy makers to whom the apparent predictive value of his work was most attractive. Brenner had promised his approach could provide an accurate estimate of the social cost (measured by total and disease-specific mortality rates, as well as rates for homicide and suicide) associated with the various unemployment rates produced by alternative economic policies (2). But given the prevailing skepticism about Brenner's work, policy analysts must turn instead to the myriad of micro-level studies on health and unemployment. Here they must attempt to isolate those areas upon which an epidemiological consensus exists as a sound foundation for policy recommendations.

PLANT CLOSURE STUDIES

One particularly promising micro-level alternative to aggregate time-series analysis is studies that focus on plant closures. Workers rendered unemployed as a group through no fault of their own may be assumed to be reasonably healthy before redundancy, and changes in status after job loss easily identified. A longitudinal study of 1,816 Dutch shipyard workers, despite a problem of study drop-outs, demonstrated significantly more chest pain and hypertension among those who became unemployed, as well as increased emotional upset (21, 22). While rates of hospitalization for the unemployed fell for causes such as accidents and musculoskeletal disease, the rate of admissions for cardiovascular disease increased (23). An additional Swedish shipyard study documented the stress associated with the anticipation of closure and the differential effect of closure according to age. In contrast to younger workers, those over 55 revealed increased sick-role behavior, isolation, alcohol use, and depression (24). Perhaps reflecting the incapacitating effect of unemployment on some workers, a 10-year prospective study of redundant workers at a Norwegian cannery found the cumulative disability pension rate (awarded strictly for medical reasons) was three times higher than among controls (25). A Finnish study documented that redundant male wood-processing workers, but not female colleagues, demonstrated lower mental well-being scores than did a control group (26). A British general practice study of former workers at a meat-producing plant also documented an increased incidence of chronic disease and an accompanying increase in visits to both family doctors and hospital outpatient departments (27, 28). A Canadian study of 183 redundant workers followed over a 16-month period found unemployment had a negative impact on sense of well-being and life satisfaction, but only to a very modest degree (29). A further Canadian study in which 310 employees lost jobs found increased levels of stress among male blue-collar workers, and similar symptoms were present in spouses. While there was some evidence of increased ill-health after closure for both employees and spouses, this appeared to represent an exacerbation of previous health problems (30). Unfortunately, most studies of plant closure follow relatively small numbers of employees over short time spans and have difficulty finding truly comparable control groups (31). Nevertheless, the findings are sufficiently uniform to be persuasive that plant closures adversely affect the physical and particularly the mental health of former workers.

MORTALITY AND MORBIDITY ANALYSIS

The factory closure model, however, has not provided definitive insight (32) into the relationship between health and unemployment. This approach must be supplemented by a variety of other methodologies to which mortality investigations make an important contribution. Several studies in Great Britain fail to confirm Brenner's belief that mortality is intimately linked to unemployment. Studying Scotland for a 28-year period, McAvinchey (33) found unemployment to decrease mortality for women up to age 65 and men up to 45. Men over that age were subject to increased mortality rates. A second Scottish study, covering a 22-year period, found a link between unemployment and mortality for older men in the short term and a stronger link when only ischemic heart disease was considered (34). Males aged 15 to 64 unemployed in England and Wales in 1971 and 1981 have been studied using data from the Office of Population Censuses and Surveys Longitudinal Study (35, 36). Interestingly, as in a Canadian plant closure study (30), findings also applied generally to the spouses of these males. A high rate of mortality, particularly from lung cancer, suicide, and ischemic heart disease, was found for the unemployed. This ill-health was not a cause of the unemployment, and a portion of it may be explained by low socioeconomic status. The authors conclude that 20 to 30 percent of the excess mortality rate suffered by unemployed males may be ascribed to job loss. A study of 91 local health authorities in Sweden for a 5-year period confirmed that death from ischemic heart disease in males correlated strongly with unemployment, regardless of other social variables (37). It seems clear, then, that for selected groups, for selected causes, in several nations, unemployment accounts for at least some increase in mortality rate.

For many persons, death is preceded for a variable length of time by morbidity. Given that job loss seems to increase mortality, evidence should exist as to a greater than expected rate of antecedent physical illness. Though the evidence is fragmentary, a number of conclusions appear justified. First, several studies document a lack of serious prior illness for the male unemployed, thereby discrediting the notion that sickness causes job loss rather than the converse (38, 39). Second, in several U.S. studies individuals anticipating or experiencing job loss, when compared with controls who remained employed, showed elevation of uric acid, cholesterol, and norepinephrine and a minor increase in blood pressure, all of which appeared to revert to normal when employment was found (40–42). Whether these transient and often small changes are clinically relevant may be difficult to establish. Third, the unemployed have a higher incidence of self-reported illness, physical symptoms, and medical attention seeking than do job-holders (43–46). Fourth, a Canadian study has documented that though the unemployed report levels of physical activity comparable with those of the employed, at all levels of activity they are less healthy than job-holders even after adjustments are made for age, sex, and family income (47).

Finally, and most importantly, several studies have suggested an increased incidence of physician-diagnosed disease in the unemployed compared with the employed. The rate of admission to medical and surgical wards in a Danish study was twice as high for the unemployed as the employed (48). A study using data from the 1981 Canada Health Survey showed the unemployed had a much greater chance of being diagnosed with heart disease, high blood pressure, or arthritic problems than did the employed (43). In the British Regional Heart Study, men experiencing job loss in the period 1978–1980 revealed markedly higher rates of ischemic heart disease, bronchitis, and chronic obstructive lung disease (49). In a large British survey unemployment was found to function accurately as a proxy for more detailed deprivation indicators and was correlated with a number of morbidity measures, especially depression and respiratory diseases (50). A general-practice-based study in Britain demonstrated that upon becoming unemployed, male patients developed significantly more chronic diseases, especially elevated blood pressure and coronary artery disease, when compared with an employed control group (51). It is reasonably well documented, then, that unemployment, at least among males, has an adverse effect on physical health, particularly with reference to the cardiovascular system.

MENTAL HEALTH

If one examines the effect of unemployment on mental health, the relationship again emerges as complex and contingent upon prevailing social or medical resources. A time-series study in Illinois from 1970 to 1985 found inpatient admissions correlated with unemployment at a 1- and 6-month lag, while out-patient utilization peaked at a 3-month lag (52). In contrast, a study in England and Wales from 1950 to 1976 found a correlation of first admission rates only for men aged 25 to 44 and women aged 20 to 54. Neither group revealed a time-lag response, perhaps reflecting the more ready accessibility of the National Health Service (53). A study at a major Toronto psychiatric facility found, at a 6-month lag, rising unemployment correlated with diminishing admissions and discharges. Since, like Great Britain, Canada has universal medicare, this trend was thought to reflect not inaccessibility but limitations of hospital capacity and changing criteria for admission (54). Clearly, the medical assets of the country in which unemployment occurs influence the correlation with psychiatric hospitalization.

A population at risk for serious emotional disturbance in recessionary times is identifiable in the literature. In a study of eight Missouri public psychiatric hospitals over a 100-month period no relationship was found for the general population between unemployment and first admission rates. However, a correlation was found between readmissions and unemployment, suggesting former psychiatric patients experience increased economic vulnerability. As well, persons unemployed at the time of a recession did show a high correlation with first admissions, again indicating economic marginality predisposed to psychiatric institutionalization (55). This contention was supported by a study of two mental health centers in St. Louis for a 5-year period in which a significant relationship was found between economic decline and first admissions for the unemployed as well as a group composed of housewives, students, and retirees (56). A Scottish study of male parasuicide for 1968 to 1982 found that those out of work for more than a year were roughly 19 times more likely to harm themselves deliberately than were employed men (57). An additional Scottish study found that unemployment discriminated those with a history of repeated suicide attempts from those with no such history and also predicted repetition within a year of the initial episode (58). It is clear, then, that unemployment during a period of recession shows a firm correlation with significant psychiatric morbidity as defined by hospitalization or self-destructive behavior. Yet even here caveats may exist: for example, a British study of 954 men revealed that the unemployed from areas of chronically high unemployment showed lower emotional distress than did those from areas of low unemployment (59). Once again, community norms and circumstances appear to mediate the impact of unemployment.

Figures dealing with catastrophic events such as attempted suicide or institutionalization, however, fail to capture the more general emotional impact of unemployment. Using self-reported survey measures in Kansas City, Catalano and Dooley (60) found that unemployment was highly correlated in the general population with both mood disturbances and increases in stressful life events. An important prospective study of 300 Miami men aged 35 to 60 over a 5-year period clearly demonstrated that those who became unemployed had higher levels of depression, anxiety, and somatization than those who remained employed. A German study of unemployed men over the age of 45 found similar psychological distress and noted that symptoms regressed with reemployment or formal retirement (62). The German findings were found to hold for Finnish males of all ages, a pattern that appeared less pronounced among female workers (63). Unemployment, then, clearly has an adverse effect on the mental health of many in the community who never came in contact with formal psychiatric care.

WOMEN, FAMILIES, AND YOUNG PERSONS

The studies cited in the preceding discussion of mortality and physical and mental health, diverse though they are, share a common characteristic: they focus almost exclusively on males, doubtless reflecting the traditional dominance of the workplace by men. However, some investigations dealing with women are available. A Massachusetts study of 844 women in the 45 to 54 age group clearly established that the employed perceive fewer health problems and report less illness behavior than the unemployed. In contrast to studies on men's unemployment, it appears that for a portion of the unemployed women ill-health caused job loss rather than the converse (64). This may reflect better compensation benefits for male workers or perhaps greater pressures to return to the work force despite illness. Similarly, the 1979 U.S. National Health Interview Survey studied 20,764 white women aged 18 to 55 without chronic disorders. The employed, judged by self-reported health and illness behavior, were healthier than the unemployed and, in particular, the recently nonemployed (65). Both these studies confirm research documenting the health-conferring nature of employment for women (66, 67), though a recent study of 536 women over a 15-year period failed to correlate discontinuities in either employment or marital status with increased morbidity (68). Even when differences in national social institutions are taken into account, this relationship appears to persist. In Sweden, where social support for the unemployed largely removes financial worries, unemployed women still reveal diminished psychological well-being, especially in terms of stress and depression, when compared with job-holders (69). Thus, while individual personality traits doubtless influence an individual's response to job loss (70), it is clear that most women suffer some adverse mental and physical effects.

What of the families of the men and women who become unemployed? A Canadian study documented a high correlation between physical abuse of women and unemployment for the male partner (71). A Glasgow study of 655 births documented that, after controlling for social class, children born to families in which the male was unemployed were of lower birth weight by 4.5 percent (72). The size of this deficit is comparable to the effect of maternal smoking during pregnancy. While other British studies have found similar correlations between birth weight and parental unemployment (73), a more recent U.S. investigation of New York City birth weights over a 17-year period could find no evidence that the unemployment rate had a negative impact on infant health (74). Despite the use of a time-series approach, this study failed to substantiate Brenner's earlier work on a national level (75). More alarming is the finding that as infants progress in age, they appear to remain at risk. A study comparing children from deprived areas in Glasgow with those from more affluent areas found the former were nine times more likely to be admitted to hospital (76). The family variables most closely correlated were overcrowded houses and parental unemployment. Compared with these factors, the protective effect of immunization against measles and whooping cough was insignificant. Less dramatic than hospitalization but still significant is the increase in general practice consultations which, in a British study, rose substantially for families in which male workers became unemployed (77). The existing literature, then, while deficient in many areas (78), is strongly suggestive of a pathological impact for unemployment on the children and families of the unemployed.

As children grow up, all too soon they may face unemployment themselves. A prospective Swedish study of 1,083 final-year students with a 2-year follow-up clearly demonstrated the adverse consequences for those who failed to find employment (79). When compared with their employed peers, they revealed increased psychosomatic symptomatology, decreased social activities, increased drug and alcohol use, and increased utilization of health services. A Finnish study of 2,000 young people in the 17- to 20-year age group revealed unemployment had a significant adverse impact on mental health over a 5-year period (80). Results similar to the Swedish study were found for two groups of school-leavers in Leeds at a 2-year follow-up (81), and for 1,150 17-year-olds from 11 urban areas of England with a 1-year follow-up (82). In the latter study gender and race appeared to modify certain aspects of the findings. Several studies have shown that unemployment is a significant risk factor for self-harm among adolescents. For example, a British study documented that 28 percent of 16- to 18-year-old parasuicides in the Oxford area were unemployed, compared with 7 percent unemployed in the general population (83). Finally, an ambitious Irish longitudinal study of 16- to 25-year-olds has shown differences in physical health between the unemployed and job-holders (84). The former were more likely to have experienced previous ill-health, to have had an accident in the 12 months before the study, and to use tobacco and illicit drugs. Unemployed females were less likely to engage in preventive medical measures, and both sexes were more likely to ascribe health status to chance or external agency rather than to their own actions. Like their elders, then, it is clear that adolescents and young adults experience both physical and especially mental ill-health as a result of unemployment.

CONCLUSION: A ROLE FOR HEALTH POLICY

The foregoing review clearly demonstrates that the literature on the relationship between unemployment and health is complex and sometimes contradictory. The variable results of these studies depend not simply on the differing methodological preferences of their authors but on the age and sex of the population studied, the locale of the study population, the symptoms of interest, and doubtless many other factors. Yet certain generalizations seem warranted. First, the highest risk groups for adverse effects of unemployment appear to be middle-aged men, youth who have recently left school, the economically marginal such as women attempting reentry to the labor force, and children in families in which the primary earner is unemployed. Second, the most consistently documented disorders associated with job loss appear to be stress manifested by symptoms ranging from relatively mild anxiety and depression to suicide; cardiovascular disease, especially ischemic heart disease and hypertension; and respiratory disease. Finally, unemployment engenders increased utilization of medical services, particularly primary care, in those countries where access is not dependent on personal finances.

How may one explain this apparent relationship between unemployment and ill-health? The literature surveyed in this chapter does not provide a persuasive model. Brenner, it will be recalled, argued that job loss induces poverty, psychological stress, and inappropriate coping techniques such as excess alcohol consumption, which in aggregate prove pathogenic. Few if any of the micro-level studies cited advance beyond the task of establishing a connection between a particular population and adverse health outcomes to consider etiological issues. Clearly, the critical link between jobs and health must be sought elsewhere.

A promising though tentative model may emerge from the important work of Marmot (85). By following the health status of thousands of British civil servants over almost two decades, he was able to show a remarkably precise relationship between employment grade and age-standardized mortality. These individuals were not the socially marginal; they were, rather, steadily employed, reasonably remunerated, and in receipt of a comprehensive benefit scheme. Poverty, in short, could not explain the observed differences. When a specific cause of death such as coronary artery disease was examined in detail, the common risk factors such as elevated blood pressure, cholesterol levels, or smoking behavior could account for less than half the observed differences between groups. Some other factor was clearly operative, in the words of Robert Evans, "*something* that powerfully influences health and that is correlated with hierarchy per se" (86, p. 6).

It is this notion of hierarchy—of economic power, political authority, and social position—that is particularly heuristic for the health of the unemployed. Deprived of income and the employment-derived identity that defines social roles under contemporary capitalism, the unemployed are consigned by both themselves and society to the bottom of the national hierarchy. Here, like the lowest grade of Whitehall civil servant, their vulnerability to disease begins to climb relative to those who remain employed. If the precise pathophysiological mechanism of this enhanced risk remains as yet an arcane corner of psychoneuroimmunology (87), its applicability to the health of the unemployed does not seem premature. Indeed, the model may well serve to explain the larger observations that the physical quality of life is higher in socialist, that is, nonhierarchical, countries than in capitalist countries at comparable levels of economic development (88) and that standard measures of health outcomes in general favor high levels of democracy and left-wing regimes over right-wing regimes (89).

This persuasive theoretical position cannot, however, be allowed to obscure important conceptual constraints that significantly inhibit both the study of unemployment and health and the creation of relevant social policy. It must be recognized, first, that unemployment is not one objective state, the stuff of official statistics (90), but an existential phenomenon that differs according to the identity of those who experience it. A man who is the family's sole wage-earner, a middle-aged woman seeking a return to the work force after many years at home, a teenager searching for a first job, or a worker on the brink of retirement—all experience and, in health terms, react to unemployment in very different ways.

Second, the venue in which the unemployed find themselves may significantly influence the health consequences of being jobless. In nations such as Sweden, Britain, or Canada where access to publicly funded health care is universal, the apparent health consequence may differ from the U.S. experience where the vulnerable working poor may be virtually without access to care. Again, the level and comprehensiveness of a nation's unemployment insurance and retraining programs govern the financial stress and degree of future pessimism experienced by the unemployed. In effect, then, there is not one international experience of unemployment but many individual national experiences, and the measurable health responses would thus be expected to show an equal variability.

Third, in order to make convincing statements about the health impact of unemployment, data over a long time period are required. Yet paradoxically—and this is a criticism of several of Brenner's studies—the longer the period studied, the more likely the meaning and implications of unemployment itself will dramatically change. In the first quarter of the 20th century, for example, the scientific management theories of Taylor and the mass production techniques of Ford created in the United States an industrial work force of interchangeable laborers. These workers required scant training, had no role in planning production, experienced high rates of turnover, and were required only to focus on small specialized tasks. Such workers displaced an earlier generation of more costly and highly skilled craftsmen (91). The now-obsolete artisans were not simply unemployed: a way of life for the elite of the working class completely disappeared. The psychological implications of that transformation of role and status must have been as painfully obvious to the participants as they are opaque to a later generation of observers.

In ways as yet to be studied, unemployment in the Taylorite era may differ from today's experience of unemployment. The era of Fordism, characterized by mass production, relatively high wages, and liberal credit to fuel consumption, has faced accelerating erosion over the last two decades. In both Europe (92) and the United States (93) two factors—globalization of production so as to locate in the least expensive labor environment and technological change, especially the revolution in information transfer—have created yet another wave of unemployment. The same interchangeable workers integral to Fordism are now facing a future of insecure, part-time, low-skilled, and poorly paid work. New to this contemporary unemployment process has been the dramatic impact on middle managers. Following the restructuring of traditional corporate pyramids into more horizontal organizations and the introduction of sophisticated information-processing technology, these white-collar workers enter the post-Fordist era facing the same deskilling and low pay as former plant workers (94). How the new unemployment differentially affects the health of these two distinct groups of workers and how these effects compare with the impact on victims of earlier periods of large-scale job loss remains entirely unknown. It is clear, however, that a constant effect cannot be simply assumed.

Despite such conceptual constraints, policy planners must begin to face the reality of a linkage between unemployment and ill-health and to forge a gradual response to it. In so doing, a number of specific pitfalls must be avoided (95). First, policy must not medicalize unemployment: it is ultimately a social process, not merely a disorder suffered by unfortunate individuals. Second, the long-term goal of policy is not the normalization of unemployment by making it more comfortable for its victims. Comfort is a legitimate short-range objective; the abolition of unemployment individually and socially is the long-term intent. Finally, in identifying job loss as a cause of ill-health, one must not forget that employment is also a major cause of morbidity and mortality. Indeed, a recent Australian study of young workers concluded that the quality of work was more important in determining health status than was unemployment (96).

The initial area of policy concerns is short-term responses dedicated to defining and enhancing awareness of the relationship between health and unemployment. First, studies of two types must be undertaken. The precise health consequences of job loss in specific national or subnational jurisdictions must be investigated by large-scale, longitudinal studies, including appropriate control groups and continuing for at least 10 years to allow for long-term pathological outcomes. The results of such studies should form the basis of a second level of investigation that would compare the human and financial cost of ill-health with that of various interventions such as job-training schemes. Second, the health sector must be made aware of the pathogenicity of unemployment. Physicians and other health care providers must be taught early in their training the effects of joblessness on individual health and methods of intervening (97–99). Similarly, local health authorities must be made aware of the alterations in resource utilization, especially mental health facilities and family physician's services, likely to accompany rising unemployment and must be given tools to plan accordingly (100, 101).

In the medium term, policy must be directed at ameliorating the probably adverse effects of unemployment. First, high-risk groups must be identified and efficacious interventions tailored to their needs. For example, from the existing literature, middle-aged men and teenagers appear at significant risk. The former suffer from increased cardiovascular disease, which might benefit from dietary assistance, exercise programs, and smoking cessation. The latter are at risk for parasuicide and drug use, both of which would benefit from accessible counseling services. Second, stress management and realistic job-search programs, perhaps funded jointly by government, unions, and industry, have been shown to reduce anxiety and enhance the possibility of reemployment (52, 102–106). Third, a series of specific measures might, as discussed in the European Economic Community since the mid-1980s, create a social guarantee with respect to work. That is, individuals would be assured the right to employment or appropriate vocational training after a certain period of joblessness (107). Such measures would be accompanied by incentives for job sharing, maternity/paternity leave, early retirement, or remunerated community service.

Finally, long-term policy would address the complex issue of work, unemployment, and health in the 21st century (97, 108, 109). While it would demand little less than a basic restructuring of the relationship between work and the state, exactly such a consequence grew from the last period of prolonged economic crisis, the Depression, resulting in the contemporary welfare state. Some such changes—pay equity, for example—are already in progress, while other innovations, such as limiting lifetime working hours, are very much a future consideration. Perhaps the most promising area of policy development focuses on severing the link between income and employment.

Social policy in most western nations, dedicated to ending poverty, has been subordinated to economic policy that has chosen economic growth as a priority, arguing that the end result would be increased welfare for all. Yet the swelling ranks of the poor or unemployed suggest the economists' goal will not be achieved (110). The unemployment benefit schemes in most countries were designed during postwar situations of full employment and were intended to provide reasonably well for a small group of temporarily jobless workers. For the small number of permanently unemployed, social assistance schemes provide subsistence benefits. Many European countries, largely excluding the Mediterranean rim, have a minimum income system designed to cover very basic expenses for all citizens based on a means test. Unfortunately, the social reality of work, especially in the last decade, has shown these programs to be out-dated. They are unable to cope with swelling and chronic unemployment and impoverishing underemployment. As production jobs gravitate to cheaper labor markets in developing countries and technology simplifies both production and clerical tasks, employment is permanently lost and not at all balanced by the creation of a miniscule number of technology-related positions (111). Retraining for nonexistent jobs or the paper guarantee of the right to meaningful employment, seen in this light, is an anachronism.

The most promising solution to this expanding problem appears to be a dramatic break with the past. Income maintenance schemes traditionally top up employment-generated income and thus carry the assumption that citizen entitlement is work-related. In contrast, a basic income program carries quite a different connotation by guaranteeing subsistence for all irrespective of whether they work. Not only does this approach provide income to secure basic necessities but, more significantly, it replaces the state paternalism of existing programs with a right of citizenship, analogous to education or health care in many countries, unrelated to employment status. This is not, of course, to suggest an inactive citizenry. Many social services in the caring and nurturing sector of society, activities in creative arts, or in areas related to the assurance of environmental integrity have recently been downsized or eliminated by parsimonious governments. This nonpaid third-sector work cries out for the attention of those with time to contribute. Under a basic income program, then, the hierarchical implications of job loss become dramatically reduced and, it is to be hoped, so too are the attendant adverse implications for health (93, 94, 112).

The great epidemiologists of the 19th century were painfully aware of the connection between the grinding poverty of the working class and ill-health (113, 114). Within this class none were more pitiable than the submerged tenth, the chronically unemployed or unemployable. Living in unimaginable squalor, their health and longevity were commensurately circumscribed. In the late 20th century, protected by the general prosperity of developed nations and their attendant social support systems, we have lost touch with the insights of investigators like Villermé or Chadwick. Overshadowed by developments in technology, social medicine has been swept from a significant position on the medical agenda. Yet we have recently been forced to concede how relatively little community health status is influenced by medical diagnosis and treatment (115). Attention is again shifting from individual patients and their biological upsets to large populations and the pathogenicity of social conditions. This chapter has presented evidence that unemployment deserves to be considered a significant social cause of ill-health. It remains for policy planners to find first the bandage and then the cure.

Acknowledgment — I am grateful to Bill Bryce for sharing his personal and bibliographical knowledge of contemporary working-class America.

REFERENCES

1. Wilson, S., and Walker, G. Unemployment and health: A review. *Public Health* 107: 153–162, 1993.
2. Brenner, M. H. Health costs and benefits of economic policy. *Int. J. Health Serv.* 7: 581–623, 1977.
3. Brenner, M. H. Mortality and the economy: A review, and the experience of England and Wales, 1936–1976. *Lancet* ii: 568–573, 1979.
4. Brenner, M. H., and Mooney, A. Unemployment and health in the context of economic change. *Soc. Sci. Med.* 17: 1125–1138, 1983.
5. Brenner, M. H. Relation of economic change to Swedish health and social well-being, 1950–1980. *Soc. Sci. Med.* 25: 183–195, 1987.
6. Brenner, M. H. Economic change, alcohol consumption and heart disease mortality in nine industrialized countries. *Soc. Sci. Med.* 25: 119–132, 1987.
7. Lee, A., et al. Cigarette smoking and employment status. *Soc. Sci. Med.* 33: 1309–1312, 1991.
8. Claussen, B., and Aasland, O. The alcohol use disorders identification test (Audit) in a routine health examination of long-term unemployed. *Addictions* 88: 363–368, 1993.

9. Morris, J., Cook, D., and Shaper, A. Non-employment and changes in smoking, drinking, and body weight. *B.M.J.* 304: 536–541, 1992.

10. Eyer, J. Review of *Mental Illness and the Economy. Int. J. Health Serv.* 6: 139–148, 1976.

11. Eyer, J. Prosperity as a cause of death. *Int. J. Health Serv.* 7: 125–168, 1977.

12. Eyer, J. Does unemployment cause the death rate peak in each business cycle? A multifactor model of death rate change. *Int. J. Health Serv.* 7: 625–662, 1977.

13. Smith, R. He never got over losing his job: Death on the dole. *B.M.J.* 291: 1492–1495, 1985.

14. Kasl, S. V. Mortality and the business cycle: Some questions about research strategies when utilizing macro-social and ecological data. *Am. J. Public Health* 69: 784–788, 1979.

15. Spruit, I. Unemployment and health in macro-social analysis. *Soc. Sci. Med.* 16: 1903–1917, 1982.

16. Gravelle, H., Hutchinson, G., and Stern, J. Mortality and unemployment: A critique of Brenner's time-series analysis. *Lancet* ii: 657–679, 1981.

17. Lew, E. A. Mortality and the business cycle: How far can we push an association? *Am. J. Public Health* 69: 782–783, 1979.

18. Colledge, M. Economic cycles and health: Towards a sociological understanding of the impact of the recession on health issues. *Soc. Sci. Med.* 16: 1919–1927, 1982.

19. Cohen, S., Ginsberg, A., and Vladeck, B. The effect of unemployment and inflation on hospital-based ambulatory care. *Am. J. Public Health* 68: 1219–1221, 1978.

20. Bunn, A. Ischemic heart disease mortality and the business cycle in Australia. *Am. J. Public Health* 69: 772–781, 1979.

21. Iversen, L., and Sabroe, S. Plant closures, unemployment, and health: Danish experiences from the declining ship-building industry. In *Unemployment, Social Vulnerability and Health in Europe*, edited by D. Schwefel, P. Svenson, and H. Zoller, pp. 31–47. Springer-Verlag, Berlin, 1987.

22. Iversen, L., and Sabroe, S. Participation in a follow-up study of health among unemployed and employed people after a company closedown: Drop outs and selection bias. *J. Epidemiol. Community Health* 42: 396–401, 1988.

23. Iversen, L., Sabroe, S., and Damsgaard, M. Hospital admissions before and after shipyard closure. *B.M.J.* 299:1073–1076, 1989.

24. Joelson, L., and Wahlquist, L. The psychological meaning of job insecurity and job loss: Results of a longitudinal study. *Soc. Sci. Med.* 25: 179–182, 1987.

25. Westin, S., Schlesselman, J., and Korper, M. Long-term effects of a factory closure: Unemployment and disability during ten years' follow-up. *J. Clin. Epidemiol.* 42: 435–441, 1989.

26. Koskela, V., Arnkill, N., and Tikkanen, J. Unemployment and mental wellbeing: A factory closure study in Finland. *Act. Psychiatr. Scand.* 88: 429–433, 1993.

27. Beale, N., and Nethercott, S. The nature of unemployment morbidity. 1. Recognition. *J. R. Coll. Gen Pract.* 38: 197–199, 1988.

28. Beale, N., and Nethercott, S. The health of industrial employees four years after compulsory redundancy. *J. R. Coll. Gen. Pract.* 37: 390–394, 1987.

29. Burke, R. The closing at Canadian Admiral: Correlates of individual well-being sixteen months after shutdown. *Psychol. Rep.* 55: 91–98, 1984.

30. Grayson, J. The closure of a factory and its impact on health. *Int. J. Health Serv.* 15: 69–93, 1985.

31. Morris, J., and Cook, D. A critical review of the effects of factory closures on health. *Br. J. Ind. Med.* 48: 1–8, 1991.
32. Bartley, M., and Fagin, L. Hospital admissions before and after shipyard closure. *Br. J. Psychiatry* 156: 421–424, 1990.
33. McAvinchey, I. Economic factors and mortality, some aspects of the Scottish case 1950–1978. *J. Pol. Econ.* 31: 1–27, 1978.
34. Forbes, J., and McGregor, A. Unemployment and mortality in post-war Scotland. *J. Health Econ.* 3: 239–257, 1984.
35. Moser, K., Fox, A., and Jones, D. Unemployment and mortality in the OPCS Longitudinal Study. *Lancet* ii: 1324–1329, 1984.
36. Moser, K., et al. Unemployment and mortality: Comparison of the 1971 and 1981 longitudinal study census samples. *B.M.J.* 294: 86–90, 1987.
37. Starrin, B., Larsson, G., and Brenner, S.-O. Regional variations in cardiovascular mortality in Sweden—Structural vulnerability in the local community. *Soc. Sci. Med.* 27: 911–917, 1988.
38. Briggs, J., et al. The effects of the recession on the health of the people in two underprivileged areas of Oldham. *Public Health* 104: 437–447, 1990.
39. Westcott, G. The effect of unemployment on health in Scunthorpe and related health risk factors. *Public Health* 101: 399–416, 1987.
40. Kasl, S., Cobb, S., and Brooks, G. Changes in serum uric acid and cholesterol levels in men undergoing job loss. *JAMA* 206: 1500–1507, 1968.
41. Kasl, S., and Cobb, S. Blood pressure changes in men undergoing job loss: A preliminary report. *Psychosom. Med.* 32: 19–38, 1970.
42. Cobb, S. Physiological changes in men whose jobs were lost. *J. Psychosom. Res.* 18: 245–258, 1974.
43. D'Arcy, C., and Siddique, C. Unemployment and health: An analysis of "Canada Health Survey" data. *Int. J. Health Serv.* 15: 609–635, 1985.
44. Kasl, S., Gore, S., and Cobb, S. The experience of losing a job: Reported changes in health, symptoms and illness behaviour. *Psychosom. Med.* 37: 106–122, 1975.
45. Ahmad, W., Kernohan, E., and Baker, M. Influence of ethnicity and unemployment on the perceived health of a sample of general practice attenders. *Community Med.* 11: 148–156, 1989.
46. McKenna, S., and Payne, R. Comparison of the General Health Questionnaire and the Nottingham Health Profile in a study of unemployed and re-employed men. *Fam. Pract.* 6: 3–8, 1989.
47. Grayson, P. Health, physical activity level, and employment status in Canada. *Int. J. Health Serv.* 23: 743–761, 1993.
48. Lajer, M. Unemployment and hospitalization among bricklayers. *Scand. J. Soc. Med.* 10: 3–10, 1982.
49. Cook, et al. Health of unemployed middle-aged men in Great Britain. *Lancet* i: 1290–1294, 1982.
50. Payne, J., et al. Are deprivation indicators a proxy for morbidity? A comparison of the prevalence of arthritis, depression, dyspepsia, obesity and respiratory symptoms with unemployment rates and Jarman scores. *J. Public Health Med.* 15: 161–170, 1993.
51. Beale, N., and Nethercott, S. The nature of unemployment morbidity. 2. Description. *J. R. Coll. Gen. Pract.* 38: 200–202, 1988.

52. Kiernan, M., et al. Economic predictors of mental health service utilization: A time-series analysis. *Am. J. Community Psychol.* 17: 801–820, 1989.

53. Stokes, G., and Cochrane, R. The relationship between national levels of unemployment and the rate of admission to mental hospitals in England and Wales, 1950–1976. *Soc. Psychiatry* 19: 117–125, 1984.

54. Trainor, J., Boydell, K., and Tibshirami, R. Short-term economic change and utilization of mental health facilities in a metropolitan area. *Can. J. Psychiatry* 32: 379–383, 1987.

55. Ahr, P., Gorodezky, M., and Cho, D. Measuring the relationship of public psychiatric admissions to rising unemployment. *Hosp. Community Psychiatry* 32: 398–401, 1981.

56. Barling, P., and Handal, P. Incidence of utilization of public mental health facilities as a function of short-term economic decline. *Am. J. Community Psychol.* 8: 31–39, 1980.

57. Platt, S., and Kreitman, N. Trends in parasuicide and unemployment among men in Edinburgh, 1968–82. *B.M.J.* 289: 1029–1032, 1984.

58. Morton, M. Prediction of repetition of parasuicide: With special reference to unemployment. *Int. J. Soc. Psychiatry* 39: 87–99, 1993.

59. Jackson, P., and Warr, P. Mental health of unemployed men in different parts of England and Wales. *B.M.J.* 295: 525, 1987.

60. Catalano, R., and Dooley, C. Economic predictors of depressed mood and stressful life events in a metropolitan community. *J. Health Soc. Behav.* 18: 292–307, 1977.

61. Linn, M., Sandifer, R., and Stein, S. Effects of unemployment on mental and physical health. *Am. J. Public Health* 75: 502–506, 1985.

62. Frese, M., and Mohr, G. Prolonged unemployment and depression in older workers: A longitudinal study of intervening variables. *Soc. Sci. Med.* 25: 173–178, 1987.

63. Lahelma, E. Unemployment and mental well-being: Elaboration of the relationship. *Int. J. Health Serv.* 22: 261–274, 1992.

64. Jennings, S., Mazaik, C., and McKinlay, S. Women and work: An investigation of the association between health and employment in middle-aged women. *Soc. Sci. Med.* 19: 423–431, 1984.

65. Anson, O., and Anson, J. Women's health and labour force status: An inquiry using a multi-point measure of labour force participation. *Soc. Sci. Med.* 25: 57–63, 1987.

66. Nathanson, C. Social roles and health status among women: The significance of employment. *Soc. Sci. Med.* 14A: 463–471, 1980.

67. Wheeler, A., Lee, E., and Loe, H. Employment, sense of well-being and use of professional services among women. *Am. J. Public Health* 73: 908–911, 1983.

68. Hibbard, J., and Pope, C. Health effects of discontinuities in female employment and marital status. *Soc. Sci. Med.* 36: 1099–1104, 1993.

69. Brenner, S.-O., and Lennart, L. Long-term unemployment among women in Sweden. *Soc. Sci. Med.* 25: 153–161, 1987.

70. Starrin, B., and Larsson, G. Coping with unemployment—A contribution to the understanding of women's unemployment. *Soc. Sci. Med.* 25: 163–171, 1987.

71. Ratner, P. The incidence of wife abuse and mental health status in abused wives in Edmonton, Alberta. *Can. J. Public Health* 84: 246–249, 1983.

72. Cole, T., Donnet, M., and Standfield, J. Unemployment, birthweight, and growth in the first year. *Arch. Dis. Child.* 58: 717–721, 1983.

73. Brennan, M., and Lancashire, R. Association of childhood mortality with housing and unemployment. *J. Epidemiol. Community Health* 32: 28–33, 1978.
74. Joyce, T. A time-series analysis of unemployment and health: The case of birth outcomes in New York City. *J. Health Econ.* 8: 419–436, 1989.
75. Brenner, M. Fetal, infant and maternal mortality during periods of economic instability. *Int. J. Health Serv.* 3: 145–159, 1973.
76. Maclure, A., and Stewart, G. Admission of children to hospitals in Glasgow: Relation to unemployment and other deprivation variables. *Lancet* ii: 682–685, 1984.
77. Beale, N., and Nethercott, S. Job-loss and family morbidity: A study of a factory closure. *J. R. Coll. Gen. Pract.* 35: 510–514, 1985.
78. Smith, R. "We get on each other's nerves": Unemployment and the family. *B.M.J.* 291: 1707–1710, 1985.
79. Hammarstrom, A., Urban, J., and Theorell, T. Youth unemployment and ill health: Results from a 2-year follow-up study. *Soc. Sci. Med.* 26: 1025–1033, 1988.
80. Hammar, T. Unemployment and mental health among young people: A longitudinal study. *J. Adolesc.* 16: 407–420, 1993.
81. Banks, M., and Jackson, P. Unemployment and risk of minor psychiatric disorder in young people. *Psychol. Med.* 12: 789–798, 1982.
82. Warr, P., Banks, M., and Ullah, P. The experience of unemployment among black and white urban teenagers. *Br. J. Psychol.* 76: 75–87, 1985.
83. Hawton, K., et al. Adolescents who take overdoses: Their characteristics, problems and contacts with helping agencies. *Br. J. Psychiatry* 140: 118–123, 1982.
84. Cullen, J., et al. Unemployed youth and health: Findings from the pilot phase of a longitudinal study. *Soc. Sci. Med.* 25: 133–146, 1987.
85. Marmot, M. G. Social inequalities in mortality: The social environment. In *Class and Health: Research and Longitudinal Data*, edited by R. G. Wilkinson, pp. 21–33. Tavistock, London, 1986.
86. Evans, R. G. Introduction. In *Why Are Some People Healthy and Others Not? The Determinants of Health of Populations*, edited by R. G. Evans, M. L. Barer, and T. R. Marmor, pp. 3–26. Aldine de Gruyter, New York, 1994.
87. Hertzman, C., Frank, J., and Evans, R. G. Heterogeneities in health status and the determinants of population health. In *Why Are Some People Healthy and Others Not? The Determinants of Health of Populations*, edited by R. G. Evans, M. L. Barer, and T. R. Marmor, pp. 67–92. Aldine de Gruyter, New York, 1994.
88. Lena, H. F., and London, B. The political and economic determinants of health outcomes: A cross-national analysis. *Int. J. Health Serv.* 23: 585–602, 1993.
89. Cereseto, S., and Waitzkin, H. Capitalism, socialism, and the physical quality of life. *Int. J. Health Serv.* 16: 643–658, 1986.
90. Ezzy, D. Unemployment and mental health: A critical review. *Soc. Sci. Med.* 37: 41–52, 1993.
91. Waring, S. P. *Taylorism Transformed: Scientific Management Theory since 1945.* University of North Carolina Press, Chapel Hill, 1991.
92. Taylor-Gooby, P. Citizenship, dependency, and the welfare mix: Problems of inclusion and exclusion. *Int. J. Health Serv.* 23: 455–474, 1993.
93. Aronowitz, S., and DiFazio, W. *The Jobless Future, Sci-tech and the Dogma of Work.* University of Minnesota Press, Minneapolis, 1994.

94. Rifkin, J. *The End of Work: The Decline of the Global Labor Force and the Dawn of the Post-market Era*. G. P. Putnam's Sons, New York, 1995.

95. Miles, I. Some observations on "unemployment and health" research. *Soc. Sci. Med.* 25: 223–225, 1987.

96. Graetz, B. Health consequences of employment and unemployment: Longitudinal evidence for young men and women. *Soc. Sci. Med.* 36: 715–724, 1993.

97. Smith, R. Improving the health of the unemployed: A job for health authorities and health workers. *B.M.J.* 292: 470–472, 1986.

98. Abraham, I., and Krowchuk, H. Unemployment and health: Health promotion for the jobless male. *Nurs. Clin. North Am.* 21: 37–47, 1986.

99. Claussen, B. A clinical follow up of unemployed II: Sociomedical evaluations as predictors of re-employment. *Scand. J. Prim. Health Care* 11: 234–240, 1993.

100. Harris, C., and Smith, R. What are health authorities doing about the health problems caused by unemployment? *B.M.J.* 294: 1076–1079, 1987.

101. Svensson, P.-G. International social and health policies to prevent ill health in the unemployed: The World Health Organization perspective. *Soc. Sci. Med.* 25: 201–204, 1987.

102. Manuso, J. Coping with job abolishment. *J. Occup. Med.* 19: 598–602, 1977.

103. Frese, M. Alleviating depression in the unemployed: Adequate financial support, hope and early retirement. *Soc. Sci. Med.* 25: 213–215, 1987.

104. Caplan, R., et al. Job seeking, reemployment, and mental health: A randomized field experiment in coping with job loss. *J. Appl. Psychol.* 74: 759–769, 1989.

105. Jones, L. The health consequences of economic recessions. *J. Health Soc. Pol.* 3: 1–14, 1991.

106. Liem, R. Unemployment and mental health implications for human service policy. *Policy Stud. J.* 10: 350–364, 1981.

107. Kieselbach, T. Youth unemployment and health effects. *Int. J. Soc. Psychiatry* 34: 83–94, 1988.

108. Cahill, J. Structural characteristics of the macro-economy and mental health: Implications for primary prevention research. *Am. J. Community Psychol.* 11: 553–571, 1983.

109. Olafsson, O., and Svensson, P.-G. Unemployment-related lifestyle changes and health disturbances in adolescents and children in the western countries. *Soc. Sci. Med.* 22: 1105–1113, 1986.

110. Walker, A. The persistence of poverty under welfare states and the prospects for its abolition. *Int. J. Health Serv.* 22: 1–17, 1992.

111. Abrahamson, P. E. Welfare and poverty in the Europe of the 1990s: Social progress or social dumping? *Int. J. Health Serv.* 21: 237–264, 1991.

112. Handy, C. *The Future of Work: A Guide to a Changing Society*. Basil Blackwell, Oxford, 1985.

113. Coleman, W. *Death Is a Social Disease: Public Health and Political Economy in Early Industrial France*. University of Wisconsin Press, Madison, 1982.

114. Eyler, J. *Victorian Social Medicine: The Ideas and Methods of William Farr*. Johns Hopkins University Press, Baltimore, Md., 1979.

115. Townsend, P., and Davidson, N. *Inequalities in Health: The Black Report*. Penguin Books, Harmondsworth, 1982.

CHAPTER 9

Man-Made Medicine and Women's Health: The Biopolitics of Sex/Gender and Race/Ethnicity

Nancy Krieger and Elizabeth Fee

Glance at any collection of national health data for the United States, whether pertaining to health, disease, or the health care system, and several obvious features stand out (1–5). First, we notice that most reports present data in terms of race, sex, and age. Some races are clearly of more interest than others. National reports most frequently use racial groups called "white," and "black," and increasingly, they use a group called "Hispanic." Occasionally, we find data on Native Americans, and on Asians and Pacific Islanders. Whatever the specific categories chosen, the reports agree that white men and women, for the most part, have the best health, at all ages. They also show that men and women, across all racial groups, have different patterns of disease: obviously, men and women differ for conditions related to reproduction (women, for example, do not get testicular cancer), but they differ for many other conditions as well (for example, men on average have higher blood pressure and develop cardiovascular disease at an earlier age). And, in the health care sector, occupations, just like diseases, are differentially distributed by race and sex.

All this seems obvious. But it isn't. We know about race and sex divisions because this is what our society considers important. This is how we classify people and collect data. This is how we organize our social life as a nation. This is therefore how we structure our knowledge about health and disease. And this is what we find important as a subject of research (6–9).

It seems so routine, so normal, to view the health of women and men as fundamentally different, to consider the root of this difference to be biological sex, and to think about race as an inherent, inherited characteristic that also affects health (10). The work of looking after sick people follows the same categories. Simply walk into a hospital and observe that most of the doctors are white men, most of the registered nurses are white women, most of the kitchen and laundry workers are black and Hispanic women, and most of the janitorial staff are black and Hispanic men. Among the patients, notice who has appointments with private clinicians and who is getting care in the emergency room; the color line is obvious. Notice who provides health care at home: wives, mothers, and daughters. The gender line at home and in medical institutions is equally obvious (11–15).

These contrasting patterns, by race and sex, are longstanding. How do we explain them? What kinds of explanations satisfy us? Some are comfortable with explanations that accept these patterns as natural, as the result of natural law, as part of the natural order of things. Of course, if patterns are that way by nature, they cannot be changed. Others aim to understand these patterns precisely in order to change them. They look for explanations suggesting that these patterns are structured by convention, by discrimination, by the politics of power, and by unreasonable law. These patterns, in other words, reflect the social order of people.

In this chapter, we discuss how race and sex became such all-important, self-evident categories in 19th and 20th century biomedical thought and practice. We examine the consequences of these categories for our knowledge about health and for the provision of health care. We then consider alternative approaches to studying race/ethnicity, gender, and health. And we address these issues with reference to a typically suppressed and repressed category: that of social class.

THE SOCIAL CONSTRUCTION OF "RACE" AND "SEX" AS KEY BIOMEDICAL TERMS AND THEIR EFFECT ON KNOWLEDGE ABOUT HEALTH

In the 19th century, the construction of "race" and "sex" as key biomedical categories was driven by social struggles over human inequality. Before the Civil War, the dominant understanding of race was as a natural/theological category—black–white differences were innate and reflected God's will (16–19). These differences were believed to be manifest in every aspect of the body, in sickness and in health. But when abolitionists began to get the upper hand in moral and theological arguments, proponents of slavery appealed to science as the new arbiter of racial distinction.

In this period, medical men were beginning to claim the mantle of scientific knowledge and assert their right to decide controversial social issues (20–22). Recognizing the need for scientific authority, the state of Louisiana, for example, commissioned one prolific proponent of slavery, Dr. Samuel Cartwright, to prove the natural inferiority of blacks, a task that led him to detail every racial difference imaginable—in texture of hair, length of bones, vulnerability to disease, and even color of the internal organs (23–25). As the Civil War changed the status of blacks from legal chattel to bona fide citizens, however, medical journals began to question old verities about racial differences and, as importantly, to publish new views of racial similarities (26, 27). Some authors even attributed black–white differences in health to differences in socioeconomic position. But by the 1870s, with the destruction of reconstruction, the doctrine of innate racial distinction again triumphed. The scientific community once again deemed "race" a fundamental biological category (28–32).

Theories of women's inequality followed a similar pattern (33–36). In the early 19th century, traditionalists cited scripture to prove women's inferiority. These authorities agreed that Eve had been formed out of Adam's rib and that all women had to pay the price of her sin—disobeying God's order, seeking illicit knowledge from the serpent, and tempting man with the forbidden apple. Women's pain in childbirth was clear proof of God's displeasure.

When these views were challenged in the mid-19th century by advocates of women's rights and proponents of liberal political theory, conservatives likewise turned to the new arbiters of knowledge and sought to buttress their position with scientific facts and medical authority (37, 38). Biologists busied themselves with measuring the size of women's skulls, the length of their bones, the rate of their breathing, and the number of their blood cells. And considering all the evidence, the biologists concluded that women were indeed the weaker sex (39–41).

Agreeing with this stance, medical men energetically took up the issue of women's health and equality (42–45). They were convinced that the true woman was by nature sickly, her physiological systems at the mercy of her ovaries and uterus. Because all bodily organs were interconnected, they argued, a woman's monthly cycle irritated her delicate nervous system and her sensitive, small, weak brain. Physicians considered women especially vulnerable to nervous ailments such as neurasthenia and hysteria. This talk of women's delicate constitutions did not, of course, apply to slave women or to working-class women—but it was handy to refute the demands of middle-class women whenever they sought to vote or gain access to education and professional careers. At such moments, many medical men declared the doctrine of separate spheres to be the ineluctable consequence of biology.

At the same time, 19th century medical authorities began to conceptualize class as a natural, biological distinction. Traditional, pre-scientific views held class hierarchies to be divinely ordained; according to the more scientific view that emerged in the early 19th century, class position was determined by innate, inherited ability. In both cases, class was perceived as an essentially stable, hierarchical ranking. These discussions of class usually assumed white or Western European populations and often applied only to males within those populations.

With the impact of the industrial revolution, classes took on a clearly dynamic character. As landowners invested in canals and railroads, as merchants became capitalist entrepreneurs, and as agricultural workers were transformed into an industrial proletariat, the turbulent transformation of the social order provoked new understandings of class relationships (46). The most developed of these theories was that of Karl Marx, who emphasized the system of classes as a social and economic formation and stressed the contradictions between different class interests (47). From this point onward, the very idea of social classes in many people's minds implied a revolutionary threat to the social order.

In opposition to Marxist analyses of class, the theory of Social Darwinism was formulated to suggest that the new social inequalities of industrial society reflected natural law (48–51). This theory was developed in the midst of the economic depression of the 1870s, at a time when labor struggles, trade union organizing, and early socialist movements were challenging the political and economic order. Many scientists and medical men drew upon Darwin's idea of "the struggle for survival," first expressed in the *Origin of the Species* in 1859 (52), to justify social inequality. They argued that those on top, the social elite, must by definition be the "most fit" because they had survived so well. Social hierarchies were therefore built on and reflected real biological differences. Poor health status simultaneously was sign and proof of biological inferiority.

By the late 19th century, theories of race, gender, and class inequality were linked together by the theory of Social Darwinism, which promised to provide a scientific basis for social policy (48–51). In the realm of race, for example, proponents of Social Darwinism blithely predicted that the "Negro question" would soon resolve itself—the "Negro" would naturally become extinct, eliminated by the inevitable workings of "natural selection" (29, 53). Many public health officers—particularly in the southern states—agreed that "Negroes" were an inherently degenerate, syphilitic, and tubercular race, for whom public health interventions could do little (54–57). Social Darwinists also argued that natural and sexual selection would lead to increasing differentiation between the sexes (34, 48, 58). With further evolution, men would become ever more masculine and women ever more feminine. As proof, they looked to the upper classes, whose masculine and feminine behavior represented the forefront of evolutionary progress.

Over time, the Social Darwinist view of class gradually merged into general American ideals of progress, meritocracy, and success through individual effort. According to the dominant American ideology, individuals were so mobile that fixed measures of social class were irrelevant. Such measures were also un-American. Since the Paris Commune, and especially since the Bolshevik revolution, discussions of social class in the United States were perceived as politically threatening. Although fierce debates about inequality continued to revolve around the axis of nature versus nurture, the notion of class as a social relationship was effectively banished from respectable discourse and policy debate (48, 59). Social position was once again equated only with rank, now understood as socioeconomic status.

In the early 20th century, Social Darwinists had considerable influence in shaping public views and public policy (48, 59–64). They perceived two new threats to American superiority: the massive tide of immigration from eastern and southern Europe, and the declining birth rate—or "race suicide"—among American white women of Anglo-Saxon and Germanic descent. Looking to the fast-developing field of genetics, now bolstered by the rediscovery of Gregor Mendel's laws and by T. H. Morgan's fruit fly experiments (65–68), biological determinists regrouped under the banner of eugenics. Invoking morbidity and mortality data that showed a high rate of tuberculosis and infectious disease among the immigrant poor (69–71), they declared "ethnic" Europeans a naturally inferior and sickly stock and thus helped win passage of the Immigration Restriction Act in 1924 (72–74). This legislation required the national mix of immigrants to match that entering the United States in the early 1870s, thereby severely curtailing immigration of racial and ethnic groups deemed inferior. "Race/ ethnicity," construed as a biological reality, became ever more entrenched as the *explanation* of racial/ethnic differences in disease; social explanations were seen as the province of scientifically illiterate and naive liberals, or worse, socialist and Bolshevik provocateurs.

Other developments in the early 20th century encouraged biological explanations of sex differences in disease and in social roles. The discovery of the sex chromosomes in 1905 (75–77) reinforced the idea that gender was a fundamental biological trait, built into the genetic constitution of the body. That same year, Ernest Starling coined the term "hormone" (78) to denote the newly characterized chemical messengers that permitted one organ to control—at a distance— the activities of another. By the mid-1920s, researchers had isolated several hormones integral to reproductive physiology and popularized the notion of "sex hormones" (79–83). The combination of sex chromosomes and sex hormones was imbued with almost magical powers to shape human behavior in gendered terms; women were now at the mercy of their genetic limitations and a changing brew of hormonal imperatives (84, 85). In the realm of medicine, researchers turned to sex chromosomes and hormones to understand cancers of the uterus and breast and a host of other sex-linked diseases (86–90); they no longer saw the need to worry about environmental influences. In the workplace, of course, employers said that sex chromosomes and hormones dictated which jobs women could—and could not—perform (45, 91, 92). This in turn determined the occupational hazards to which women would be exposed—once again, women's health and ill-health was really a matter of their biology.

Within the first few decades of the 20th century, these views were institutionalized within scientific medicine and the new public health. At this time, the training of physicians and public health practitioners was being recast in modern, scientific terms (93–95). Not surprisingly, biological determinist views of racial/ethnic and sex/gender differences became a natural and integral part of the curriculum, the research agenda, and medical and public health practice. Over time, ethnic differences in disease among white European groups were downplayed and instead, the differences between whites and blacks, whites and Mexicans, and whites and Asians were emphasized. Color was now believed to define distinct biological groups.

Similarly, the sex divide marked a gulf between two completely disparate groups. Within medicine, women's health was relegated to obstetrics and gynecology; within public health, women's health needs were seen as being met by maternal and child health programs (8, 45, 96). Women were perceived as wives and mothers; they were important for childbirth, childcare, and domestic nutrition. Although no one denied that some women worked, women's occupational health was essentially ignored because women were, after all, only temporary workers. Outside the specialized realm of reproduction, all other health research concerned men's bodies and men's diseases. Reproduction was so central to women's biological existence that women's nonreproductive health was rendered virtually invisible.

Currently, it is popular to argue that the lack of research on white women and on men and women in nonwhite racial/ethnic groups resulted from a perception of white men as the norm (97–99). This interpretation, however, is inaccurate. In fact, by the time that researchers began to standardize methods for clinical and epidemiological research, notions of difference were so firmly embedded that whites and nonwhites, women and men, were rarely studied together. Moreover, most researchers and physicians were interested only in the health status of whites and, in the case of women, only in their reproductive health. They therefore used white men as the research subjects of choice for all health conditions other than women's reproductive health and paid attention to the health status of nonwhites only to measure degrees of racial difference. For the most part, the health of women and men of color and the nonreproductive health of white women was simply ignored. It is critical to read these omissions as evidence of a logic of difference rather than as an assumption of similarity.

This framework has shaped knowledge and practice to the present. In the United States, vital statistics present health information in terms of race and sex and age, conceptualized only as biological variables—ignoring the social dimensions of gender and ethnicity. Data on social class are not collected. At the same time, public health professionals are unable adequately to explain or to change inequalities in health between men and women and between diverse racial/ethnic groups. We now face the question: Is there any alternative way of understanding these population patterns of health and disease?

ALTERNATIVE WAYS OF
STUDYING RACE, GENDER, AND HEALTH:
SOCIAL MEASURES FOR SOCIAL CATEGORIES

The first step in creating an alternative understanding is to recognize that the categories we traditionally treat as simply biological are in fact largely social. The second step is to realize we need social concepts to understand these social categories. The third step is to develop social measures and appropriate strategies for a new kind of health research (10).

With regard to race/ethnicity, we need to be clear that "race" is a spurious biological concept (100–102). Although historical patterns of geographic isolation and migration account for differences in the distribution of certain genes, genetic variation within so-called racial groups far exceeds that across groups. All humans share approximately 95 percent of their genetic makeup (100, p. 155). Racial/ethnic differences in disease thus require something other than a genetic explanation.

Recognizing this problem, some people have tried to substitute the term "ethnicity" for "race" (103, 104). In the public health literature, however, "ethnicity" is rarely defined. For some, it apparently serves as a polite way of referring to what are still conceptualized as "racial"/biological differences. For others, it expresses a new form of "cultural" determinism, in which ethnic differences in ways of living are seen as autonomous "givens" unrelated to the social status of particular ethnic groups within our society (105, 106). This cultural determinism makes discrimination invisible and can feed into explanations of health status as reductionist and individualistic as those of biological determinism.

For a different starting point, consider the diverse ways in which racism operates, at both an institutional and interpersonal level (107–109). Racism is a matter of economics, and it is also more than economics. It structures living and working conditions, affects daily interactions, and takes its toll on people's dignity and pride. All of this must be considered when we examine the connection between race/ethnicity and health.

To address the economic aspects of racism, we need to include economic data in all studies of health status (110, 111). Currently, our national health data do not include economic information—instead, racial differences are often used as indicators of economic differences. To the extent that economics are taken into account, the standard approach assumes that differences are either economic or "genetic." So, for those conditions where racial/ethnic differences persist even within economic strata—hypertension and preterm delivery, for example—the assumption is that something biological, something genetic, is at play. Researchers rarely consider the noneconomic aspects of racism or the ways in which racism continues to work within economic levels.

Some investigators, however, are beginning to consider how racism shapes people's environments. Several studies, for example, document the fact that toxic dumps are most likely to be located in poor neighborhoods and are disproportionately located in poor neighborhoods of color (112–114). Other researchers are starting to ask how people's experience of and response to discrimination may influence their health (115–118). A recent study of hypertension, for example, found that black women who responded actively to unfair treatment were less likely to report high blood pressure than women who internalized their responses (115). Interestingly, the black women at highest risk were those who reported *no* experiences of racial discrimination.

Countering the traditional practice of always taking whites as the standard of comparison, some researchers are beginning to focus on other racial/ethnic groups to better understand why, within each of the groups, some are at higher risk than others for particular disease outcomes (119–121). They are considering whether people of color may be exposed to specific conditions that whites are not. In addition to living and working conditions, these include cultural practices that may be positive as well as negative in their effects on health. Some studies, for example, point to the importance of black churches in providing social support (122–124). These new approaches break with monolithic assumptions about what it means to belong to a given racial/ethnic group and consider diversity *within* each group. To know the color of a person's skin is to know very little.

It is equally true that to know a person's sex is to know very little. Women are often discussed as a single group defined chiefly by biological sex, members of an abstract, universal (and implicitly white) category. In reality, we are a mixed lot, our gender roles and options shaped by history, culture, and deep divisions across class and color lines. Of course, it is true that women, in general, have the capacity to become pregnant, at least at some stages of their lives. Traditionally, women as a group are defined by this reproductive potential. Usually ignored are the many ways that gender as a social reality gets into the body and transforms our biology—differences in childhood expectations about exercise, for example, affect our subsequent body build (38, 125).

From a health point of view, women's reproductive potential does carry the possibility of specific reproductive ills ranging from infertility to preterm delivery to cervical and breast cancer. These reproductive ills are not simply associated with the biological category "female," but are differentially experienced according to social class and race/ethnicity. Poor women, for example, are much more likely to suffer from cervical cancer (119, 126). By contrast, at least among older women, breast cancer is more common among the affluent (126, 127). These patterns, which at times can become quite complex, illustrate the general point that, even in the case of reproductive health, more than biological sex is at issue. Explanations of women's reproductive health that ignore the social patterning of disease and focus only on endogenous factors are thus inadequate.

If we turn to those conditions that afflict both men and women—the majority of all diseases and health problems—we must keep two things simultaneously in mind. First are the differences and similarities among diverse groups of women; second are the differences and similarities between women and men.

For a glimpse of the complexity of disease patterns, consider the example of hypertension (128, 129). As we mentioned, working-class and poor women are at greater risk than affluent women; black women, within each income level, are more likely to be hypertensive than white women (5). The risks of Hispanic women vary by national origin: Mexican women are at lowest risk, Central American women at higher risk, and Puerto Rican and Cuban women at the highest risk (130, 131). In what is called the "Hispanic paradox," Mexican-American women have a higher risk profile than Anglo-American women, yet experience lower rates of hypertension (132). To further complicate the picture, the handful of studies of Japanese and Chinese women in the United States show them to have low rates, while Filipina women have high rates, almost equal those of African Americans (130, 133, 134). Rates vary across different groups of Native American women; those who live in the Northern plains have higher rates than those in the Southwest (130, 135). From all this, we can conclude that there is enormous variation in hypertension rates among women.

If we look at the differences between women and men, we find that men in each racial/ethnic group have higher rates of hypertension than women (129). Even so, the variation among women is sufficiently great that women in some racial/ethnic groups have higher rates than men in other groups. Filipina women, for example, have higher rates of hypertension than white men (5, 133). Obviously, the standard biomedical categories of race and sex cannot explain these patterns. If we want to understand hypertension, we will have to understand the complex distribution of disease among real women and men; these patterns are not merely distracting details but the proper test of the plausibility of our hypotheses.

As a second example, consider the well-known phenomenon of women's longer life expectancy. This difference is common to all industrialized countries, and amounts to about seven years in the United States (136, 137). The higher mortality of men at younger ages is largely due to higher accident rates, and at older ages, to heart disease.

The higher accident rates of younger men are not accidental. They are due to more hazardous occupations, higher rates of illicit drug and alcohol use, firearms injuries, and motor vehicle crashes—hazards related to gender roles and expectations (136, 137). The fact that men die earlier of heart disease—the single most common cause of death in both sexes—may also be related to gender roles. Men have higher rates of cigarette smoking and fewer sources of social support, suggesting that the masculine ideal of the Marlboro man is not a healthy one. Some contend that women's cardiovascular advantage is mainly biological, due to the protective effect of their hormone levels (138). Interestingly, however, a study carried out in a kibbutz in Israel, where men and women were engaged in comparable activities, found that the life expectancy gap was only four and a half years—just over half the national average (139). While biological differences between men and women now receive much of the research attention, it is important to remember that men are gendered beings too.

Clearly, our patterns of health and disease have everything to do with how we live in the world. Nowhere is this more evident than in the strong social class gradients apparent in almost every form of morbidity and mortality

(110, 140–143). Yet here the lack of information and the conceptual confusion about the relationship between social class and women's health is a major obstacle. As previously noted, in this country, we have no regular method of collecting data on socioeconomic position and health. Even if we had such data, measures of social class generally assume male heads of households and male patterns of employment (111, 144). This, indeed, is one of the failures of class analyses—that they do not deal adequately with women (144–147).

Perhaps the easiest way to understand the problems of class measurements and women's health is briefly to mention the current debates in Britain, a country that has long collected social class data (148, 149). Men and unmarried women are assigned a social class position according to their employment; married women, however, are assigned a class position according to the employment of their husbands. As British feminist researchers have argued, this traditional approach obscures the magnitude of class differences in women's health (149). Instead, they are proposing measures of household class that take into account the occupations of both women and their husbands, and also other household assets.

Here in the United States, we have hardly any research on the diverse measures of social class in relation to women's health. Preliminary studies suggest we also would do well to distinguish between individual and household class (150, 151). Other research shows that we can partly overcome the absence of social class information in U.S. medical records by using census data (126, 152). This method allows us to describe people in terms of the socioeconomic profile of their immediate neighborhood. When coupled with individual measures of social class, this approach reveals, for example, that working-class women who live in working-class neighborhoods are somewhat more likely to have high blood pressure than working-class women who live in more affluent neighborhoods (152). We thus need conceptually to separate three distinct levels at which class operates: individual, household, and neighborhood.

As a final example of why women's health cannot be understood without reference to issues of sex/gender, race/ethnicity, and social class, consider the case of AIDS (153–155). The definition of disease, the understanding of risk, and the approach to prevention are shaped by our failure to grasp fully the social context of disease. For the first decade, women's unique experiences of AIDS were rendered essentially invisible. The first definition of AIDS was linked to men, because it was perceived to be a disease of gay men and those with a male sex-linked disorder, hemophilia. The very listing of HIV-related diseases taken to characterize AIDS was a listing based on male experience of infection. Only much later, after considerable protest by women activists, were female disorders—such as invasive cervical cancer—made part of the definition of the disease (156, 157).

Our understanding of risk is still constrained by the standard approaches. AIDS data are still reported only in terms of race, sex, and mode of transmission; there are no data on social class (158). We know, however, that the women who have AIDS are overwhelmingly women of color. As of July 1993, of the nearly 37,000 women diagnosed with AIDS, over one half were African American, another 20 percent were Hispanic, 25 percent were white, and about 1 percent were Asian, Pacific Islander, or Native American (158). What puts these women at risk? It seems clear that one determinant is the missing variable, social class. Notably, the women at highest risk are injection drug users, the sexual partners of injection drug users, and sex workers (154). The usual listing of behavioral and demographic risk factors, however, fails to capture the social context in which the AIDS epidemic has unfolded. Most of the epidemiological accounts are silent about the blight of inner cities, the decay of urban infrastructure under the Reagan–Bush administrations, unemployment, the drug trade, prostitution, and the harsh realities of everyday racism (159, 160). We cannot gain an adequate understanding of risk absent a real understanding of people's lives.

Knowledge of what puts women at risk is of course critical for prevention. Yet, just as the initial definitions of AIDS reflected a male-gendered perspective, so did initial approaches to prevention (161). The emphasis on condoms assumed that the central issue was knowledge, not male–female power relations. For women to use condoms in heterosexual sex, however, they need more than bits of latex; they need male assent. The initial educational materials were created without addressing issues of power; they were male-oriented and obviously white—in both the mode and language of presentation. AIDS programs and services, for the most part, still do not address women's needs, whether heterosexual, bisexual, or lesbian. Pregnant women and women with children continue to be excluded from most drug treatment programs. And when women become sick and die we have no remotely adequate social policies for taking care of the families left behind.

In short, our society's approach to AIDS reflects the larger refusal to deal with the ways in which sex/gender, race/ethnicity, and class are inescapably intertwined with health. This refusal affects not only what we know and what we do about AIDS, but also the other issues we have mentioned—hypertension, cancer, life expectancy—and many we have not (162). As we have tried to argue, the issues of women's health cannot be understood in only biological terms, as simply the ills of the female of the species. Women and men are different, but we are also similar—and we both are divided by the social relations of class and race/ethnicity. To begin to understand how our social constitution affects our health, we must ask, repeatedly, what is different and what is similar across the social divides of gender, color, and class. We cannot assume that biology alone will provide the answers we need; instead, we must reframe the issues in the context of the social shaping of our human lives—as both biological creatures and historical actors. Otherwise, we will continue to mistake—as many before us have done—what is for what must be, and leave unchallenged the social forces that continue to create vast inequalities in health.

REFERENCES

1. National Center for Health Statistics. *Health, United States, 1991*. DHHS Pub. No. (PHS) 92-1232. U.S. Public Health Service, Hyattsville, Md., 1992.
2. National Center for Health Statistics. *Vital Statistics of the United States—1988. Vol. I, Natality*. DHHS Pub. No. (PHS) 90-1100. U.S. Government Printing Office, Washington, D.C., 1990.
3. National Center for Health Statistics. *Vital Statistics of the United States—1987. Vol. II, Mortality, Part A*. DHHS Pub. No. (PHS) 90-1101. U.S. Government Printing Office, Washington, D.C., 1990.
4. National Center for Health Statistics. *Vital Statistics of the United States—1988. Vol. II, Mortality, Part B*. DHHS Pub. No. (PHS) 90-1102. U.S. Government Printing Office, Washington, D.C., 1990.
5. U.S. Department of Health and Human Services. *Health Status of Minorities and Low-Income Groups*, Ed. 3. U.S. Government Printing Office, Washington, D.C., 1991.
6. Krieger, N. The making of public health data: Paradigms, politics, and policy. *J. Public Health Policy* 13: 412–427, 1992.
7. Navarro, V. Work, ideology, and science: The case of medicine. In *Crisis, Health, and Medicine: A Social Critique*, edited by V. Navarro, pp. 142–182. Tavistock, New York City, 1986.
8. Fee, E. (ed.). *Women and Health: The Politics of Sex in Medicine*. Baywood, Amityville, N.Y., 1983.
9. Tesh, S. *Hidden Arguments: Political Ideology and Disease Prevention Policy*. Rutgers University Press, New Brunswick, N.J., 1988.
10. Krieger, N., et al. Racism, sexism, and social class: Implications for studies of health, disease, and well-being. *Am. J. Prev. Med.* 9(Suppl. 2): 82–122, 1993.
11. Butter I., et al., *Sex and Status: Hierarchies in the Health Workforce*. American Public Health Association, Washington, D.C., 1985.
12. Sexton, P. C. *The New Nightingales: Hospital Workers, Unions, New Women's Issues*. Enquiry Press, New York, 1982.
13. Melosh, B. *The Physician's Hand: Work, Culture and Conflict in American Nursing*. Temple University Press, Philadelphia, 1982.
14. Wolfe, S. (ed.). *Organization of Health Workers and Labor Conflict*. Baywood, Amityville, N.Y., 1978.
15. Feldman, P. H., Sapienza, A. M., and Kane, N. M. *Who Cares for Them? Workers in the Home Care Industry*. Greenwood Press, New York, 1990.
16. Krieger, N. Shades of difference: Theoretical underpinnings of the medical controversy on black/white differences in the United States, 1830–1870. *Int. J. Health Serv.* 17: 256–278, 1987.
17. Stanton, W. *The Leopard's Spots: Scientific Attitudes Towards Race in America, 1815–59*. University of Chicago Press, Chicago, 1960.
18. Stepan, N. *The Idea of Race in Science, Great Britain, 1800–1860*. Archon Books, Hamden, Conn., 1982.
19. Jordan, W. D. *White Over Black: American Attitudes toward the Negro, 1550–1812*. University of North Carolina Press, Chapel Hill, 1968.
20. Rosenberg, C. E. *No Other Gods: On Science and American Social Thought*. Johns Hopkins University Press, Baltimore, Md., 1976.
21. Daniels, G. H. The process of professionalization in American science: The emergent period, 1820–1860. *Isis* 58: 151–166, 1967.

22. Rothstein, W. G. *American Physicians in the 19th Century: From Sects to Science.* Johns Hopkins University Press, Baltimore, Md., 1972.
23. Cartwright, S. A. Report on the diseases and physical peculiarities of the Negro race. *New Orleans Med. Surg. J.* 7: 691–715, 1850.
24. Cartwright, S. A. Alcohol and the Ethiopian: Or, the moral and physical effects of ardent spirits on the Negro race, and some accounts of the peculiarities of that people. *New Orleans Med. Surg. J.* 15: 149–163, 1858.
25. Cartwright, S. A. Ethnology of the Negro or prognathous race—A lecture delivered November 30, 1857, before the New Orleans Academy of Science. *New Orleans Med. Surg. J.* 15: 149–163, 1858.
26. Reyburn, R. Remarks concerning some of the diseases prevailing among the Freedpeople in the District of Columbia (Bureau of Refugees, Freedmen and Abandoned Lands). *Am. J. Med. Sci.* (n.s.) 51: 364–369, 1866.
27. Byron, J. Negro regiments—Department of Tennessee. *Boston Med. Surg. J.* 69: 43–44, 1863.
28. Foner, E. *Reconstruction: America's Unfinished Revolution, 1863–1877.* Harper & Row, New York City, 1988.
29. Haller, J. S. Jr. *Outcasts from Evolution: Scientific Attitudes of Racial Inferiority, 1859–1900.* University of Illinois Free Press, Urbana, 1971.
30. Stocking, G. W. *Race, Culture, and Evolution: Essays in the History of Anthropology.* Free Press, New York, 1968.
31. Lorimer, D. *Colour, Class and the Victorians.* Holmes & Meier, New York, 1978.
32. Gamble, V. N. (ed.). *Germs Have No Color Line: Blacks and American Medicine, 1900–1940.* Garland, New York, 1989.
33. Barker-Benfield, G. J. *The Horrors of the Half-Known Life: Male Attitudes toward Women and Sexuality in Nineteenth-Century America.* Harper & Row, New York, 1976.
34. Fee, E. Science and the woman problem: Historical perspectives. In *Sex Differences: Social and Biological Perspectives,* edited by M. S. Teitelbaum, pp. 175–223. Anchor/Doubleday, New York, 1976.
35. Jordanova, L. *Sexual Visions: Images of Gender in Science and Medicine between the Eighteenth and Twentieth Centuries.* University of Wisconsin Press, Madison, 1989.
36. Ehrenreich, B., and English, D. *Complaints and Disorders: The Sexual Politics of Sickness.* The Feminist Press, Old Westbury, N.Y., 1973.
37. Russett, C. E. *Sexual Science: The Victorian Construction of Womanhood.* Harvard University Press, Cambridge, Mass., 1989.
38. Hubbard, R. *The Politics of Women's Biology.* Rutgers University Press, New Brunswick, N.J., 1990.
39. Fee, E. Nineteenth-century craniology: The study of the female skull. *Bull. Hist. Med.* 53: 415–433, 1979.
40. Smith-Rosenberg, C., and Rosenberg, C. E. The female animal: Medical and biological views of woman and her role in 19th century America. *J. Am. Hist.* 60: 332–356, 1973.
41. Gould, S. J. *The Mismeasure of Man.* W. W. Norton, New York, 1981.
42. Smith-Rosenberg, C. Puberty to menopause: The cycle of feminity in nineteenth-century America. *Feminist Stud.* 1: 58–72, 1973.
43. Smith-Rosenberg, C. *Disorderly Conduct: Visions of Gender in Victorian America.* Knopf, New York, 1985.
44. Haller, J. S., and Haller, R. M. *The Physician and Sexuality in Victorian America.* University of Illinois Press, Urbana, 1974.

45. Apple, R. D. (ed.). *Women, Health, and Medicine in America: A Historical Handbook*. Rutgers University Press, New Brunswick, N.J., 1990.
46. Williams, R. *Culture & Society: 1780–1950*, revised edition. Columbia University Press, New York, 1983 [1958].
47. Marx, K. *Capital*, vol. I. International Publishers, New York, 1967 [1867].
48. Hofstadter, R. *Social Darwinism in American Thought*. Beacon Press, Boston, 1955.
49. Young, R. M. *Darwin's Metaphor: Nature's Place in Victorian Culture*. Cambridge University Press, Cambridge, U.K., 1985.
50. Kevles, D. J. *In the Name of Eugenics: Genetics and the Uses of Human Heredity*. Knopf, New York, 1985.
51. Chase, A. *The Legacy of Malthus: The Social Costs of the New Scientific Racism*. Knopf, New York, 1977.
52. Darwin, C. *On the Origin of Species by Means of Natural Selection, or the Preservation of Favoured Races in the Struggle for Life*. Murray, London, 1859.
53. Anderson, M. J. *The American Census: A Social History*. Yale University Press, New Haven, Conn., 1988.
54. Hoffman, F. L. *Race Traits and Tendencies of the American Negro*. American Economic Association, New York, 1896.
55. Harris, S. Tuberculosis in the Negro. *JAMA* 41: 827, 1903.
56. Allen, L. C. The Negro health problem. *Am. J. Public Health* 5: 194, 1915.
57. Beardsley, E. H. *A History of Neglect: Health Care for Blacks and Mill Workers in the Twentieth-Century South*. University of Tennessee Press, Knoxville, 1987.
58. Geddes, P., and Thompson, J. A. *The Evolution of Sex*. Walter Scott, London, 1889.
59. Ludmerer, K. M. *Genetics and American Society: A Historical Appraisal*. Johns Hopkins University Press, Baltimore, Md., 1972.
60. Higham, H. *Strangers in the Land: Patterns of American Nativism, 1860–1925*. Rutgers University Press, New Brunswick, N.J., 1955.
61. Haller, M. H. *Eugenics: Hereditarian Attitudes in American Thought*. Rutgers University Press, New Brunswick, N.J., 1963.
62. Pickens, D. K. *Eugenics and the Progressives*. Vanderbilt University Press, Nashville, Tenn., 1968.
63. King, M., and Ruggles, S. American immigration, fertility, and race suicide at the turn of the century. *J. Interdisciplinary Hist.* 20: 347–369, 1990.
64. Degler, C. N. *In Search of Human Nature: The Decline and Revival of Darwinism in American Social Thought*. Oxford University Press, Oxford, 1991.
65. Allen, G. E. *Life Science in the Twentieth Century*. Cambridge University Press, Cambridge, U.K., 1978.
66. Castle, W. E. The beginnings of Mendelism in America. In *Genetics in the Twentieth Century*, edited by L. C. Dunn, pp. 59–76. Macmillan, New York, 1951.
67. Wilkie, J. S. Some reasons for the rediscovery and appreciation of Mendel's work in the first years of the present century. *Br. J. Hist. Sci.* 1: 5–18, 1962.
68. Morgan, T. H. *The Theory of the Gene*. Yale University Press, New Haven, 1926.
69. Kraut, A. M. *The Huddled Masses: The Immigrant in American Society, 1800–1921*. Harlan Davison, Arlington Heights, Ill., 1982.
70. Stoner, G. W. Insane and mentally defective aliens arriving at the Port of New York. *N. Y. Med. J.* 97: 957–960, 1913.
71. Solis-Cohen, S. T. The exclusion of aliens from the United States for physical defects. *Bull. Hist. Med.* 21: 33–50, 1947.

72. Ludmerer, K. Genetics, eugenics, and the Immigration Restriction Act of 1924. *Bull. Hist. Med.* 46: 59–81, 1972.
73. Barkan, E. Reevaluating progressive eugenics: Herbert Spencer Jennings and the 1924 immigration legislation. *J. Hist. Biol.* 24: 91–112, 1991.
74. Kraut, A. M. Silent travelers: Germs, genes, and American efficiency, 1890–1924. *Soc. Sci. Hist.* 12: 377–393, 1988.
75. Farley, J. *Gametes & Spores: Ideas About Sexual Reproduction, 1750–1914*. Johns Hopkins University Press, Baltimore, Md., 1982.
76. Allen, G. Thomas Hunt Morgan and the problem of sex determination. *Proc. Am. Philos. Soc.* 110: 48–57, 1966.
77. Brush, S. Nettie M. Stevens and the discovery of sex determination by chromosomes. *Isis* 69: 163–172, 1978.
78. Starling, E. The Croonian lectures on the chemical correlation of the functions of the body. *Lancet* 2: 339–341, 423–425, 501–503, 579–583, 1905.
79. Lane-Claypon, J. E., and Starling, E. H. An experimental enquiry into the factors which determine the growth and activity of the mammary glands. *Proc. R. Soc. London [Biol.]* 77: 505–522, 1906.
80. Marshall, N. *The Physiology of Reproduction*. Longmans, Green and Co., New York, 1910.
81. Oudshoorn, N. Endocrinologists and the conceptualization of sex. *J. Hist. Biol.* 23: 163–187, 1990.
82. Oudshoorn, N. On measuring sex hormones: The role of biological assays in sexualizing chemical substances. *Bull. Hist. Med.* 64: 243–261, 1990.
83. Borrell, M. Organotherapy and the emergence of reproductive endocrinology. *J. Hist. Biol.* 18: 1–30, 1985.
84. Long, D. L. Biology, sex hormones and sexism in the 1920s. *Philos. Forum* 5: 81–96, 1974.
85. Cobb, I. G. *The Glands of Destiny (A Study of the Personality)*. Macmillan, New York, 1928.
86. Allen, E. (ed.). *Sex and Internal Secretions: A Survey of Recent Research*. Williams & Wilkins, Baltimore, Md., 1939.
87. Frank, R. *The Female Sex Hormone*. Charles C Thomas, Springfield, Ill., 1929.
88. Lathrop, A. E. C., and Loeb, L. Further investigations of the origin of tumors in mice. III. On the part played by internal secretions in the spontaneous development of tumors. *J. Cancer Res.* 1: 1–19, 1916.
89. Lane-Claypon, J. E. *A Further Report on Cancer of the Breast, With Special Reference to its Associated Antecedent Conditions. Reports on Public Health and Medical Subjects, No. 32.* Her Majesty's Stationery Office, London, 1926.
90. Wainwright, J. M. A comparison of conditions associated with breast cancer in Great Britain and America. *Am. J. Cancer* 15: 2610–2645, 1931.
91. Chavkin, W. (ed.). *Double Exposure: Women's Health Hazards on the Job and at Home*. Monthly Review Press, New York, 1984.
92. Ehrenreich, B., and English, D. *For Her Own Good: 150 Years of the Experts' Advice to Women*. Anchor Books, Garden City, N.Y., 1979.
93. Starr, P. *The Social Transformation of American Medicine*. Basic Books, New York, 1982.
94. Fee, E. *Disease and Discovery: A History of the Johns Hopkins School of Hygiene and Public Health*. Johns Hopkins University Press, Baltimore, Md., 1987.
95. Fee, E., and Acheson, R. M. (eds.). *A History of Education in Public Health: Health that Mocks the Doctors' Rules*. Oxford University Press, Oxford, 1991.

96. Meckel, R. *Save the Babies: American Public Health Reform and the Prevention of Infant Mortality, 1850–1920.* Johns Hopkins University Press, Baltimore, Md., 1990.
97. Rodin, J., and Ickovics, J. R. Women's health: Review and research agenda as we approach the 21st Century. *Am. Psychol.* 45: 1018–1034, 1990.
98. Healy, B. Women's health, public welfare. *JAMA* 266: 566–568, 1991.
99. Kirchstein, R. L. Research on women's health. *Am. J. Public Health* 81: 291–293, 1991.
100. Lewontin, R. *Human Diversity.* Scientific American Books, New York, 1982.
101. King, J. C. *The Biology of Race.* University of California Press, Berkeley, 1981.
102. Cooper, R., and David, R. The biological concept of race and its application to epidemiology. *J. Health Polit. Policy Law* 11: 97–116, 1986.
103. Cooper, R. Celebrate diversity—or should we? *Ethnicity Dis.* 1: 3–7, 1991.
104. Crews, D. E., and Bindon, J. R. Ethnicity as a taxonomic tool in biomedical and biosocial research. *Ethnicity Dis.* 1: 42–49, 1991.
105. Mullings, L. Ethnicity and stratification in the urban United States. *Ann. N.Y. Acad. Sci.* 318: 10–22, 1978.
106. Feagin, J. R. *Racial and Ethnic Relations,* Ed. 3. Prentice-Hall, Englewood Cliffs, N.J., 1989.
107. Feagin, J. R. The continuing significance of race: Anti-black discrimination in public places. *Am. Sociol. Rev.* 56: 101–116, 1991.
108. Essed, P. *Understanding Everyday Racism: An Interdisciplinary Theory.* Sage Publications, Newbury Park, Calif., 1991.
109. Krieger, N., and Bassett, M. The health of black folk: Disease, class and ideology in science. *Monthly Review* 38: 74–85, 1986.
110. Navarro, V. Race or class versus race and class: Mortality differentials in the United States. *Lancet* 2: 1238–1240, 1990.
111. Krieger, N., and Fee, E. What's class got to do with it? The state of health data in the United States today. *Socialist Rev.* 23: 59–82, 1993.
112. Polack, S., and Grozuczak, J. *Reagan, Toxics and Minorities: A Policy Report.* Urban Environment Conference, Washington, D.C., 1984.
113. Commission for Racial Justice, United Church of Christ. *Toxic Wastes and Race in the United States: A National Report on the Racial and Socioeconomic Characteristics of Communities with Hazardous Waste Sites.* United Church of Christ, New York, 1987.
114. Mann, E. *L.A.'s Lethal Air: New Strategies for Policy, Organizing, and Action.* Labor/Community Strategy Center, Los Angeles, 1991.
115. Krieger, N. Racial and gender discrimination: Risk factors for high blood pressure? *Soc. Sci. Med.* 30: 1273–1281, 1990.
116. Armstead, C. A., et al. Relationship of racial stressors to blood pressure and anger expression in black college students. *Health Psychol.* 8: 541–556, 1989.
117. James, S. A., et al. John Henryism and blood pressure differences among black men. II. The role of occupational stressors. *J. Behav. Med.* 7: 259–275, 1984.
118. Dressler, W. W. Social class, skin color, and arterial blood pressure in two societies. *Ethnicity Dis.* 1: 60–77, 1991.
119. Fruchter, R. G., et al. Cervix and breast cancer incidence in immigrant Caribbean women. *Am. J. Public Health* 80: 722–724, 1990.
120. Kleinman, J. C., Fingerhut, L. A., and Prager, K. Differences in infant mortality by race, nativity, and other maternal characteristics. *Am. J. Dis. Child.* 145: 194–199, 1991.

121. Cabral, H., et al. Foreign-born and US-born black women: Differences in health behaviors and birth outcomes. *Am. J. Public Health* 80: 70–72, 1990.
122. Taylor, R. J., and Chatters, L. M. Religious life. In *Life in Black America*, edited by J. S. Jackson, pp. 105–123. Sage, Newbury Park, Calif., 1991.
123. Livingston, I. L., Levine, D. M., and Moore, R. D. Social integration and black intraracial variation in blood pressure. *Ethnicity Dis.* 1: 135–149, 1991.
124. Eng, E., Hatch, J., and Callan, A. Institutionalizing social support through the church and into the community. *Health Ed. Q.* 12: 81–92, 1985.
125. Lowe, M. Social bodies: The interaction of culture and women's biology. In *Biological Woman—The Convenient Myth*, edited by R. Hubbard, M. S. Henefin, and B. Fried, pp. 91–116. Schenkman, Cambridge, Mass., 1982.
126. Devesa, S. S., and Diamond, E. L. Association of breast cancer and cervical cancer incidence with income and education among whites and blacks. *J. Natl. Cancer Inst.* 65: 515–528, 1980.
127. Krieger, N. Social class and the black/white crossover in the age-specific incidence of breast cancer: A study linking census-derived data to population-based registry records. *Am. J. Epidemiol.* 131: 804–814, 1990.
128. Krieger, N. The influence of social class, race and gender on the etiology of hypertension among women in the United States. In *Women, Behavior, and Cardiovascular Disease*, proceedings of a conference sponsored by the National Heart, Lung, and Blood Institute, Chevy Chase, Md., September 25–27, 1991. U.S. Government Printing Office, Washington, D.C., 1994, in press.
129. U.S. Department of Health and Human Services. *Report of the Secretary's Task Force on Black & Minority Health, Volume IV: Cardiovascular and Cerebrovascular Disease, Part 2.* Washington, D.C., 1986.
130. Martinez-Maldonado, M. Hypertension in Hispanics, Asians and Pacific Islanders, and Native Americans. *Circulation* 83: 1467–1469, 1991.
131. Caralis, P. U. Hypertension in the Hispanic-American population, *Am. J. Med.* 88(Suppl. 3b): 9s–16s, 1990.
132. Haffner, S. M., et al. Decreased prevalence of hypertension in Mexican-Americans. *Hypertension* 16: 255–232, 1990.
133. Stavig, G. R., Igra, A., and Leonard, A. R. Hypertension and related health issues among Asians and Pacific Islanders in California. *Public Health Rep.* 103: 28–37, 1988.
134. Angel, A., Armstrong, M. A., and Klatsky, A. L. Blood pressure among Asian Americans living in Northern California. *Am. J. Cardiol.* 54: 237–240, 1987.
135. Alpert, J. S., et al. Heart disease in Native Americans. *Cardiology* 78: 3–12, 1991.
136. Waldron, I. Sex differences in illness, incidence, prognosis and mortality: Issues and evidence. *Soc. Sci. Med.* 17: 1107–1123, 1983.
137. Wingard, D. L. The sex differential in morbidity, mortality, and lifestyle. *Annu. Rev. Public Health* 5: 433–458, 1984.
138. Gold, E. (ed.). *Changing Risk of Disease in Women: An Epidemiological Approach.* Colbamore Press, Lexington, Mass., 1984.
139. Leviatan, V., and Cohen, J. Gender differences in life expectancy among kibbutz members. *Soc. Sci. Med.* 21: 545–551, 1985.
140. Syme, S. L., and Berkman, L. Social class, susceptibility and sickness. *Am. J. Epidemiol.* 104: 1–8, 1976.
141. Antonovsky, A. Social class, life expectancy and overall mortality. *Milbank Mem. Fund Q.* 45: 31–73, 1967.

142. Townsend, P., Davidson, N., and Whitehead, M. *Inequalities in Health: The Black Report and The Health Divide.* Penguin, Harmondsworth, U.K., 1988.
143. Marmot, M. G., Kogevinas, M., and Elston, M. A. Social/economic status and disease. *Annu. Rev. Public Health* 8: 111–135, 1987.
144. Roberts, H. (ed.). *Women's Health Counts.* Routledge, London, 1990.
145. Dale, A., Gilbert, G. N., and Arber, S. Integrating women into class theory. *Sociology* 19: 384–409, 1985.
146. Duke, V., and Edgell, S. The operationalisation of class in British sociology: Theoretical and empirical considerations. *Br. J. Sociol.* 8: 445–463, 1987.
147. Charles, N. Women and class—A problematic relationship. *Sociol. Rev.* 38: 43–89, 1990.
148. Morgan, M. Measuring social inequality: Occupational classifications and their alternatives. *Community Med.* 5: 116–124, 1983.
149. Moser, K. A., Pugh, H., and Goldblatt, P. Mortality and the social classification of women. In *Longitudinal Study: Mortality and Social Organization. Series LS, No. 6,* edited by P. Goldblatt, pp. 146–162. Her Majesty's Stationery Office, London, 1990.
150. Krieger, N. Women and social class: A methodological study comparing individual, household, and census measures as predictors of black/white differences in reproductive history. *J. Epidemiol. Community Health* 45: 35–42, 1991.
151. Ries, P. Health characteristics according to family and personal income, United States. *Vital Health Stat.* 10(147). DHHS Pub No. (PHS) 85-1575. National Center for Health Statistics. U.S. Government Printing Office, Washington, D.C., 1985.
152. Krieger, N. Overcoming the absence of socioeconomic data in medical records: Validation and application of a census-based methodology. *Am. J. Public Health* 82: 703–710, 1992.
153. Carovano, K. More than mothers and whores: Redefining the AIDS prevention needs of women. *Int. J. Health Serv.* 21: 131–142, 1991.
154. PANOS Institute. *Triple Jeopardy: Women & AIDS.* Panos Publications, London, 1990.
155. Anastos, K., and Marte, C. Women—The missing persons in the AIDS epidemic. *HealthPAC,* Winter 1989, pp. 6–13.
156. Centers for Disease Control. 1993 Revised classification system for HIV infection and expanded surveillance case definition for AIDS among adolescents and adults. *MMWR* 41: 961–962, 1992.
157. Kanigel, R. U.S. broadens AIDS definition: Activists spur change by Centers for Disease Control. *Oakland Tribune,* January 1, 1993, p. A1.
158. Centers for Disease Control and Prevention. *HIV/AIDS Surveillance Rep.* 5: 1–19, July 1993.
159. Drucker, E. Epidemic in the war zone: AIDS and community survival in New York City. *Int. J. Health Serv.* 20: 601–616, 1990.
160. Freudenberg, N. AIDS prevention in the United States: Lessons from the first decade. *Int. J. Health Serv.* 20: 589–600, 1990.
161. Fee, E., and Krieger, N. Thinking and rethinking AIDS: Implications for health policy. *Int. J. Health Serv.* 23: 323–346, 1993.
162. Fee, E., and Krieger, N. Understanding AIDS: Historical interpretations and the limits of biomedical individualism. *Am. J. Public Health* 83: 1477–1486, 1993.

Interpreting the Evidence:
Competing Paradigms and the Emergence
of Lesbian and Gay Suicide as a "Social Fact"

Kathleen Erwin

The removal of homosexuality from the Diagnostic and Statistical Manual in 1973 signaled that the American Psychiatric Association no longer considered homosexuality a psychopathology. Despite this change in definition, however, studies continue to show significantly higher rates of depression, substance abuse, and attempted suicide among lesbians and gay men than among heterosexuals in the United States. This apparent contradiction has been explained in terms of "the myth and fact of gay suicide" (1, 2). The "myth" refers to the discredited but still popular belief that the inherent psychopathology of gay people makes them suicidal; the "fact," to the more contemporary belief that self-destructive behavior among many gays and lesbians in the United States is due to social isolation and the internalization of negative stereotypes.

What are the origins of the myth of gay pathology in U.S. and Western European societies, and how did it come to be widely accepted as an explanation for gay and lesbian psychological distress? What were the forces that revealed this explanation as mythical, and how have new explanations, which view the causal agent as external to the individual, come to be formulated in Western societies? This chapter attempts to address these questions in order to illuminate how historical and political forces have shaped our contemporary social and medical understanding of, and response to, gay and lesbian psychological distress, and how emerging explanations offer new hope for prevention of mental "dis-ease" among gays and lesbians.

INDICATORS OF PSYCHOLOGICAL DISTRESS
AMONG GAYS AND LESBIANS

Rates of attempted suicide and suicide mortality among gays and lesbians in the United States are extremely difficult to ascertain, due to incomplete and inaccurate reporting. Many gays and lesbians are not "out" as gay and, even among those who are, their deaths may not be reported as suicide due to the stigma attached to both homosexuality and suicide.[1] Because of this invisibility and underreporting, studies of suicide and attempted suicide among gays and lesbians make no claims to be representative of the gay population nationwide, in terms of gender, age, ethnicity, or distribution. Nevertheless, the accumulated evidence, summarized below, indicates that self-destructive behavior is disturbingly—and disproportionately—high among American gays and lesbians.

In 1977, Jay and Young (3) conducted a study of over 5,000 lesbians and gay men in the United States and Canada, ranging in age from 14 to 82. They reported that 40 percent of gay men and 39 percent of lesbians had attempted or seriously considered suicide; of those who attempted suicide, 53 percent of the men and 33 percent of the women said their homosexuality was a factor (3, p. 729). Another study, published in 1978 by Bell and Weinberg (4), surveyed 575 white gay men, 111 black gay men, 229 white lesbians, and 64 black lesbians. Bell and Weinberg found that significantly higher percentages of gays than heterosexuals had attempted or seriously considered suicide. The figures were consistent across race and gender: 37 percent of white gay men compared to 13 percent of white heterosexual men; 24 percent of black gay men compared to 2 percent of black heterosexual men; 41 percent of white lesbians compared to 26 percent of white heterosexual women; and 25 percent of black lesbians compared to 19 percent of black heterosexual women (4, p. 451).

The proportion of suicides and attempted suicides among gay youth is especially startling. In the Bell and Weinberg study, over half of the lesbians and gay men who had attempted suicide had done so at age 20 years or younger; 36 percent of the black lesbians' and 32 percent of the black gay men's attempts occurred before age 17, while 21 percent of the white lesbians' and 27 percent of the white gay men's occurred by that age (4). More recently, in 1989, Gibson (5) found suicide to be the main cause of death among gay and lesbian youth, accounting for at least 30 percent of all adolescent suicides (while gays are generally estimated to represent only 10 percent of the population). Gibson and others have calculated the risk of suicide among gay and lesbian youth to be three to six times that of heterosexual adolescents (2, 5, 6).

High rates of alcoholism and other drug abuse are also reported among gays and lesbians, and have been associated with many of the suicide attempts. Studies indicate that approximately 30 percent of gay men and lesbians could be considered "alcoholic," "heavy" or "excessive" drinkers, or "alcohol dependent"

---

[1] The terms "lesbian" and "gay" are culturally and historically specific terms that should not be applied uniformly to all people who engage is same-sex sexual relations. In Europe and North America, from the 19th century to the present, the term "homosexual" came to refer to people engaging primarily in same-sex sexual relations. In this chapter, I use the terms "gay" and "lesbian" to refer to male and female "homosexuals" in contemporary American society.

(7, 8). In a 1973 study of 230 white middle-class people, including 89 gay men, 57 lesbians, 40 heterosexual men, and 44 heterosexual women, Saghir and Robins (8) found that 35 percent of lesbians and 30 percent of gay men were alcohol dependent at some point in their lives, compared with 5 percent of heterosexual women and 20 percent of heterosexual men. Gays and lesbians also frequently report feelings of self-hatred, isolation, depression, and low self-esteem (1–10).

These data point to high levels of emotional distress among gays and lesbians, but they do not explain the origin of the distress. Up to the contemporary period, such findings were seen as evidence that homosexuality was immoral and inherently pathological; feelings of self-hatred and self-destructiveness result from recognition of one's own immorality or pathology. Charges of immorality were drawn from early Judeo-Christian writings, which were interpreted as condemning same-sex relations. Theories of homosexual pathology became dominant in the 19th and early 20th centuries as part of a larger shift from religious to "scientific" explanations of human behavior. In the last quarter century, researchers and gay and lesbian activists have challenged the religious and medical explanations, proposing instead that oppressive social conditions are the root cause of gay and lesbian suicide and psychological distress. Critically examining these competing paradigms demonstrates how historical, social, and political forces have been instrumental in shaping the scientific and medical response to gay and lesbian psychological distress to the present day.

HOMOSEXUALITY AND SUICIDE AS SIN

In the Judeo-Christian tradition, homosexuality has long been seen as sinful and immoral, but not for the reasons often invoked today. The Jewish proscription on homosexuality in ancient times was directed specifically at males, who faced the death penalty for homosexual acts, while female homosexuality seemed unproblematic. This distinction arose because the proscription was not aimed at eliminating homosexuality, per se, but rather at discouraging Jews from attending Canaanite temples where the holy men engaged in sexual acts with other men who came to worship. Because the Canaanite holy women engaged in heterosexual acts, lesbianism was not similarly problematized in early Judaism (11). By 1270 A.D., however, these religious proscriptions had become naturalized, and French legal codes included laws prohibiting both male and female homosexual acts, upon penalty of death (11, 12).

Religious and secular laws against homosexual acts, which are still widely enforced today throughout many parts of the world, imply that sinful or weak people *choose* to engage in homosexual acts due to lasciviousness and immorality. Suicide within this framework, then, results when the person—faced with burning at the stake, public humiliation, or personal shame—chooses instead a second immoral act, that of taking his or her own life (1, p. 3). While the religious model does not medicalize or pathologize homosexuality, Judeo-Christian tenets have nevertheless strongly influenced the response by the modern medical, psychiatric, and public health professions to both homosexuality and the psychological distress with which it is associated.

HOMOSEXUAL SUICIDE AND SCIENTIFIC INQUIRY IN THE 19th CENTURY

The religious interpretation of homosexuality and homosexual suicide first began to be challenged in the 19th century. Fueling the challenges were rapid social and economic changes, including a shift to industry as the primary mode of production. The consequent influx of single men and women into urban areas led to greater exploration of alternative lifestyles, growth of female and male prostitution, and the establishment of specific geographically defined homosexual neighborhoods. The increasing visibility of homosexual behavior led to a new intellectual dialogue regarding the causes of male homosexuality in particular. These inquiries shifted the focus from viewing homosexuality as a religious concern to viewing it as a medical and biological one, and led to the emergence of the "homosexual" as a social category and topic of scientific discourse. This shift can be seen as part of a larger social trend of secular institutions using "reason" to actively challenge the dominance of the Christian church in a variety of areas newly investigated by "science" (13–17).

Competing for supremacy in late 19th century European thought were two main theories of homosexuality. One posited that homosexuality was a non-pathological, "natural," and harmless variation, and the other labeled it a mental disorder, or "sickness," in which suicidal tendencies were not uncommon. Both of these perspectives challenged the idea that homosexual acts were "chosen sin" or criminal, and thus contested the dominance of the Christian church over sexual matters (13, 14). Moreover, both drew upon prevailing notions of biological determinism. Thus, even though the "homosexuality as harmless" proponents intended to diminish the stigmatization of homosexuals, they subscribed to the biological premise that also lay at the heart of the sickness hypothesis.

Beginning in the 1860s, the theory of homosexuality as an innate, nonpathological variation was promoted by social reformers such as Karl Ulrichs, Havelock Ellis, Edward Carpenter, Edward Stevenson, and Magnus Hirschfeld (18–23). Karl Ulrichs, himself a homosexual and an attorney, did not see homosexuality itself as a cause of psychological distress or suicide (14). Indeed, he saw homosexuals (whom he termed "Urnings") as mentally healthy, and believed they not only were harmless, but perhaps even particularly valuable for their combined male and female qualities (13, 14). Later, Ellis, Hirschfeld, Carpenter, and Stevenson embraced these views and joined Ulrichs in advocating the repeal of laws prohibiting homosexual acts.

The competing formulation, viewing mental distress and suicidality as manifestations of homosexual pathology, found one of its strongest advocates in the well-respected Austrian psychiatrist Richard von Krafft-Ebing. A leading proponent of the medical model, Krafft-Ebing believed a heritable defect resulting in an abnormal nervous system could be traced in sexually "pathological" individuals. This pathology resulted in higher rates of mental abnormalities, suicide, and violence among sexual "perverts" than among other men (1, p. 6). Thus, Krafft-Ebing argued, for their own protection and that of society, perverts should be institutionalized in asylums.

As a psychiatrist who studied homosexuality among the mentally ill, rather than in the general population, it is not surprising that Krafft-Ebing came to these conclusions—nor was it surprising to his contemporary adversaries. Ulrichs, critiquing the medical-pathological theories advocated by such heterosexual doctors, complained in 1879: "My scientific opponents are mostly doctors of the insane . . . for example, Westphal, v. Krafft-Ebing, Stark. They have observed Urnings in lunatic asylums. They have apparently never seen mentally healthy Urnings. The published views of the doctors for the insane are accepted by others" (14, p. 108).

Despite Ulrichs' protestations, the medical-pathological interpretation had become dominant by the early 20th century. It dovetailed with the then-popular Darwinian view of sexual intercourse as evolving purely for the purposes of reproduction (16). Moreover, it did not pose a direct threat to religious proscriptions against homosexual acts. Supported by medical doctors and scientists, Krafft-Ebing's theories held sway over the "unscientific" theories advocated by homosexuals and other "social reformers."

Although these two competing formulations, both presupposing the fundamentally individual nature of homosexuality, took center stage in the scientific and social debates of the late 19th century, the seeds of an alternative formulation were also being sown. Emile Durkheim's (24) landmark sociology treatise, *Suicide*, published in 1897, posited that suicide was not an individual phenomenon, but a "social fact" that could be explicated through sociological methods (25). Despite its importance to the development of sociology, Durkheim's thesis was not extended to the question of homosexual suicide, which came to be viewed as a medical and psychological "fact" rather than a social one. It took nearly three-quarters of a century before the social facts underlying homosexual suicide received serious scientific attention.

PSYCHOANALYTIC THEORY AND HOMOSEXUAL SUICIDE

It was in this highly charged context of competing theories and contested disciplinary boundaries that Sigmund Freud, in the early 20th century, proposed his still controversial psychoanalytic theories of homosexuality and psychopathology. Challenging the biological basis of mental conditions, Freud proposed that sexuality, and in turn homosexuality, was primarily the product of early psychological development and familial relations, rather than neurological defects. While he conceded that in some cases homosexuality could be inborn, he contended that when psychoanalytic facts were considered, "the supposition that nature in a freakish mood created a 'third sex' falls to the ground" (26, p. 158).

Freud believed that certain neuroses were associated with homosexuality, and could be traced to abnormal psychological development and the reversal of the Oedipal complex for both men and women (13, 26–30). With regard to homosexual suicide specifically, in "The Psychogenesis of a Case of Homosexuality in a Woman," published in 1920, Freud noted that an attempted suicide was the precipitating event leading to the woman's therapy. While the woman attributed her suicide attempt to rejection by another woman, Freud interpreted it as "wish-fulfillment" and "self-punishment." That is, he saw the suicide attempt as motivated by the frustrated wish of the girl to have a child by her father, and a death wish for one or both of her parents that had been turned upon herself (26, p. 149). Thus, the suicide attempt was neither a manifestation of an innate neurological defect (as Krafft-Ebing might have supposed), nor an expression of the woman's deep grief; rather, it demonstrated the continuing enactment of the Oedipal drama gone awry in a female homosexual.

Initially, Freud's theories on human sexuality were sharply criticized as unscientific. However, over time, psychoanalytic theory became widely accepted, and by the 1930s in the United States, it had become the foundation for seeing homosexuality as psychopathological (31).[2] This interpretation derived from the strong Christian tradition in the United States, as well as the American emphasis on individualism, that is, the belief that individuals' conditions are largely determined by their individual characteristics. Moreover, medicalization, rather than criminalization, was considered a much more humane and liberal treatment of social deviants, as it still is in many quarters today. It was in response to many of Freud's basic tenets that more recent alternative theories to the concept of homosexuality as sickness have been developed.

CHALLENGING THE PATHOLOGICAL MODELS
OF GAY SUICIDE

The political upheavals of the 1960s and 1970s created a new social and intellectual climate for challenging the pathological basis of "deviance" and

---

[2]There is some controversy over whether or not Freud saw homosexuality as inherently pathological, and indeed Freud's writings are somewhat contradictory on this point (26–28, 32). Freud argued that everyone was innately bisexual and had at least some latent homosexual desires, and that homosexual acts should be decriminalized. However, his belief that homosexuality resulted from childhood trauma, and should be cured through psychoanalysis, has been pointed to as evidence that Freud did see homosexuality as pathological.

psychological distress among many oppressed groups. With respect to homosexual suicide specifically, these challenges led to a shift from emphasis on pathology to a focus on the social conditions that produce psychological distress among homosexuals.

The gay liberation movement that developed in the United States in the 1970s was largely responsible for the development of the concept of a "gay identity," based on the status of being a sexual minority (15, 33, 34). Activists strove to challenge the widely accepted psychoanalytic notion that homosexuality was a sickness resulting from childhood trauma. Instead, echoing Ulrichs' and Ellis's 19th century theories, many claimed that homosexuality was a healthy, natural outcome on the spectrum of sexual possibilities. Thus, homosexuality itself—whether innate or fixed early in a child's development—is neither a sin nor a sickness, and cannot be forcibly changed or cured. These claims were supported by the findings of Kinsey and other sex researchers in the 1950s and 1960s, who found a wide range of diversity in sexual behavior, and found bisexual and homosexual behavior to be much more common than previously believed (28, 31).

Gay activists and medical professionals recognized that gays and lesbians suffer from high rates of suicide and attempted suicide, substance abuse, and other self-destructive behavior. Given these same facts, what is striking is that they reframed the issue of psychological distress and self-destructiveness as one in which the proximate cause was feelings of isolation and self-hatred, and the ultimate cause lay in society's intolerance. The feelings of self-hatred come from both internalized and external homophobia, that is, negative attitudes toward homosexuality and gay people (1, 5, 6, 10, 35, 36). Thus, echoing Durkheim's thesis of the previous century, homosexual suicide was reframed as a "social fact," rather than an individual psychological one (37).

THE SOCIAL FACTS:
PSYCHOLOGICAL EFFECTS OF HETEROSEXISM

According to this construction, gays and lesbians grow up in a homophobic society in which they learn that homosexuality is immoral and sick, concepts drawn from the religious and early medical-psychological theories. At some point in their lives, varying from person to person, they come to realize they are different from most other people based on their erotic and emotional attractions to people of the same biological sex. By this time, however, they have already internalized society's homophobia. As role models, most gays and lesbians have only the media's negative stereotypes of sick, sinful, "effeminate" men or "masculine" women. When they try to tell their families, they are often rejected and/or sent to psychotherapy to be "cured." Moreover, they must continue to "come out" throughout their lives, if they want themselves and their significant relationships recognized. They may face discrimination in the workplace, in housing, and in other social and economic arenas. Faced with lack of role models, fear of public disclosure, negative self-image, familial rejection and, most recently, fear and deep grief in the face of the AIDS epidemic, many become self-destructive (1, 5, 35, 36, 38–40).

Although the term "homophobia" is still commonly used to refer to isolated or individual-level demonstrations of negativism toward gays and lesbians, more recently, the term "heterosexism" has begun to replace homophobia in describing the myriad ways in which society discriminates against sexual minorities. Hetero-sexism incorporates both the idea of dislike of homosexuality and gay people, and the societal and institutional-level discrimination against gays and lesbians. It shifts the focus from blaming prejudiced individuals for their "homophobia" to placing the onus on larger social institutions and values. In addition, this term draws a parallel with other forms of discrimination, like racism and sexism (35, 36).

Viewing heterosexism as the primary underlying cause of mental distress among gays and lesbians holds two implications for "treatment." The first is that the ultimate cause of the disease, heterosexism, must be actively addressed through efforts to change the laws, institutions, and attitudes that oppress homo-sexuals. The second is that the proximate causes of mental distress—that is, feelings of isolation, shame, negative parental response, and other manifestations of stigmatization—must be addressed through responsive forms of individual, group, and family counseling, which recognize not only the environmental causes of the distress but also that all aspects of psychological distress may *not* neces-sarily be related to one's experience as gay (5, 41, 42).

Despite the removal of homosexuality from the Diagnostic and Statistical Manual III, many medical professionals continue to have heterosexist atti-tudes that impede their ability to recognize and correctly diagnose psychological problems among gay and lesbian clients (7, 9, 41, 42). Others continue to seek evidence of neurological abnormalities to explain the "cause" of homosexuality.[3] As a result of these attitudes and ingrained biomedical beliefs, the psychological problems of many gay and lesbian clients continue to go untreated or mistreated. In a study of psychiatrists, Kourany found that "the magnitude of [psychiatrists'] lack of exposure to [homosexual youth] suggested that they either did not recog-nize or did not want to treat these patients" (9, p. 114). Moreover, lesbians and gay men continue to cite fear of heterosexist response as a primary reason for not getting adequate health care (47).

---

[3] See, for example, the recent controversial research of LeVay (43) and Allen and Gorski (44). Both studies hypothesize causal links between homosexuality and structures in the brains of gay men who died of AIDS. Although some medical researchers argue that proof of a biological basis for homo-sexuality would reduce prejudice against lesbians and gays (45, 46), critics counter that "scientific" evidence of biological difference would lead only to renewed efforts to "cure" the "deformed" brains of gays (and lesbians?).

ONGOING CHALLENGES TO EXPLICATING
GAY AND LESBIAN SUICIDE

Even among those who accept the premise that psychological distress among gays and lesbians results from societal heterosexism, many find this formulation a necessary, but insufficient, explanation for gay and lesbian suicide. This critique is based on the recognition of the immense social, economic, and cultural diversity among lesbians, gays, and others who engage in same-sex sexual activity in the United States. Thus, the formulation of heterosexism as the sole root of psychological distress is too narrow, and ignores other kinds of oppression experienced by many sexual minorities. Moreover, continuing research in the field of sexuality shows that not even all lesbians and gay men agree on what it means to themselves to be "homosexual" or "gay"—despite restrictive legal definitions focused specifically on particular behaviors. These critiques form the basis for continuing exploration of the social determinants of gay and lesbian suicide.

Lesbians and the Women's Movement

Throughout the modern period, theories of causation regarding female homosexuality, also used to explain psychological distress among lesbians, have for the most part been patterned after the theories developed by men to explain male homosexuality and psychological distress. Thus, both Ulrichs and Krafft-Ebing believed that female homosexuals were the mirror images of the male homosexuals upon whom they based their theories. Along similar lines, Freud's theory of human sexuality, both heterosexual and homosexual, relies on the male-centered notion of "penis envy," which differentially affected men and women. This conflation has served not only to obscure the existence of lesbians in history, but more importantly, for the purposes of understanding lesbian suicidality, it has also obscured the social conditions that contribute to psychological distress among lesbians.

Recognizing this oversight, lesbians, particularly white lesbian feminists, have challenged both the long-standing conflation of lesbianism with male homosexuality, as well as the notion that heterosexism alone accounts for the oppression and psychological distress they may experience in this society. They argue that their identity as women is as central to their life experience as their identity as lesbians. Some have sought more fluid definitions of their sexuality, such as "woman-identified women" and "political lesbians" (48–50). Rich (49) argues that lesbians see their oppression as linked to men's control over women's sexuality and reproduction.

In the realm of lesbian mental health, these arguments suggest that the economic and social oppression lesbians experience as women is as critical to their feelings of self-worth as is their experience as lesbians. This point is graphically illustrated in the alarming statistics on suicide attempts among women (as compared with men) cited earlier in this chapter. It implies that prevention of psychological distress among lesbians must come through addressing sexist attitudes and structures, as well as heterosexist ones.

Gay and Lesbian People of Color

For people of color in the United States, membership in particular ethnic minority groups may be central to their identity, and they often feel marginalized by racism in both the gay movement and the larger society. They may come from families and communities where the norms and expectations of men and women are different from those in the dominant culture. These cultural norms have also shaped their experiences with heterosexism and psychological distress.

When youth of color experience racism in the larger society, they often turn to their families and communities for support and role models (51). However, gay and lesbian youth of color are frequently rejected by their families when they "come out." Moreover, some youth come from cultures that have even stricter sex role expectations than does the dominant culture. In order to "come out," these youth must leave their families and reject their cultures to fit into the predominantly white gay culture of urban America. The psychological stress of familial rejection and cultural alienation in an already hostile social environment often leads to increased levels of psychological distress (5, 37, 51–53).

Alternative Constructions of Sexuality

Cultural differences can also provide an avenue for exploring dominant constructions of sexuality, and for creating, or recreating, alternative understandings of sexual diversity that challenge heterosexism. For example, recent scholarship by anthropologists and Native Americans, especially gay and lesbian American Indians, has rekindled interest in the traditional "berdache" and "amazon" roles found in many Native American tribes (53–56).[4] The berdache was a biological male who expressed "feminine" attributes that were understood to be endowed by the Creator in a dream or vision. Girls might also express the "masculine" attributes of amazons. A child found to have these special attributes was given special social roles and responsibilities throughout life, including, in many cases, that of the marital or sexual partner of others of the same biological sex (who were not berdache or amazon). Recent research has indicated

---

[4]The anthropological term "berdache" was introduced by early French observers, who borrowed it from the Persian word for passive homosexual. Williams and others have used the term "amazon" to describe the female berdache (53, 56). These Euro-American terms are used here for the sake of convenience. Roscoe (56) has compiled a comprehensive list of indigenous terms.

that these beliefs have not died out among Native Americans and, in fact, in some cases are reemerging along with the resurgence of Indian identity and pride (53, 54, 57). Many other cultural groups maintain traditional attitudes and values regarding identity and sexuality that differ greatly from the Western European religious, medical, and psychological views dominant in the United States (58–62). These varying cultural constructions of same-sex relationships both provide alternative possibilities for understanding same-sex relations and highlight the significant role of social attitudes in shaping identity, self-esteem, and mental health.

The very definitions of lesbian and gay "identity" in contemporary Euro-American culture have also been challenged by the now burgeoning research on sexuality in many disciplines and by the self-proclaimed sex radicals of the 1990s; these alternative constructions likewise have implications for mental health (35, 36). For instance, although the terms "gay" and "lesbian" generally refer to people whose primary emotional and erotic attachments are to people of the same biological sex, often a disjuncture exists between people's behavior and their identity. The distinction between behavior and identity raises important questions with respect to the impact of heterosexism on mental health. For instance, does a married man who occasionally engages in homosexual sex, but considers himself straight, face the same kind of oppression as a self-identified gay man? Does a woman who is celibate and "passes as straight," but considers herself a lesbian, face the same kind of oppression as a lesbian who is engaged in an openly gay relationship? Do gays and lesbians whose behavior challenges dominant gender roles experience more psychological distress and opposition than those who conform to dominant gender roles? How these identities, as well as behaviors, differently impact the mental health of different individuals is still very poorly understood (5, 6, 35–37, 62).

Most recently, the term "queer," utilized to ridicule homosexuals in the past, has been reclaimed by many radicals. Popularized by the radical gay organization, Queer Nation, "queer" has become a challenge to restrictive categories such as "lesbian," "gay," or "bisexual," which are seen as separating and marginalizing people rather than highlighting their shared oppression. Instead, queer includes all people who have been marginalized by society, and who refuse to assimilate to mainstream norms (63, p. 12), again introducing the concept of "choice" into the notion of sexual orientation.

As for its implications for mental health, the 1990s radicals' view of oppression as inclusive of all marginalized groups, rather than fragmented among different groups, is useful, since it draws attention to the need for broad social change to address feelings of low self-worth, isolation, and suicide affecting many marginalized groups in the United States. At the same time, it is necessary to acknowledge that different forms of oppression do affect groups and individuals differently, as evidenced by the racism, sexism, and heterosexism experienced by lesbians of color, for instance.

NEW DIRECTIONS FOR PUBLIC HEALTH
AND SOCIAL SCIENCE RESEARCH

Research in sexuality and sexual identity, and their implications for mental health, is still relatively new, especially research that takes into account social intolerance as the ultimate causal agent in psychological distress. The continuing challenges to this formulation highlight the historical, social, and cultural specificity, as well as fluidity, of current conceptions of homosexual suicide.

One problematic arena concerns the kind of published research that informs theory and practice. Although homosexuality is increasingly becoming a topic of academic research and debate, there is a noticeable paucity of reference to gay suicide in the public health and mental health literature (41, 64). Despite the occasional token article found in many journals, the vast majority of articles examining the relationship between sexual identity, mental health, and suicide appear in such journals as *The Journal of Homosexuality*. Research on suicide among gay people of color and lesbians is especially scant (2, 6, 37), as most articles on homosexual suicide focus primarily on the experiences of white gay men. Given the high rates of gay and lesbian suicide, the neglect of gay and lesbian suicide in academic journals points to a high degree of heterosexism (37, 65, 66).

A second topic for critical reflection by social scientists, practitioners, and researchers involves the definitions, assumptions, and methodologies that form the foundations of scientific inquiry, and shape our understanding of human behavior. In the area of gay and lesbian suicide, this means continually questioning underlying assumptions about the relationships between mental health and sexual identity, and exploring new methods of understanding the complexity of human behavior and its changing cultural meanings. Such exploration raises new challenges and questions for researchers, including: How does one measure the impact of heterosexism on a person's mental health, and how does one measure the cumulative effects of multiple oppressions? Can the effect of one oppression ever be separated from another oppression among people who are multiply oppressed? How do cultural ideas about gender and gender roles differently affect the mental health of those who challenge those roles and of those who do not—even if both are "gay," or if *neither* identifies as gay? Moreover, how can we better understand the cultural and social institutions or individual qualities and action that mitigate the effects of oppression? Research in the fields of sociology, anthropology, social epidemiology, and social psychology has begun to tackle these questions through predominantly qualitative methods and approaches that more actively involve community members in research design and implementation (5, 36, 50, 51, 53, 67–69). Efforts in this direction must be developed and expanded in order to broaden the base of knowledge that informs social, scientific, and public health theories.

CONCLUSION

The phenomenon of disturbingly high rates of homosexual suicide and psychological distress has long been recognized, although only in recent decades has it come to be studied as such. In order to better understand the social and medical response to this public health issue, this chapter has examined contending theories of gay and lesbian suicide, from biblical times to the present, that have dominated European, and later North American, thought. The religious, medical, and psychological theories share a common emphasis on problematizing *individual* psychology or physiology as the root cause of homosexual suicide. In contrast, more contemporary social theories that emerged in the 1970s have located the cause of gay and lesbian suicide and psychological distress in the oppressive forces of an unjust and intolerant society.

These strikingly divergent approaches to explaining high rates of lesbian and gay psychological distress highlight the extent to which scientific research and theories are shaped by historical, political, social, and cultural processes. Placing the religious and medical theories in their historical context and critically examining their underlying assumptions illuminates the origins of the myth of homosexual suicide and the reasons for its persistence in some quarters today. Similarly, the historical and political forces of the last two decades have led to the emergence of new theories that challenge the myth of gay and lesbian suicide, and begin to incorporate issues of gender, cultural, and class diversity into our understanding of gay and lesbian mental health. Adopting this latter framework calls for a radical restructuring of the fields of psychology and public health, away from the blame-the-victim approach that sees psychological problems as rooted in the individual, rather than in society. Moreover, critical reflection on these contemporary views points toward provocative new directions for social science and public health research.

Acknowledgments — Special thanks to Nancy Krieger and Karen Franklin for their inspiration, assistance, and thoughtful editing, and to Vern Bullough and an anonymous reviewer for their helpful comments in revising this chapter.

REFERENCES

1. Rofes, E. *"I Thought People Like That Killed Themselves:" Lesbians, Gay Men and Suicide.* Grey Fox Press, San Francisco, 1983.
2. Schneider, S. G., Farberow, N. L., and Kruks, G. Suicidal behavior in adolescent and young adult gay men. *Suicide Life Threat. Behav.* 19(4): 381–394, 1989.
3. Jay, K., and Young, A. *The Gay Report: Lesbians and Gay Men Speak Out About Sexual Experiences and Lifestyles,* pp. 729–731. Summit Books, New York, 1979.
4. Bell, A. P., and Weinberg, M. S. *Homosexualities,* pp. 195–216, 450–457. Simon & Schuster, New York, 1987.

5. Gibson, P. Gay male and lesbian youth suicide. In *Report of the Secretary's Task Force on Youth Suicide, Volume 3: Prevention and Interventions in Youth Suicide.* DHHS Publication No. 89-1623. U.S. Government Printing Office, Washington, D.C., 1989.
6. Remafedi, G., Farrow, J. A., and Deisher, R. W. Risk factors for attempted suicide in gay and bisexual youth. *Pediatrics* 87(6): 869–875, 1991.
7. Kus, R. J. Alcoholism and non-acceptance of gay self: The critical link. *J. Homosex.* 15(½): 25–41, 1988.
8. Saghir, M. T., and Robins, E. *Male and Female Homosexuality: A Comprehensive Investigation*, pp. 118–119, 276–277. Williams & Wilkins, Baltimore, 1973.
9. Kourany, R. F. C. Suicide among homosexual adolescents. *J. Homosex.* 13(4): 111–117, 1987.
10. Martin, A. D. Learning to hide: The socialization of the gay adolescent. *Adolesc. Psychiatry* 10: 52–65, 1982.
11. Crompton, L. The myth of lesbian impunity: Capital laws from 1270 to 1791. *J. Homosex.* 6(½): 11–22, 1980/81.
12. Bullough, V. L., and Bullough, M. *Sin, Sickness and Sanity.* Garland Publishing, New York, 1977.
13. Bullough, V. L. *Homosexuality: A History.* Garland STPM Press, New York, 1979.
14. Kennedy, H. C. The 'third sex' theory of Karl Heinrich Ulrichs. *J. Homosex.* 6(½): 103–111, 1980/81.
15. Weeks, J. *Sex, Politics and Society: The Regulation of Sexuality Since 1800.* Longman Group, New York, 1981.
16. Weeks, J. *Sexuality and Its Discontents*, pp. 61–95. Routledge & Kegan Paul, London, 1985.
17. Lewontin, R. C., Rose, S., and Kamin, L. J. *Not in Our Genes: Biology, Ideology and Human Nature*, pp. 37–51. Pantheon Books, New York, 1984.
18. Ulrichs, K. H. *Inclusa: Anthropological Studies in the Sexual Love Between Men*, translated by M. Lombardi. Urania Manuscripts, Los Angeles, 1979.
19. Ellis, H. *Sexual Inversion*, F. A. Davis, Philadelphia, 1901.
20. Carpenter, E. *Homogenic Love and Its Place in Free Society.* Redundancy Press, London, 1980.
21. Carpenter, E. *The Intermediate Sex: A Study of Some Transitional Types of Men and Women.* Mitchell Kennedy Press, New York, 1912.
22. Stevenson, E. *The Intersexes: A History of Similisexualism as a Problem in Social Life.* Arno Press, New York, 1975.
23. Hirschfeld, M. *Sexual Anomalies and Perversions, Physical and Psychological Development and Treatment. A Summary of the Works of Professor Dr. Magnus Hirschfeld, Compiled as a Humble Memorial by his Pupils.* Torch, London, 1948.
24. Durkheim, E. *Suicide.* Free Press, New York, 1951 [1897].
25. Selkin, J. The legacy of Emile Durkheim. *Suicide Life Threat. Behav.* 13(1): 3–14, 1983.
26. Freud, S. The psychogenesis of a case of female homosexuality. In *Sexuality and the Psychology of Love*, edited by P. Rieff, pp. 133–159. Macmillan, New York, 1963 [1920].
27. Freud, S. Certain neurotic mechanisms in jealousy, paranoia and homosexuality. In *Sexuality and the Psychology of Love*, edited by P. Rieff, pp. 160–170. Macmillan, New York, 1963 [1922].
28. Altman, D. *The Homosexualization of America.* Beacon Press, Boston, 1982.

29. Hall, C. S., and Lindzey, G. *Theories of Personality*, Chapt. 2: Freud's Classical Psychoanalytic Theory, pp. 31–73. John Wiley & Sons, New York, 1978.
30. Chodorow, N. *The Reproduction of Mothering, Psychoanalysis and the Sociology of Gender*. University of California Press, Berkeley, 1978.
31. Klaitch, D. *Woman to Woman*. Simon & Schuster, New York, 1978.
32. Lewes, K. *The Psychoanalytic Theory of Male Homosexuality*. Simon & Schuster, New York, 1988.
33. Faderman, L. *Odd Girls and Twilight Lovers: A History of Lesbian Life in Twentieth Century America*. Columbia University Press, New York, 1991.
34. D'Emilio, J. *Sexual Politics, Sexual Communities: The Making of a Homosexual Minority in the United States, 1940–1970*. University of Chicago Press, Chicago, 1983.
35. Herek, G. Beyond 'homophobia': A social psychological perspective on attitudes toward lesbians and gay men. *J. Homosex.* 10(½): 1–21, 1984.
36. Herek, G. The context of anti-gay violence: Notes on cultural and psychological heterosexism. *J. Interpersonal Violence* 5(3): 316–334, 1990.
37. Saunders, J., and Valente, S. M. Suicide risk among gay men and lesbians: A review. *Death Stud.* 11: 1–23, 1987.
38. Martin, A. D., and Hetrick, E. S. The stigmatization of the gay and lesbian adolescent. *J. Homosex.* 15(½): 163–183, 1988.
39. Savin-Williams, R. C. Coming out to parents and self-esteem among gay and lesbian youth. *J. Homosex.* 18(½): 1–35, 1989.
40. Schneider, S. G., et al. AIDS-related factors predictive of suicidal ideation of low and high intent among gay and bisexual men. *Suicide Life Threat. Behav.* 21(4): 313–328, 1991.
41. Fowler, R. D. (ed.). Section on psychology in the public forum. *Am. Psychol.* 46(9): 947–974, 1991.
42. Simon, R. (ed.). Special feature on gays and lesbians in therapy. *Fam. Ther. Networker* 15(1): 26–60, 1991.
43. LeVay, S. A difference in hypothalamic structure between heterosexual and homosexual men. *Science* 253: 1034–1037, 1991.
44. Allen, L. S., and Gorski, R. A. Sexual orientation and the size of the anterior commissure in the human brain. *Proc. Natl. Acad. Sci. USA* 89: 7199–7202, 1992.
45. Perlman, D. Brain cell study finds link to homosexuality, tissue differs between gay and straight men. *San Francisco Chronicle*, August 30, 1991, p. A1.
46. Petit, C. Evidence of difference in brains of gay men, study bolsters biological basis of sex roles. *San Francisco Chronicle*, August 1, 1992, p. A1.
47. Stevens, P. E., and Hall, J. M. A critical historical analysis of the medical construction of lesbianism. *Int. J. Health Serv.* 21(2): 291–307, 1991.
48. Marotta, T. *The Politics of Homosexuality*. Houghton Mifflin, Boston, 1987.
49. Rich, A. Compulsory heterosexuality and the lesbian existence. In *The Signs Reader: Women, Gender and Scholarship*, edited by E. Abel and E. Abel, pp. 139–168. University of Chicago Press, Chicago, 1983.
50. Golden, C. Diversity and variability in women's sexual identity. In *Lesbian Psychologies: Explorations and Challenges*, edited by Boston Lesbian Psychologies Collective, pp. 19–34. University of Illinois Press, Urbana, 1987.
51. Tremble, B., Schneider, M., and Appathurai, C. Growing up gay or lesbian in a multicultural context. *J. Homosex.* 17(3/4): 253–267, 1989.
52. Riggs, M. Tongues Untied. Video recording. Frameline, San Francisco, 1989.

53. Williams, W. L. *The Spirit and the Flesh: Sexual Diversity in American Indian Culture.* Beacon Press, Boston, 1986.
54. Roscoe, W. (ed.). *Living the Spirit: A Gay American Indian Anthology.* St. Martin's Press, New York, 1988.
55. Blackwood, E. Sexuality and gender in certain Native American tribes: The case of cross-gender females. *Signs: J. Women Culture Soc.* 10(1): 27–42, 1984.
56. Roscoe, W. Bibliography of berdache and alternative gender roles among North American Indians. *J. Homosex.* 14(3/4): 81–171, 1987.
57. Erwin, K. Mental Health Issues in the Context of Culture, Race and Sexuality: A Preliminary Study of Gay and Lesbian Native Americans. Unpublished paper. University of California, Berkeley, May 1991.
58. Nanda, S. *Neither Man Nor Woman: The Hijras of India.* Wadsworth Publishing, Belmont, Calif., 1990.
59. Robertson, J. Gender-bending in paradise: Doing 'female' and 'male' in Japan. *Genders* 5: 50–69, 1989.
60. Caplan, P. (ed.), *The Cultural Construction of Sexuality.* Tavistock, London, 1987.
61. Blackwood, E. (ed.). *Anthropology and Homosexual Behavior.* Haworth Press, New York, 1986. [Reprint of special issue of *J. Homosex.* 11(3/4), 1986.]
62. Ross, M. W., Paulsen, J. A., and Stalstrom, O. W. Homosexuality and mental health: A cross-cultural review. *J. Homosex.* 15(½): 131–152, 1988.
63. Berube, A., and Escoffier, J. Queer Nation. *Out/Look: Natl. Gay Lesbian Q.,* Winter 1991, pp. 12–14.
64. McGinnis, J. M. Suicide in America—moving up the public health agenda. *Suicide Life Threat. Behav.* 17(1): 18–30, 1987.
65. Fikar, C. R., and Koslap-Petraco, M. Pediatric Forum: What about gay teenagers? *Am. J. Dis. Child.* 145: 252, 1991.
66. Herek, G., et al. Avoiding heterosexist bias in psychological research. *Am. Psychol.* 46(9): 957–963, 1991.
67. Herdt, G. Representations of homosexuality: An essay on cultural ontology and historical comparison, Parts I and II. *J. Hist. Sex.* 1(3): 481–504; 1(4): 603–632, 1991.
68. Krieger, N. Racial and gender discrimination: Risk factors for high blood pressure? *Soc. Sci. Med.* 30(12): 1273–1281, 1990.
69. Roscoe, W. Making history: The challenge of gay and lesbian studies. *J. Homosex.* 15(3/4): 1–40, 1988.

CHAPTER 11

Disability Theory and Public Policy: Implications for Critical Gerontology

Jae Kennedy and Meredith Minkler

The concentration of disability in older age groups is an epidemiological fact so widely recognized by researchers, policy analysts, and service providers that it is often seen as truistic. Indeed, this relationship is the empirical basis of the "decline and loss" paradigms of aging (1) and, when combined with current population trends, leads to the sort of crisis thinking described by Robertson (2) as "apocalyptic demography." In the public service sector, "the aged and disabled" are frequently treated as a single target population, and with good reason—recent census data indicate that although less than 16 percent of the total adult non-institutionalized population is over age 65, this subgroup accounts for over 60 percent of all adults who report need for assistance with the most basic activities of daily living (3).

Yet there has been an ongoing effort on the part of aging advocates and analysts to distinguish disability from aging, stressing that covariance is not equivalence (e.g., 4). They point out that much of the "normal" functional decline associated with aging is due to poor health behaviors (5) and statistical aggregation of internally heterogeneous age groups (6). This has led some researchers to contrast "successful aging" (i.e., avoiding functional limitation through exercise, diet, and appropriate medical care) with "usual aging" (7). Although this distinction is a useful one—for example, in underscoring the importance of health promotion over the life course—a problematic consequence of this sort of dichotomy involves the potential for further stigmatization of older persons with disabilities (8).

In the area of disability studies, there has likewise been a tendency to distinguish disability from aging. This is due primarily to the centrality of workforce participation in both disability theory and policy. Disability is seen as a discrete categorical workforce exemption for groups otherwise expected to participate in the labor market—that is, young and middle-aged adults. A large and multifaceted rehabilitation industry has grown around the provision of various private and public disability services to this group, and benefit eligibility is typically related to employment status (9). Crucial "non-wage-earning" populations—children, homemakers, and the elderly—are therefore acknowledged only in passing in most prominent critical analyses of disability policy (10, 11), despite the fact that they make up the bulk of the disabled population, at least in industrial and postindustrial societies.

This lack of conceptual crossover is unfortunate, particularly for those working in critical gerontology. Perhaps because advocates have played such a vocal and consistent role in the development of disability studies, the field as a whole is considerably more familiar with, and willing to employ, the general theoretical frameworks of political and moral economy. Indeed, one might argue that the independent living movement was in large part a backlash against traditional biomedical conceptions of disability. Much of the current theoretical work in this area explicitly recognizes the role of economic systems and social values in the construction and reproduction of disability.

Toward the end of applying a critical gerontology framework to aging and disability, we begin by examining different definitions and models of disability, stressing the contribution of newer approaches that give prominence to the role of broader environmental factors in the disablement process. We then turn to the social production and distribution of disability, using both epidemiology and political economy as conceptual frameworks. The linkage of disability and work impedance is then examined and the consequences in disability programming explored, with special consideration to inherent age, gender, and racial biases. Some of the historical antecedents of disability stigma in aging populations are also identified. We conclude by suggesting that analysts develop the principles put forth by the independent living movement, as well as recent work on the moral economy of interdependency over the life course, to broaden our ways of thinking about and addressing disability and aging.

DEFINING DISABILITY

Disability, or more accurately, the disablement process, is a dynamic social phenomenon that has as much to do with cultural norms and socioeconomic status as it does with individual physiological conditions (12, 13). While disease (particularly chronic disease) and injury are often related to disability, they are neither sufficient nor necessary causes. Perhaps the most influential theorist in this area, sociologist Saad Nagi, defines disability as "an inability or limitation in performing roles and tasks expected within a social environment" (14). This is an explicitly relational perspective, dependent on the social environment that defines the parameters of normal activity.

This relational perspective is evident in current typologies of disablement such as the World Health Organization's International Classification of Impairments, Disabilities, and Handicaps (ICIDH), a supplement to the International

Classification of Diseases (ICD) (15). The ICIDH defines specific classes of disease, impairment, disability, and handicap (note that the latter term is controversial in North America, for reasons that we will discuss later in this section). Disablement, according to this model, starts within the individual's body and ends in her sociocultural environment. There is a recognition that disease or injury can lead to a loss of individual physiological function (impairment), which may in turn affect capacity or performance on a number of levels. Yet there is an important distinction between difficulty in performing basic tasks (disability) and the social, economic, and interpersonal consequences of that deficit (handicap). Despite the fact that aging increases the likelihood of disease, impairment, disability, and handicap, age per se plays no direct part in the disablement process.

A crucial feature of stage typologies such as the ICIDH is that the progression between stages is not viewed as inevitable, allowing a more precise discussion of cause and effect, and therefore a more coherent analysis of potential interventions. Thus, it is observed that medical treatment may prevent active pathologies from causing impairments, and effective rehabilitation may reduce or eliminate disabilities resulting from impairments. Assistive devices can moderate the effects of impairments and disabilities. Environmental modifications such as the reduction of physical barriers can reduce or prevent handicap, and so can anti- discrimination laws such as the 1990 Americans with Disabilities Act.[1] Indeed, an individual may actually skip steps in the disablement process. For example, a disfiguring impairment may not lead to any disability, but if it negatively affects a person's social interactions or opportunities, it constitutes a handicap. Likewise, various "hidden" conditions such as diabetes or epilepsy may have few social or economic consequences, although they can cause significant disability.

Models like the ICIDH have been criticized on various grounds. As noted earlier, the use of the term "handicap" (the etiology of which is explicitly linked to dependency—beggars with hand-in-cap) is so offensive to many North American disability activists as to render the whole exercise suspect (17). Other critics detect a clinical bias. Zola (18) observes that, because stage frameworks originate disablement within the individual, they invariably downplay the pivotal role of the sociopolitical environment. Such models are thus sociological extensions of a standard biomedical model (which views disability as an individual deficit to be ameliorated by professional intervention). Analysts such

---

[1] The Americans with Disabilities Act prohibits discriminatory treatment of persons with disabilities in employment, transportation, and public accommodation. In the employment area, for example, organizations making hiring and promotion decisions are required to consider the qualifications of employees or potential employees independent of their disability status. Federal enforcement of the Act has been uneven to date, as private businesses and public agencies struggle with implementation issues (16).

as Hahn, in contrast, describe disability as an oppressed minority group status (19, pp. 46–47):

> All facets of the environment are molded by public policy and government policies reflect widespread social attitudes and values; as a result, existing features of architectural design, job requirements, and daily life that have a discriminatory impact on disabled citizens cannot be viewed merely as happenstance or coincidence. On the contrary, they seem to signify conscious or unconscious sentiments supporting a hierarchy of dominance and subordination between nondisabled and disabled segments of the population that is fundamentally incompatible with the legal principles of freedom and equality.

In defense of the ICIDH, authors have noted that the framework in no way posits the primacy of disease, impairment, disability, or handicap (20), and indeed that the acknowledged discontinuities between these stages allow emphasis of different parts of the disablement process, including sociopolitical critiques of handicap status (21, 22). By integrating the clinical and social aspects of disability, the ICIDH and similar disability typologies offer analysts the opportunity to refine discussion of individual and environmental factors affecting the production and distribution of disability within a population. As suggested in the next section, one possible extension of this approach, and one that complements a political economy perspective, explicitly incorporates the population focus of social epidemiology in the study of disability across age groups.

THE SOCIAL PRODUCTION AND DISTRIBUTION
OF DISABILITY

The fundamental premise of social epidemiology is that illness is generated by the interaction of the physical and cultural environment with the biophysiological properties of individuals within a population (23, 24). Consider the example of chronic respiratory disease. The prevalence of such disease in a community is determined not only by individual factors (e.g., age, sex, hereditary predisposition, smoking behavior, diet, and exercise) but by a host of interrelated factors in the physical and biological environment (e.g., climate, air pollution, and prevalence of viral and bacterial agents) and the sociocultural environment (e.g., general socioeconomic level of the community and distribution of resources within the community, availability of medical and social services, lifestyle norms, and workplace conditions) (25–27).

A similar, but not identical, approach can be taken to describe the production of disability. A higher prevalence of conditions such as respiratory disease thus would lead to a higher rate of disability within a community. The production of disability is also mediated by various environmental factors, but these are not necessarily the same factors as those which produce disease and impairment. As Albrecht observes (9, p. 35):

> Diseases and impairments are organically based, whereas disability is more strongly influenced by the environment. For many persons with disabilities, public attitudes, emotions, stigma, stereotypes, lack of access to rehabilitation, and occupational barriers are more limiting than the physical impairment. Hence we speak of the disabling environment. This concept places the locus of disability not solely within individuals who have impairments but also in the social, economic, and political environment. By this argument, people are impaired but the environment is disabling. In truth, disability is constituted both by impairments and the disabling environment. The concept of disabling environment, however, forces us to acknowledge that disabilities are physically based but socially constructed. Societies, then, produce disabilities differently from impairments.

Disabling environments vary among and within cultures and communities, and the production of disability appears to be closely linked to the dominant means of production and distribution of resources. This is, of course, the axiomatic premise of the political economy framework. A nomadic hunter-gatherer society, for example, would presumably deem a modest mobility impairment as considerably more disabling than would a stable agrarian society with greater role division and food surplus. In industrial and postindustrial societies, disability is constructed primarily as an impedance to wage labor. We will return to the policy consequences of this employment-based construction of disability; but the point here is that a condition is truly disabling only if the individual's community perceives it as such.

The fact that disability is unequally distributed within cultures also indicates a distinct sociogenic component to disability. There is compelling evidence that the prevalence of disability, like morbidity (28–31) and mortality (32–34), varies inversely with socioeconomic factors such as income, employment status, and education (35–37).

Again, the causal linkage of socioeconomic status and disability is different from the linkage of socioeconomic status and disease. Aside from exposure to various health risks leading to higher levels of physical and/or cognitive impairment, persons of low socioeconomic status presumably lack both the external and internal resources to prevent or minimize the transformation of impairment to disability and disability to handicap. There are, of course, the obvious financial barriers to medical, rehabilitative, and support services and technologies which disproportionately affect persons of low socioeconomic status (i.e., the uninsured and underinsured), but there are multiple human capital constraints that may also limit the ability to cope with changes in functional capacity. Indeed, the experience of poverty itself could be described as disabling or, to use the more precise ICIDH terminology, *handicapping*, in the general sense of imposing grave social disadvantage. In any case, descriptive analyses indicate that disability, like age, race, and gender, is a cumulative marker of social stratification (38).

An environmental perspective is useful for describing another important phenomenon: the steady rise in the total incidence and prevalence of disability in developed nations (39–44). Zola (18) attributes this rise to three general factors: (a) the development and widespread application of life-prolonging treatments and technologies, which may increase morbidity while decreasing mortality; (b) the relative and absolute growth of elderly populations; and (c) political, economic, and social pressures to expand the categorization of people as disabled. In other words, technological and demographic transformations affect the production of impairment and disability, while changes in definitions affect the construction of disability. Industrialized countries share not only a rise in disability rates, but a rise in the level of publicly voiced concern among policymakers and social critics about this growth (9). A rhetoric of crisis pervades policy discussions of disability and disability programming which mirrors the Cassandraesque vision of aging described by Robertson (2) and suggests a common ontology.

In most public policy discourse, the "problem of disability" is described in terms of economic costs. These include direct expenditures for acute medical care, institution-based long-term care, and various rehabilitative and support services and technologies. They may also include indirect economic costs such as diminished labor force participation on the part of persons with disabilities and the family and friends who support them. So defined, disability is indeed a staggering expense: LaPlante and his colleagues (45), updating Chirikos's (46) assay, estimate total social costs of disability in the United States (including work and productivity loss) at roughly $150 billion per year. But these superficial economic descriptions do not address the underlying symbolic and structural role of disability status within the modern welfare state. We next review the theoretical work linking disability to labor market participation, and the problems this approach presents for our thinking about aging and disability.

THE CONSTRUCTION OF DISABILITY CATEGORIES

The ICIDH and similar theoretical models define disability as a disruption or violation of "normal" roles, but define those roles fairly broadly. However, not all roles are equally important to the larger social system. Using Mills's (47) distinction, role discontinuities become public problems rather than private troubles only when they are seen as directly or indirectly incurring public costs (monetary or otherwise). Disability is deemed a problem when it causes persons to consume rather than produce economic surplus. This can occur directly, through consumption of publicly funded services, and indirectly, through failure to participate in the wage labor market. The latter problem is the typical focus of most disability theorists working within a political economy framework.

Persons with disabilities, insofar as their impairments limit or preclude workforce participation, present a challenge to the standard exchange relationships within the capitalist economic system. They are unable to sell their labor, and therefore unable to access the goods and services they need to survive. The modern state has traditionally responded to disability in the so-called "working-aged" population in one of two ways. It either compensates those deemed unable to participate in the workforce, or provides training and rehabilitation to prepare persons with disabilities to enter or re-enter the labor market. A third option, regulating the workplace directly by defining the rights of persons with disabilities as employees, is a relatively recent policy development typified by the 1990 Americans with Disabilities Act.

Underlying all government disability programs is an elaborate control apparatus, setting multiple barriers to accessing benefits and defining narrow eligibility categories. From a political economy perspective, the state has a great stake in containing the total proportion of persons deemed unable to work. The challenge for the state is to ensure that only the most desperate take advantage of nonwork allocations—simultaneously maintaining a needs-based distributional system and an array of institutional and structural barriers designed to discourage its use.

The main ways to contain the utilization of the state's welfare systems involve making the resources unappealing or unattainable. This may include subjecting needs-based claims to various social sanctions and a host of legal and administrative requirements that make accessing resources difficult and demeaning. Perhaps the most common and straightforward approach is to narrowly define categories of legitimate need, thereby making the resources unattainable to the majority of the population (10). As Stone suggests, old age, youth, widowhood, and sickness have evolved as categories "granted social exemption from participation in the work-based distributive system." It is these *categories*, rather than older or disabled *individuals*, which "have a legitimate claim on social aid. . . . the categories thus act as boundaries between the primary, work-based distributive system and the secondary, needs-based system" (10).

For categories to fulfill this boundary function, they must: (*a*) coincide with widely accepted norms of control and responsibility with regard to workforce participation; (*b*) be readily identifiable; and (*c*) be relatively stable conditions that are not easily feigned. Old age (arbitrarily designated as 65 or older in U.S. policy) and youth have become the primary categories for workforce exemption, in part because they are stable and easily measured states. In contrast, the category of disability (the modern policy formulation of illness), like that of single motherhood (the modern policy formulation of widowhood), is the subject of constant debate and regular reformulation by policymakers.

There are clearly intertwined moral and economic dimensions to the public definition of disability categories. The moral issues have to do with individual volition—are people "really" unable to participate in the labor market or do they simply choose not to? The work-based distribution system is buttressed by a powerful set of public attitudes about the social obligation to work. Persons who opt out of the labor force to seek public benefits may therefore be subject to considerable stigma. The legitimacy of needs-based claims is imputed on the basis of the perceived capacity for work and on the degree to which life choices influence this capacity.

The economic issues focus mainly on public expenditure containment. The crafting of the ill-fated U.S. Health Security Act in 1993, for example, included a heated debate over whether limitations in two or three or more activities of daily living (ADLs) constituted grounds for covered services. Cost considerations appeared to be most persuasive in this debate, since use of the more liberal definition of disability (difficulty with two ADLs) would have added more than 900,000 disabled people to the rolls of those eligible for services (48).

The following section explores the consequences of the programmatic linkage of disability to workforce participation, focusing particularly on those groups already marginalized by the wage labor market.

GENDER, RACE, CLASS, AND AGE BIASES IN DISABILITY PROGRAMS

The primacy of work can be readily observed in U.S. disability programs, which can be broken down into two major classes: social insurance (e.g., Social Security Disability Insurance or SSDI, worker's compensation, and state disability), and social assistance or welfare (e.g., Supplemental Security Income or SSI). Eligibility for both types of programs is explicitly linked with the work-based distributional system. This linkage is positive for social insurance programs, in that benefit eligibility is dependent on current employment or prior work history, and negative for social assistance programs, for which benefit eligibility is dependent on nonparticipation in the workforce. As we will discuss below, gender, race, age, and class considerations play an important role in influencing program eligibility and the nature of the assistance received.

Social insurance disability programs such as SSDI are modeled after private insurance, and are subject to some of the same shortcomings. They are intended to be self-financing, so they usually cover only those workers who are currently contributing or have contributed to the program fund. Benefit levels are often tied to contribution level (i.e., salary) instead of severity of disability. The biomedical eligibility criteria employed by these programs tend to favor acute conditions and injuries rather than the chronic conditions that are more prevalent in older workers.

While social insurance programs help protect workers from impoverishment resulting from the sudden onset of disability, they also function as a stop-loss mechanism for industry. Worker's compensation programs, for example, were developed during the middle of the industrial revolution (after rudimentary worker protection laws were enacted) to help shield manufacturers from unpredictable and potentially costly lawsuits from employees injured or killed on the job. Social insurance programs also function to reproduce and reinforce the economic and social disparities among workers after withdrawal from the workforce by linking benefit levels to work history and contribution level. For example, Social Security is effective at maintaining income levels after retirement, but because of the enormous wage inequalities in the United States, the program helps perpetuate social class differences and high levels of relative economic vulnerability among large subgroups of the elderly (49).

In contrast, social assistance programs such as SSI, Medicaid, and food stamps are supported by general government funds, and eligibility is not directly tied to employment. They offer significantly less generous benefits than their social insurance counterparts (lest they serve as disincentives to workforce participation), and eligibility criteria assess family income and assets as well as long-term impairment. Benefits are usually targeted to those at or below the federal poverty line, and often consist of direct services rather than cash transfers. The needs that are addressed are defined in the most basic survival terms. Resources are targeted for subsistence—that is, direct provision or indirect payments for food, housing, or medical care. Because programs are funded directly by the state, caseloads and costs are closely monitored and controlled. For most people with disabilities, public assistance is limited to this latter class of programs.

An analysis of modern welfare policy suggests that disability, defined as inability to participate in the workforce due to a physical or mental impairment, is only one of a series of complex and nondiscrete social categories bounding the labor market. These categories segment the population into wage-payers, wage-earners, and dependents, thereby facilitating the concentration of political and economic power.

One of the primary ways that the state (and the dominant economic institutions it supports) enforces the boundaries of the wage labor market is by defining a huge class of important social maintenance activities, and the persons who perform them, as outside the sphere of paid work. Gender has historically been the main criterion used to separate these spheres of public and private responsibility. The social roles of wife, mother, and daughter carry overt and significant expectations for unpaid labor: the care of children, spouses, and elderly or disabled parents (50).

Leaving aside the broader critique of the social inequity inherent in such a system, it is important to stress the consequence of these gender expectations for disability policy. Impairment or disability among family members can and does dramatically increase the time and effort required to fulfill the caregiving responsibilities "normally" assigned to women as wives, mothers, and daughters (51). Since these support activities are devalued to begin with, the additional caregiving demands (and concomitant stress and impedance to workforce participation) are typically not recognized, at least as a public problem worthy of policy remediation or compensation.

Disability within non-wage-earning groups, including, importantly, the elderly, is thus generally construed as a family problem rather than an individual problem. The physical support and maintenance of family members with disabilities become a public rather than private concern only when caregivers are unable or unwilling to provide adequate unpaid assistance. The institutional and community-based long-term care services in the United States therefore function as a secondary support system. Because this system is conceptually and programmatically linked to failures of family supports, it also tends to be devalued and therefore chronically underfunded.

Consider the case of a typical Medicaid-funded program, providing older disabled clients with a modest level of personal assistance and household chores on a daily basis. Eligibility for such a program would be based not only on medically verifiable impairment, but on availability of unpaid family support and on family income. Only in rare cases would family members or other "informal caregivers" be paid by such a program to assist their disabled relatives.

Although women are more likely to become disabled and require assistance, their unpaid caregiving activities limit their access to public supports. Insofar as family care responsibilities constrain workforce participation, they serve as a barrier to accessing the benefits of the wage market. If a woman designated as an unpaid caregiver becomes disabled herself, she will not be eligible for work-based social insurance.

Social assistance programs for non-wage-earning groups are embedded in the needs-based distributional system, with all of its accompanying barriers discouraging utilization of benefits (i.e., social stigma, access hurdles, and limited direct services rather than cash benefits). Such programs are directly targeted to the poor, and indirectly targeted to women. In the absence of any individual earned income, means-testing shifts the unit of analysis from the person with a disability to her family. Fraser notes that there is an overt gender subtext to such program eligibility requirements (52, p. 149):

> The system as a whole is a two-tiered one. . . . One set of programs is oriented to individuals and tied to participation in the paid work force . . . [and] is designed to supplement and compensate for the primary market in paid labor power. A second set of programs is oriented to households and tied to combined household income . . . [and] is designed to compensate for what are considered family failures, in particular the absence of a male breadwinner. What integrates the two sets of programs is a common core set

of assumptions regarding the sexual division of labor, domestic and non-domestic. It is assumed that families do or should contain one primary breadwinner who is male and one unpaid domestic worker (homemaker and mother) who is female.

This institutional gender bias is carried into old age through contribution-based retirement programs such as Social Security and means-tested health and long-term care programs such as Medicaid. Moreover, because of differences in the demography of aging, morbidity, and mortality (53), women are more likely to rely on such programs for longer periods of time (54).

Race, like gender, also has profound implications for the definition and experience of disability in old age. People of color are at elevated risk both for experiencing disability and for having their impairments "treated" and managed for long periods of time, often through public programs. Although most of the research on race differences in disability among the elderly tends to be limited to comparisons of whites and African Americans, even this narrow literature is revealing.

While African American adults have a lower mean adult age than whites, they report significantly higher rates of activity limitation: 5.1 percent of the African American population, as opposed to 3.7 percent of the white population (3). Moreover, as Gibson (55) notes, many African Americans aged 55 and over appear to constitute a new type of retiree—the "unretired retired." She suggests that a significant portion of this population opts out of the workforce before the Social Security retirement threshold of 65, choosing to rely on modest federal disability benefits such as SSI rather than equally modest wages. According to this argument, the status of disabled worker is economically and psychologically preferable to that of marginal worker, particularly in communities where employment opportunities are extremely limited. Further research is needed to explicate the degree to which race may be, in part, a proxy for social class in relation to the phenomenon of the "unretired retired," but the latter's importance as a descriptively accurate category for many older African Americans underscores the value of taking it into account in retirement planning and policy development.

Although the emphasis on employment in disability programs differentially affects populations already facing social and structural barriers to workforce participation (i.e., women and people of color), it also creates some distinct age biases. Because the primary objective of most disability support services and cash transfers is to establish or restore independence, typically defined in a narrow financial sense of economic self-sufficiency, older persons already given a permanent exemption from the workforce are often excluded, even if they could benefit from those services.

The limited social insurance benefits available to disabled seniors focus almost entirely on the avoidance or postponement of costly institution-based services. As Estes (56) has noted, the primary beneficiaries of programs for the elderly (and we would add, the disabled elderly in particular) have often tended to be service providers, rather than elders themselves. These programs embody the "decline and loss" paradigm of disability and aging which pervades much of geriatrics and gerontology. In the next section we will briefly discuss the evolution of this perspective of aging and disability.

AGE, DISABILITY, AND STIGMA: CONTEMPORARY AND HISTORICAL PERSPECTIVES

A decline and loss paradigm often ignores the broader needs and aspirations of older people with disabilities, reinforcing the biomedicalization of aging (57) and the marginalization of disabled seniors. In the latter regard, as noted earlier, recent attempts to stress "healthy" and "successful" aging have sometimes had the effect of reinforcing negative attitudes toward those elders who are in fact disabled. Arguing that it is "ageist" to equate old age with disability, gerontologists and aging advocates sometimes wittingly or unwittingly help transfer fears about aging to fears of disability. Cohen observes that the accompanying prejudice against disabled elders, which he called "the elderly mystique,"[2] is not infrequently shared by older people: "the elderly themselves have concluded that when disability arrives, hope about continued growth, self realization and full participation in family and society must be abandoned so that all energy can be directed toward the ultimate defeat, which is not death but institutionalization" (59, p. 25).

There is a growing appreciation of the potential for reaching goals of autonomy, growth, participation, and high life satisfaction on the part of the non-disabled elderly, but these goals tend to be recalibrated dramatically downward for those elders who become disabled. Where "access" and "full participation" have become key concepts for the younger disabled population, the sights of families and professionals, and of older disabled persons themselves, tend to be far more circumscribed. In this way, aging professionals, elders, and society in general appear to have traded earlier, limited views of aging for an even more limited view of what it means to be old and disabled (1).

Although a thorough discussion of this phenomenon is beyond the scope of this chapter, it is interesting to speculate about the roots of our current tendency to "split" old age into healthy or successful on the one hand, and unhealthy or unsuccessful—with little chance of autonomy and participation—on the other. Historian Thomas Cole, for example, has suggested that this tendency may be

---

[2] The term "elderly mystique" was coined by Rosenfelt (58) in 1965 in reference to a more general negative view of aging and the elderly held by young and old alike. While Cohen resurrected and used the term more than 20 years later, he has defined it more specifically as prejudice against the disabled elderly. It is the latter conceptualization that is employed in the current discussion.

"part of an historical pattern based on splitting or dichotomizing the 'negative' from the 'positive' aspects of aging and old age" (60, p. 18):

> The primary virtues of Victorian morality—independence, health, success—required constant control over one's body and physical energies. The decay of the body in old age, a constant reminder of the limits of self control, came to signify precisely what bourgeois culture hoped to avoid: dependence, disease, failure and sin.

The view of a dichotomized old age, and of the virtuous and benevolent execution of one life stage as heavily influencing one's happiness in the next, was further reinforced in the spheres of health and medicine. Since many prescriptions for a moral life were also the maxims for good health, physicians of the early 1800s often stressed a life of righteousness as a means of achieving a good and healthy/non-disabled old age (61).

Beginning in the late 1800s, a variety of political, economic, and other social forces resulted in a gradual movement away from a dichotomized view of old age and toward a general devaluation and medicalization of this life stage. As Cole notes, for example, in both the United Kingdom and the United States, "the word 'senile' itself was transformed . . . from a general term signifying old age to a medical term signifying the inevitably debilitated condition of the aged" (62). By equating old age with disability, reformers in many European countries provided additional momentum in the movement to enact old-age pension schemes. While their motives were often laudable, the effect of this "compassionate ageism" (63) was much the same as its earlier, less compassionate version: the elderly were systematically devalued and aging became interestingly synonymous with disease, disability, and decline.

Missing from both the earlier, Victorian-era notions of a dichotomized old age and later emphasis on a decline and loss paradigm is, of course, a dialectical vision of aging—one that truly respects its diversity and its place as part of a natural and unified lifetime. A dialectical vision of aging would acknowledge both able-bodiedness and disability as valid parts of the aging experience. By holding both visions simultaneously, moreover, it would enable a more thoughtful approach to meeting the needs of those elders who are or become disabled (1). A useful framework for moving in this direction may be found in the disability literature, in the latter's concept of independent living.

INDEPENDENT LIVING AND INTERDEPENDENCE: AN ALTERNATIVE VIEW OF THE DISABILITY EXPERIENCE

The independent living movement is a loose coalition of persons with disabilities and their allies (advocates and analysts sympathetic to the aims of the movement) who pursue public policies that minimize segregation and maximize autonomy. The movement has proven remarkably effective in advancing its political agendas, and the philosophy of independent living is increasingly influential in disability theory and research. According to Ratzka, the principles of independent living assert (64):

> The right of all persons, regardless of age, type or extent of disability, to live in the community, as opposed to living in an institution; have the same range of choices as everyone else in housing, transportation, education, and employment; participate in the social, economic, and political life of their communities; have a family; live as responsible, respected members of their communities, with all the duties and privileges that entails; and unfold their potential.

The independent living perspective suggests that the condition of the body is, or rather should be, irrelevant to the economic, social, and family life of the individual. This does not deny the need for support services and technologies; indeed, it implies that considerable resources should be directed toward the full integration of persons with disabilities. But these services and technologies must be, to the fullest extent possible, under the direct control of the recipient. In the words of Judy Heumann, director of the U.S. Department of Education's Office of Special Education and Rehabilitation, "Independent living is not doing things by yourself, it is being in control of how things are done" (quoted in 65).

In the wake of the passage of the Americans with Disabilities Act, an increasing number of leaders of the disability movement have assumed positions of power or influence in various facets of the U.S. policymaking apparatus. Independent living concepts are therefore becoming more central to various federal policy and research initiatives across a variety of domains, including education, housing, employment, and health care. As these individuals continue to grow in influence and in chronological age, one can expect the philosophy of independent living to affect aging services and policies as well.

The independent living philosophy has important implications for our consideration of the aging and disabled. First, as noted earlier, it provides an important counterpoint to conceptual and programmatic approaches to disability in old age which stress avoidance of institutionalization as a necessary and sufficient goal of maintenance or rehabilitation efforts. Second, and relatedly, it reminds us that even in advanced old age, "Life is more than simply the sum of a list of activities of daily living. There must be room for experiencing a fluid, unpredictable story line unfolding over time" (66, p. 278).

Finally, the philosophy of the independent living movement extends gerontology's concerns with "aging in place" by underscoring the importance of minimizing not only geographical disruptions, but also social and economic ones, as well as disruptions in the sense of control that we now know to be an important component of well-being across the life course (67–70).

Despite its emphasis on the language of independence, the independent living movement is philosophically very much in tune with the notion of a "moral economy of interdependence" (71). As Robertson points out, the elderly (and, we would add, people with disabilities), are often "caught between a social ethic of independence on the one hand and a service ethic which constructs them as dependent on the other" (71). Getting beyond this dilemma means embracing a deeper sense of the relationship between individuals with disabilities and the larger community, stressing reciprocity, but a reciprocity far removed from narrow marketplace conceptualizations of giving and getting in return.

Applied to people with disabilities and the broader community, a moral economy of interdependence would stress creating conditions within which the former exercise control over their lives and participate equally in the larger society. It would stress that people with disabilities and people without disabilities are intimately tied to one another and that the needs of the disabled are, in a real sense, shared by all of us. The independent living philosophy and related conceptualizations of interdependence, in short, have a great deal to offer those concerned with developing broader and more empowering approaches to aging and disability.

IMPLICATIONS OF DISABILITY THEORY AND RESEARCH FOR CRITICAL GERONTOLOGY

Although substantial portions of the older population are free of disability at any given time, disability is a typical part of the individual aging process. As Zola points out, "the issue of disability for individuals . . . is not whether but when, not so much which one, but how many and in what combination" (18). Most of the theoretical work to date in both gerontology and disability studies has failed to adequately acknowledge this fact. By creating artificial distinctions based on chronological age and government retirement policies, we risk overlooking common service needs and desires for personal autonomy which bridge age groups.

We have proposed several directions for researching policy and practice to help break down these artificial walls and promote a common ground. First, there is a continued need for the development of models of disability and aging that underscore the broader environmental contexts within which the disablement process takes place. By stressing that disabilities are indeed physically based but socially constructed, we can better understand the political and moral economic forces that help explain the distribution and meaning of disability within and across diverse groups and society.

Second, in the light of the disproportionate representation of disability among the old, the definitional and programmatic linking of disability to workforce participation merits careful reconsideration. We have argued that such a linkage not only reinforces the valuing of people primarily in economic terms, but further marginalizes groups such as caregivers and the elderly, who are already excluded from the labor force.

Third, and relatedly, the gender, race, class, and age biases inherent in existing programs serving the elderly and disabled are in need of further research and policy attention. The two-tier system of financial assistance works to the systematic disadvantage of elders who are low-income, women, people of color, and/or disabled. Such populations are disproportionately represented in second tier programs such as SSI. These social insurance programs tend to have "a low compassion index" (72), providing miserly benefits and stigmatizing beneficiaries.

Recent policy proposals that would tighten program eligibility would further disadvantage these groups. Likewise, proposals to increase normal retirement age to 67 or 70 would penalize those groups most likely to leave the workforce early due to disability and/or caregiving responsibilities (i.e., women, low-income elders, and elders of color). Research and policy efforts must recognize and address the differential impacts of such "reforms." The current biases against caregivers merit particular scrutiny, as the aging of the population and the rapid spread of managed care and other cost-containment approaches promise to increase reliance on informal family support for the elderly and disabled in the years ahead.

Finally, as noted earlier, concepts such as healthy and successful aging, while useful in pointing up the importance of health promotion and disease prevention across the life course, need to be used with considerable caution for the many elders who are or will become disabled. Idealized "one hoss shay" notions of old age in which the elderly, like the master's horse in Oliver Wendell Holmes's (73) poem, live out a full and long life with little or no impairment and then simply die are both realistic and potentially victim blaming. A dialectical vision of old age, which appreciates the diversity of the aging experience and makes room for both able-bodied and disabled elders, is an important one to bear in mind as we plan for unprecedented numbers of elders in the decades ahead.

The spirit and philosophy of the independent living movement, which stresses choice, participation, and the minimization of the economic and social disruptions associated with the onset or aggravation of disability, provide an important framework for analysis and action. Yet as Robertson (71) suggests, of at least equal importance is movement toward a moral economy of interdependence, which moves beyond narrow conceptualizations of needs, rights, and entitlements to focus instead on a broad vision of reciprocity. Instead of segmenting the needs of the elderly and disabled, we should acknowledge as a society the "webs of interdependence" in which all members of the national community live. Aging and disability are facts of life that ultimately confront most human beings, and recognition of this fact may help form the basis of a more caring and civilized society.

Acknowledgments — The authors would like to recognize the formative role that the staff and advisors of the World Institute on Disability have had on our understanding of disablement in general and of disability policy in particular. The insights of Ed Roberts, Judy Heumann, Simi Litvak, Devva Kasnitz, Irv Zola, and Mitch LaPlante helped inspire and inform this analysis.

REFERENCES

1. Minkler, M. Aging and disability: Behind and beyond the stereotypes. *J. Aging Stud.* 4(3): 245–260, 1990.
2. Robertson, A. The politics of Alzheimer's disease: A case study in apocalyptic demography. In *Critical Perspectives on Aging*, edited by M. Minkler and C. L. Estes. Baywood, Amityville, N.Y., 1991.
3. Kennedy, J., and LaPlante, M. A profile of adults needing assistance with activities of daily living. *Disabil. Stat. Rep.* 9, 1998, in press.
4. Riley, M., and Bond, K. Beyond ageism: Postponing the onset of disability. In *Aging in Society: Selected Reviews of Recent Research*, edited by M. Riley, B. Hess, and K. Bond. Lawrence Erlbaum, Hillsdale, N.J., 1983.
5. Gorman, K., and Posner, J. Benefits of exercise in old age. *Clin. Geriatr. Med.* 4: 181–192, 1988.
6. Bortz, W. Disuse and aging. *JAMA* 248: 1203–1208, 1982.
7. Rowe, J., and Kahn, R. Human aging: Usual and successful. *Science* 237: 143–149, 1987.
8. Minkler, M. Critical perspectives on aging: New challenges for gerontology. *Ageing and Soc.* 16: 467–487, 1996.
9. Albrecht, G. *The Disability Business: Rehabilitation in America.* Sage Library of Social Research, Newbury Park, Calif., 1992.
10. Stone, D. *The Disabled State.* Temple University Press, Philadelphia, 1984.
11. Bickenbach, J. *Physical Disability and Social Policy.* University of Toronto Press, Toronto, 1993.
12. Haber, L. Identifying the disabled: Concepts and methods in the measurement of disability. *Soc. Sec. Bull.* 12: 17–34, 1967.
13. Nagi, S. Some conceptual issues in disability and rehabilitation. In *Sociology and Rehabilitation*, edited by M. Sussman. American Sociological Association, Washington, D.C., 1965.
14. Nagi, S. An epidemiology of disability among adults in the United States. *Milbank Q.* 54: 439–467, 1976.
15. World Health Organization. *International Classification of Impairments, Disabilities, and Handicaps.* Geneva, 1980.
16. West, J. *Federal Implementation of the Americans with Disabilities Act, 1991–1994.* Milbank Memorial Fund, New York, 1994.
17. Pfeiffer, D. The problem of disability definition. *J. Disabil. Policy Stud.* 4(2): 23–28, 1993.
18. Zola, I. Disability statistics, what we count and what it tells us: A personal and political analysis. *J. Disabil. Policy Stud.* 4(2): 10–39, 1993.

19. Hahn, H. The political implications of disability definitions and data. *J. Disabil. Policy Stud.* 4(2): 11–17, 1993.
20. Wood, P. The language of disablement: A glossary relating to disease and its consequences. *Int. Rehabil. Med.* 2(2): 86–92, 1980.
21. Wood, P. Maladies imaginaires: Some common misconceptions about ICIDH. *Int. Disabil. Stud.* 9(3): 125–128, 1987.
22. Brown, S. *Defining Persons with Disabilities: A Lack of Science.* Society for Disability Studies Annual Conference, Seattle, 1992.
23. Kleinbaum, D., Kupper, L., and Morgenstern, H. *Epidemiologic Research: Principles and Quantitative Methods.* Lifetime Learning Publishers, Belmont, Calif., 1982.
24. Gordis, L. *Epidemiology.* Saunders, Philadelphia, 1996.
25. Stehr, D., Klein, B., and Murata, G. Emergency department return visits in chronic obstructive pulmonary disease—The importance of psychosocial factors. *Ann. Emerg. Med.* 20(10): 1113–1116, 1991.
26. Weinberger, S. *Principles of Pulmonary Medicine,* Ed. 2. Saunders, Philadelphia, 1992.
27. Baum, G. L. (ed.). *Textbook of Pulmonary Disease.* Little Brown, Boston, 1994.
28. Adler, N., et al. Socioeconomic status and health: The challenge of the gradient. *Am. Psychologist* 49(1): 15–24, 1994.
29. National Center for Health Statistics. Health characteristics by occupation and industry. *Vital and Health Statistics* 10(170), 1989.
30. Syme, S., and Berkman, L. Social class, susceptibility and sickness. *Am. J. Epidemiol.* 104(1): 1–8, 1976.
31. Syme, S., Hyman, M., and Enterline, P. Some social and cultural factors associated with the occurrence of coronary heart disease. *J. Chron. Dis.* 17: 277–289, 1964.
32. Antonovsky, A. Social class, life expectancy, and overall mortality. *Milbank Mem. Fund Q.* 45: 31–73, 1967.
33. Frey, R. The socioeconomic distribution of mortality rates in Des Moines, Iowa. *Public Health Rep.* 97: 545–549, 1982.
34. Kitigawa, E., and Hauser, P. *Differential Mortality in the United States: A Study in Socioeconomic Epidemiology.* Harvard University Press, Cambridge, Mass., 1973.
35. Chirikos, T., and Nickel, J. Socioeconomic determinants of continuing functional disablement from chronic disease episodes. *Soc. Sci. Med.* 22(12): 1329–1335, 1986.
36. Ficke, R. *Digest of Data on Persons with Disabilities.* NIDRR, Washington, D.C., 1992.
37. Rice, D., and LaPlante, M. Chronic illness, disability, and increasing longevity. In *The Economics and Ethics of Long-Term Care and Disability,* edited by S. Sullivan and M. Lewin. American Enterprise Institute, Washington, D.C., 1988.
38. LaPlante, M. The demographics of disability. *Milbank Q.* 2: 55–77, 1991.
39. Colvez, A., and Blanchet, M. Disability trends in the United States population 1966–1976: Analysis of reported causes. *Am. J. Public Health* 71(5): 454–471, 1981.
40. LaPlante, M. Trends in Survival of Persons with Severe Disability, U.S. 1970–85, and Implications for the Future. Paper presented at the 21st National Meeting of the Public Health Conference on Records and Statistics, Hyattsville, Md., 1987.
41. Manton, K. The dynamics of population aging: Demography and policy analysis. *Milbank Q.* 69(2): 309–338, 1991.

42. Verbrugge, L. Recent, present, and future health of American adults. *Annu. Rev. Public Health* 10: 333–361, 1989.
43. Ycas, M. Trends in the incidence and prevalence of work disability. In *Disability in the United States: A Portrait From National Data*, edited by S. Thompson-Hoffman and I. Storck. Springer, New York, 1991.
44. Zedlewski, S., and McBride, T. The changing profile of the elderly: Effects on future long-term care needs and financing. *Milbank Q.* 70(2): 247–275, 1992.
45. LaPlante, M., et al. *Briefing on Employment and Disability.* Disability Statistics Rehabilitation Research and Training Center, San Francisco, 1994.
46. Chirikos, T. Aggregate economic losses from disability in the United States: A preliminary assay. *Milbank Q.* 67: 59–91, 1989.
47. Mills, C. *The Power Elite.* Oxford University Press, New York, 1956.
48. Kennedy, J. Americans Needing Assistance with Activities of Daily Living: Current Estimates and Policy Implications. Dissertation, University of California, Berkeley, 1996.
49. Myles, J. Postwar capitalism and the extension of social security into a retirement wage. In *Critical Perspectives on Aging: The Political and Moral Economy of Growing Old*, edited by M. Minkler and C. Estes. Baywood Publishing Company, Amityville, N.Y., 1991.
50. Abel, E. Man, woman, chore boy: Transformations in the antagonistic demands of work and care on women in the 19th and 20th centuries. *Milbank Q.* 73(2): 187–211, 1995.
51. Abel, E. *Who Cares for the Elderly? Public Policy and the Experience of Adult Daughters.* Temple University Press, Philadelphia, 1991.
52. Fraser, N. *Unruly Practices: Power, Discourse, and Gender in Contemporary Social Theory.* University of Minnesota Press, Minneapolis, 1989.
53. Seigel, J. *A Generation of Change: A Profile of America's Older Population.* Russel Sage Foundation, New York, 1993.
54. Butler, R. On behalf of older women: Another reason to protect Medicare and Medicaid. *N. Engl. J. Med.* 334(12): 794–796, 1996.
55. Gibson, R. The subjective retirement of Black Americans. *J. Gerontol. Soc. Sci.* 46: S204–S209, 1991.
56. Estes, C. *The Aging Enterprise.* Jossey-Bass, San Francisco, 1979.
57. Estes, C., and Binney, L. The biomedicalization of aging: Dangers and dilemmas. *Gerontologist* 29: 587–596, 1989.
58. Rosenfelt, R. The elderly mystique. *J. Soc. Iss.* 21: 37–43, 1965.
59. Cohen, E. The elderly mystique: Constraints on the autonomy of the elderly with disabilities. *Gerontologist* 28: 24–31, 1988.
60. Cole, T. The specter of old age: History, politics and culture in an aging America. *Tikkun* 3: 14–18, 93–95, 1988.
61. Achenbaum, W. *Images of Old Age in America, 1790 to the Present.* Institute of Gerontology, University of Michigan and Wayne State University, Ann Arbor and Detroit, 1978.
62. Cole, T. Aging, history and health: Progress and paradox. In *Health and Aging*, edited by J. J. F. Schroots, J. Birren, and A. Svanborg. Springer, New York, 1988.

63. Binstock, R. The oldest old: A fresh perspective or compassionate ageism revisited? *Milbank Mem. Fund Q.* 63: 420–541, 1983.
64. Ratzka, A. The user cooperative model in personal assistance: The example of STIL, the Stockholm Cooperative for Independent Living. In *PAS in Europe and America: Report of an International Symposium*, edited by B. Duncan and S. Brown. Rehabilitation International, New York, 1994.
65. Kennedy, J., Litvak, S., and Zukas, H. Independent living and personal assistance services: The research, training and technical assistance programs at the World Institute on Disability. *OSERS* 3: 43–49, 1994.
66. White, H. Disabled elderly: You can't run, but you can hide. *Gerontologist* 31(2): 278, 1991.
67. Langer, E. Old age: An artifact? In *Aging: Biology and Behavior*, edited by J. McGough and S. Kiesler. Academic Press, New York, 1981.
68. Schultz, R. Aging and control. In *Human Helplessness: Theory and Applications*, edited by J. Garber and M. Seligman. Academic Press, New York, 1980.
69. Seeman, T. Personal control and coronary artery disease: How generalized expectancies about control may influence disease risk. *J. Psychosom. Res.* 35: 661–669, 1991.
70. Syme, S. Control and health: An epidemiological perspective. In *Stress, Personal Control and Health*, edited by A. Steptoe and A. Appels. Wiley, New York, 1989.
71. Robertson, A. Beyond apocalyptic demography: Toward a moral economy of interdependence. *Ageing and Soc.*, 1998, in press.
72. Margolis, A. *Risking Old Age in America.* Westview, San Francisco, 1990.
73. Holmes, O. *The Deacon's Masterpiece on the Wonderful "One Hoss Shay."* Houghton Mifflin, Cambridge, Mass., 1881.

SECTION II

Empirical Investigation:
Social Epidemiology at Work

Preface to Section II

It is one thing to have social epidemiologic theories of disease distribution. It is another to apply them to concrete analysis of population distributions of disease and social inequalities in health. Examples of how this can be done are provided by the chapters in the three parts of *Section II,* which empirically investigate inequities in health in relation to work, income, physical hazards, violence, discrimination, and access to health services.

Yet, while the investigations in *Section II* consider various societal determinants of diverse health outcomes, appropriately none attempt the impossible task of addressing all the possible pathways leading to embodiment of inequality for any given outcome. The point of social epidemiologic theories is not to imply that all pathways should be investigated in any one study. Instead, what these theories can do is enable researchers to think through, systematically, choices about what to measure (and how) and to identify what are likely to be important unmeasured covariates. With this knowledge, investigators can better understand the meaning and limitations of the analytic findings our studies generate as well as identify the partners with whom we need to work to achieve sustainable advances in meeting the goal of social equity in health.

Part 1, concerned with "Dying for a Living: Income, Work, and Health," includes four empirical analyses focused on outcomes involving social inequalities in both health and health care. The first, in Chapter 12, by Carles Muntaner and P. Ellen Parsons, concerns "Income, Social Stratification, Class, and Private Health Insurance: A Study of the Baltimore Metropolitan Area" and was first published in *International Journal of Health Services* in 1996 (2). Emphasizing that societal conditions affecting generation and distribution of income, and not just income itself, are relevant to explaining social inequities in the distribution of health insurance, the authors empirically demonstrate the salience of incorporating "theory-driven indicators of social stratification such as human capital, labor market segmentation, and control over productive assets" into analyses of access to health care. Next, highlighting the importance of poverty as a determinant of population health. is a national study conducted by Robert Hahn and colleagues, on "Poverty and Death in the United States," presented in Chapter 13 and first published in *International Journal of Health Services* in 1996 (3). Illustrating the need to consider effect modification by race/ethnicity and gender, this investigation found that while poverty was associated with increased risk of mortality in all groups, the greatest excess risk of mortality associated with poverty occurred among black men and the least among white women. Moreover, standard "risk factors" (e.g., smoking, cholesterol levels, and physical inactivity) contributed to explaining the excess risk associated with poverty only among women, not men, which raised important questions about conventional explanations for the patterning of mortality by poverty.

Providing another, cross-national vantage on links between class, gender inequality, and health is the investigation reported in Chapter 14, by Ossi Rahkonen and colleagues, on "Understanding Income Inequalities in Health among Men and Women in Britain and Finland," first published *International Journal of Health Services* in 2000 (4). Relevant findings included the greater salience of household, compared to individual, income for understanding the population distribution of self-rated health among women compared to men; and, related, the stronger income gradients evident in Britain compared to Finland, likely reflective of the latter's higher social wage. Further illustrating the relevance of a lifecourse perspective on work, Chapter 15, by Sarah Arber, takes on the topic of "Integrating Nonemployment into Research on Health Inequalities" (5). In this analysis, first published in *International Journal of Health Services* in 1996, Arber demonstrated the importance of including the non-employed in analysis of class inequalities in health, especially older women and men, if accounts of the working class burden of ill-health are to be adequately estimated.

Part 2 in turn addresses social inequalities in health as they pertain to "Physical Hazards: Work, Violence, and Safety," with its three chapters considering workers' injuries and health in a globalizing economy, gender and occupational health, and associations between state-mandated safety regulations and injury mortality. Chapter 16, by Hector Balcazar and colleagues, on "Factors Associated with Work-Related Accidents and Sickness among Maquiladora Workers: The Case of Nogales, Sonora, Mexico," was first published in *International Journal of Health Services* in 1995 (6). Revealing the high prevalence of occupational injuries and illness among these workers, this study also importantly obtained data on work-policies implicated in these hazards, including whether the employer offered information about occupational hazards or ensured the presence of a doctor or nurse on-site in the plant. Next, highlighting discrepancies between gender ideology and gendered realities of work, an innovative study by Karen Messing and colleagues, reported in Chapter 17, analyzes "Sugar and Spice and Everything Nice: Health Effects of the Sexual Division of Labor among Train Cleaners" (7). First published in *International Journal of Health Services* in 1993, its principal finding was that while "women's work" typically is portrayed as cleaner and less hazardous than "men's work," in the case of French train cleaners, the reverse was true. Specifically, women's assignment to the "womanly" tasks of cleaning toilets and human waste resulted in their having more physically hazardous, demanding, and dirtier jobs than their male counterparts. Chapter 18, in turn, by Phil Brown and colleagues, presents a study that analyzed "State-Level Clustering of Safety Measures and Its Relationship to Injury Mortality" (8). First published in *International Journal of Health Services* in 1997, this investigation interestingly found that while associations often existed between state injury mortality rates and state regulations pertaining to firearms and speed limits, associations with state-level socioeconomic indicators, e.g., percent of the population receiving food stamps, were even more stronger. Pointing to the complexities of analyzing the health impacts of policies, this study likewise underscores the necessity of reckoning with social disparities in health for any outcome studied.

Finally, bringing together diverse etiologic pathways at diverse levels involving diverse aspects of social injustice, Part 3 includes four chapters addressing "Embodied Connections: Cumulative Interplay of Inequalities and Physical and Mental Health." Chapter 19, by Marthe R. Gold and Peter Franks, first published in *International Journal of Health Services* in 1990 concerns "The Social Origin of Cardiovascular Risk: An Investigation in a Rural Community" (9). Delineating pervasive yet complex relationships between diverse measures of socioeconomic position and both measures of conventional cardiovascular risk factors plus measured blood pressure and serum cholesterol, this investigation illustrates how actual patterns of social inequalities in health can pose vital and constructive tests of etiologic hypotheses. Likewise emphasizing the importance of analyzing social disparities in disease distribution, and not just disease mechanisms, is Chapter 20, by Marsha Lillie-Blanton and colleagues, on "Latina and African American Women: Continuing Disparities in Health," which was first published in *International Journal of Health Services* in 1993 (10). Linking evidence on racial/ethnic and economic disparities in hazardous social and physical exposures, e.g., urban crowding, pollution, and unsafe jobs, this chapter underscores how policy efforts addressing racial/ethnic inequalities in health must tackle structural determinants, including but not limited to income level and distribution. The salience of homelessness and both sexual and physical violence to women's risk of HIV is then analyzed in Chapter 21, by Barbara Fisher and colleagues, on "Risks Associated with Long-Term Homelessness among Women: Battery, Rape, and HIV Infection" (11). This analysis, first published in *International Journal of Health Services* in 1995, exemplifies why victim-blaming narratives, of the type critiqued by Crawford in Chapter 3, are especially misleading when analyzing the health of persons subjected to multiple forms of social and economic deprivation and coercion. Finally, Chapter 22, by Nancy Krieger and Steve Sidney, on "Prevalence and Health Implications of Anti-Gay Discrimination: A Study of Black and White Women and Men in the CARDIA Cohort. Coronary Artery Risk Development in Young Adults," provides a useful reminder that people live and embody all aspects of their social position, simultaneously, across the lifecourse, not just one piece at a time (12). First published in *International Journal of Health Services* in 1997, this analysis constituted the first population-based study to link anti-gay discrimination to a somatic health outcome and to consider its impact in relation to socioeconomic position, gender, and racial discrimination.

In summary, as suggested by the diverse chapters in *Section II*, putting epidemiology to work via investigating determinants of social disparities in health requires grappling, conceptually, operationally, and analytically, with the realities of embodied biologic expressions of social inequality. It is not as if someone is, say, one day working class, another day a woman, another day Latina, and still another day heterosexual, or someone else is one day a professional, another day a man, another day African American, and another day gay. That said, while theory can help us appreciate interconnections between these aspects of lived experience and their implications for health, it is ultimately an empirical question as to whether all, some, or none of these aspects of social position is actually relevant to the health outcome under study. Hence the rationale for putting social epidemiology to work.

REFERENCES

1. Krieger, N. Theories for social epidemiology in the 21st century: An ecosocial perspective. *Int. J. Epidemiol.* 30: 668–677, 2001.
2. Muntaner, C., and Parsons, P. E. Income, social stratification, class, and private health insurance: A study of the Baltimore metropolitan area. *Int. J. Health Serv.* 26: 655–671, 1996.
3. Hahn, R. A., et al. Poverty and death in the United States. *Int. J. Health Serv.* 26: 673–690, 1996.
4. Rahkonen, O., et al. Understanding income inequalities in health among men and women in Britain and Finland. *Int. J. Health Serv.* 30: 27–47, 2000.
5. Arber, S. Integrating nonemployment into research on health inequalities. *Int. J. Health Services* 26: 445–481, 1996.
6. Balcazar, H., Denman, C., and Lara, F. Factors associated with work-related accidents and sickness among maquiladora workers: The case of Nogales, Sonora, Mexico. *Int. J. Health Serv.* 25: 489–502, 1995.
7. Messing, K., Doniol-Shaw, G., and Haentjens, C. Sugar and spice and everything nice: Health effects of the sexual division of labor among train cleaners. *Int. J. Health Serv.* 23: 133–146, 1993.
8. Brown, P., et al. State-level clustering of safety measures and its relationship to injury mortality. *Int. J. Health Serv.* 27: 347–357, 1997.
9. Gold, M. R., and Franks, P. The social origin of cardiovascular risk: An investigation in a rural community. *Int. J. Health Serv.* 20: 405–416, 1990.
10. Lillie-Blanton, M., et al. Latina and African American women: Continuing disparities in health. *Int. J. Health Serv.* 23: 555–584, 1993.
11. Fisher, B., et al. Risks associated with longterm homelessness among women: Battery, rape, and HIV infection. *Int. J. Health Serv.* 25: 351–369, 1995.
12. Krieger, N., and Sidney, S. Prevalence and health implications of anti-gay discrimination: A study of black and white women and men in the CARDIA cohort. Coronary Artery Risk Development in Young Adults. *Int. H. Health Serv.* 27: 157–176, 1997.

PART 1

Dying for a Living:
Income, Work, and Health

Income, Social Stratification, Class, and Private Health Insurance: A Study of the Baltimore Metropolitan Area

Carles Muntaner and P. Ellen Parsons

The availability of health insurance is a critical component in determining access to the U.S. health care system (1, 2). Lack of health insurance is associated with substandard medical care (3, 4) and with increased risk of subsequent morbidity and mortality (5).

During the 1970s and 1980s, private health insurance, which in 1985 covered three-quarters of the population under 65 years of age (6), became increasingly unavailable for the employed population (7, 8). Although the majority of the insured in the United States obtain private health insurance through their workplace, most of the uninsured are also employed but are tied to a job that does not provide health insurance (9, 10). As a result, knowledge of employment status alone is not sufficient to determine access to private health insurance. The character of that employment—the nature of the work (e.g., industry versus service), the terms of the employment (e.g., part- versus full-time), the size of the firm, and the position of the individual in the hierarchy—is critical to the question of whether health insurance is offered (10). Moreover, individual and family characteristics influence acceptance of workplace insurance offers. Such characteristics include age, family composition, health status of the employee or other family members, availability of other insurance plans, and family income.

The assessment of employment status and relevant employment characteristics must take into account the social as well as the personal context of that employment (or nonemployment). Employed and unemployed persons live in social situations that provide them more or less of the economic resources needed to obtain private health insurance. Retired persons and persons otherwise not in the

This research was funded by the Intramural Research Program at the National Institute of Mental Health, National Institutes of Health.

labor force may have historical or familial relationships with the workplace that provide them with health insurance, even if their income levels are reduced. These factors are not measured directly by employment status alone. Employment, albeit a central determinant, is but one of many social determinants of private health insurance status.

In an era when access to health insurance can be a matter of life and death, the study of the social determinants of private health insurance coverage will inform the effort to understand U.S. inequalities in access to health care and consequent inequalities in health status.

Health services research tends to focus on private health insurance as the major mode of access to health care (e.g., 11–15). Although some large governmental surveys provide a rich source of descriptive data without explicit theoretical frameworks (e.g., 16, 17), most studies of private health insurance lean toward using a single indicator of social stratification as determinant of coverage, usually income (e.g., 11–15) and, on rare occasions, wealth (18). Given that there are multiple measures of social stratification, reliance on a single indicator may be insufficient to characterize the social determinants of private health insurance coverage.

Although income can be conceptualized as an indicator of social stratification, social scientists often consider income as the dependent variable to be explained by sociological models (19–22). For example, some sociological models try to explain which characteristics of persons or positions in the social structure determine income differentials, because relative income alone does not explain how a person was able to gain her or his share of the social product (23). Positions in the social structure are associated with various kinds of income (e.g., income derived from renting land versus wages derived from being an employee), differentials in wealth (e.g., value of assets owned), and social resources (e.g., personal networks) (24–26). Thus reliance on income as the sole indicator of social stratification may overlook differentials in resources such as wealth or benefits associated with type of employment that may affect the availability of access to health care.

As opposed to the pragmatic considerations that might lead to the choice of income and poverty indicators among health service researchers, social epidemiologists tend to ascribe a more theoretical relevance to social stratification in the determination of health and disease (e.g., 27). Social epidemiologists and medical sociologists have developed a number of theory-driven indicators of position in the social structure to characterize populations (2, 27–32).

The distinct approaches to social stratification in studies of inequalities in health taken by social epidemiology and by health services research might have several explanations. For example, availability of health insurance is largely determined by ability to pay (7), although the relationship between health status and income is mediated by many social and behavioral factors (e.g., 32). Most important, health services research is an applied science and thus is less concerned with the social causes of inequalities in access to health care than with effective action toward their reduction. Although the relevance of social theory (e.g., class analysis) to health insurance research has been recently highlighted (33), no studies have presented empirical analyses of the relative utility of different models of social stratification for explaining the availability of private health insurance.

It is our aim to provide such analyses in this study by using a variety of theory-driven indicators of social stratification and assessing the relative strength of the association between these indicators and private health insurance. Next, we will evaluate the implications of these analyses for choosing among alternative models of social stratification in health services research.

A small number of epidemiological studies have compared the ability of different indicators of social stratification to predict health status (e.g., 34, 35). In adopting a more theoretical approach to the prediction of health insurance status, we selected indicators of social stratification corresponding to alternative sociological models. We define social stratification as the ordering of individuals according to one or several dimensions aimed at explaining inequalities in social resources (i.e., economic, political, and cultural (36)). Next, we present our selected indicators in the context of the social theories from which they are drawn.

Human capital theory posits that education increases the value of an individual's contribution to the productive process, which translates into greater social rewards (37). Other models of social stratification are not based on individual differences but emphasize social structure instead (e.g., 38, 39). That is, the reward-relevant properties of jobs derive from their location in the hierarchical structure of the workplace as defined not by the workers' education but by the unequal distribution of authority rights over human and physical resources (20). Among these models we find *incentive contract* (40) and *hierarchy theory* (41), which maintain that managerial/professional occupations obtain higher wages as a compensation for self-monitoring, thus making job loss due to shirking more costly than it would be otherwise (22).

Class analysis is an alternative approach to social stratification (24, 25).[1] Class analysis maintains that several relational mechanisms (i.e., employer versus employee, manager versus worker, skilled versus nonskilled worker) generate inequalities in social resources. In Wright's (42) individual-level approach to social class, certain class locations (nominally defined employers, managers, and skilled workers) are thought to generate inequalities in income as a result of differential appropriation of the social surplus: employers sell the

---

[1] According to certain definitions of social class (i.e., control over productive assets), it should not be defined as a measure of social stratification because class entails relations between individuals rather than there mere stratification. However, even within a relational approach, the appropriation of social surplus entails an implicit hierarchy of wealth and power (24).

products produced by their workers, managers obtain higher wages because of a "loyalty dividend" received in compensation for their supervisory function, and skilled workers obtain higher wages from a "credential rent" because their skills are kept in short supply in the labor market (24, 25). Social class has also been defined according to *production and nonproduction* work (43). This conceptualization divides the work force between work aimed at producing commodities and work providing services. Another social class framework is *labor market segmentation* (44), which holds that, as a consequence of the evolution of employment relations and the evolution of the U.S. economic structure, workers employed in large firms enjoy higher wages and more job security and benefits than do those working for small employers.

METHODS

The study sample was based on a 1993 telephone survey of the population of white residents between the ages of 21 and 89 living in the Baltimore Metropolitan Statistical Area (MSA; Baltimore and surrounding counties). The Waksberg telephone sampling method (45) was used and thought to be appropriate for the following reasons: (*a*) the Baltimore MSA has high availability of telephones (95.3 percent of households have telephones (46)); (*b*) the study was not targeted toward poor populations (47); and (*c*) it ensured the inclusion of unlisted numbers (27.5 percent of households in the Baltimore MSA (46)). We obtained 397 respondents using this method, with a response rate of 69 percent and a refusal rate of 1 percent. An effort rate of up to eight calls at different times on different days per prospective respondent was employed.

A telephone interview was administered that included questions on sociodemographic characteristics, work, and health insurance. Sociodemographic characteristics included the respondent's age, gender, and marital status (recorded as "married or having a live-in partner"). Questions on work inquired about employment status, occupation, industry, income, full-time work, firm size, self-employment, number of employees supervised, and degree of involvement in policy-making at work.

Employment status was recorded as working for pay or not. Working full-time was coded as working 35 hours or more per week. Occupation and industry were ascertained verbatim, later coded according to the Bureau of the Census Classification of Occupations by trained coders, and operationalized as a dichotomous variable for occupation (i.e., managerial/professional occupations versus others) and industry (i.e., agriculture, mining, construction, manufacturing, transportation, and services versus trade, finance, business services, and government). These two dichotomous variables were then combined to create an indicator designating workers in production industries, workers in nonproduction industries (i.e., services), and a residual category of managers/professionals. Educational credentials were coded as attaining less than a bachelor's degree versus attaining a bachelor's degree or more. Wright's social class locations of ownership and organizational control were measured with three categorical variables that assessed self-employment, as well as supervision and policy-making functions in the workplace (25). Owners were defined as self-employed persons who supervised employees. Managers were defined as persons who supervised employees and participated in policy-making decisions at work. Social class as measured by skills/credentials was ascertained with the aforementioned questions on occupation and education and coded according to Wright's (42) scheme: professionals and managers or technicians with a bachelor's degree or more were considered "experts." Firm size was coded as less than 50 employees, between 50 and 499 employees, and 500 or more employees. Income was ascertained as gross household income per year and coded in four intervals ranging from $25,000 or less to more than $65,000. The median of this income variable was used to create a dichotomous variable for multi-variate analyses.

Health insurance was coded as "any private health insurance" (i.e., through self-pay or through an employer) and "public insurance only or uninsured," following the categorization of the National Medical Expenditure Survey (48). "Public insurance only or uninsured" were combined because of sample size considerations.

We used logistic regression to estimate the association between indicators of social stratification and private insurance coverage. Bivariate relations were examined first. The second step of model building involved adjustment for gender, age, and marital status. This adjustment dealt not only with the possible association of these sociodemographic variables, social stratification, and health insurance (e.g., poor single women with children are eligible for Medicaid coverage), but also with the corresponding potential biases introduced by telephone surveys (49). Next, those indicators of social stratification that signaled a strong and significant association with private insurance were added to the sociodemographic model. Indicators that did not reach statistical significance and did not have an appreciable influence on the coefficients of the other variables (50) were dropped from the last model.

RESULTS

The distributions of sociodemographic variables (age, gender, marital status) and indicators of social stratification (employment status, full-time work, education, occupation, household income, firm size, production work, ownership, organizational and skills assets) by type of health insurance are presented in Table 1. Participants who were employed, worked full-time, had a bachelor's

Table 1

Distribution of a sample of the white population in the
Baltimore Metropolitan Statistical Area with private health
insurance by sociodemographic characteristics and
indicators of social stratification

	Private insurance (n = 338) No. (%)	Other insurance (n = 59) No. (%)
Age, yr[a]		
21–30	93 (27.52)	25 (42.38)
31–40	121 (35.80)	15 (25.42)
41–60	86 (25.44)	10 (16.95)
61–89	38 (11.24)	9 (15.25)
Gender		
Men	155 (45.86)	26 (44.07)
Women	183 (54.14)	33 (55.93)
Marital status[a]		
Married or having a live-in partner	203 (60.06)	27 (45.76)
Other	135 (39.94)	32 (54.24)
Employment status		
Employed	269 (79.82)	39 (66.10)
Unemployed	68 (20.18)	20 (33.90)
Full-time work[a]		
≥35 hr/week	231 (85.87)	28 (71.79)
<35 hr/week	38 (14.13)	11 (28.21)
Education[a]		
<Bachelor's degree	211 (62.43)	49 (84.48)
≥Bachelor's degree	127 (37.57)	9 (15.52)
Occupation		
Managers/professionals	47 (18.36)	12 (30.77)
Other	209 (81.64)	27 (69.23)
Household income[b]		
≤$25,000	69 (22.48)	19 (45.24)
$26,000–$40,000	94 (30.62)	9 (21.43)
$41,000–$65,000	93 (30.29)	9 (21.43)
>$65,000	51 (16.61)	5 (11.90)

Table 1   (Cont'd.)

	Private insurance (n = 338) No. (%)	Other insurance (n = 59) No. (%)
Wright's class typology		
Ownership assets		
Owner	31 (11.52)	5 (12.82)
Non-owner (wage earner)	238 (88.48)	34 (87.18)
Organizational assets[a]		
Manager	72 (26.87)	5 (12.82)
Non-manager	196 (73.13)	34 (87.18)
Skill/credential assets		
High skills/credentials[c]	43 (16.41)	3 (7.69)
Low skills/credentials	219 (83.59)	36 (92.31)
Firm size[a]		
≥50 employees	94 (79.66)	168 (91.80)
<50 employees	24 (20.34)	15 (8.20)
Production work[a]		
Workers[d] in production industries	107 (31.66)	15 (25.42)
Workers[d] in service industries	156 (46.15)	38 (64.41)
Managers/professionals	75 (22.19)	6 (10.17)

[a]Chi-square test for age $\chi^2 = 7.49$, $P = .05$; marital status $\chi^2 = 4.21$, $P = .04$; employment status $\chi^2 = 5.47$, $P = .01$; full-time work $\chi^2 = 5.05$, $P = .02$; education $\chi^2 = 10.68$, $P = .001$; organizational assets $\chi^2 = 3.57$, $P = .05$; firm size $\chi^2 = 9.38$, $P = .002$; production/nonproduction work $\chi^2 = 7.62$, $P = .02$.
[b]Mantel-Haenszel chi-square test for trend for income $\chi^2 = 5.88$, $P = 0.01$.
[c]High skills/credentials workers are called "experts" in Wright's model (25).
[d]Except managers/professionals.
Note: In some instances the total number of participants does not add up to 397 due to missing values in the independent variable.

degree or more, lived in higher income households, worked in larger firms, and worked in production industries were more likely to be covered by private health insurance than were participants in other social stratification positions. Similarly, participants who were owners or managers of the firms in which they worked were more likely to be covered by private health insurance than were wage laborers and non-managers.

The unadjusted estimates of the odds of being covered versus not covered by private health insurance are given in Table 2 for each indicator of social

Table 2

Odds ratios (O.R.) and 95 percent confidence intervals (C.I.) of being covered by private health insurance for indicators of social stratification among white residents in the Baltimore Metropolitan Statistical Area: Results from logistic regression analysis, unadjusted and adjusted[a] estimates

	Private health insurance					
	Unadjusted estimates			Adjusted estimates		
Independent variables	O.R.	95% C.I.	P value	O.R.	95% C.I.	P value
Employment status						
Unemployed	1.00[b]			1.00		
Employed	2.03	1.11, 3.70	.02	2.16	1.13, 4.12	.02
Full-time work						
<35 hr/week	1.00			1.00		
≥35 hr/week	2.39	1.09, 5.19	.03	1.88	0.81, 4.35	.13
Education						
<Bachelor's degree	1.00			1.00		
≥Bachelor's degree	3.28	1.56, 6.90	.001	3.54	1.67, 7.51	.001
Occupation						
Other	1.00			1.00		
Managers/professionals	1.98	0.93, 4.18	.07	1.73	0.78, 3.82	.17

	OR	95% CI	p	OR	95% CI	p
Household income						
≤$25,000	1.00			1.00		
>$25,000	7.34	2.83, 19.01	.0001	7.48	2.77, 20.17	.0001
Wright's class typology						
Ownership and organizational assets[c]						
Non-manager and non-owner (wage laborer)	1.00			1.00		
Owner or manager	2.51	1.04, 6.10	.04	2.34	0.95, 5.81	.06
Skill/credential assets						
Non-experts	1.00			1.00		
Experts	2.36	0.69, 7.99	.16	2.19	0.63, 7.60	.21
Firm size						
<50 employees	1.00			1.00		
≥50 employees	2.86	1.43, 5.72	.003	2.81	1.39, 5.68	.004
Production/nonproduction work						
Workers in service industries	1.00			1.00		
Workers in production industries	1.74	0.91, 3.32	.09	1.74	0.90, 3.37	.09
Managers/professionals	1.45	1.10, 1.96	.01	1.43	1.06, 1.96	.03

[a]Adjusted for age, gender, and marital status.
[b]Indicates reference category.
[c]Due to the small number of owners, the categories "managers" and "owners" were combined. Although Wright's model differentiates between ownership and control of businesses (42), top managers derive more of their wealth from ownership of shares of stock than from wages.

stratification.[2] Participants in households with annual incomes above $25,000 were seven times as likely to be covered by private health insurance as were those in households with annual incomes equal to or below $25,000. Participants with a bachelor's degree or more were more than three times as likely to have private insurance as were those with less than a bachelor's degree. Participants working in primary labor markets (i.e., in larger firms) were almost three times as likely to be privately insured as were those working in small firms. Owners and managers were more than twice as likely to benefit from a private health insurance plan as were wage earners and nonmanagement workers. Finally, employed participants were twice as likely to be privately insured as were the unemployed. The results from the logistic regression models with adjustment for age, gender, and marital status are also outlined in Table 2. Odds ratios were in general similar to the bivariate analyses, with some positive confounding shown for the full-time work indicator.

The effects of adding social stratification indicators of education and labor market segmentation to the household income model are shown in Table 3 (p. 666). The addition of indicators of human capital (i.e., education) and labor market segmentation (i.e., size of firm) improved the prediction of the household income model (difference $\chi^2_{(2)} = 11.86$, $P < .01$). Over and above the effect of income, education and size of firm were significant predictors of private health insurance.

DISCUSSION

Our results show that different models of social stratification can predict the availability of private health insurance among the white population of the Baltimore MSA. In particular, indicators of human capital and labor market segmentation were significant predictors of private health insurance even after the effect of income had been taken into account. Because of the important relationship between access to health care (i.e., health insurance coverage) and positive health outcomes, our findings suggest that the inclusion of indicators of social stratification would be beneficial in studies of the determinants of inequalities in health status as well as in studies of inequalities in access to care.

Studies of social inequalities in health often rely on health insurance status as a social class marker, which is used alone or in combination with one or more socioeconomic characteristics (10). However, the role of the state in the provision of health care coverage for particular categories of poor persons (e.g., the elderly, those with disabilities, and members of single-parent families), and of

---

[2] The weighting of the sample to the population (close to 2.5 million inhabitants according to the Bureau of the Census projections for 1992) would yield statistical significance for all our parameters. Therefore we choose not to weight the sample.

Table 3

Adjusted[a] odds ratios (O.R.) and 95 percent confidence intervals (C.I.) of being covered by private health insurance for indicators of income, education, and labor market position among white residents in the Baltimore Metropolitan Statistical Area: Results from multiple logistic regression analysis

	Private health insurance					
	Model I[b]			Model II[c]		
Independent variables	O.R.	95% C.I.	P value	O.R.	95% C.I.	P value
Household income						
≤$25,000	1.00[d]			1.00		
>$25,000	7.48	2.77, 20.17	.0001	8.87	2.04, 38.54	.003
Education						
<Bachelor's degree				1.00		
≥Bachelor's degree				4.92	1.41, 17.17	.01
Labor market segmentation: Firm size						
≥50 employees				1.00		
<50 employees				2.40	1.03, 5.61	.04

[a]Adjusted for age, gender, and marital status.
[b]Model I includes age, gender, marital status, and income.
[c]Model II includes age, gender, marital status, income, education, and firm size.
[d]Reference category.
Note: Model chi-square (df) = 18.37 (4) for Model I; model chi-square (df) = 30.23 (6) for Model II. Difference $\chi^2_{(2)}$ = 11.86, P < .01.

nearly universal Medicare coverage for those 65 years of age and over, mediates the relationship between social class and ill-health (10).

Because not all poor persons have public coverage and most persons 65 and older are not poor, health care coverage status is an inadequate proxy for social class. The Medicaid program, which targets the poor and disabled as well as poor single-parent families (usually headed by women), covers only 40 percent of the poor (3).

Moreover, many poor persons categorically eligible for public programs that provide health care coverage are by definition more likely to be ill. Generally, persons with public coverage are much more likely to be in fair or poor health than are persons with private coverage. Among working-age adults, women with public coverage are four times more likely to be in fair or poor health than are those with private coverage and twice as likely as those with no coverage at all (51). Among persons 65 and over, those with Medicare and public coverage are twice as likely as those with Medicare and private coverage to be in fair or poor health and nearly twice as likely as those with Medicare only (51). Persons with public coverage, though poor, do not adequately represent the poor as a whole because they are disproportionately likely to be sick compared with poor persons who have some other coverage or no coverage at all. The inclusion of class variables that influence state-mediated health insurance status is therefore a necessary step to understand the social determinants of access to health care.

It is important to note that our inferences are limited to the white population in the Baltimore MSA. The fact that our population consisted of whites exclusively precluded the search for interactions between racism and social stratification. We already know that blacks and Hispanics are more likely to be uninsured (7), to work in secondary labor markets (44), and to control fewer assets (52). The potential bias introduced by selecting out households without telephones, although affecting only 5 percent of Baltimore MSA households (46), might have also attenuated our estimates. It seems probable that, because non-telephone households are more likely to include residents who are low-income, manual workers, less educated, and unemployed, they would also be found more often among those working in secondary labor markets and among those with less productive assets.

Although alternative models of social stratification generate different interpretations of results, some models yield similar indicators (24). For example, variables used in the measure of human capital (i.e., education) are similar to variables used in the measure of Wright's skills/credentials assets (a combination of education and occupational categories (44)). Conversely, one could interpret the results obtained with education, the indicator of human capital, as support for Wright's skills/credentials assets theory. In addition, the measurement of "incentive contract," although theoretically closer to "organizational assets," is similar to the measurement of "skills/credentials assets." Finally, employment status and full-time work could be interpreted as indicators of labor market segmentation (44), thus providing additional support for the labor market segmentation model. Individuals employed in primary labor markets provide a skilled, "expensive" form of labor that larger corporations are more interested in keeping (53). Therefore, these workers might be more likely to receive private health insurance than are those in secondary labor markets, who are largely part-time, nonunionized service and clerical workers whose employers are less likely to provide insurance (54, 55).

Class location according to ownership of productive and organizational assets was not the main predictor of private health insurance. This result is a partial refutation of Wright's model because ownership relations are thought to produce the largest inequalities in social resources (19, 42). However, it has already been underscored that Wright's nominal class measures are implicitly continuous (for example, ownership is measured with regard to the number of employees (22)). The use of gross nominal categories may mask what is actually a class gradient (22). Moreover, the ability to capture class differences is limited by the characteristics of our sample. General population samples such as our Baltimore MSA sample might not include enough owners of large firms to produce a meaningful difference in private health insurance coverage between owners and non-owners. We therefore recommend that future studies of social class and health insurance oversample these ownership locations (20, 39).

Our results also point toward a need to outline multilevel models in the study of the social determinants of health insurance coverage. A firm belongs to a supraindividual (i.e., organizational) level of analysis because firms are composed of groups of individuals (56). Thus, a limitation of the present study is that it cannot assess whether different firms of the same size have different relations to health insurance coverage. Future studies should assess the relationship between firm characteristics and health insurance in the context of multilevel analyses.

Several specific recommendations can be made for future studies on the determinants of health insurance status. Researchers might use a number of theory-driven indicators of social stratification and class (e.g., education, firm size, ownership, and management) leading to different explanations (e.g., labor market segmentation, relations of production, human capital) and a better prediction of health care insurance status. The availability of multiple class indicators will depend, nonetheless, on the state agencies' capacity to collect data reflecting different theoretical orientations. This is not an easy task. Several authors have given compelling accounts of the political struggles involved in the selection of class indicators in government-funded surveys and statistical reports (57–59).

Future studies might build on our results by exploring the relation between stratification, class, and several forms of discrimination (e.g., based on "race/ ethnicity," sexual orientation, gender) and adding new class indicators (e.g., wealth).

Finally, specific hypotheses concerning class and social stratification need to be tested to strengthen our understanding of the determinants of health insurance coverage (e.g., 60). Given the findings in this study, future investigations on the determinants of private health insurance can benefit, both theoretically and empirically, from testing contending models of social stratification, such as human capital, labor market segmentation, and differential control over productive assets. Such research will be necessary to fully comprehend inequalities in health insurance coverage.

REFERENCES

1. Glaser, W. A. The United States needs a health system like other countries. *JAMA* 270: 980–984, 1993.
2. Susser, M. Health as a human right: An epidemiologist's perspective on the public health. *Am. J. Public Health* 83: 418–426, 1993.
3. Aday, L. A. *At Risk In America: The Health and Health Care Needs of Vulnerable Populations in the US.* Jossey-Bass, San Francisco, 1993.
4. Burstin, H. R., Lipsitz, S. R., and Brenna, T. A. Socioeconomic status and risk for substandard medical care. *JAMA* 268: 2383–2387, 1992.
5. Franks, P., Clancy, C. M., and Gold, M. R. Health insurance and mortality: Evidence from a National Cohort. *JAMA* 270: 737–741, 1993.
6. Last, J. M., and Wallace, R. B. *Public Health and Preventive Medicine*, Ed. 13. Appleton and Lange, Norwalk, Conn., 1992.
7. Friedman, E. The uninsured: From dilemma to crisis. *JAMA* 265: 2491–2495, 1991.
8. Levit, K. R., Olin, G. L., and Letsch, S. W. Americans' health insurance coverage, 1980–91. *Health Care Financ. Rev.* 14: 31–57, 1992.
9. Foley, J. D. *Sources of Health Insurance and Characteristics of the Uninsured: Analysis of the March 1992 Current Population Survey.* SR-16, Issue Brief No. 133. Employee Benefit Research Institute, Washington, D.C., 1993.
10. Weissman, J. S., and Epstein, A. M. *Falling Through the Safety Net: Insurance Status and Access to Health Care.* Johns Hopkins University Press, Baltimore, 1994.
11. Cantor, J. C. Expanding health insurance coverage: Who will pay? *J. Health Polit. Policy Law* 15: 755–778, 1990.
12. Davis, K., Gold, M., and Makuc, D. Access to health care for the poor: Does the gap remain. *Ann. Rev. Public Health* 2: 159–182, 1981.
13. Fether, J., Hadley, J., and Mullner, R. Falling through the cracks: Poverty, insurance coverage and hospital care for the poor, 1980–1982. *Milbank Q.* 62: 544–566, 1984.
14. Hayward, R. A., et al. Inequities in health services among insured Americans: Do working-age adults have less access to medical care than the elderly? *N. Engl. J. Med.* 318: 1507–1512, 1988.
15. Marquis, M. S., and Buchanan, J. L. How will changes in health insurance tax policy and employer health plan contributions affect access to health care and health care costs? *JAMA* 271: 939–944, 1994.
16. Short, P., Monheit, A., and Beauregard, K. *A Profile of Uninsured Americans.* DHHS Publ. No. (PHS) 89-3443. National Medical Expenditure Survey Research Findings 1. National Center for Health Services Research and Health Care Technology Assessment, Rockville, Md., 1989.
17. Swartz, K. Dynamics of people without health insurance: Don't let the numbers fool you. *JAMA* 271: 64–66, 1994.

18. Mutchler, J. E., and Burr, J. A. Racial differences in health and health service utilization in later life: The effect of SES. *J. Health Soc. Behav.* 32: 342–356, 1991.
19. Wright, E. O. *Class Structure and Income Determination.* Academic Press, New York, 1979.
20. Robinson, R. V., and Kelley, J. Class as conceived by Marx and Dahrendorf: Effects on income inequality, class consciousness, and class conflict in the U.S. and Great Britain. *Am. Sociol. Rev.* 55: 827–841, 1979.
21. Smith, M. R. What is new in "new structuralist" analyses of earnings? *Am. Sociol. Rev.* 55: 827–841, 1990.
22. Halaby, C. N., and Weakliem, D. L. Ownership and authority in the earnings function: Nonnested tests of alternative specifications. *Am. Soc. Rev.* 58: 16–30, 1993.
23. Calinicos, A., and Harman, C. *The Changing Working Class.* Bookmarks, Chicago, 1989.
24. Wright, E. O. Typologies, scales, and class analysis: A comment on Halaby and Weakliem. *Am. Sociol. Rev.* 58: 31–34, 1993.
25. Wright, E. O., and Cho, D. The relative permeability of class boundaries to cross-class friendships: A comparative study of the United States, Canada, Sweden and Norway. *Am. Sociol. Rev.* 57: 85–102, 1992.
26. Muntaner, C., et al. Psychotic inpatients' social class and their admission to state or private psychiatric Baltimore hospitals. *Am. J. Public Health* 84: 287–289, 1994.
27. Krieger, N., et al. Racism, sexism, and social class: Implications for studies of health, disease, and well-being. *Am. J. Prev. Med.* 9(Suppl. 6): 82–122, 1993.
28. Navarro, V. Race or class versus race and class: Mortality differentials in the United States. *Lancet* 336: 1238–1240, 1990.
29. Liberatos, P., Link, B. G., and Kelsey, J. L. The measurement of social class in epidemiology. *Epidemiol. Rev.* 10: 87–121, 1988.
30. Susser, M., Watson, W., and Hopper, K. *Sociology in Medicine,* Ed. 3. Oxford University Press, New York, 1985.
31. Pappas, G., et al. The increasing disparity in mortality between socioeconomic groups in the United States, 1960–1986. *N. Engl. J. Med.* 329: 103–109, 1993.
32. Williams, D. Socioeconomic differentials in health: A review and a reformulation. *Soc. Psychol. Q.* 53: 81–99, 1990.
33. Navarro, V. *The Politics of Health Policy: The U.S. Reforms, 1980–1994.* Blackwell, Cambridge, Mass., 1994.
34. Winkleby, M. A., et al. How education, income and occupation contribute to risk factors for cardiovascular disease. *Am. J. Public Health* 82: 816–820, 1992.
35. Leigh, J. P., and Fries, J. F. Occupation, income, and education as independent covariates for arthritis in four national probability samples. *Arthritis Rheum.* 34: 984–995, 1991.
36. Kohn, M. L., and Schooler, C. *Work and Personality: An Inquiry into the Impact of Social Stratification.* Ablex, Norwood, N.J., 1983.
37. Becker, G. S. *The Economic Approach to Human Behavior.* University of Chicago Press, Chicago, 1976.
38. Kalleberg, A., and Griffin, L. Class, occupation and inequality in job rewards. *Am. J. Sociol.* 83: 731–768, 1980.
39. Marshall, G., et al. *Classes in Modern Britain.* Hutchinson, London, 1988.
40. Lazear, E. J. Incentive contracts. In *Allocation, Information and Markets,* edited by J. Eatwell, M. Milgate, and P. Newman, pp. 152–162. W. W. Norton, New York, 1989.
41. Calvo, G. A., and Wellisz, S. Hierarchy, ability, and income distribution. *J. Polit. Econ.* 87: 991–1010, 1979.

42. Wright, E. O. *Classes.* Verso, London, 1985.
43. Kohn, M. L., et al. Position in the class structure and psychological functioning in the United States, Japan, and Poland. *Am. J. Sociol.* 95: 964–1008, 1990.
44. Gordon, D. M., Edwards, R., and Reich, M. *Segmented Work, Divided Workers: The Historical Transformation of Labor in the United States.* Cambridge University Press, Cambridge, Mass., 1982.
45. Waksberg, J. Sampling methods for random digit dialing. *J. Am. Stat. Assoc.* 73: 40–46, 1978.
46. Survey Sampling, Inc. *Unlisted Rates of the Top 100 MSAs for 1990.* Fairfield, Conn., 1991.
47. Olson, S. H., et al. Evaluation of random digit dialing as a method of control selection in case-control studies. *Am. J. Epidemiol.* 135: 210–222, 1992.
48. Hahn, B., and Lefkowitz, D. *Annual Expenses and Sources of Payments for Health Care Services.* AHCPR Publ. No. 93-0007. National Medical Expenditure Survey Research Findings 14. Agency for Health Care Policy and Research, Public Health Service, Rockville, Md., 1992.
49. Smith, T. W. Phone Home? An Analysis of Household Telephone Ownership. Paper presented at the International Conference on Telephone Survey Methodology, Charlotte, N.C., November 1987.
50. Greenland, S. Modeling and variable selection in epidemiologic analysis. *Am. J. Public Health* 79: 340–349, 1989.
51. Breen, C., and Parsons, P. E. How the health care system influences access to care. *Ann. Epidemiol.* 1996, in press.
52. Mishel, L., and Bernstein, J. *The State of Working America 1992–1993.* M. E. Sharpe, New York, 1993.
53. Schor, J. B. *The Overworked American.* Basic Books, New York, 1992.
54. Field, M. J., and Shapiro, H. T. *Employment and Health Benefits: A Connection at Risk.* Institute of Medicine, National Academic Press, Washington, D.C., 1993.
55. Renner, C., and Navarro, V. Why is our population of uninsured and underinsured persons growing? The consequences of the "deindustrialization" of the United States. *Int. J. Health Serv.* 19: 433–442, 1989.
56. Ostroff, C. The relationship between satisfaction, attitudes, and performance: An organizational level analysis. *J. Appl. Psychol.* 77: 963–974, 1992.
57. Krieger, N., and Fee, E. Social class: The missing link in U.S. health data. *Int. J. Health Serv.* 24: 25–44, 1994.
58. Alonso, W., and Starr, P. *The Politics of Numbers.* Russell Sage Foundation, New York, 1987.
59. Lacey, M. J., and Furner, M. O. *The State and Social Investigation in Britain and the United States.* Woodrow Wilson Series, Washington, D.C., 1994.
60. Navarro, V. Why Congress did not enact the health care reform. *J. Health Polit. Policy Law* 20: 455–462, 1995.

CHAPTER 13

Poverty and Death in the United States

Robert A. Hahn, Elaine D. Eaker, Nancy D. Barker,
Steven M. Teutsch, Waldemar A. Sosniak,
and Nancy Krieger

Low socioeconomic position is widely recognized as a risk factor for morbidity and mortality (1–10). Researchers have reported dose-response associations with mortality for many socioeconomic characteristics, including education (11–22), occupation and occupational status (11, 12, 19, 22–29), employment (27, 30–32), health insurance (33, 34), income (11–13, 19, 35), poverty or residence in a poverty area (36, 37), and regional economic conditions and trends (11, 38–42). Socioeconomic effects exist for total mortality and several specific causes of death. Socioeconomic position is also associated with morbidity, disability, and decreased survival (7, 43–46), and accounts for a substantial proportion of the excess mortality of blacks compared with whites in the United States (47, 48). Several studies have indicated socioeconomic effects on mortality in the United States, England and other European countries, New Zealand, and Japan (8, 17, 18, 26, 28–30). In the United States and England, although socioeconomic differences in mortality declined earlier in the 20th century, these differences have generally increased in recent decades (13, 14, 26, 40, 49).

Despite the documented association between poverty and mortality, no recent study has examined the proportion of mortality associated with poverty in the United States, partly because national vital statistics rarely include socioeconomic data (49–52). Additionally, few studies have assessed the extent to which multiple biological and behavioral risk factors contribute to observed socioeconomic gradients in mortality. Because knowledge about the societal effect and causes of social inequalities in health is important for health policy and health planning to redress these inequalities (53), we conducted a study to estimate the proportion of mortality attributable to poverty on a national scale and to assess the extent to which this excess might be explained by major known risk factors.

Several studies have focused on the association of socioeconomic position and mortality in the U.S. population. Pappas and colleagues (13) compared U.S. mortality differentials by income and education with differentials reported by Kitagawa and Hauser (11) two decades earlier; other risk factors were not controlled for. Rogot, Sorlie, and Johnson (12) assessed the effect of income, education, and employment status on life expectancy, but only whites were examined and findings were adjusted only for age and smoking status. Only the classic study of Kitagawa and Hauser has estimated the magnitude of socioeconomically related mortality—292,000 deaths—for the population in 1960; the only associated risk factors considered were age, race, sex, education, and income (11).

Three published studies have used the first National Health and Nutrition Examination Survey (NHANES-I) and NHANES-I Epidemiologic Follow-up Study (NHEFS) to examine socioeconomic effects on mortality in the United States. Feldman and colleagues (14) studied education as a relatively unchanging marker of adult socioeconomic position; they found little confounding by several behavioral risk factors, but did not report the effect of adjustment for income or residence in a poverty area. Franks, Clancy, and Gold (33) found an effect of lack of health insurance on black and white mortality adjusted for initial health, employment status, income, education, and several other behavioral and physical risk factors. Finally, Williams and Lepkowski (36) examined poverty as a risk factor for mortality, adjusted for health insurance status, medical care, and various physical and behavioral risk factors; unlike Feldman and associates (14) and Franks and associates (33), Williams and Lepkowski used an analytic approach (i.e., logistic regression) that did not account for follow-up time. Although all these studies demonstrate the effects of socioeconomic position on mortality, none estimates the proportion of U.S. mortality attributable to low socioeconomic position.

We examined poverty as a risk factor for mortality in the NHANES-I and NHEFS sample of the U.S. population 25 to 74 years of age. We first assessed the overall association of poverty and mortality and determined whether this association differed by age, black and white race/ethnicity, and gender. On the basis of these factors, we estimated the proportion of U.S. mortality attributable to poverty among black and white men and women during the 1971–1984 study period and in 1991. Finally, to determine the characteristics of poverty that contribute to its effect, we assessed behavioral and physical risk factors that might either confound the association of poverty and mortality or result from poverty and lead to mortality.

METHODS

Data Sources

From 1971 through 1975, as part of the NHANES-I, a probability sample of 14,407 adults 25 to 74 years of age from the noninstitutionalized U.S. civilian population was interviewed and examined (54, 55). During the initial survey period (i.e., 1971–1974), persons who lived in poverty areas, persons of older age, and women of childbearing age were oversampled. During 1974–1975, an additional sample was drawn to increase the total sample size; this supplement was not oversampled.

From 1981 through 1984, extensive efforts were made in the NHEFS to recontact, reinterview, and briefly reexamine the NHANES-I survey population (55). Follow-up information was available for 13,318 (92.4 percent) of the original sample; of these initial respondents, 2,022 (15.2 percent) had died. Death certificates were acquired for 1,935 (95.7 percent) of decedents. Success in follow-up differed by several risk factors, but differed only slightly by annual income (i.e., from 91 percent among persons with incomes <$4,000 to 95 percent among persons with incomes ≥$10,000) (55). The population analyzed in this study includes NHEFS subjects with known risk factor and follow-up status. Risk factors examined in the study are those assessed at initial examination, when information was available (55). When subjects were disabled or had died, proxies provided follow-up information.

We examined the following biological risk factors: serum cholesterol level (≥200 mg/dL versus <200 mg/dL), systolic blood pressure (≥160 mm Hg versus <160 mm Hg), and body-mass index (≥31.1 for men and ≥32.3 for women versus <31.1 for men and <32.3 for women); for women, we also examined natural versus surgical menopause, and ever versus never use of replacement hormones. We examined the following behavioral factors: smoking (current versus never or prior smoking), lack of physical activity at work or in recreation, and daily alcohol consumption (≥1 oz versus <1 oz). In addition to income, we considered the following demographic and socioeconomic variables: age (25–44, 45–64, and 65–74 years at initial interview), black and white race/ethnicity, marital status (married versus not married), and education (>12th grade versus ≤12th grade). Because only 172 NHANES-I participants were neither black nor white and because only 19 of these persons had died, we restricted our analysis to blacks and whites (i.e., 98.7 percent of the follow-up cohort).

For the purposes of this study, we refer to persons at or below the poverty level when first interviewed as "poor," and to persons living above this level as "nonpoor." NHANES-I used the Bureau of the Census definition of poverty, which accounts for family size and monetary income (56). Poverty threshold levels are adjusted annually using the Consumer Price Index. In 1973, the poverty threshold for a family of four persons was $4,540; in 1991, the threshold was $13,924.

Analysis

We used Cox proportional hazards methods to analyze the relative survival time for nonpoor versus poor persons, controlling for other variables (57). We first assessed the proportional hazards assumption that underlies Cox proportional hazards analysis by evaluating the parallelism of a natural logarithmic transformation of survival curves for poverty and for each study covariate, using the Lifetest Procedure in the Statistical Analysis System (SAS), version 6.07 (58). Continuous variables were categorized into two or three levels. We included variables that satisfied the proportional hazards assumption in subsequent models and stratified models by variables that did not satisfy the assumption.

Next, we compared the hazard of dying among the poor with the hazard of dying among the nonpoor. We calculated hazard ratios (59) using the proportional hazards procedure (PROC PHREG) in SAS. To determine whether the association of poverty and mortality differed by age and black–white race/ethnicity, we compared survival models that included both age–poverty and race/ethnicity–poverty interaction terms with survival models without each of these terms, one at a time. Comparison models also included terms for race/ethnicity, age, and poverty alone, as well as all potential confounders (as listed above). We tested gender–poverty interaction separately, excluding two reproductive variables relevant only to women: hysterectomy and use of estrogen replacement hormones.

Each model included only NHANES-I subjects for whom information was available on all risk factors in that model. We used the likelihood ratio test to assess the significance of interaction terms. To determine whether the association between poverty and mortality in the study cohort might result from illness existing at the outset of the study, we compared the analysis of all cohort subjects with analysis of a cohort excluding subjects for the first two follow-up years (i.e., who were at increased risk for death because of recent illness).

We then assessed the numbers of deaths and mortality rates attributable to poverty (i.e., the population attributable risk (PAR)) for persons 25–74 years of age in the United States. Relative hazards of mortality associated with poverty were applied to estimates of the prevalence of poverty in the U.S. population in 1973, the mid-year of the NHANES-I (60). We calculated attributable mortality in persons 35–84 years of age in 1982 (61) (the mid-year of the follow-up period) because the NHANES cohort had aged by a mean of approximately 10 years during the study interval (i.e., 1971–1984) and subjects are at risk of death between 35 and 84 years of age. Poverty attributable mortality rates were calculated by dividing poverty attributable mortality (e.g., for black men, 35–74 years of age) by the population at risk. To calculate PARs, we used hazard ratios adjusted for age and race/ethnicity, but not for the other risk factors examined, because the other risk factors were likely to be intermediate variables in the association between poverty and mortality.

PAR was calculated for each sex–race group by summing the contributions of each age stratum weighted by the proportion of deaths in the age group compared with all deaths in this sex–race group (62). Age-specific PARs were calculated by the following standard method:

$$PAR_i = \frac{(P_i)\times(RR_i-1)}{1+[(P_i)\times(RR_i-1)]}$$

where P_i is the prevalence of a risk factor in age stratum i (e.g., poverty among persons 25–44 years of age) associated with an outcome of interest (e.g., all-cause mortality), and RR_i is the relative risk (or hazard ratio) of the outcome associated with exposure to this risk factor. Thus, PAR is a function of the prevalence of contributing exposures and the risk for the outcome associated with those exposures. The magnitude of the effect of the exposure on the outcome (e.g., the number of deaths) is estimated by multiplying the PAR by the number of outcome events in the population.

To determine recent proportions of mortality attributable to poverty in the United States, we used estimates of the prevalence of poverty in the United States in 1991 (63). We calculated attributable mortality among persons 25–84 years of age in 1991—the most recent mortality data available (64).

To determine the behavioral and physical characteristics of poverty that might contribute to its effect on mortality, we then assessed confounding by study risk factors in the NHANES-I study period. After first examining the distribution of study risk factors among persons who were poor and who were nonpoor, we compared survival models that included all potential confounders with models in which a single potential confounder was removed (65). If removal of the single potential confounder substantially altered the hazard ratio for poverty, the confounder was retained in the model; other potential confounders were eliminated. We arbitrarily considered a change in the hazard ratio of 20 percent or more to be a substantial change. We repeated this procedure until we had eliminated all nonconfounders in the study from the model. Because two study covariates (i.e., hysterectomy and use of estrogen replacement hormones) applied to women subjects only, we examined potential confounding separately for men and women.

The software currently available to analyze the data from complex sample surveys (SUDAAN) does not allow for variables that do not meet the proportional hazards assumption. Because several variables in our analysis did not meet this assumption, we were unable to use weighted estimates or to account for study design. Nevertheless, we evaluated the effects of not accounting for the study design and weights in our analysis. For models in which study variables did meet the proportional hazards assumption, we compared the analysis in SUDAAN that accounted for design with the unweighted analysis produced by SAS.

RESULTS

NHANES-I provided follow-up information on 1,670 poor persons and 8,182 nonpoor persons in the cohort; 458 (27.4 percent) of poor persons and 1,221 (14.9 percent) of nonpoor persons had died during the follow-up interval. The median follow-up time was 9.9 years. Fifty-two percent of decedents had died from cardiovascular diseases, 23 percent from cancers, and 4 percent from injuries; the distribution of causes of death did not differ substantially by poverty status.

1. *Proportional hazards assumption*: We confirmed the proportional hazards assumption for poverty and for age, gender, race/ethnicity, marital status, exercise, smoking, drinking, and hypertension, but not for education, body-mass index, cholesterol, natural or surgical menopause, or use of estrogen replacement hormones. We thus included the former in subsequent models and the latter as stratifying variables. For models incorporating variables that satisfied the proportional hazards assumption, comparison of analyses using SUDAAN and SAS indicated close approximation of most point estimates, thus indicating good approximation by unweighted analysis.

2. *Race/ethnicity, gender, and age interaction in the association of poverty and mortality*: The effect of poverty on mortality did not differ substantially for blacks and whites or males and females. The relative hazards effect of poverty on mortality did not differ substantially by age among women, but did differ by age among men, declining from 3.0 among men 25–44 years of age to 2.2 among men 45–64 and 1.5 among men 65–74 (Table 1). Subsequent analyses for men thus included an interaction term for age. For women, the hazard ratio for all ages was 2.0; adjusted for age and race/ethnicity, the hazard ratio for mortality among women was 1.4.

3. *Mortality attributable to poverty*: In the United States in 1973, the mid-year of the NHANES-I data collection period, 9.2 percent of black and white persons 25–74 years of age lived in poverty (Table 2). The prevalence of poverty differed greatly by gender and race/ethnicity; poverty was lowest among white men, and increasingly higher among white women, black men, and black women (Table 2). Thirty percent of black women 25–75 years of age lived in poverty—a proportion 5.3 times that for white men. Overall, poverty was twofold greater among persons |65 years of age than among persons 25–44 years of age.

During 1973, 86,571 deaths, that is, 6.0 percent of all U.S. mortality among black and white persons 25–84 years of age was attributable to poverty (Table 3). Rates of death attributable to poverty differed by race/ethnicity and gender and were lowest for white women, 2.4 times as high for white men, 2.8 times as high for black women, and 6.5 times as high for black men (Table 3).

During 1991, the prevalence of poverty among black and white adults 25–74 years of age was 10.3 percent (Table 2). The prevalence of poverty differed substantially by race/ethnicity and gender (Table 2). Compared with white men, the prevalence of poverty was 1.5 times as high among white women, 2.6 times as high among black men, and 4.4 times as high among black women. There was no consistent association of age and the prevalence of poverty.

Overall, 5.9 percent of U.S. mortality among black and white men and women 25–84 years of age during 1991 (i.e., 91,136 deaths) was attributable to poverty (Table 3). White women had the lowest rate of mortality attributable to poverty;

Table 1

The effects of poverty on mortality, by age, NHANES-I Epidemiologic
Follow-up Study, 1971–1984, relative hazard for poverty
(95% confidence limits)

Age group, yrs	Unadjusted	Adjusted for:	
		Race/ethnicity	Race/ethnicity, all potential confounders[a]
Men			
25–44	3.0 (1.5, 6.0)	2.9 (1.4, 5.9)	2.9 (1.4, 5.9)
45–64	2.2 (1.6, 2.9)	2.1 (1.5, 2.9)	1.6 (1.1, 2.2)
65–74	1.5 (1.2, 1.7)	1.4 (1.2, 1.7)	1.2 (1.0, 1.5)
		Adjusted for:	
		Race/ethnicity and age	Race/ethnicity, age, all potential confounders[a]
Women			
All ages	2.0 (1.7, 2.9)	1.4 (1.1, 1.8)	1.2 (0.9, 1.5)

[a]Potential confounders include serum cholesterol, systolic blood pressure, body-mass index, smoking, lack of physical activity, alcohol consumption, marital status, black or white race/ethnicity, education, and, for women, natural or surgical menopause and use of estrogen replacement hormones.

white men had a rate 2.2 times the rate of white women, black women 3.6 times, and black men 8.6 times.

4. *Confounding in the association of poverty and mortality*: Compared with nonpoor persons, poor persons were more likely to be female, black, older, less educated, and unmarried (Table 4). Poor persons were more likely to have elevated blood pressure and to be physically inactive, but less likely to drink heavily. The prevalence of smoking and high cholesterol levels did not differ substantially between poor and nonpoor subjects. Poor women were less likely to have had a hysterectomy and only half as likely to have taken estrogen replacement hormones as nonpoor women (Table 4).

Table 2

Prevalence of poverty among persons 25–75 years of age,
by race/ethnicity, United States, 1973, 1991

Ages, yrs	Poverty, %, 1973	Poverty, %, 1991
White men		
25–44	4.6	7.4
45–64	5.0	6.1
65–74	10.4	5.6
25–74	5.6	6.8
Black men		
25–44	12.4	17.0
45–64	19.8	17.0
65–74	32.4	26.1
25–74	17.4	17.9
White women		
25–44	7.2	10.7
45–64	7.7	8.5
65–74	17.2	10.4
25–74	9.3	10.0
Black women		
25–44	28.0	30.7
45–64	28.0	25.2
65–74	40.5	38.3
25–74	29.8	29.8
Total		
25–44	7.6	11.0
45–64	8.1	8.9
65–74	16.2	10.5
25–74	9.2	10.3

Among men, controlling for all potential confounders reduced the hazard ratio (from a model including only poverty) by 3 percent for men 25–44 years of age, 27 percent for men 45–64 years of age, and 20 percent for men 65–74 years of age (Table 1). Among women aged 25–74 years, controlling for potential confounders reduced the hazard ratio (from a model including only poverty) by 42 percent. No single potential confounder contributed a change of 20 percent or greater in the hazard ratio for either men or women.

Table 3

Population attributable risk (PAR) among persons 25–75 years of age:
Annual attributable deaths and death rates for U.S. population,
1971–1984 and 1991, by race/ethnicity and gender

	PAR (%)		Annual poverty attributable deaths[a]		Poverty attributable death rates[a]	
	1971–84	1991	1971–84	1991	1971–84	1991
Men						
White	5.2	5.7	37,432	41,941	93.7	89.6
Black	16.8	15.1	15,995	18,079	256.1	354.7
Women						
White	4.5	3.6	24,655	21,645	39.6	41.4
Black	11.2	10.3	8,488	9,471	111.0	147.3
Total	6.0	5.9	86,571	91,136	74.5	82.3

[a]Deaths and death rates (per 100,000 person years in the age range 25–84 years) are calculated for 1982, the mid-year of the follow-up period. Deaths for the 75–84 age group are included to allow for the 10-year follow-up period.

From 1973 through 1991, the prevalence of poverty among blacks and whites ≥25 years of age increased by 12 percent; the greatest increases were among whites and among men (Table 2). During this period, the poverty-associated PAR increased among men and decreased among women (Table 3). Mortality rates attributable to poverty increased among white men but declined among white women and among black men and women.

DISCUSSION

During the early 1970s, 6.0 percent of U.S. mortality among black and white adults 25–74 years of age was attributable to poverty; in 1991, 5.9 percent of U.S. mortality among adults was attributable to this factor. If poverty were listed as a cause of death (using 1991 mortality data), it would rank as the third leading cause of death among black men, the fourth leading cause among black women, the sixth leading cause among white men, and the eighth leading cause among white women (66).

Rates of mortality attributable to poverty were substantially higher for men than for women and for blacks than for whites; in 1991, rates ranged from a low of 41.4 per 100,000 for white women to a high of 354.7 for black men. Differences in attributable mortality rates reflect both differences in the prevalence of

Table 4

Vital status, risk factor prevalence by poverty status:
NHANES-I Epidemiologic Follow-up Study, 1971–1984

Characteristics	Nonpoverty, number (%)		Poverty, number (%)		P value[a]
Total	8,182		1,670		
Vital status					
Dead	1,221	(14.9)	458	(27.4)	0.001
Age group, yrs					
25–44	3,620	(44.2)	555	(33.2)	0.001
45–64	2,213	(27.1)	356	(21.3)	
65–75	2,349	(28.7)	759	(45.5)	
Race/ethnicity					
White	7,248	(88.6)	1,004	(60.1)	0.001
Black	934	(11.4)	666	(39.9)	
Gender					
Men	3,324	(40.6)	584	(35.0)	0.001
Women	4,858	(59.4)	1,086	(65.0)	
Marital status[b]					
Married	6,521	(79.7)	848	(50.8)	0.001
Education[b]					
<12th grade	5,837	(73.6)	1,510	(95.3)	0.001
Exercise[b]					
None	4,079	(49.9)	1,015	(60.9)	0.001
Current smoking[b]					
Yes	2,283	(29.8)	426	(28.3)	0.046
Alcohol consumption					
<1 oz/day	7,506	(91.7)	1,585	(94.9)	0.001
≥1 oz/day	676	(8.3)	85	(5.1)	
Hypertension					
Systolic ≥160 mm Hg	1,289	(15.8)	464	(27.8)	
Body-mass index					
≥31.1 (men) ≥32.3 (women)	814	(10.0)	270	(16.2)	0.001
Cholesterol					
≥200 mg/dL	5,374	(65.7)	1,103	(66.1)	0.773
Hysterectomy[b]					
Yes	1,264	(40.9)	245	(33.2)	0.019
Estrogen replacement[b]					
Yes	880	(27.1)	113	(14.6)	0.001

[a]Chi-square test.
[b]Information not available for entire cohort.

poverty and differences in mortality rates. Because poverty, as measured in this study, did not include nonmonetary "transfers" (e.g., Medicaid, Medicare, food stamps, or subsidized housing), the effects of poverty can be assumed to occur despite these benefits.

This analysis of a sample of black and white adults 25–75 years of age in the United States indicates that the association of poverty and death among women is partially explained by the differential distribution of major risk factors for mortality combined, but is not substantially explained by the distribution of any single risk factor. For men, the lack of confounding of the association by risk factors examined in this study implies that other consequences of poverty must explain the increased rates of mortality among the poor compared with the nonpoor. The strong association between poverty and numerous behavioral and biological risk factors for mortality remains a critical area for investigation.

When interpreting these results, several caveats must be considered. First, socioeconomic position may be examined by diverse measures (10). Poverty as assessed in NHANES-I is a useful measure of socioeconomic position because it accounts for not only family income but also living conditions (e.g., household size and number of children ≤18 years of age). Poverty was analyzed in this study because it captured basic notions of inadequate resources and because it corresponded to available standard census information for both 1973 and 1991.

Second, the measure of poverty was modified once between the time of its assessment in NHANES-I and the more recent time period for which we estimated the population effect of poverty on mortality. The effect of these changes on the estimation of the prevalence of poverty in the population was minimal, adding 0.2 percent to the estimated 13.0 percent overall prevalence of poverty in the United States in 1980 (67).

Third, although we designated persons who were classified as below the poverty threshold in 1973 as "poor" and those at or above the threshold as "nonpoor," poverty and nonpoverty status are not fixed personal characteristics. For example, from 1987 through 1988, 4.5 million nonpoor persons (2.2 percent of the nonpoor population) became poor and 6.4 million poor persons (25.7 percent of the poor population in 1987) became nonpoor (68). The transition into or out of poverty was associated with characteristics such as race/ethnicity, age, income, type of residence, and work experience. Thus, it was likely that a substantial portions of persons classified as poor at their initial interview in NHANES-I subsequently became nonpoor, and vice versa (in smaller proportion, but larger numbers). An effect of poverty was demonstrated in this study despite possible misclassification. The effect of poverty on mortality ascertained in the study may have been greater among persons who remained poor during the follow-up period than among those who became nonpoor; however, NHEFS data do not allow assessment of this hypothesis. In addition, including persons near the poverty threshold with those at higher income levels is likely to yield a conservative estimate of the effect of poverty on mortality. The absence of historical data on poverty levels precluded the analysis of trend.

Fourth, while we considered the effect of poverty during the early 1970s on mortality during the follow-up period in 1982, we examined the effect of poverty in 1991 on mortality in the same year. We used mortality in 1991 because data from this year were the most current. Because mortality rates have declined steadily over recent decades, the mortality rates attributable to poverty in 1991 will most likely be lower than our estimates, and the increase in attributable mortality since 1973 will similarly be smaller.

Fifth, in comparing the PAR of poverty on mortality for 1971–1984 with that for 1991, we assumed that the effect of poverty on mortality was constant over this period. Several studies, however, have indicated that the disparity in mortality by socioeconomic position (as measured by income and education) has increased in recent decades (13, 14). Thus, our analysis probably underestimates the effect of poverty on mortality in the more recent period and is likely to be a conservative estimate of PAR in 1991.

Sixth, whereas we found a strong association of poverty and all-cause mortality, our study did not allow determination of the causal pathway connecting poverty and death. Morbidity occurring prior to the NHANES-I may have led both to poverty and to subsequent mortality. The relative importance of this hypothesis depends on the proportion of mobility between upper and lower socioeconomic classes and on the proportion of mobility caused by health status. Evidence from other studies indicates that although "downward social mobility" associated with poor health does occur (69), poor health contributes relatively little to poverty; the direction of causation is primarily from poverty to poor health to mortality (70–72). Moreover, in the NHANES-I cohort, poverty was assessed a mean of 10 years before the follow-up survey; thus, it was likely that illness ultimately resulting in death contributed to poverty rather than the reverse situation. Our finding of minimal difference in analytic results excluding study subjects followed up within two years indicates little effect of early sickness on the association of poverty and mortality.

Seventh, we were unable to consider risk factors not assessed in NHEFS (e.g., environmental exposures). These factors may partially explain the association of poverty and mortality. Although overall utilization of health care was not assessed in NHANES-I or NHEFS, data suggest that utilization differs substantially by poverty status. Compared with nonpoor persons in the NHANES-I cohort in 1973, persons living in poverty were 2.1 times more likely to report never having had a medical check-up. A recent study of the NHANES-I cohort found that, independent of income, an excess mortality of 25 percent occurred among persons who did not have private insurance coverage in comparison with persons who did have such insurance coverage, indicating that this barrier to health care is associated with a substantial increase in mortality (33).

Eighth, we examined mortality only among persons 25–75 years of age. In 1991, persons ≥25 years of age constituted 65.0 percent of the U.S. population, but included only 48.3 percent of persons below the poverty level (56). Nevertheless, deaths among persons 25–75 years of age accounted for ≥95 percent of mortality in the United States; thus, even if lower income fully explained mortality among younger persons, it would account for less than 5 percent of overall U.S. mortality. Because, compared with older persons, younger persons commonly die at different rates, from different causes, and in association with different risk factors, the effect of poverty on the mortality of the younger population is likely to differ substantially from that found in this study; this issue merits separate study.

In summary, although the NHANES-I and the NHEFS did not allow detailed analysis of the associations among poverty and diverse risk factors for mortality and their changes over time, these surveys did provide a useful estimate of the overall effect of poverty on mortality in the United States. Moreover, they allowed us to examine the association of poverty and numerous observer-measured and self-reported risk factors and to consider the role of risk factors—some of which had not been examined previously—as confounders of the association between poverty and mortality.

The reduction of excess mortality among poor persons may require the development of programs of employment, welfare, or other support. The decline of poverty rates by more than 50 percent from 1959 to 1973 and the subsequent increase of these rates by more than 30 percent indicate the possibility of change. The complex association of poverty, risk factors, and mortality among adults in the United States indicates a need to examine in greater detail the causes of risk factor distributions among populations at different income levels (10). Several complementary approaches to this question are reasonable:

1. Ethnographic studies on the role of specific ways of living and socialization—linked to conditions at work, at home, and in neighborhoods—among communities defined by poverty.

2. A comparative study of poor and nonpoor persons with high (and low) risk behavior profiles to determine the meaning, role, and origins of risk behaviors in the lives of these persons.

3. A study of precursors of risk factors of interest; for example, a case-control study in which "cases" are persons who are hypertensive or sedentary, and the exposures to be examined include conditions at home and in the workplace, economic conditions, parental risk behavior, educational sources, local societal norms related to the risk factors, and access to media and public health information.

4. Longitudinal studies to assess how specified levels of poverty and wealth are linked to spending on food, shelter, health care, education, transportation, and other aspects of daily life, and the reasons people give for spending both essential and "discretionary" income.

5. Contextual studies of the links among regional economies; job opportunities; state and local budgets for welfare, health, education, and other social programs; and patterns of poverty, wealth, and disease.

A combination of approaches to the association of poverty, risk, and mortality may lead to the development of interventions that substantially reduce not only poverty, but also its consequent inequalities in health.

Acknowledgments — We thank Anne Haddix, Ph.D., of the Centers for Disease Control and Prevention (CDC), and Lydia Rogers of the Income Statistics Branch, Housing Division, Bureau of the Census, for assistance in deciphering economic reports, and David G. Kleinbaum, Ph.D., of Emory University and the CDC, for methodologic advice.

Note — This chapter is a revised version of a paper published in *Epidemiology* 6: 490–497, 1995. See also Letter to the Editor and Authors' Response, *Epidemiology* 7: 453–454, 1996.

REFERENCES

1. Antonovsky, A. Social class, life expectancy and overall mortality. *Milbank Mem. Fund Q.* 45: 31–73, 1967.
2. Antonovsky, A., and Bernstein, J. Social class and infant mortality. *Soc. Sci. Med.* 11: 453–470, 1977.
3. Marmot, M. G., Kogevinas, M., and Elston, M. A. Social/economic status and disease. *Ann. Rev. Public Health* 8: 111–135, 1987.
4. Williams, D. R. Socioeconomic differentials in health: A review and redirection. *Soc. Psychol. Q.* 53: 81–99, 1990.
5. Kaplan, G. E., and Keil, J. E. Socioeconomic factors and cardiovascular disease: A review of the literature. *Circulation* 88: 1973–1998, 1993.
6. Adler, N. E., et al. Socioeconomic inequalities in health: No easy solution. *JAMA* 269: 3140–3145, 1993.
7. Haan, M. N., and Kaplan, G. A. The contribution of socioeconomic position to minority health. In *Report of the Secretary's Task Force on Black and Minority Health, Volume II: Crosscutting Issues in Minority Health*. U.S. Department of Health and Human Services, Washington, D.C., 1985.
8. Black, D., et al. *Inequalities in Health: The Black Report*. Penguin Books, Harmondsworth, Middlesex, 1982.
9. Whitehead, M. *The Health Divide*. Penguin Books, Harmondsworth, Middlesex, 1987.
10. Krieger, N., et al. Racism, sexism, and social class: Implications for studies of health, disease, and well-being. *Am. J. Prev. Med.* 9: 82–122, 1993.
11. Kitagawa, E. M., and Hauser, P. M. *Differential Mortality in the United States: A Study in Socioeconomic Epidemiology*. Harvard University Press, Cambridge, Mass., 1973.
12. Rogot, E., Sorlie, P. D., and Johnson, N. J. Life expectancy by employment status, income, and education in the National Longitudinal Mortality Study. *Public Health Rep.* 107: 457–461, 1992.

13. Pappas, G., et al. The increasing disparity in mortality between socioeconomic groups in the United States, 1960 and 1986. *N. Engl. J. Med.* 329: 103–109, 1993.
14. Feldman, J. J., et al. National trends in educational differentials in mortality. *Am. J. Epidemiol.* 129: 919–933, 1989.
15. Ries, P. Educational differences in health status and health care. *Vital Health Stat. Ser. 10* 179: 1–66, 1991.
16. Guralnik, J. M., et al. Educational status and active life expectancy among older blacks and whites. *N. Engl. J. Med.* 329: 110–116, 1993.
17. Doornbos, G., and Kromhout, D. Educational level and mortality in a 32-year follow-up study of 18-year old men in the Netherlands. *Int. J. Epidemiol.* 19: 374–379, 1990.
18. Kunst, A. E., and Mackenbach, J. P. The size of mortality differences associated with educational level in nine industrialized countries. *Am. J. Public Health* 84: 932–937, 1994.
19. Slater, C. H., Lorimor, R. J., and Lairson, D. R. The independent contributions of socioeconomic status and health practices to health status. *Prev. Med.* 14: 372–378, 1985.
20. Liu, K., et al. Relationship of education to major risk factors and death from coronary heart disease, cardiovascular diseases and all causes. *Circulation* 66: 1308–1314, 1982.
21. Keil, J. E., et al. Mortality rates and risk factors for coronary disease in black as compared with white men and women. *N. Engl. J. Med.* 329: 73–78, 1993.
22. Seltzer, C. C., and Jablon, S. Army rank and subsequent mortality by cause: 23-year follow-up. *Am. J. Epidemiol.* 105: 559–566, 1977.
23. Guralnick, L. Mortality by occupation and industry among men 20 to 64 years of age: United States, 1950. *Vital Stat. Special Rep.* 53(2): 47–A43, 1962.
24. Marmot, M. G., Shipley, M. J., and Rose, G. Inequalities in death—Specific explanations of a general pattern? *Lancet* 1(8384): 1003–1006, 1984.
25. Cooper, S. P., Buffler, P. A., and Cooper, C. J. Health characteristics by occupation and industry of longest employment. *Vital Health Stat. Ser. 10* 168: 1–105, 1989.
26. Pamuk, E. R. Social class inequality in mortality from 1921 to 1972 in England and Wales. *Popul. Stud.* 39: 17–31, 1985.
27. Fox, J., Goldblatt, P., and Jones, D. Social class mortality differentials: Artifact, selection or life circumstances? In *Longitudinal Study, Mortality and Social Organization*, edited by P. Goldblatt. Her Majesty's Stationery Office, London, 1985.
28. Kagamimori, S., Iibuchi, Y., and Fox, J. A comparison of socioeconomic differences in mortality between Japan and England and Wales. *World Health Stat. Q.* 36: 119–128, 1983.
29. Pearce, N. E., et al. Mortality and social class in New Zealand II: Male mortality by major disease groupings. *N.Z. Med. J.* 96: 711–716, 1983.
30. Iverson, L., et al. Unemployment and mortality in Denmark, 1970-80. *BMJ* 295: 879–884, 1987.
31. Sorlie, P. D., and Rogot, E. Mortality by employment status in the National Longitudinal Mortality Study. *Am. J. Epidemiol.* 132: 983–992, 1990.
32. Moser, K. A., Fox, A. J., and Jones, D. R. Unemployment and mortality in the OPCS Longitudinal Study. *Lancet* 2: 1324–1329, 1984.
33. Franks, P., Clancy, C. M., and Gold, M. R. Health insurance and mortality. *JAMA* 270: 737–741, 1993.
34. Office of Technology Assessment. *Does Health Insurance Make a Difference?* Background paper, OTA-BP-H-99. Washington, D.C., 1992.

35. Kaplan, G. A., et al. Socioeconomic status and health. In *Closing the Gap*, edited by R. W. Amler and H. B. Dull, pp. 125–129. Oxford University Press, New York, 1987.

36. Williams, D. R., and Lepkowski, J. M. Poverty and health: A national study of the determinants of excess mortality. In *Proceedings of the 1991 Public Health Conference on Records and Statistics*, pp. 217–222. Washington, D.C., 1991.

37. Haan, M., Kaplan, G. A., and Camacho, T. Poverty and health: Prospective evidence from the Alameda County Study. *Am. J. Epidemiol.* 125: 989–998, 1987.

38. Forsdahl, A. Are poor living conditions in childhood and adolescence an important risk factor for arteriosclerotic heart disease? *Br. J. Prev. Soc. Med.* 31: 91–95, 1977.

39. Brenner, M. H. Mortality and economic instability: Detailed analysis for Britain and comparative analysis for selected industrialized countries. *Int. J. Health Serv.* 13: 563–619, 1983.

40. Wing, S., et al. Socioeconomic characteristics associated with the onset of decline of ischemic heart disease mortality in the United States. *Am. J. Public Health* 78: 923–926, 1988.

41. Yeracaris, C. A., and Kim, J. H. Socioeconomic differentials in selected causes of death. *Am. J. Public Health* 68: 342–351, 1978.

42. Wilkinson, R. G. Income distribution and life expectancy. *BMJ* 304: 165–168, 1992.

43. Newacheck, P. W., et al. Income and illness. *Med. Care* 18: 1165–1176, 1980.

44. Centers for Disease Control, National Center for Health Statistics. Current estimates from the National Health Interview Survey, 1991. *Vital Health Stat. Ser. 10* 184: 1–232, 1992.

45. Lundberg, O. Class and health: Comparing Britain and Sweden. *Soc. Sci. Med.* 23: 511–517, 1986.

46. Baquet, C. R., et al. Socioeconomic factors and cancer incidence among blacks and whites. *J. Natl. Cancer Inst.* 83: 551–557, 1991.

47. Otten, M. W., et al. The effect of known risk factors on the excess mortality of black adults in the United States. *JAMA* 263: 845–850, 1990.

48. Rogers, R. G. Living and dying in the U.S.A.: Sociodemographic determinants of death among blacks and whites. *Demography* 29: 287–303, 1992.

49. Marmot, M. G., and McDowall, M. E. Mortality decline and widening social inequalities. *Lancet* 2: 274–276, 1986.

50. Krieger, N., and Fee, E. Social class: The missing link in U.S. health data. *Int. J. Health Serv.* 24: 25–44, 1994.

51. Krieger, N. Overcoming the absence of socioeconomic data in medical records: Validation of a census-based methodology. *Am. J. Public Health* 82: 703–710, 1992.

52. Navarro, V. Race or class versus race and class: Mortality differentials in the United States. *Lancet* 336: 1238–1240, 1992.

53. Hurowitz, J. C. Toward a social policy for health. *N. Engl. J. Med.* 329: 130–134, 1993.

54. National Center for Health Statistics. *Plan and Operation of the Health and Nutrition Examination Survey, United States, 1971-73. Vital Health Stat. Ser. 1* 10a. DHEW Publication (HRA)76-1310. U.S. Department of Health, Education, and Welfare, Rockville, Md., 1976.

55. Cohen, B. B., et al. (Centers for Disease Control and Prevention, National Center for Health Statistics). Plan and operation NHANES-I Epidemiologic Followup Study 1982-84. *Vital Health Stat. Ser. 1* 22. DHHS publication (PHS)87-1342. U.S. Public Health Service, Washington, D.C., 1987.

56. Bureau of the Census. Poverty in the United States: 1991. *Curr. Popul. Rep. Ser. P-60* 181, 1992.
57. Kleinbaum, D. M. *Survival Analysis: A Self-Instruction Approach.* Springer-Verlag, New York, 1995.
58. SAS Institute. *SAS Technical Report P-229. SAS/STAT Software: Changes and Enhancements.* SAS Institute Inc., Cary, N.C., 1983.
59. Cox, D. R., and Oakes, D. O. *Analysis of Survival Data.* Chapman & Hall, London, 1984.
60. Bureau of the Census. Consumer Income. Characteristics of the low-income population: 1973. *Curr. Popul. Rep. Ser. P-60* 98, 1975.
61. Centers for Disease Control and Prevention, National Center for Health Statistics. *Vital Statistics of the United States. 1982, Volume II—Mortality, Part A.* U.S. Department of Health and Human Services, Hyattsville, Md., 1986.
62. Walter, S. D. Estimation and interpretation of attributable risk in health research. *Biometrics* 32: 829–849, 1976.
63. Bureau of the Census. Poverty in the United States: 1991. *Curr. Popul. Rep. Ser. P-60* 181, 1992.
64. Centers for Disease Control and Prevention. Advance report of final mortality statistics, 1991. *Monthly Vital Stat. Rep.* 42: 1–64, 1993.
65. Kleinbaum, D. G., Kupper, L. L., and Morgenstern, H. *Epidemiologic Research.* Lifetime Learning Publications, Belmont, Calif., 1982.
66. Centers for Disease Control and Prevention. *Health United States 1991 and Prevention Profile.* U.S. Public Health Service, Hyattsville, Md., 1992.
67. Bureau of the Census. Changes in the definition of poverty. *Curr. Popul. Rep.* 133: 60, 1991.
68. Bureau of the Census. Transitions in income and poverty status: 1987–88. *Curr. Popul. Rep. Ser. P-70* 24, 1991.
69. Wadsworth, M. E. J. Serious illness in childhood and its association with later-life achievement. In *Class and Health: Research and Longitudinal Data,* edited by R. G. Wilkinson, pp. 50–74. Tavistock, New York, 1986.
70. Blane, D. An assessment of the Black Report's explanation of health inequalities. *Sociol. Health Illness* 7: 423–445, 1985.
71. Fox, A. J., Goldblatt, P. O., and Jones, D. R. Social class mortality differentials: Artefact, selection or life circumstances? *J. Epidemiol. Commun. Health* 39: 1–8, 1985.
72. Wilkinson, R. G. Socio-economic differences in mortality: Interpreting the data on their size and trends. In *Class and Health: Research and Longitudinal Data,* edited by R. G. Wilkinson, pp. 1–20. Tavistock, New York, 1986.

CHAPTER 14

Understanding Income Inequalities in Health among Men and Women in Britain and Finland

Ossi Rahkonen, Sara Arber, Eero Lahelma,
Pekka Martikainen, and Karri Silventoinen

Controversy continues over the relationship between income and health. Macro-level analyses have shown an association between income inequality and life expectancy: the larger the income differences in a country the shorter the life expectancy, and vice versa (1–8). For example, Wilkinson (1) argues that the direct effects of poverty on mortality are less important than the psychosocial consequences in terms of stress and lack of social cohesion. His thesis has been criticized on methodological grounds (9–11), and several cases that poorly fit Wilkinson's hypothesis have been identified. In particular, Finnish men contradict Wilkinson's findings; Finland is one of the most egalitarian societies as measured by income equality (12), yet life expectancy of Finnish men is lower than in many other countries with larger income inequalities. Irrespective of whether an association between income inequality and health has been found in previous studies, the pathways through which income inequality is linked to mortality and ill-health have yet to be convincingly established.

Ecological studies often omit confounding factors that operate at the individual level. In a nationally representative U.S. sample, family income, but not community income inequality, independently predicted mortality (9). There are only a few ecological studies on morbidity. However, Kennedy and colleagues (7) reported that after adjusting for several individual variables such as family income, educational attainment, and smoking, inequalities in the state-wide distribution of income within the United States were associated with lower

This study was supported by the Academy of Finland.

self- perceived health. They also found a strong association between household income and perceived health.

Wilkinson's research, and the many other recent studies on the association between income and health, have involved aggregate-level analysis. But we also need studies at the individual level to examine the relationship between a person's individual income or household income and health. It has been postulated that societies with high levels of inequality in the distribution of income have larger health status differences associated with income measured at the household or individual level (7).

Recent studies have reported an inverse association between individual income and health (13–15) and that income level is a predictor of mortality (16, 17) and morbidity even after adjusting for several socioeconomic factors such as employment status, education, social class, and housing tenure (15, 18, 19).

A key issue is to examine whether the association between income and health is entirely explained by social class and employment status. It is well-known that health status among the lower occupational classes is poorer than among the higher classes and that those who are disabled have lower income levels than those with better health. Both a causal association and reverse causality are possible (20). Education, occupation, and employment status influence both health and income, but the direction of the relationship between income and health may be less clear cut (21, 22).

Two previous comparative studies examined income-related health inequalities in several industrial countries, including Britain and Finland, using data from the 1980s and early 1990s (22, 23). In both studies the income measure used was net household income per equivalent adult. Both studies found clear income-related health differences in each country. The differences were large in the United States and Britain and small in Finland (22, 23). Again, the size of income-related inequalities in health decreased substantially when education, social class, and employment status were adjusted (22).

Nevertheless, these studies have some shortcomings. For example, only one indicator of income is used, usually household income. It is important to use both household and individual income. There has also been a lack of attention to gender differences in the relationship between income and health, and little research has specifically addressed how women's health differs by income. The relationship between income and health among women may vary between countries, depending on the nature and pattern of women's employment participation in a society.

Employment Status and Income Differences of
Men and Women in Britain and Finland

Britain and Finland are two western welfare states with both similarities and differences. According to Esping-Andersen's (24) typology of welfare state regimes, Finland belongs to the Scandinavian "social democratic" or "institutional" welfare states characterized by universal social benefits. Britain represents the "liberal" (24) or "residual" welfare state (25), characterized by means-tested benefits and modest social insurance schemes.

The "Scandinavian Model" (26) is based on high male and female employment participation and on universal social benefits underpinned by publicly subsidized daycare and parental leave (27). The Scandinavian welfare model has been regarded as "woman-friendly" (28) because it supports women's combining motherhood and paid employment. It is a special feature of the Finnish labor market that women's full-time employment participation is very high, comparable with that of Finnish men (29).

However, Finland experienced a sudden and deep economic recession in the early 1990s when unemployment skyrocketed to nearly 20 percent, with unemployment rates somewhat higher for men than women (30). During the first half of the 1990s, welfare cuts and some new taxes and fees were introduced and the number of people receiving social assistance payments increased rapidly (31–33).

The British welfare state regime deviates from the Scandinavian one, providing fewer incentives to support women's participation in the labor force and minimal publicly funded daycare facilities (34). Consequently, British women are often dependent on male breadwinners, and lone mothers are often dependent on means-tested social benefits (35). In 1996, 45 percent of British female employees were working part-time (36); in Finland the corresponding figure was below 10 percent. In 1994, 22 percent of women aged 25 to 64 in Britain were housewives, three times the percentage in Finland (37). Differences in women's employment participation form the most striking structural disparity between the two countries: fewer women are employed in Britain than in Finland, and when British women's higher level of part-time employment is taken into account, British women's opportunities for financial independence are much poorer than those of Finnish women. Previous research (21) has shown that in Britain, health among housewives is poorer than that of full-time and part-time employed women. Part-time employed women generally have a much lower individual income than full-time employed women. Nonemployed British women have a very low or nonexistent individual income, but are likely to be much more heterogeneous in terms of their husbands' class and household income.

Both in Finland and Britain, income inequalities have become more marked over the last decade. In Finland, this has taken place particularly in the mid-1990s because of the labor market crisis. However, the change has been a relatively minor one (38) because all income groups, including the highest ones, were economically affected during the recession. Although income inequality in Finland has increased somewhat since the mid 1990s, income differences are still smaller than in many other OECD countries. In contrast, income inequalities and inequalities associated with employment status in Britain have gradually widened over the 1980s and 1990s (36). The two countries clearly differ by income distribution; income differences in Finland are among the smallest in the world, while in Britain income differences are very pronounced (12, 39). Indeed, a variety of previous studies have shown an inverse relationship between health and social class and education in Finland and Britain (29, 40, 41), with larger health inequalities in Finland than in Britain.

Aims of the Study

Gender differences in the labor market in Finland and Britain, together with greater income disparities in Britain than in Finland, led to the hypothesis that relative health differences between income groups would be larger in Britain for men but smaller for women, especially according to individual income. We used two income measures: individual income and household equivalent income. We expected that different income measures would give different results, especially among British women. Since a higher proportion of British than Finnish women are housewives or work part-time, we expected a less clear health gradient by individual income for British than for Finnish women. Household equivalent income was expected to show a more linear pattern than individual income among men and women in both countries.

The aims of this study were:

1. to compare the extent and pattern of health differences by income among men and women in Britain and Finland;
2. to study whether the relationship between income and health could be explained by employment status, education, and occupational class in Britain and in Finland; and
3. to examine whether the pattern and strength of the relationship between income and health differed for men and women when using alternative ways of measuring income: gross individual income and net household equivalent income.

DATA AND METHODS

Sample

The key to comparative research is that data sets are as similar as possible and that the data from different countries come from the same time period. This study used broadly comparable interview surveys conducted in Britain and Finland during the same year, 1994. The British data set derives from the nationwide General Household Survey (GHS), collected annually by the governmental Office of National Statistics (42). This nationally representative government survey interviews personally all adults aged 16 and over in the household. The number of respondents was 18,237 and the response rate for both men and women was 81 percent. The Finnish data set is drawn from the nationwide Survey on Living Conditions (SLC), collected by the government statistical authorities, Statistics Finland (43). This nationally representative government survey interviewed personally people aged 15 and over. The number of respondents was 8,650 and the response rate was 74 percent for women and 72 percent for men. Both samples satisfactorily represent adults living in private households. In this study we analyzed data for 25- to 64-year-old men and women.

Measurement of Health

Self-perceived health was measured by asking each respondent to describe his or her health. In the Finnish data set the answer categories were excellent, good, average, poor, or very poor. In the British survey the answer categories were good, fairly good, or not good. We analyzed perceived health as *less than good*; that is average, poor, or very poor health in Finland, and fairly good and not good health in Britain.

Perceived health incorporates a variety of physical, emotional, and personal components of health, which taken together comprise individual "healthiness." As such, self-assessed health is a broad indicator of health-related well-being (44) and represents a robust, global summary measure of health status (45). It reflects different dimensions of health in a very similar way for both women and men in different cultural areas, at least within western Europe (46). Indeed, in prospective studies, poor self-assessed health has proved to be a strong predictor of mortality (47), and a WHO report has recently recommended use of the self-perceived health measure for comparative purposes (48).

Measurement of Sociodemographic Variables

Income was investigated using quintiles of net household income and gross individual income, both of which provide measures of relative rather than absolute income. A Swedish study compared the impact of both absolute and relative income on health and found broadly similar results using both income measures (13). In our study, household income was equivalized for household composition to yield "net household equivalent income." This was done by adjusting income by household composition using the following formula: first adult = 1, second adult = 0.7, and child below 18 years old = 0.5 (38). For example, the total household income is divided by 1.7 for a married couple and by 2.7 for a couple with two children. According to this scale, a couple with two children needs 2.7 times as much household income as a single-person household in order to achieve a similar standard of living (38). Income quintiles were calculated separately for both men and women and for each country. There is a notable difference in the way that income was measured in these two data sets. In Britain, household income was aggregated from each adult giving information about his or her own income from all sources, with information on income asked from each adult in the household during the interview. This procedure resulted in missing income data for 9 to 16 percent of respondents in this survey. In Finland, income was obtained by linking the survey data with the official tax registry and no income data were missing.

Employment status classification was based on the respondent's main activity during the week preceding the interview in both countries. The categories included full-time employed, part-time employed, unemployed, housewives, retired, and others. The unemployed included all respondents who were out of paid work but available for work and looking for a job. Housewives included those who were keeping house for themselves and at least one other family member and did not have any paid job; male housewives were very few and were omitted from the analysis. The retired group included those who had retired prematurely because of disability or chronic illness, or were permanently sick and unable to work. Small groups of full-time students, members of the armed forces, conscripts, and unclassifiable were categorized as "other."

Social class was based on the respondent's own occupation coded as upper white-collar, lower white-collar, manual workers, entrepreneurs (Finland)/ self-employed (Britain), and farmers (Finland only) plus those who had never worked. If not currently employed, the respondent's social class was determined using his or her previous occupation.

Education in Finland was derived from a national register of educational degrees at Statistics Finland linked to the Finnish survey. In Britain, information on education was self-reported. The occupational and educational classifications in Finland and Britain were harmonized according to our previous study (40, 41) and categorized into three levels: higher, secondary, and basic education.

The main purpose of this study was to analyze health differences according to relative income levels, not to make strict comparisons of absolute levels of health in each income group. Therefore, minor differences in the question formulations, which may affect the observed levels of self-perceived health, are less important in this study where the focus is to examine relative differences.

Statistical Methods

Prevalence percentages of less-than-good health were calculated using direct age-standardization with five-year age groups, using the population of Finland as the standard population. To examine the pattern and magnitude of health inequalities in the two countries, further analysis used multivariate logistic regression models (49). Models were fitted using the GLIM statistical package (50). The results of the models are presented as odds ratios (OR). The highest income quintile serves as the reference category, with an OR of 1.0. Model 1 is adjusted for age in single years; model 2 also included employment status; and model 3 additionally included education and social class.

To summarize the extent of the health differences, we also calculated a slope, the estimated OR of less-than-good perceived health per one unit increase on the five-level income variable, obtained by entering the income variable into the logistic regression model as a continuous variable. We tested the statistical significance ($P < 0.05$) of this slope (in this chapter called a "linear" effect), as well as testing the significance for income as a categorical variable (quintiles) while adjusting for the slope (test for "nonlinearity). In addition to the slope, several other summary indices can be calculated, each with a different interpretation as well as advantages and disadvantages (51).

RESULTS

Descriptive Data on Health by Socioeconomic Background

Table 1 shows the age-standardized prevalence of reporting less-than-good self-perceived health by socioeconomic background. Clear differences are evident using all four socioeconomic variables, and the patterns between countries are very similar. Manual workers reported poorer health than nonmanual workers, and farmers' health, especially women farmers' health, was particularly poor. The socioeconomic differences among women were slightly larger than those among men. Unemployed men and women reported poorer health than the full-time employed. The health of the part-time employed was similar to that of the full-time employed with the exception of British part-time employed men, whose health was poorer than their full-time employed counterparts. Health among housewives was generally poorer than that of the unemployed. The pattern by educational attainment is clear: the lower the educational level, the poorer the self-reported health in both countries.

A clear association between income and health is usually evident; each step down the income scale is related to an increased prevalence of less-than-good health. Almost half (47 percent) of the Finnish men in the lowest quintile of individual income reported less-than-good health, compared with only 21 percent in the highest income quintile. Among British men, the health difference between the highest (16 percent) and lowest (42 percent) income quintiles was similarly large. Health differences were larger by individual income than by household income, with the exception of British women, for whom the lowest quintile by individual income was little different from the fourth and third income quintiles. In contrast, among Finnish women, the health differences measured by individual income show a clear gradient, with the top income quintile much healthier than the lowest quintile, which had much poorer health than the intermediate quintiles. In Finland, health differences were especially large between the two

Table 1

Age-adjusted prevalence of self-perceived health as less than good,
by socioeconomic background in Finland and Britain, percent

	Finland		Britain	
	Men	Women	Men	Women
Employment status				
Full-time employed	28%	25%	24%	28%
Part-time employed	28	24	31	26
Unemployed	37	33	31	33
Housewife	—	31	—	38
Retired	79	75	83	82
Other	—	—	44	58
Social class				
Upper white-collar	21	20	21	26
Lower white-collar	30	26	31	31
Worker	36	36	36	37
Entrepreneur	33	27	29	31
Farmer	35	40	—	—
Never worked	36	29	30	55
Education				
Upper	21	17	21	24
Middle	32	28	31	32
Lower	37	35	37	39
Missing	—	—	40	50
Gross individual income quintile				
Highest	21	17	16	24
2nd	27	27	24	31
3rd	34	29	29	37
4th	32	32	37	35
Lowest	47	38	42	34
Missing	—	—	27	34
Net household income quintile per consumption unit				
Highest	23	19	22	24
2nd	30	28	22	29
3rd	33	31	29	33
4th	34	33	37	37
Lowest	37	32	39	41
Missing	—	—	27	33

highest income groups measured by household income, but leveled off when moving downward through income levels.

Explaining the Association between Income and Health

The association between income and less-than-good self-perceived health was clarified using logistic regression analysis. First, we examined self-perceived health by gross individual income among men (Table 2, Figure 1). The first model (model 1) confirmed the results in the prevalence table (Table 1). In both Britain and Finland, men from the lowest income quintile were four times more likely to report their health as less than good than those in the highest income quintile. In Finland, the pattern was slightly curvilinear, with the fourth quintile having somewhat better health than the third quintile. Even when income was used as a continuous variable, the slope was similar in both countries: 1.36 in Finland and 1.43 in Britain. There were no statistically significant differences in the slope between the two countries.

However, after employment status was included in the model (model 2), the income differences decreased, especially in the lowest quintile, many of whom are currently not in paid employment. Nevertheless, health differences by income quintiles remained statistically significant, while the slopes of this relationship were statistically significant in Britain and Finland. After including education and social class (model 3), the health differences between income quintiles further narrowed. In Britain, the other income quintiles differed from the highest and the linear gradient remained. But in Finland, only the lowest income quintiles reported significantly poorer health. In Finland the curvilinear association and in Britain the linear association remained, but each was much weaker after adjusting for the other socioeconomic variables. The slope between countries also remained statistically significant. In both countries, men in the lowest income quintile were almost twice as likely to report their health as less than good than were their counterparts in the highest income quintile, even after adjusting for employment status, education, and social class (Figure 1).

The age-adjusted association in model 1 between individual income and self-perceived health was weaker among women than among men, and was clearly stronger in Finland than in Britain (Table 2, Figure 1). Finnish women in the lowest income quintile were more than three times more likely to report less-than-good health than were women in the highest income quintile. In Britain, the association was curvilinear; the health of the lowest income quintile was slightly better than that of the third and fourth income quintiles. In model 2, when employment status was included, the ORs decreased, especially in Finland. But the health of the highest quintile remained better than that of all lower income quintiles. In Britain, the OR for the health of the lowest income quintile decreased markedly and was very similar to that of the highest income quintile. When education and social class were included (model 3), in Finland only the

Table 2

Logistic regression analysis of income differences in perceived health in Britain and Finland: gross individual income, men and women, odds ratios (OR)

	Men			Women		
	Model 1: age	Model 2: model 1 + employment status	Model 3: model 2 + education + social class	Model 1: age	Model 2: model 1 + employment status	Model 3: model 2 + education + social class
Finland						
Slope	1.361	1.221	1.116	1.313	1.232	1.109
P^a	0.0001	0.0001	0.0145	0.0001	0.0001	0.0304
Highest	1.00	1.00	1.00	1.00	1.00	1.00
2nd	1.60*	1.55*	1.16	1.77*	1.71*	1.24
3rd	2.09*	2.01*	1.36	2.05*	1.95*	1.30
4th	1.77*	1.46*	1.00	2.25*	2.02*	1.35
Lowest	4.34*	2.68*	1.77*	3.54*	2.49*	1.64*
P^b	0.0001	0.0007	0.0063	0.0724	0.0784	0.8292

Britain					
Slope					
1.428	1.292	1.183	1.125	0.996	0.922
p^a					
0.0001	0.0001	0.0001	0.0001	0.8837	0.0107
Highest					
1.00	1.00	1.00	1.00	1.00	1.00
2nd					
1.58*	1.53*	1.30*	1.40*	1.39*	1.15
3rd					
2.22*	2.16*	1.63*	1.92*	1.74*	1.31*
4th					
3.17*	2.46*	1.77*	1.80*	1.43*	1.06
Lowest					
4.27*	2.71*	1.96*	1.64*	1.06	0.79
p^b					
0.7391	0.0492	0.5325	0.0001	0.0001	0.0002
p^c					
0.1489	0.0040	0.0122	0.0001	0.0010	0.0001

^{a}P-value of slope.

^{b}P-value of categorized income when slope is adjusted.

^{c}P-value of difference in slopes between Finland and Britain.

*Statistically significant difference from the reference category at the 5% level.

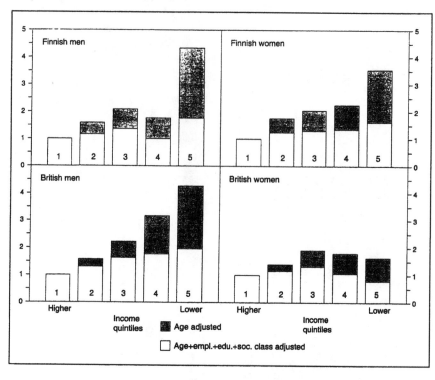

Figure 1. Odds ratios for income differences measured by gross individual income in perceived health among men and women in Britain and Finland; both age-adjusted figures and figures adjusted for age, employment status, education, and social class. Income quintiles from highest (1) to lowest (5).

lowest income quintile differed from the highest quintile among Finnish men. In Britain, the health of the third income quintile was significantly poorer than that of the highest income quintile. Indeed, in this model (model 3), the lowest income quintile in Britain reported the best health (OR = 0.79). Meanwhile, there was a statistically significant difference in the slope between countries in all models indicating that the association between health and individual income for women was different in the two countries.

The association between net household equivalent income and self-perceived health was similar to that for individual income among men (Table 3, Figure 2). However, the age-adjusted model (model 1) showed that the patterns between the countries were different: the association in Finland was not linear, whereas in Britain the association was linear. In Finland, the difference was especially large between the two highest income quintiles (OR = 1.0 versus OR = 1.98). When employment status was included in model 2, the health differences by income narrowed and the differences in the slope between the countries were no longer statistically significant. After the adjustment of all four variables (model 3), the income differences in health narrowed further, although in Finland all income quintiles remained different from the highest one. In Britain, only the two lowest income quintiles differed from the highest one, while the slope was similar in both countries, 1.09.

Among women, the association between age-adjusted health and net household income was clear and linear in both countries (Table 3, Figure 2). After controlling for women's employment status (model 2), the differences narrowed but remained statistically significant. When education and social class were included (model 3), the association remained linear in both countries, although in Finland none of the income quintiles differed from the highest quintile. There were no health differences by income among Finnish women by household income, but differences remained significantly linear among British women.

SUMMARY AND DISCUSSION

We found health differences by income in both Finland and Britain. However, low income was associated with poor health in different ways in these two contrasting welfare states. Among men the pattern was similar whether individual income or household equivalent income was used. Health differences by income were clear, but attenuated after adjusting for employment status, education, and social class. Most of the association between low income and health for men in both countries was therefore due to their low class, low educational level, and greater chance of nonemployment. Much of the poor health of those in the lowest income quintile results from the high proportion not in employment, many no doubt for health-related reasons.

For women the pattern in the two countries was dissimilar. Among Finnish women, similar health differences were found when measured by individual income and by household income after adjusting for age and employment status. However, the household income differences largely disappeared after adjusting for education and social class, and the remaining association between individual income and health was quite small. Among British women, the association between health and household equivalent income remained strong and linear after adjusting for other variables. However, when gross individual income was used as a measure of income, the pattern was curvilinear and the healthiest women in Britain were those in the highest and lowest income quintiles, after adjusting for other variables.

The use of cross-sectional data on income and health, as in this study, makes it difficult to disentangle the direction of causality. When education, social class, and especially employment status were adjusted, at least part of the reverse causality might have been removed. Much of the association between income and health is explained by the differences in employment status. Nevertheless,

Table 3

Logistic regression analysis of income differences in perceived health in Britain and Finland:
net household equivalent income, men and women, odds ratios (OR)

	Men			Women		
	Model 1: age	Model 2: model 1 + employment status	Model 3: model 2 + education + social class	Model 1: age	Model 2: model 1 + employment status	Model 3: model 2 + education + social class
Finland						
Slope	1.225	1.169	1.089	1.216	1.163	1.067
P^a	0.0001	0.0001	0.0167	0.0001	0.0001	0.0890
Highest	1.00	1.00	1.00	1.00	1.00	1.00
2nd	1.98*	1.77*	1.52*	1.49*	1.39*	1.16
3rd	2.37*	2.00*	1.60*	1.96*	1.73*	1.35
4th	2.24*	1.84*	1.41*	2.23*	1.82*	1.34
Lowest	2.79*	2.27*	1.68*	2.22*	1.89*	1.31
P^b	0.0008	0.0076	0.0538	0.0844	0.2464	0.5871

Britain

Slope	1.295	1.179	1.092	1.268	1.219	1.161
P^a	0.0001	0.0001	0.0030	0.0001	0.0001	0.0001
Highest	1.00	1.00	1.00	1.00	1.00	1.00
2nd	1.46*	1.45*	1.22	1.36*	1.36*	1.25*
3rd	1.52*	1.40*	1.09	1.72*	1.67*	1.48*
4th	2.36*	1.95*	1.47*	2.21*	2.03*	1.72*
Lowest	2.87*	1.95*	1.41*	2.59*	2.22*	0.81*
P^b	0.1600	0.0845	0.1641	0.7168	0.3927	0.6041
P^c	0.0087	0.1909	0.3230	0.0008	0.0026	0.0062

^{a} P-value of slope.
^{b} P-value of categorized income when slope is adjusted.
^{c} P-value of difference in slopes between Finland and Britain.
*Statistically significant difference from the reference category at the 5% level.

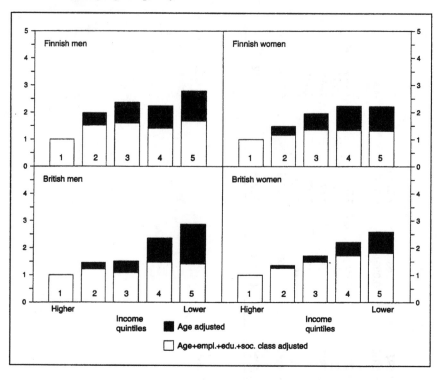

Figure 2. Odds ratios for income differences measured by net household equivalent income in perceived health among men and women in Britain and Finland; both age-adjusted figures and figures adjusted for age, employment status, education, and social class. Income quintiles from highest (1) to lowest (5).

the association remained statistically significant even after adjusting for employment status, education, and social class, except for Finnish women when using household income as the measure of income. This suggests that level of income may have some independent effect on health.

The relationship between income and health was linear among women in both countries and for both income measures, with the exception of British women when using individual income. Among British men the association was also linear. For Finnish men the association was nonlinear when measured by individual income but approached linearity when using household equivalent income and adjusting for the other variables.

An important finding from the present study is that the association between health and income does not appear to have a threshold in the sense that only people in poverty are in poorer health than others. The shape of the association was mainly linear, health worsening on movement down the income ladder.

However, it is still possible that those with a very low income, such as those at the lowest 5 or 10 percent of the income distribution, have extremely poor health.

Another major finding of our study is that the relationship between health and income existed using both income measures, individual income and household income. However, the relationship was different for the two measures, particularly for British women. Using individual income, the health of the lowest income quintile among British women was especially good after adjusting for employment status and other variables. This group mainly consists of housewives and part-time employed women. According to the age-adjusted prevalence, the health of housewives was somewhat poorer than that of employed women. However, there were no health differences between full-time employed and part-time employed women in either country. This seemingly contradictory finding disappeared when household income was examined. The curvilinear relationship between individual income and health could be explained by the gendered labor market in Britain. Fewer women are employed full-time in Britain than in Finland. Part-time employed women are at the lower end of the income distribution, but their health seems to be as good as that of women in the higher income quintile. In addition, many British women who have no individual income are housewives married to men belonging to a higher income group. Unfortunately, the Finnish survey has no data on husband's income, education, and occupation and we could not investigate husband's socioeconomic status as a confounder for health differences by income among women.

Our results indicate that using only one measure for income gives a limited picture of the association between income and health, especially among women. Household equivalent income is more strongly and consistently associated with health than is individual income, and therefore is suggested as a more appropriate indicator for income. It is also clearly important to investigate the association between health and income separately for men and women. Our findings suggest that in future studies on income and health, household equivalent income should be used and employment status should be adjusted. This is especially important for women because of their varying levels of labor market participation in different societies.

Acknowledgments — We thank George Ellison and an anonymous referee for helpful comments on an earlier version of this chapter.

Note — Earlier versions of this chapter have been presented at the Nordic Conference on Social Medicine, Helsinki, Finland, September 1997; the European Public Health Association Annual Meeting, Pamplona, Spain, November 1997; the International Sociological Association World Conference, Montréal, Canada, July 1998; and the XV International Scientific Meeting of the International Epidemiological Association, Florence, Italy, September 1999.

REFERENCES

1. Wilkinson, R. G. *Unhealthy Societies: The Afflictions of Inequality.* Routledge, London, 1996.
2. McIsaac, S. J., and Wilkinson, R. G. Income distribution and cause specific mortality. *Eur. J. Public Health* 7: 45–53, 1997.
3. Wilkinson, R. G. Income inequality summarises the health burden of individual deprivation. *BMJ* 314: 1727–1728, 1997.
4. Rogers, G. B. Income and inequality as determinants of mortality: An international cross-section analysis. *Popul. Stud.* 33: 343–351, 1979.
5. Kaplan, G. A., et al. Inequality in income and mortality in the United States: Analysis of mortality and potential pathways. *BMJ* 312: 999–1003, 1996.
6. Kawachi, I., and Kennedy, B. P. Health and social cohesion: Why care about income inequality? *BMJ* 314: 1037–1040, 1997.
7. Kennedy, B. P., et al. Income distribution, socioeconomic status, and self rated health in the United States: Multilevel analysis. *BMJ* 317: 917–921, 1998.
8. Lynch, J. W., et al. Income inequality and mortality in metropolitan areas of the United States. *Am. J. Public Health* 88: 1074–1080, 1988.
9. Fiscella, K., and Franks, P. Poverty or income inequality as predictor of mortality: Longitudinal cohort study. *BMJ* 314: 1724–1727, 1997.
10. Judge, K., Mulligan, J.-O., and Benzeval, M. Income inequality and population health. *Soc. Sci. Med.* 46: 567–579, 1998.
11. Gravelle, H. How much of the relation between population mortality and unequal distribution of income is a statistical artefact? *BMJ* 316: 382–385, 1998.
12. Atkinson, A., Rainwater, L., and Smeeding, T. *Income Distribution in OECD Countries.* Social Policy Studies No. 18. OECD, Paris, 1995.
13. Lundberg, O., and Fritzell, J. Income distribution, income change and health: On the importance of absolute and relative income for health status in Sweden. In *Economic Change, Social Welfare and Health in Europe,* edited by L. S. Levin, L. McMahon, and E. Ziglio, pp. 37–58. WHO Regional Publications, European Series, No. 54. Finland, 1994.
14. Der, G., et al. The relationship of household income to a range of health measures in three age cohorts from the west of Scotland. *Eur. J. Public Health* 9, 1999, in press.
15. Blaxter, M. *Health and Lifestyle.* Tavistock/Routledge, London, 1990.
16. McDonough, P., et al. Income dynamics and adult mortality in the United States, 1972 through 1989. *Am. J. Public Health* 87: 1476–1483, 1997.
17. Marmot, M. G., et al. Contribution of psychosocial factors to socioeconomic differences in health. *Milbank Q.* 76: 403–448, 1998.
18. Ecob, R., and Davey Smith, G. Income and health: What is the nature of the relationship? *Soc. Sci. Med.* 48: 693–705, 1999.
19. Stronks, K., et al. The interrelationship between income, health and employment status. *Int. J. Epidemiol.* 26: 592–600, 1997.
20. Kitagawa, E. M., and Hauser, P. M. *Differential Mortality in the United States: A Study in Socioeconomic Epidemiology.* Harvard University Press, Cambridge, Mass., 1973.

21. Arber, S. Comparing inequalities in women's and men's health: Britain in the 1990s. *Soc. Sci. Med.* 44: 773–787, 1997.
22. Cavelaars, A., et al. Differences in self-reported morbidity by income level in six European countries. 1998.
23. van Doorslaer, E., et al. Income-related inequalities in health: Some international comparisons. *J. Health Econ.* 16: 93–112, 1997.
24. Esping-Anderson, G. *Three Worlds of Welfare Capitalism.* Polity Press, Oxford, 1990.
25. Titmus, R. *Essays on the Welfare State.* Allen and Unwin, London, 1958.
26. Erikson, R., et al. (eds.). *The Scandinavian Model: Welfare States and Welfare Research.* M. E. Sharpe, Armonk, N.Y., 1987.
27. Esping-Andersen, G., and Kolberg, J. E. Welfare states and employment regimes. In *Between Work and Social Citizenship,* edited by J. E. Kolberg, pp. 3–36. Sharpe, Armonk, N.Y., 1992.
28. Hernes, H. The welfare state citizenship of Scandinavian women. In *The Political Interests of Gender: Developing Theory and Research with a Feminist Face,* edited by K. B. Jones and A. G. Jonasdottir, pp. 187–213. Sage, London, 1988.
29. Lahelma, E., and Arber, S. Health inequalities among men and women in contrasting welfare states: Britain and three Nordic countries compared. *Eur. J. Public Health* 4: 227–240, 1994.
30. Statistics Finland, 1998. Available from: httt://www.stat.fi
31. Stephens, J. D. The Scandinavian welfare states: Achievements, crisis, and prospects. In *Welfare States in Transition,* edited by G. Esping-Andersen, pp. 32–65. Sage, London, 1996.
32. Heikkilä, M., and Uusitalo, H. (eds). *The Costs of Cuts.* National Research and Development Centre for Welfare and Health, Helsinki, 1997.
33. Kautto, M., et al. (eds). *Nordic Social Policy: Changing Welfare States.* Routledge, London, 1999.
34. Joshi, H., and Davies, H. *Child Care and Mothers Lifetime Earnings: Some European Comparisons.* Discussion paper No. 600. Centre for Economic Policy Research, London, 1992.
35. Arber, S., and Gilbert, N. Re-assessing women's working lives. In *Women and Working Lives: Divisions and Change,* edited by S. Arber and N. Gilbert. Macmillan, London, 1991.
36. Church, J., and Whyman, S. A review of recent social and economic trends. In *Health Inequalities: Decennial Supplement,* edited by F. Drever and M. Whitehead, pp. 29–43. HMSO, London, 1997.
37. Lahelma, E., et al. Widening or narrowing inequalities in health? Comparing Britain and Finland from the 1980s to 1990s. *Soc. Health Illness,* 2000, in press.
38. Uusitalo, H. Four years of recession: What happened to income distribution? In *The Costs of Cuts,* edited by M. Heikkilä and H. Uusitalo, pp. 101–118. National Research and Development Centre for Welfare and Health, Helsinki, 1997.
39. Gottschalk, P., and Smeeding, T. M. Cross-national comparisons of earnings and income inequality. *J. Econ. Lit.* 35: 633–687, 1997.
40. Arber, S., and Lahelma, E. Inequalities in women's and men's illhealth: Britain and Finland compared. *Soc. Sci. Med.* 37: 1055–1068, 1993.

41. Rahkonen, O., Arber, S., and Lahelma, E. Health inequalities in early adulthood: A comparison of young men and women in Britain and Finland. *Soc. Sci. Med.* 41: 163–171, 1995.

42. Bennett, N., et al. *Living in Britain: Results from the 1994 General Household Survey.* OPCS, HMSO, London, 1996.

43. Ahola, A., et al. *Elinolotutkimus 1994: Aineiston keruu* (Survey on Living Conditions 1994: Collecting the Data). Statistics Finland, Helsinki, 1994.

44. Segovia, J., Bartlett, R. F., and Edwards, A. C. An empirical analysis of the dimensions of health measures. *Soc. Sci. Med.* 29: 761–768, 1989.

45. Manderbacka, K. Examining what self-rated health question is understood to mean by respondents. *Scand. J. Soc. Med.* 26: 145–153, 1998.

46. Jylhä, M., et al. Is self-rated health comparable across cultures and genders? *J. Gerontol. Soc. Sci.* 53B: S144–S152, 1998.

47. Idler, E. L., and Benyamini, Y. Self-rated health and mortality: A review of twenty-seven community studies. *J. Health Soc. Behav.* 38: 21–37, 1997.

48. Bruin, A. de, Pichavet, H. S. J., and Nossikov, A. *Health Interview Surveys: Towards International Harmonisation of Methods and Instruments.* WHO Regional Publications, Copenhagen, 1996.

49. Fienberg, S. E. *The Analysis of Cross-Classified Categorical Data.* The MIT Press, Cambridge, Mass., 1980.

50. Francis, B., Green, M., and Payne, C. (eds). *The GLIM System: Release 4 Manual.* Clarendon Press, Oxford, 1994.

51. Kunst, A. *Cross-national Comparisons of Socio-economic Differences in Mortality.* CIP-Gegevens Koninklijke Bibliotheek, Den Haag, 1997.

CHAPTER 15

Integrating Nonemployment
into Research on Health Inequalities

Sara Arber

Until the late 1980s, the British debate on inequalities in health was dominated by a concern with men of working age, focusing on class based on the man's current occupation (1–6). Latterly, more attention has been paid to inequalities in women's health (7–14). There has been extensive research on the link between unemployment and health (15–19), but less attempt to integrate the latter with research on class inequalities.

In this chapter I argue that we cannot neglect the nonemployed in our analyses of inequalities in health, first, because of demography—nonemployed people represent a very significant and increasing proportion of all adults in the population. Second, decisions about whether to include the nonemployed in analyses of class inequalities in health influence the magnitude of reported inequalities and the extent to which inequalities widen or diminish over time. Third, an understanding of measuring inequalities in health among those not in paid work throws light on more general conceptual issues relating to inequalities in health.

The demographic situation is shown in Table 1. Only 57 percent of British adults aged over 18 are in paid employment. It is inappropriate to exclude the 43 percent of nonemployed adults from analyses of inequalities in health. The largest nonemployed group is retired people (19 percent of all adults), followed by full-time housewives (13 percent) and unemployed people (6 percent). Despite the size of the retired population and concerns with the health care costs of this growing section of the population, there is still little research on inequalities in older people's health (20–22). People over 65 are almost all outside the formal labor market, therefore issues about how to measure class inequalities among the nonemployed are particularly salient in relation to later life.

This chapter begins with a discussion of issues relating to measuring class inequalities for different groups of nonemployed people, then turns to the relationship between class and employment participation, analyzing whether inequalities in health are comparable between the nonemployed and the employed. I use

Table 1

Self-assessed employment status of British men and women aged 18
and over, 1991–1992[a]

	Men	Women	All
Employed	66%	49%	57%
Full-time	62	27	43
Part-time	4	22	14
Not employed	34%	51%	43%
Retired	20	19	19
Housewife	1	24	13
Unemployed	8	3	6
Other not employed (including disabled, student, temporarily sick)	6	5	5
	100%	100%	100%
N	17,493	19,466	36,964
Row %	47%	53%	

[a]Source: Data from *General Household Survey, 1991–92*, author's analysis.

the British General Household Survey to disentangle the independent effects on health of occupational class, educational qualifications, and employment status, focusing on both employed and nonemployed men and women.

MEASURING THE CLASS OF THE NONEMPLOYED

When measuring the class of the nonemployed, it is obviously impossible to use their *current* occupation. The main alternatives are:

1. To use the individual's *last* main occupation.
2. To use the current occupational class of the head of household or the person in the household with the highest income or occupational status.
3. To measure class based on some other unchanging characteristic of the individual, which is not influenced by the person's employment status, such as educational qualifications or age at which the person left full-time education.
4. To use measures relating to the individual's material resources, income, housing, or car ownership.

Different approaches have conventionally been used according to age and the reasons for nonemployment, but these conventions have varied among countries:

1. *Nonemployed working-age men.* In Britain, working-age men who are unemployed, or not working because of long-term disability or temporary sickness, have mainly been classified by their last occupation. In this way all men have been included in class analyses of health (3–6). However, in other countries the practice has been to assign them to a separate status as nonemployed, for example in Finland and Sweden (23, 24). In the latter case, these men have often been grouped as if they were homogeneous on account of their lack of current employment. Many countries do not routinely collect data on last occupation for those not currently in paid employment, so are unable to classify the nonemployed by their last occupation.

2. *Working age women who are full-time housewives.* The conventional approach in Britain has been to categorize full-time housewives by the occupational class of their husband (7–10). In government statistics and most British health research, all married women have been classified by their husband's occupational class irrespective of the wife's employment status or whether she has a higher or lower socioeconomic status than her husband. This practice is increasingly anachronistic when three-quarters of working-age married women are in paid employment. An extensive debate has raged about the wisdom of continuing with the "conventional" approach or adopting the alternative individualistic approach of classifying all women by their current (or last) occupation (7, 8, 25, 26). In the Nordic countries, the practice of classifying women by their husband's occupation was abandoned in the 1960s in favor of using their current occupation—the individualistic approach (23). In these countries data are not routinely collected about a woman's partner, so it is not possible to evaluate the merits of alternative approaches.

3. *Full-time students.* The majority of researchers interested in inequalities in young people's health have classified them according to their father's occupational class and sometimes also their mother's socioeconomic characteristics, that is, their class of origin (27, 28). Classifying by parent's class implicitly treats full-time students as dependents and has analogies with the classification of women as a dependent of their husband. Where full-time students no longer live in the parental home this practice is problematic.

4. *Retired people.* Much research treats older people as a homogeneous group, often not making conceptual distinctions except for demographic variables such as sex, age, marital status, and race. In the United States there is extensive research on the health of elderly people, but an almost total absence of work on how health inequalities relate to socioeconomic position (29). This absence partly reflects the paucity of data sets containing information on both health and the older person's previous labor market position. Where inequalities in health have been studied, older people have primarily been classified by their current material circumstances, such as income and housing. Many countries have adopted this strategy because no information is routinely collected about the previous occupation of older people.

Thus, alternative ways of classifying the nonemployed have been adopted depending on the reasons for nonemployment and on the individual's sex and age. The different solutions are premised on alternative assumptions and are likely to lead to varying conclusions about both the extent of class inequality among different groups and its visibility as a policy issue.

EMPLOYMENT STATUS AND HEALTH

This chapter argues for the importance of basing class analyses on occupation as the primary determinant of an individual's labor market position. Using such a classification we need to decide how to incorporate nonemployment, since half of women and a third of men are nonemployed (Table 1). The proposal is that last occupation should be used to measure class for all people not currently in paid work, including for women who have not been in paid work for many years and for men during periods of large-scale unemployment. With increases in unemployment since the late 1970s, a large literature has developed on unemployment and health; however, few studies have linked an occupational class analysis to unemployment (15–19).

Most British studies of class inequalities in health classify men who are not currently employed by their last occupation. Since the unemployed are concentrated in lower occupational classes, what are the implications of this practice? Table 2 shows a linear gradient between being in full-time work and occupational class, based on current (or last main) occupation, for men and women under 60. Ninety-two percent of men in higher professional and managerial occupations (Class 1) are in full-time work; this falls to 71 percent among the semi-skilled and only 55 percent among unskilled men. Forty percent of unskilled men are not in employment compared with only 7 percent of Class 1 men. In all classes the majority of nonemployed men are unemployed.

The class gradient in employment participation falls even more dramatically for women, with 75 percent of Class 1 women in full-time work, compared with 28 percent among semi-skilled and only 8 percent among unskilled women (Table 2). Part-time work for women is lowest among women working in higher professional and managerial occupations (11 percent) and highest among women in unskilled occupations (55 percent). About 30 percent of women in all other classes work part-time. The class differential in full-time work reflects the increasing polarization in British women's employment, whereby only women working in professional and managerial occupations have the financial resources to pay for private child care and domestic support to enable them to continue to work full-time (30). For women, the main reason for nonemployment is being a full-time housewife, which is less likely for women in Classes 1 and 2, but varies little among women in the other classes. There is a weaker class gradient in unemployment for women than men.

Table 2

Employment status of men and women aged 20–59 by current (or last) occupational class[a]

| Employment status | Occupational class[b] | | | | | | |
| | Nonmanual | | | Manual | | | |
	1	2	3	4	5	6	All
Men							
Employed							
Full-time	92%	86%	86%	80%	70%	55%	82%
Part-time	1	4	3	2	4	5	3
Not employed							
Unemployed	4	6	7	10	16	25	9
Other reasons[c]	3	4	4	7	9	15	6
	100%	100%	100%	100%	100%	100%	100%
N	2,234	2,188	1,144	4,454	1,579	499	12,098
Women							
Employed							
Full-time	75%	52%	40%	38%	27%	8%	40%
Part-time	11	28	29	30	30	55	30
Not employed							
Housewife	9	13	22	21	30	25	21
Unemployed	3	3	5	5	6	5	4
Other reasons[c]	2	4	4	6	7	7	5
	100%	100%	100%	100%	100%	100%	100%
N	789	2,582	4,620	1,035	2,523	1,071	12,620

[a]Source: Data from *General Household Survey, 1991–92,* author's analysis.
[b]Occupational class (derived by combining socioeconomic groups):
   1. Higher professionals, employers/managers (25+ in firm)
   2. Lower professionals, employers/managers (<25 in firm)
   3. Intermediate and junior nonmanual
   4. Skilled manual, nonprofessional own account, foremen
   5. Semi-skilled manual, personal service
   6. Unskilled manual
[c]Other reasons include permanently disabled, temporarily sick, full-time students, and, for men, housewife.

The likelihood of poor health leading to job loss may be mediated by occupational class, since a given illness or disability is more likely to lead to loss of job in manual than in professional and managerial occupations. This is both because of the fitness level required to perform different types of work and because employee sickness benefits are more generous at higher levels of the class structure, often allowing employees to retain their job even after extended periods of ill-health.

Since the nonemployed are concentrated in the lower social classes, especially among men, and the nonemployed have poorer health, one would expect that social class gradients in health would be greater where the nonemployed are included in class analyses of health (classified by their last occupation) than where only employed people are analyzed. Arber (31), and Dahl (32) based on Norwegian data, showed that class differences in ill-health in the 1980s were as great among the nonemployed as the employed. This study considers whether this is the case in the 1990s for both men and women.

Measures of three major factors are needed to adequately understand an individual's position in the labor market: educational qualifications, occupational class, and employment status. Employment status is affected by both educational qualifications and occupational class. It is the labor market variable that is most likely to be the subject of reverse causation. The major issue is the extent of drift out of employment because of ill-health rather than drift down the class structure because of ill-health. The lack of evidence that health selection is responsible for inequalities according to current occupational class (3, 6) contrasts with debates on the association between unemployment and poor mental or physical health (15, 16, 33). A substantial proportion of this association is due to health selection—men with poor health are more likely to lose their jobs and less likely to obtain another job once unemployed. However, health selection is much less applicable to other groups of nonemployed people, for example, full-time students, women who are housewives, and the retired. There is a growing body of evidence that full-time housewives have poorer health than employed women (20, 23) and that this cannot be explained by health selection of women with poor health into the housewife role (34, 35).

Educational qualifications, unlike occupational class, have the advantage of being easily collected for all adults irrespective of their employment status and to be relatively unchanging throughout the life course. However, the expansion of education means that there are wide variations in qualifications between age cohorts. In Britain, educational qualifications have previously been considered of little value in analyzing inequalities in health among adults (3, 25) because a high proportion of the population has no qualifications. However, this objection may be much less valid in the 1990s. In other countries, educational qualifications have been the major socioeconomic indicator and used more extensively than occupation-based measures, for example in the United States (36) and in Scandinavia (37, 38). A disadvantage of using educational qualifications as the sole variable in analyses of inequalities in health is variation in the return on educational qualifications in terms of labor market achievement and income. For a given level of qualifications, ethnic minorities and women in the United States and United Kingdom obtain a lower occupational status and income than equally qualified white men.

It is important to have a clear conceptual model of the likely causal ordering of the three labor market variables (Figure 1). Educational qualifications are causally prior to occupational class and employment status, and there is little evidence of reverse causation, that is, poor health leading to low educational qualifications (39). Occupational class is causally prior to employment status and, as discussed earlier, those in higher occupational classes are less likely to experience unemployment and redundancy and more likely to be protected from job loss due to ill-health. There is little evidence for reverse causation of ill-health leading to a "drift" down into lower social class jobs (3, 6).

All three labor market variables have a major impact on individuals' material circumstances, such as their income, housing, and ownership of assets and consumer goods. Figure 1 suggests the predominant direction of these linkages. Where the direction of causality is unclear, double-headed arrows have been used. Within Western societies, financial and material well-being is closely tied to success in the labor market, thus material resources must be seen as causally dependent on the individual's labor market position. However, analyses based on income or material circumstances are problematic because of the likelihood of reverse causation; poor health may adversely affect employment participation and material well-being. There are financial effects of poor health in terms of increased health care costs and the added costs of living with a disability.

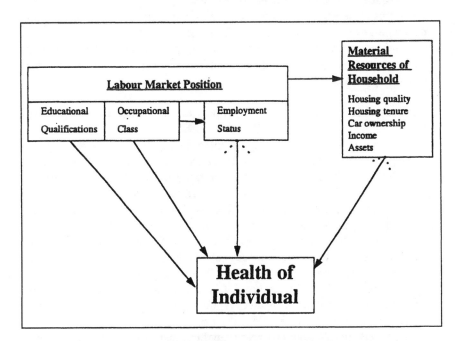

Figure 1. Model of influence of socioeconomic variables on health.

Older people's previous position in the labor market will have influenced their health during working life and is the main determinant of their income and assets after retirement, mainly through the mechanism of occupational pensions (40, 41). Most analyses of inequalities in health of older people focus on their current material circumstances such as income, housing tenure, and ownership of assets rather than on their occupational class. In this chapter I argue that it is essential to retain these two structural dimensions as conceptually distinct (Figure 1). An older person's occupational class, based on earlier position in the labor market, is logically prior to and has the primary determining influence on his or her current material resources.

DATA AND METHODS

The aims of this chapter are:

1. To clarify the independent effects of the three main components of labor market position: educational qualifications, occupational class, and employment status.
2. Because most British analyses of health inequalities classify nonemployed working-age men by their last occupational class, to examine to what extent this practice inflates the class–health gradient.
3. To compare the association between health and class for employed and for nonemployed men and women of working age.
4. For men and women aged over 60, who are in the main no longer in paid employment, to examine the association between class, based on their last occupation, and health.

The General Household Survey (GHS) provides an annual, nationally representative sample of about 10,000 British households (42). Each adult aged 16 and over living in sample households is interviewed, with an overall response rate of 82 percent in 1991–1992 (42). However, nonresponse is higher among people who are sick, including those temporarily in hospital, and the survey omits elderly people living in residential establishments. This study uses combined data from the 1991 and 1992 GHS. Most of the study focuses on working-age men and women, ages 20 to 59 inclusive, representing about 24,000 men and women. The Appendix shows that among this age group, 18 percent of men and a third of women are not employed. The final section of the chapter focuses on men and women over 60: nearly 10,000 men and women.

Two measures of ill-health are used. Chronic illness in the GHS is a self-reported measure of whether individuals report any *limiting long-standing illness* (LLI). The respondent was asked, "Have you any long-standing illness, disability or infirmity? (By long-standing I mean anything that has troubled you over a period of time or that is likely to affect you over a period of time.)" If the answer was "Yes," the respondent was asked, "Does this illness limit your activities in any way?" Those who answered "Yes" are categorized as having a "limiting long-standing illness." This measure is related to function and represents a self-assessment of the effect of any chronic ill-health on daily life.

Self-assessed health relates to the individual's personal sense of well-being. Poor self-assessed health is associated with early mortality (43, 44) and with institutionalization, after controlling for other health and age variables (45). Self-assessed health is measured by the GHS question, "Over the last 12 months, would you say your health has on the whole been good, fairly good or not good?" The analyses of self-assessed health focus on those who reported their health as "less than good" (i.e., reported "fairly good" or "not good" health).

Class is measured using current occupation, except for those not currently in paid employment who are classified by their last main job. A six-fold classification of occupations is used in most of the chapter (see Appendix). However, because of the small proportion of older women previously employed in professional occupations (Class 1), the analysis of older people groups together Classes 1 and 2 into a five-fold classification. The Appendix shows the distribution of all the variables used in the analyses separately for men and women aged 20–59, 60–69, and 70 and over.

DISENTANGLING EDUCATION, OCCUPATIONAL CLASS, AND EMPLOYMENT STATUS

Logistic regression is used to assess the relative influence on the health of working-age men and women of each of the three labor market variables: educational qualifications, occupational class, and employment status. Table 3 summarizes these models for the two health measures for men and women. The base model (Model 1) includes age (in five-year age groups) and marital status. Occupational class is added to the base model (Model 2), and educational qualifications is added to the base model (Model 3). Model 4 includes both educational qualifications and occupational class. Model 5 shows the additional effect of employment status, indicating to what extent occupational class and educational qualifications continue to have an effect after including employment status in the model.

Occupational class improves the fit of the base model to a greater extent than educational qualifications, except for women's self-assessed health—see change in log likelihood ratio (ΔLLR) when comparing Models 2 and 3 (Table 3). Model 4 shows that in each case, the inclusion of both educational qualifications and occupational class results in a statistically significant improvement in the model. The additional effect of educational qualifications barely reaches statistical significance for limiting long-standing illness but is much greater for self-assessed health. As expected, employment status has a very major association with ill-health. The reduction in LLR with the addition of employment status (in Model 5)

Table 3

Comparison of logistic regression models predicting ill-health
for working-age men and women, aged 20–59[a]

Model	Δ df	Limiting long-standing illness, ΔLLR[b]		Self-assessed health, ΔLLR[b]	
		Men	Women	Men	Women
1. Base model, LLR (age + marital)		8,854	10,342	12,647	15,446
2. 1 + class (2 – 1)	5	125**	68**	236**	192**
3. 1 + education (3 – 1)	4	76**	58**	215**	220**
4. 2 + education (4 – 2)	4	12*	22**	66**	86**
5. 4 + employment (5 – 4)	5	907**	965**	478**	494**
N		11,162	12,266	11,198	12,311

[a]Source: Data from *General Household Survey, 1991–92*, author's analysis.
[b]Significance of change in log likelihood ratio (LLR): *$P < .05$; ** $P < .01$.

is very substantial, but is much greater for limiting long-standing illness than for self-assessed health. The change in LLR with the addition of employment status to the model is much greater than the change with the inclusion of either occupational class (Model 2) or educational qualifications (Model 3).

The relative impact of each of the three labor market variables can be seen from Figures 2 through 5. (These figures are derived from Tables 4 and 5 which give the odds ratios for each of the models for men and women, respectively.) Figures 2 and 3 show how the odds ratios for occupational class (Model 2) change with the addition of educational qualifications (Model 4) and then employment status (Model 5). There is a strong unadjusted class gradient for both health measures for men, with the unskilled having three and a half times greater odds of ill-health than professional men (Figure 2). The gradient is linear across the three manual classes. Men in lower nonmanual occupations and managers have comparable odds of ill-health, which are about one and a half times greater than for professional men.

The unadjusted class gradient for women (based on their own occupation) is weaker than for men and varies between the two health measures (Figure 3). The gradient is linear for self-assessed health, but for LLI the odds are similar for women in the three manual classes—each having odds of ill-health over twice as great as for professional women. The pattern of ill-health for women according to occupational class shows little difference between women in the manual classes, unlike the pattern for men. There is a suggestion that women in skilled manual occupations have poorer health than those in other manual occupations. This is similar to Finnish findings in which women in skilled occupations have poorer health than those in semi-skilled and unskilled occupations (23).

The black area of Figures 2 and 3 shows the odds of ill-health by occupational class after adjusting for the effects of educational qualifications (Model 4 compared with Model 2). Adjusting for education reduces men's class gradient for self-assessed health more than for LLI. After adjustment, unskilled men still have a three times higher odds of LLI than professional men. For women, education also reduces the class gradient for self-assessed health to a greater extent than for LLI, showing that educational qualifications are more closely linked to self- assessed health than to LLI.

The change in class odds with the addition of employment status (Model 5 compared with Model 4) is shown by the white area in Figures 2 and 3. Employment status reduces the class gradient of LLI very substantially. The effect is greatest for unskilled men, and is somewhat less as the skill level of men in manual occupations increases. Employment status has no effect on the class gradient for men in nonmanual occupations. These findings are consistent with observations that the chances of nonemployment are greater at lower levels of the class structure. The class gradient adjusted for employment status (Model 5) is now less steep, with the unskilled having about twice the odds and other classes one and a half times the odds of ill-health compared with professional men.

Employment status has less impact on the class trend in ill-health for women and a more equal impact across the class structure, rather than being concentrated in lower manual occupations as occurs for men. This gender difference is because nonemployment for women is less likely to be health-related than for men. Employment status has a greater impact on the class trend for LLI than for self-assessed health. Women's adjusted class gradient for LLI is nonlinear. Women in Class 2 (lower professionals, technical workers, and managers and employers in small establishments) report higher levels of chronic illness than women in junior nonmanual occupations, and the adverse position of women in skilled manual occupations stands out more clearly.

Figures 4 and 5 show the odds of ill-health by educational qualifications adjusted for age and marital status (Model 3 in Tables 4 and 5). The adjustment for occupational class (Model 4) is indicated by the black area and the adjustment for employment status (Model 5) by the white area. The unadjusted educational gradient is strong and linear for self-assessed health for both men and women, with odds of poor health being three times greater for men with no qualifications than for those with a degree; the corresponding odds are two and a half times greater for women. Educational qualifications provide much less discrimination

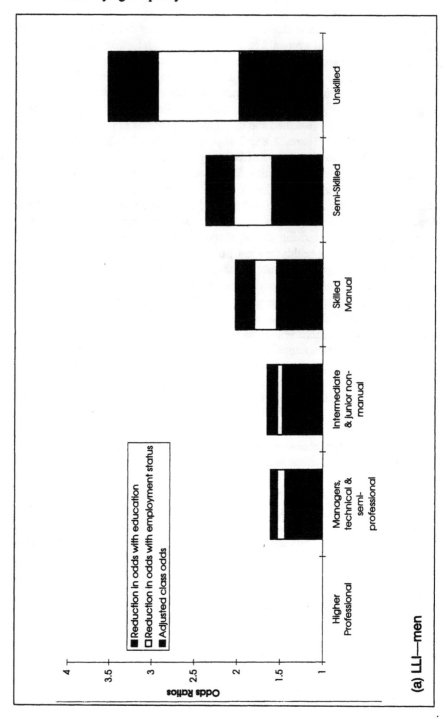

(a) LLI—men

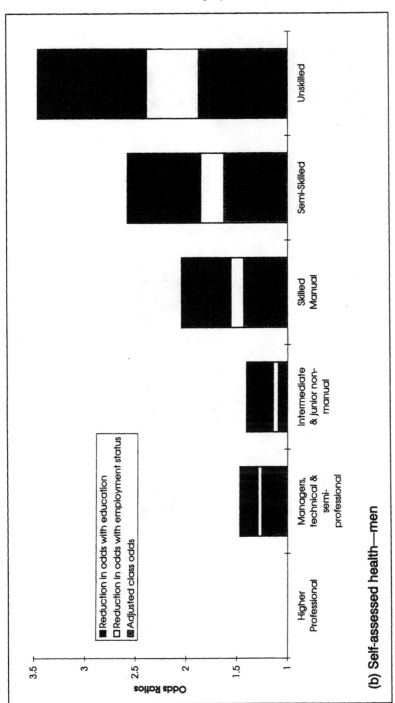

(b) Self-assessed health—men

Figure 2. Occupational class and ill-health of men: comparison of odds ratios for models. (a) Limiting long-standing illness; (b) self-assessed health.

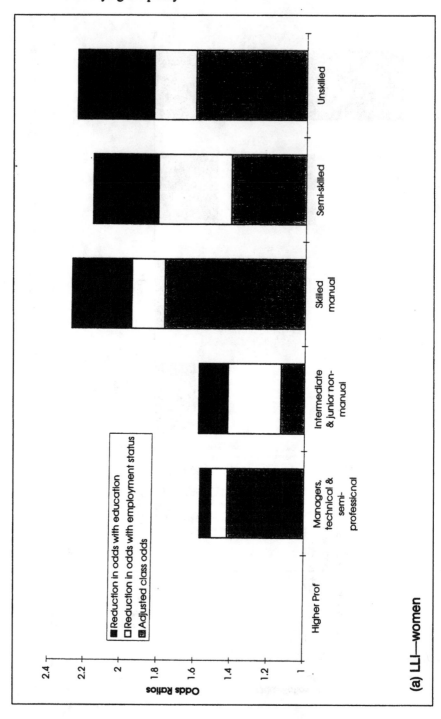

(a) LLI—women

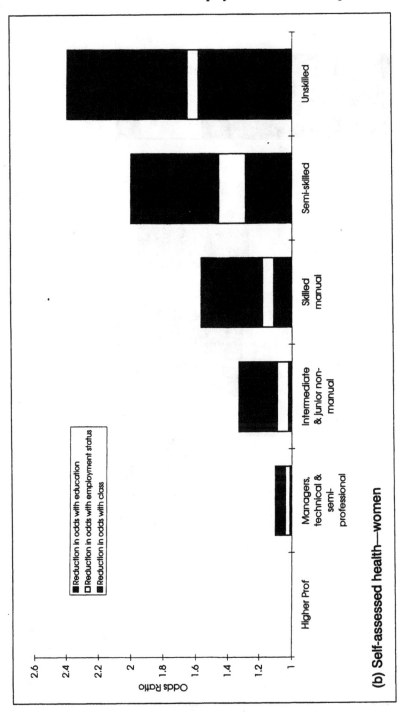

(b) Self-assessed health—women

Figure 3. Occupational class and ill-health of women: comparison of odds ratios for models. (a) Limiting long-standing illness; (b) self-assessed health.

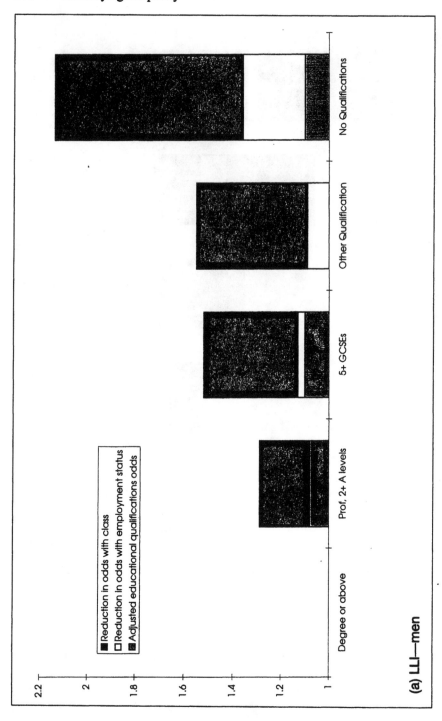

(a) LLI—men

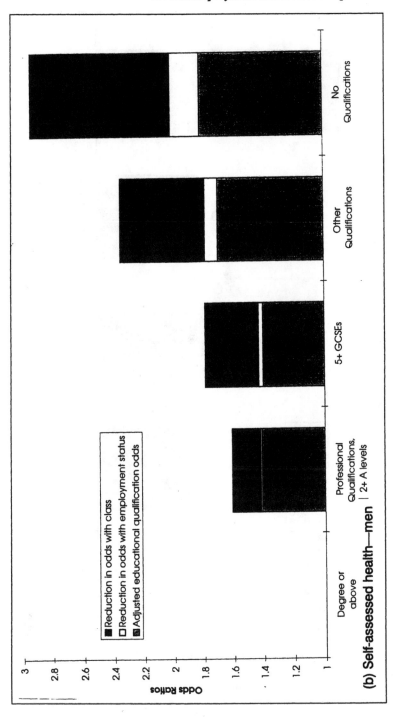

Figure 4. Educational qualifications and ill-health of men: comparison of odds ratios for models. (a) Limiting long-standing illness; (b) self-assessed health.

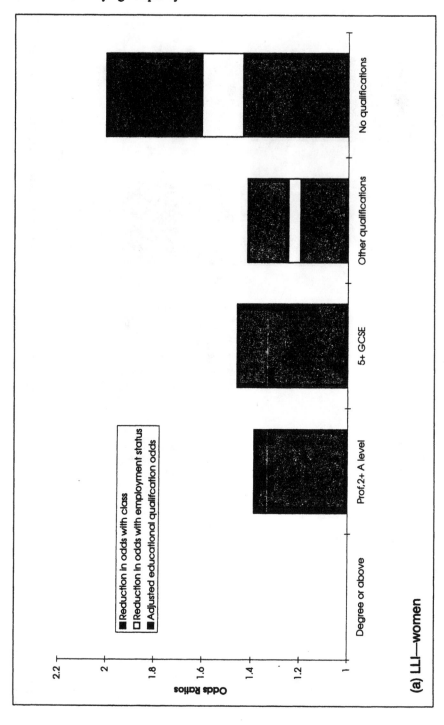

(a) LLI—women

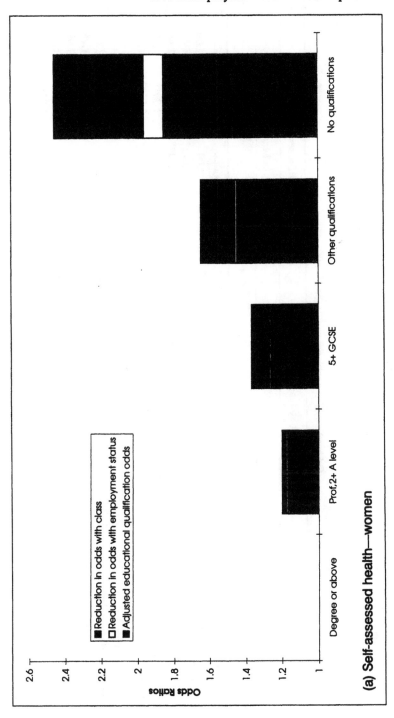

Figure 5. Educational qualifications and ill-health of women: comparison of odds ratios for models. (a) Limiting long-standing illness; (b) self-assessed health.

Table 4

Odds ratios of ill-health for men, aged 20–59[a]

	Limiting long-standing illness Models[b]				Self-assessed health Models[b]			
	2	3	4	5	2	3	4	5
Educational qualifications		+++	++	n.s.		+++	+++	+++
Degree or above		1.00	1.00			1.00	1.00	1.00
Professional qualifications, 2+ A levels		1.29*	1.08			1.61**	1.42**	1.41**
5+ GCSEs		1.52**	1.13			1.79**	1.43**	1.40**
Other qualifications		1.55**	1.09			2.36**	1.79**	1.70**
No qualifications		2.14**	1.36*			2.95**	2.02**	1.82**
Own occupational class	+++		+++	+++	+++		+++	+++
Higher professionals	1.00		1.00	1.00	1.00		1.00	1.00
Managers, lower professionals	1.61**		1.53**	1.44**	1.47**		1.29**	1.25**
Intermediate and junior nonmanual	1.65**		1.53**	1.47**	1.40**		1.14	1.09
Skilled manual, foremen	2.02**		1.80**	1.54**	2.05**		1.56**	1.43**
Semi-skilled	2.37**		2.04**	1.60*	2.59**		1.86**	1.63**
Unskilled	3.53**		2.94**	1.98**	3.48**		2.40**	1.88**

Employment status				+++				+++
Full-time				1.00				1.00
Part-time				1.51*				1.18
Unemployed				2.00**				1.61**
Retired				2.80**				1.57**
Other nonemployed				18.08**				7.55**
Model LLR^c	8,729	8,778	8,717	7,810	12,411	12,425	12,345	11,867
ΔLLR from base model	125	76	137	1,044	236	221	302	780
Δ df from base model	5	4	9	13	5	4	9	13
N	11,162				11,198			

Source: Data from *General Household Survey, 1991–92*, author's analysis.
^b Model 1, the base model, comprises age (in five-year age groups) and marital status. Significance of variable in the model: + P < .05; ++ P < .01; +++ P < .001.
Significance of difference from the reference category: * P < .05; ** P < .01; *** P < .001.
^c LLR, log likelihood ratio.

Table 5

Odds ratios of ill-health for women, aged 20–59[a,b]

| | Limiting long-standing illness | | | | Self-assessed health | | | |
| | Models | | | | Models | | | |
	2	3	4	5	2	3	4	5
Educational qualifications	+++	+++	+++	+		+++	+++	+++
Degree or above		1.00	1.00	1.00		1.00	1.00	1.00
Professional qualifications, 2+ A levels		1.39*	1.29	1.34*		1.20	1.16	1.18
5+ GCSEs		1.46**	1.31	1.34*		1.37**	1.26*	1.27*
Other qualifications		1.42**	1.24	1.20		1.65**	1.46**	1.45**
No qualifications		2.01**	1.61**	1.44*		2.47**	1.97**	1.86**
Own occupational class	+++		+++	+++	+++		+++	+++
Higher professionals	1.00		1.00	1.00	1.00		1.00	1.00
Managers, lower professionals	1.57**		1.51**	1.42*	1.10		1.04	1.01
Intermediate and junior nonmanual	1.58**		1.42*	1.13	1.33**		1.09	1.02
Skilled manual, foremen	2.28**		1.95**	1.77**	1.57**		1.18	1.11
Semi-skilled	2.17**		1.81**	1.41*	2.01**		1.46**	1.29*
Unskilled	2.26**		1.84**	1.61**	2.41**		1.66**	1.59**

Employment status				†††			†††
Full-time				1.00			1.00
Part-time				1.02			0.95
Unemployed				2.42**			1.81**
Housewife				1.93**			1.46**
Retired				2.52**			1.98**
Other nonemployed				29.11**			9.99**
Model LLR	10,274	10,284	10,252	15,254	15,226	15,168	14,674
ΔLLR from base model	68	58	90	192	220	278	772
Δ *df* from base model	5	4	9	5	4	14	22
N	12,266			12,311			

Source: Data from *General Household Survey, 1991–92*, author's analysis.
[b]See Table 4, footnotes *b* and *c*.

than occupational class for LLI. Including occupational class in the model removes the effect of education on long-standing illness for men (Model 4) and substantially reduces the effect of education on men's self-assessed health (Table 4 and Figure 4). Employment status has very little effect on the odds of ill-health by educational qualifications, unlike the major effects shown in Figures 2 and 3 for occupational class.

The association between educational qualifications and chronic illness is stronger for women than men (Figures 4a and 5a). Overall there is a weaker educational than occupational class gradient for men but less difference for women. Women and men with no qualifications have the poorest health, and those with degrees have the best health, but there is little difference in chronic illness among those with other levels of qualifications.

Employment status has a strong association with ill-health, after adjusting for occupational class and educational qualifications. Table 4 shows there is no difference in the health of women employed full-time and part-time, although part-time work for men is associated with higher levels of LLI. Unemployed women and men have over twice the odds of chronic illness compared with full-time workers. Full-time housewives also have higher levels of ill-health, confirming earlier work. The "other nonemployed" category includes people with long-term disabilities, as well as the temporarily sick, therefore this group is expected to have very high odds of chronic illness.

Employment status is very strongly associated with subjective health, but the variation in odds between the employed, unemployed, and housewives (for women) is less than for LLI. Housewives have about 50 percent higher odds of reporting poor health than employed women, and unemployed women have 81 percent higher odds. Unemployed men have 61 percent higher odds than men working full-time.

This analysis of data from the early 1990s has shown that to understand the health of working-age women and men, it is essential to clarify the interrelationships between educational qualifications, occupational class, and employment status. Educational qualifications and occupational class are strongly related to both measures of ill-health, even after including employment status in the models. Occupational class is a stronger predictor than educational qualifications of both measures of ill-health for men and of LLI for women. The class gradient is substantially weakened when employment status is included in the models, suggesting that where the nonemployed are excluded from class analyses the result will be a seeming weakening of class inequalities in health.

Educational qualifications show a sharper gradient than own occupational class for women's self-assessed health (Table 5). Educational qualifications have been largely neglected in previous research on inequalities in health in Britain, mainly because of an assumption that qualifications provide little discrimination within the population. However, the rapid expansion of higher education since the 1960s makes this supposed disadvantage no longer valid for those of working age.

Women's own class often reflects occupational downgrading following childbirth rather than their labor market potential (46–48), whereas educational qualifications are largely unchanging irrespective of childrearing and its effect on position in the labor market. Therefore, educational qualifications may be a particularly important measure of labor market potential for women and thus should be used as a complementary measure in research on inequalities in health.

INEQUALITIES IN HEALTH AMONG THE EMPLOYED AND NONEMPLOYED

This section addresses the third aim of the chapter: to assess whether class inequalities in health are as great among the nonemployed as among employed working-age people. The employed comprise full-time and part-time workers and the nonemployed comprise the unemployed, housewives, full-time students, the temporarily sick, and those not in employment because of long-term illness or disability. The occupational class of the latter group is based on their last occupation.

As shown in Table 2, nonemployed men disproportionately last worked in manual occupations, especially unskilled and semi-skilled occupations. Since the majority of working-age men who are nonemployed are either unemployed or not working because of disability, they are likely to be living on very low means-tested benefits in Britain in the 1990s. It might therefore be expected that being nonemployed will be the major determinant of ill-health, rather than the individual's previous position in the labor market measured by his or her last main occupation.

Models are contrasted for employed and nonemployed men and women using the two health measures (Tables 6 and 7). The models presented include educational qualifications and occupational class, after controlling for marital status and age (in five-year age groups) in the base model. Table 6 shows that the pattern of class inequalities in LLI differs for nonemployed and employed men. Among the nonemployed, all men previously in manual occupations have poorer health, while among those previously in nonmanual occupations there is a linear gradient. Men who were previously in manual occupations have over twice the odds of long-standing illness as men previously in higher manual occupations. This pattern contrasts with that for the employed, where the health of unskilled men stands out as very poor compared with the advantaged position of professional men, but there is little variation in the health of men currently working in other classes. Educational qualifications do not have a significant additional effect on LLI for either employed or nonemployed men.

The class gradient for men's self-assessed health is greater among the nonemployed than the employed (Table 6). Men who previously worked in manual occupations have much poorer self-assessed health than men in higher professional occupations, reflected in odds ratios that range from 2.28 for men

Table 6

Odds ratios of ill-health for employed and nonemployed men, aged 20–59[a,b]

	Limiting long-standing illness		Health "less than good"	
	Employed	Not employed	Employed	Not employed
Educational qualifications	n.s.	n.s.	+++	+
Degree or above			1.00	1.00
Professional, 2+ A levels			1.41**	1.41
5+ GCSEs			1.38**	1.68
Other qualifications			1.72**	1.81*
No qualifications			1.80**	2.12**
Own occupational class	+++	+++	+++	++
Higher professionals	1.00	1.00	1.00	1.00
Managers, lower professionals	1.54**	1.61*	1.23*	1.72*
Intermediate and junior nonmanual	1.55**	1.91*	1.06	1.83*
Skilled manual, foremen	1.53**	2.42**	1.38**	2.28**
Semi-skilled	1.66**	2.29**	1.63**	2.29**
Unskilled	2.37**	2.61**	1.98**	2.64**
Model LLR	6,040	2,122	9,776	2,253
ΔLLR from base model	32	26	149	54
Δ df from base model	5	5	9	9
N	9,404	1,777	9,436	1,781

[a]Source: Data from *General Household Survey, 1991–92,* author's analysis.
[b]See Table 4, footnotes *b* and *c*.

previously in skilled manual occupations to 2.64 for men previously in unskilled jobs. Thus, nonemployment may have a particularly detrimental effect on subjective health for men who occupy a lower position in the class structure. Such men are likely to have very few financial resources or assets to cushion their lives while nonemployed. Educational qualifications do not distinguish the long-term ill-health of employed or nonemployed men, but are associated with their subjective health.

Although occupational class inequalities are strong for nonemployed men, this is not the case for nonemployed women. Table 7 shows that a woman's last occupation does not have a statistically significant effect on her likelihood of having a long-standing illness, and for self-assessed health the effect is curved rather than linear. Women previously working in junior nonmanual occupations

Table 7

Odds ratios of ill-health for employed and nonemployed women, aged 20–59[a,b]

	Limiting long-standing illness		Health "less than good"	
	Employed	Not employed	Employed	Not employed
Educational qualifications	n.s.	++	+++	+++
Degree or above		1.00	1.00	1.00
Professional, 2+ A levels		1.61	1.14	1.30
5+ GCSEs		1.57	1.19	1.47
Other qualifications		1.43	1.43**	1.51*
No qualifications		1.96**	1.69**	2.16**
Own occupational class	++	n.s.	+++	+++
Higher professionals	1.00		1.00	1.16
Managers, lower professionals	1.47*		1.02	1.13
Intermediate and junior nonmanual	1.29		1.06	1.00
Skilled manual, foremen	1.94**		1.15	1.12
Semi-skilled	1.37		1.35*	1.33**
Unskilled	1.75**		1.57**	1.72**
Model LLR	5,707	4,049	9,940	4,932
ΔLLR from base model	19	36	116	82
Δ df from base model	5	4	9	9
N	8,477	3,789	8,506	3,805

[a]Source: Data from *General Household Survey, 1991–92,* author's analysis.
[b]See Table 4, footnotes b and c.

have the best self-assessed health, and women previously in unskilled occupations have the poorest health. The class gradient for LLI for employed women is nonlinear, with skilled manual women reporting the poorest health. Educational qualifications have a stronger effect on health for nonemployed than employed women, when included in models with occupational class.

This analysis has shown the importance of separately analyzing occupational class and employment status for both men and women. Class inequalities in health are somewhat greater for nonemployed than employed men. For nonemployed men there is evidence of a manual–nonmanual divide, whereas for employed men the poor health of the unskilled stands out sharply from other employed men. Class inequalities in health are less pronounced among women who are not in paid employment than among nonemployed men. Educational qualifications distinguish the health of nonemployed women better than previous occupational class. Thus, educational qualifications may be a better indicator of inequalities in health among nonemployed women than previous occupational class.

INEQUALITIES IN HEALTH AMONG OLDER PEOPLE

Many studies of inequalities in health entirely omit people above working age. Two factors highlight the need to consider this group in studies of health inequalities: first, the growth in the proportion of the population above state pension age, and second the trend toward earlier exit from paid employment of both women and men (49, 50), resulting in an increasing proportion of adult life spent after leaving paid employment. This section examines inequalities in self-assessed health, first for men and women aged 60–69, and then for men and women aged 70 and over. Among men in their sixties in Britain, only 22 percent work full-time and 7 percent work part-time (see Appendix). The labor force participation of women in their sixties is very low: only 4 percent work full-time and 11 percent work part-time.

Educational qualifications are generally considered to be of little value in analyzing health inequalities among older British people because two-thirds of women and 55 percent of men in their sixties have no qualifications (see Appendix). Men in their sixties are more likely to have a degree than women— 8 percent compared with 2 percent—and 8 percent of both men and women have professional qualifications or A levels (formerly, the higher level of the General Certificate of Education). When interpreting the effects of educational qualifications in these models, it is important to bear in mind the very skewed distribution of educational qualifications among this age group. The base model comprises age (in five-year age groups) and marital status (Model 1). Table 8 contrasts Model 2, which includes occupational class; Model 3, which includes educational qualifications; Model 4, which includes both occupational class and educational qualifications; and Model 5, which adds employment status.

For men and women in their sixties, there is a strong gradient with educational qualifications (Model 3). Men with no qualifications have three times the odds of poor health compared with men with a degree or professional qualifications. The gradients are stronger for women, although very few older women have higher qualifications. Occupational class has a strong effect on self-assessed health, especially for older men (Model 2). Men previously in manual occupations have over twice the odds of poor health compared with men in higher middle-class occupations.

A weaker gradient for women between occupational class and health was expected because many older women have not worked for a long period, sometimes since marriage over 40 years earlier. It is therefore remarkable that older women's own occupational class continues to have a statistically significant effect on their health. For older women the health divide is between those who previously worked in a nonmanual compared with a manual occupation.

As expected, those who continue in either full-time or part-time work in their sixties have better health than older people who are not working (Model 5). The odds of poor health are three times greater among men in their sixties who are nonemployed than among those working full-time. When employment status is included in the model, the gradient with occupational class strengthens rather than diminishes. This is because older people who are still in employment are more healthy but are disproportionately in semi-skilled and unskilled occupations (51).

For men and women over age 70, employment status is not analyzed because so few are in paid employment (see Appendix). In the General Household Survey, educational qualifications were not asked of people over age 70, so the model only contains occupational class based on the individual's last occupation, marital status, and age (in five-year age groups). Occupational class has a statistically significant effect on self-assessed health (Table 9). The gradients are particularly strong for men, with men formerly in semi-skilled and unskilled occupations having over twice the odds of poor health compared with higher middle-class men; for women the odds are over two-thirds higher for women who previously worked in semi-skilled and unskilled occupations.

Tables 8 and 9 show that class based on the older person's previous labor market position has a strong association with self-assessed health. In spite of having left the labor market a number of years earlier, men and women who previously worked in a higher occupational class continue to report better self-assessed health.

These findings suggest that an older person's previous labor market position continues to have a major influence on his or her health many years after leaving the labor market. This effect occurs for both men and women. It suggests that occupational class continues to exert an effect both through the longer term health consequences of working conditions and through the material resources associated with employment in different types of occupations, particularly receipt of occupational pensions, and the ability to accumulate other assets and wealth throughout working life.

CONCLUSION

This chapter has shown that the three measures of an individual's position in the labor market—educational qualifications, occupational class, and employment status—all have a major influence on health. This influence occurs for both men and women and continues for many years after formal retirement from the labor market. It is essential to clarify the causal ordering of these variables and to recognize that reverse causation is only likely between employment status and ill-health. Educational qualifications are closely associated with inequalities in

Table 8

Odds ratios of self-assessed health for men and women, aged 60–69[a,b]

	Men				Women			
	Models				Models			
	2	3	4	5	2	3	4	5
Educational qualifications		+++	+++	+++		+++	+++	+++
Degree or above		1.00	1.00	1.00		1.00	1.00	1.00
Professional qualifications, 2+ A levels		1.06	1.01	0.90		1.68	1.63	1.51
5+ GCSEs		1.40	1.14	1.08		2.06*	2.02*	1.87
Other qualifications		2.56**	1.88**	1.72**		2.26*	2.15*	1.90
No qualifications		3.03**	2.11**	1.91**		3.54**	3.04**	2.74**
Own occupational class	+++		+++	+++	+++		+	++
Higher middle-class	1.00		1.00	1.00	1.00		1.00	1.00
Intermediate and junior nonmanual	1.77**		1.42*	1.42*	1.22		0.97	0.94
Skilled manual, foremen	2.35**		1.73**	1.73**	2.07**		1.51*	1.47*
Semi-skilled	2.20**		1.53**	1.64**	1.65**		1.18	1.16
Unskilled	2.60**		1.76**	1.89**	2.02**		1.40*	1.53**

Employment status	+++				+++			
Full-time	1.00				1.00			
Part-time	1.04				1.15			
Not employed	2.51**				3.07**			
Model LLR	3,215	3,268	3,296	3,281	2,802	2,906	2,940	2,929
ΔLLR from base model	120	67	39	54	218	114	80	91
Δ df from base model	10	8	4	4	10	8	4	4
N				2,421				2,188

[a]Source: Data from *General Household Survey, 1991–92*, author's analysis.
[b]See Table 4, footnotes *b* and *c*.

Table 9

Odds ratios for self-assessed health as "less than good,"
men and women, aged 70 and over [a,b]

	Men	Women
Own occupational class	+++	+++
Higher middle-class	1.00	1.00
Intermediate and junior nonmanual	1.43*	0.95
Skilled manual	1.78**	1.57**
Semi-skilled	2.36**	1.76**
Unskilled	2.43**	1.68**
Model LLR	2,627	3,550
ΔLLR from base model	49	49
Δ df from base model	4	4
N	2,011	2,774

[a]Source: Data from *General Household Survey, 1991–92*, author's analysis.
[b]See Table 4, footnotes *b* and *c*.

self-assessed health and provide a powerful indicator for women. While occupational class should be the primary indicator in analyses of inequalities in health, educational qualifications should also be included, especially for women and for self-assessed health.

An increasing proportion of adults are not currently in paid work, which is more likely among those from lower occupational classes. If the nonemployed are excluded from analyses of inequalities in health, class inequalities will appear to be much smaller. Including the nonemployed in these class analyses (based on their last occupation) is advocated for *all* groups of nonemployed people. In Britain, such an approach has so far been restricted to nonemployed working-age men and has been less commonly used for other groups of nonemployed people.

The nonemployed should not be treated as homogeneous and considered as a separate group within analyses of inequalities in health. This chapter shows that there are stronger class inequalities in health among nonemployed than among employed men, but previous occupational class provides fewer clues about the health of nonemployed women. Educational qualifications are an important indicator of nonemployed women's health.

Little previous research has been devoted to examining structural inequalities in the health of older men and women, despite their representing a growing proportion of the population in all Western societies. In spite of older people having left the labor market a number of years earlier, previous employment in a higher occupational class continues to be associated with better self-assessed health.

The findings of this study support the political economy approach; class based on previous position in the labor market continues to structure the chances of active and independent life in Britain among all age groups of men and women, both inside and outside paid employment.

Acknowledgments — For access to the General Household Survey data for 1991–1992 I am indebted to the ESRC Data Archive, University of Essex, to the University of Manchester Computer Centre, and to the Office of Population Censuses and Surveys, which gave permission to use the GHS data. I am very grateful to Jay Ginn for her collaboration and for assistance with extracting the GHS data files, and to Avril Evitts for preparing the illustrations.

APPENDIX

Distribution of variables for men and women by age group (column percentages)[a]

Variable	20–59		60–69		70+	
	Men	Women	Men	Women	Men	Women
Limiting long-standing illness						
Yes	14	16	39	32	56	53
No	86	84	61	68	44	47
Self-assessed health						
Good	74	66	48	47	40	36
Fairly good or not good	26	34	52	53	60	64
Marital status						
Married or cohabiting	71	72	81	64	68	33
Never married	23	16	7	6	6	8
Previously married	6	12	12	21	26	59
Occupational class						
1. Higher professionals	19	6	17	3	17	3
2. Managers, employers, lower professionals	18	20	15	14	16	14
3. Intermediate and junior nonmanual	9	37	9	36	9	30
4. Skilled manual, own account, foremen	37	8	39	9	39	10
5. Semi-skilled, personal service	13	20	15	23	15	26
6. Unskilled	4	9	6	15	4	17
Educational qualifications[b]						
1. Degree or higher	12	7	8	2		
2. 2+ A levels, professional qualifications	16	14	8	8		
3. 5+ GCSEs	23	17	10	7		
4. Apprenticeship, other qualifications	21	29	18	13		
5. No qualifications	28	33	55	69		
Employment status						
Full-time (32+ hrs)	80	38	22	4	1	—
Part-time (under 32 hrs)	3	29	7	19	3	2
Unemployed	10	4	3	—	—	—
Full-time housewife	—	22	—	25	—	34
Retired	1	1	57	60	96	63
Other nonemployed (including disabled, temporarily ill, students)	7	5	11	1	—	1
Minimum base number						
Men	11,596		2,301		2,093	
Women	12,860		2,499		2,869	

[a]Source: Data from *General Household Survey, 1991–92,* author's analysis.
[b]GCSE, General Certificate of Secondary Education; A level, advanced level GCE.

REFERENCES

1. Hunter, D. J., and Vagero, D. (eds.), Health in 'Crisis'? Critical Problems in Health and Health Care. *Soc. Sci. Med.*, Special Issue, 32: 359–524, 1991.
2. Fox, A. J. (ed.). *Health Inequalities in European Countries.* Gower, Aldershot, 1989.
3. Department of Health and Social Security. *Inequalities in Health, The Black Report.* London, 1980.
4. Townsend, P., Davidson, N., and Whitehead, M. *Inequalities in Health and the Health Divide.* Penguin, Harmondsworth, 1988.
5. Fox, A. J., and Goldblatt, P. *Socio-Demographic Mortality Differentials from the OPCS Longitudinal Study 1971–75*, Ser. LS, No. 1. HMSO, London, 1982.
6. Davey Smith, G., Bartley, M., and Blane, D. The Black Report on socioeconomic inequalities in health 10 years on. *Br. Med. J.* 301: 373–377, 1990.
7. Arber, S. Opening the 'Black' box: Understanding inequalities in women's health. In *New Directions in the Sociology of Health*, edited by P. Abbott and G. Payne. Falmer Press, Brighton, 1990.
8. Arber, S. Class, paid employment and family roles: Making sense of structural disadvantage, gender and health status. *Soc. Sci. Med.* 32: 425–436, 1991.
9. Doyal, L. *What Makes Women Sick? Gender and the Political Economy of Health.* Macmillan, London, 1995.
10. Moser, K., Pugh, H., and Goldblatt, P. Inequalities in women's health: Looking at mortality differentials using an alternative approach. *Br. Med. J.* 296: 1221–1224, 1988.
11. Popay, J., and Bartley, M. Conditions of labour and women's health. In *Readings for a New Public Health*, edited by C. J. Martin and D. V. McQueen. Edinburgh University Press, Edinburgh, 1989.
12. Bartley, M., Popay, J., and Plewis, I. Domestic conditions, paid employment and women's experience of ill-health. *Sociol. Health Illness* 14: 313–343, 1992.
13. Macran, S., et al. Women's socio-economic status and self-assessed health: Identifying some disadvantaged groups. *Sociol. Health Illness* 16: 182–208, 1994.
14. Martikainen, P. Socioeconomic mortality differentials in men and women according to own and spouse's characteristics in Finland. *Sociol. Health Illness* 17: 353–375, 1995.
15. Stern, J. The relationship between unemployment and morbidity and mortality in Britain. *Popul. Stud.* 37: 61–74, 1983.
16. Warr, P. Twelve questions about unemployment and health. In *New Approaches to Economic Life*, edited by B. Roberts et al. Manchester University Press, Manchester, 1985.
17. Bartley, M. Unemployment and health: Causality or selection—a false antithesis? *Sociol. Health Illness* 10: 41–67, 1988.
18. Payne, R., Warr, P. B., and Hartley, J. Social class and psychological illhealth during unemployment. *Sociol. Health Illness* 6: 152–174, 1984.
19. Warr, P. B., and Jackson, P. Factors influencing the psychological impact of prolonged unemployment and re-employment. *Psychol. Med.* 15: 795–807, 1985.
20. Arber, S., and Ginn, J. *Gender and Later Life: A Sociological Analysis of Resources and Constraints.* Sage, London, 1991.
21. Arber, S., and Ginn, J. Gender and inequalities in health in later life. *Soc. Sci. Med.* 36: 33–46, 1993.
22. Arber, S., and Ginn, J. The gendered resource triangle: Health and resources in later life. In *Locating Health: Sociological and Historical Explanations*, edited by S. Platt et al. Avebury, Aldershot, 1993.
23. Arber, S., and Lahelma, E. Women, paid employment and ill-health in Britain and Finland. *Acta Sociol.* 36: 121–138, 1993.

24. Dahl, E. Inequality in health and the class position of women—the Norwegian experience. *Sociol. Health Illness* 13: 492–505, 1991.

25. Arber, S. Gender and class inequalities in health: Understanding the differentials. In *Health Inequalities in European Countries*, edited by A. J. Fox. Gower, Aldershot, 1989.

26. Goldthorpe, J. H. Women and class analysis: In defence of the conventional view. *Sociology* 17: 465–488, 1983.

27. Rahkonen, O., Arber, S., and Lahelma, E. Health inequalities in early adulthood: A comparison of young men and women in Britain and Finland. *Soc. Sci. Med.* 45: 163–171, 1995.

28. West, P. Inequalities? Social class differentials in health in British youth. *Soc. Sci. Med.* 27: 291–296, 1988.

29. Longino, C. F., Warheit, G. H., and Green, J. A. Class, aging and health. In *Aging and Health*, edited by K. S. Markides. Sage, Beverly Hills, 1989.

30. Glover, J., and Arber, S. Polarisation in mother's employment: Occupational class, age of youngest child, employment rights and work hours. *Gender, Work and Organisation* 2: 165–179, 1995.

31. Arber, S. Social class, non-employment, and chronic illness: Continuing the inequalities in health debate. *Br. Med. J.* 294: 1067–1073, 1987.

32. Dahl, E. Social inequality in health—the role of the healthy worker effect. *Soc. Sci. Med.* 33: 1077–1086, 1993.

33. Fox, A. J., Goldblatt, P., and Jones, D. R. Social class mortality differentials: Artefact, selection or life circumstances? *J. Epidemiol. Community Health* 39: 1–18, 1983.

34. Smith, K. Women, Work and Whether Occupation Matters: Differences in Mortality by Occupations in the US 1991–1987. Paper presented at the XIII World Congress of Sociology, Bielefeld, July 1994.

35. Vagero, D. Women, Work and Health. Paper presented at the XIII World Congress of Sociology, Bielefeld, July 1994.

36. Kitagawa, E. M., and Hauser, P. M. *Differential Mortality in the United States: A Study in Socioeconomic Epidemiology*. Harvard University Press, Cambridge, Mass., 1973.

37. Lahelma, E., et al. Comparison of inequalities in health: Evidence from national surveys in Finland, Norway and Sweden. *Soc. Sci. Med.* 38: 517–524, 1994.

38. Valkonen, T. Adult mortality and level of education: A comparison of six countries. In *Health Inequalities in European Countries*, edited by A. J. Fox. Gower, Aldershot, 1989.

39. Power, C., Fox, A. J., and Manor, O. *Health and Class: The Early Years*. Chapman and Hall, London, 1993.

40. Ginn, J., and Arber, S. Gender, class and income inequalities in later life. *Br. J. Sociol.* 42: 369–396, 1991.

41. Ginn, J., and Arber, S. Heading for hardship: How the British pension system has failed women. In *Social Security and Social Change: New Challenges to the Beveridge Model*, edited by S. Baldwin and J. Falkingham. Harvester Wheatsheaf, Hemel Hempstead, 1994.

42. Office of Population Censuses and Surveys. *General Household Survey, 1991*. HMSO, London, 1993.

43. Welin, L., et al. Prospective studies of social influences on mortality. *Lancet* i: 915–918, 1985.

44. Mossey, J. M., and Shapiro, E. Self-rated health: A predictor of mortality among the elderly. *Am. J. Public Health* 72: 800–808, 1982.

45. Shapiro, E., and Tate, R. Who is really at risk of institutionalization? *The Gerontologist* 28: 237–245, 1988.
46. Arber, S., and Gilbert, N. Re-assessing women's working lives. In *Women and Working Lives: Divisions and Change*, edited by S. Arber and N. Gilbert. Macmillan, London, 1991.
47. Martin, J., and Roberts, C. *Women and Employment: A Lifetime Perspective*. Department of Employment/OPCS. HMSO, London, 1984.
48. Dex, S. *Women's Occupational Mobility: A Lifetime Perspective*. Macmillan, London, 1987.
49. Kohli, M., et al. *Time for Retirement: Comparative Studies of Early Exit from the Labour Force*. Cambridge University Press, Cambridge, 1991.
50. Ginn, J., and Arber, S. Exploring mid-life women's employment. *Sociology* 29: 1–22, 1995.
51. Dale, A., and Bamford, C. Older workers and the peripheral workforce: The erosion of gender differences. *Ageing and Society* 8: 43–62, 1988.

PART 2

Physical Hazards:
Work, Violence, and Safety

Factors Associated with Work-Related Accidents and Sickness among Maquiladora Workers: The Case of Nogales, Sonora, Mexico

Hector Balcazar, Catalina Denman,
and Francisco Lara

The U.S.–Mexico border region is of great strategic importance because of the tremendous growth over the last 10 years of its population and its economic activity (1) and because of NAFTA (the North American Free Trade Agreement). The vigorous economic growth of the border area has been led by the expansion of the maquiladora industry in Mexico (1). More than 1700 maquiladora plants are currently operating on the Mexican side of the border area, employing close to 450,000 people (2).

Since the establishment of the Border Industrialization Program in 1965, Nogales has been the principal maquiladora center in the state of Sonora. In Nogales, approximately 87 plants are now in operation employing over 18,000 workers. Official estimates indicate that the maquiladora industry absorbs 36 percent of the labor force. However, this figure is probably higher than 50 percent, especially if indirect jobs are taken into account.

Due to the interconnectedness and efficiency of the highway infrastructure linking Sonoran border cities with those in Arizona, one-third of maquiladora industry contracts come from companies in the four corner states; Illinois and California occupy second and third places, respectively, as sources of maquiladora contracts in Nogales. The maquiladora industry in Nogales is comprised mostly of mid-sized plants. More than 70 percent of the plants in

The research described in this chapter was funded wholly or in part by the United States Environmental Protection Agency under assistance agreement CR 818296-01-0 to the Southwest Center for Environmental Research and Policy of Arizona State University. The chapter has not been subjected to the Agency's peer and administrative review and therefore may not necessarily reflect the views of the Agency, and no official endorsement should be inferred.

the city maintain workforce levels of below 300 employees. The most important sectors in the industry are electronic components and diverse manufacturing, which constitute 48 and 30 percent, respectively, of the maquiladora labor force.

One important aspect of the maquiladora plants in Nogales is their stability. Many of these plants have remained in the city for over 20 years and have ameliorated the effects of U.S. economic cycles on regional employment. Recently arrived migrant workers from southern Sonora and northern Sinaloa make up the main source of labor for the new positions created by expansion of the industry.

The constant economic expansion of the maquiladora industry in the border region has created a series of environmental and occupational problems (3). There is a growing environmental concern about the maquiladora industry in the U.S.–Mexico border area that can no longer be ignored, especially with NAFTA becoming operational.

This research project focuses on the health problems of maquiladora workers, specifically those who are associated with adverse working conditions in the maquiladora industry. The health of maquiladora workers in the border area has recently become an important topic of discussion from a public health perspective. One reason has been the increasing documentation of occupational health risks for workers exposed to certain types of working conditions in the maquiladora industry (4).

Earlier reports by Mexican researchers describing several health risk problems of maquiladora workers were published in the late 1970s and early 1980s (2). In the late 1980s several studies provided more specific evidence for problems in the following areas: working conditions, handling of equipment, exposure to a variety of toxic substances, lack of safety regulations for equipment use, and lack of information and instructions about handling toxic materials (2). Unfortunately, most of these studies lacked appropriate methodologies to investigate the health problems of maquiladora workers. Some of these limitations have already been described (5). Adequate sampling of workers exposed to a variety of working conditions and limitations associated with adequate reporting of health-related risks and perceptions of risks are among some of the problems that have not been sufficiently addressed. Only recently has multivariate statistical analysis been used when studying the health consequences of maquiladora work (5, 6), even though this type of methodology has been used in related studies of occupational health (7, 8).

In spite of these new studies, little information exists on the characterization of the sociodemographic profile and occupational history of maquiladora workers. The overall objective of our research was to document the occupational health problems in a sample of 497 workers of the maquiladora industry in Nogales, Sonora, Mexico. Specific objectives were to describe the sociodemographic profile, occupational history, working conditions, and health profile of maquiladora workers and to evaluate the factors (sociodemographic, occupational history, working conditions) that predict health outcomes such as accidents/diseases related to working conditions in our study sample.

METHODOLOGY

Research Design and Sampling Issues

This was a cross-sectional study of 497 maquiladora workers interviewed during the months of August and September of 1991, using a structured questionnaire. The sample was obtained from the Medical Services of Sonora (SEMESON), a health agency in charge of providing health certificates to workers that manage food, give personal services, or work in establishments employing high volumes of people, as in the maquila industry in Nogales, Sonora.

Two social workers were in charge of the recruitment of maquiladora workers who regularly attended the Medical Services of Sonora. Only workers of the maquiladora industry were selected to participate in the study. Every day, workers attended the Medical Services to obtain or renew a registration card needed by the maquiladora plants for the hiring process. By law, all maquiladora workers are required to obtain or renew a registration card before they are eligible to work in the maquila industry. The clinic hours for the provision of health screening services to get the registration card were between 6 a.m. and 10 a.m.

Maquiladora workers were selected each day during the study period. A necessary criterion for participation was that the subject had worked in the maquiladora industry within the six months prior to the interview. A letter explaining the study was given to each worker. Those who agreed to participate (the majority) were interviewed by one of the social workers. The interview lasted for 25 to 35 minutes, in which time a structured questionnaire was administered. On any given day during the data collection period an average of 12 workers were interviewed. Because of the characteristics of the study, it was not possible to sample all the workers of the maquiladora industry who attended the clinic during the study period. However, based on an average attendance rate at the clinic of 16 to 19 workers per day, more than 75 percent coverage was accomplished in this investigation for the period in question. Furthermore, based on the experience of the two social workers who conducted the interviews, there is no reason to believe that the eligible workers who were not interviewed differed from those who participated in the study.

Data Collection and Analytical Strategy

Two social workers from the community were hired and trained by the research team to administer the questionnaire. The questionnaire was standardized on a small sample of workers from the same health clinic. It included four sections related to the following areas: sociodemographic profile, occupational history, working conditions, and health profile.

The following variables were used in the bivariate analysis: gender of participant; age (<19, 20–29, ≥30); schooling (elementary incomplete, elementary complete, more than elementary); marital status (with or without partner); have children (yes/no); born in Nogales (yes/no); head of household (yes/no); number of persons sharing household food expenditures (<5, ≥5); only person providing financial support (yes/no); weekly family income (<382,363 pesos; ≥382,363 pesos); former work in other maquiladora (yes/no); number of maquiladoras previously worked in (1, 2, ≥3); other job just before working in maquiladora (yes/no); hours of work per week (<51, ≥51); extra hours worked (<15, ≥15); weekly wages (<104,228 pesos, ≥104,228 pesos); weekly wages as bonus (<25,315 pesos, ≥25,315 pesos); weekly wages extra (<64,977 pesos, ≥64,977 pesos); same task at maquiladora (yes/no); received training for performing each task (yes/no); change in task has been an improvement (yes/no); production standards in job (yes/no); production standard has changed (yes/no); agree on how problems are solved (yes/no); a doctor or nurse at place of work (yes/no); perceive some risk associated with working conditions (yes/no); plant offers information about work-related risks (yes/no); received safety equipment at the plant (yes/no); a health/safety commission at the plant (yes/no); work carries a risk for accidents (yes/no).

A detailed description of the characteristics associated with the labor force and changes in working conditions has been reported elsewhere (9).

Descriptive results are presented based on frequency distributions for selected variables of the four areas covered in the questionnaire. We performed analyses of t-tests on some of the continuous variables. The descriptive results shown in Table 1 are classified by gender. Odds ratios and 95 percent confidence intervals were calculated for those variables found to be significantly associated with the health outcome variables (accidents and disease/sickness conditions attributed to maquiladora work). We performed multivariate logistic regression analyses using variables that were statistically significant at the $P < .05$ level from the bivariate analysis. The dependent variables in the logistic regression models were the presence/absence of accidents and disease or sickness associated with working conditions. These conditions were reported by the subject at the time of the interview based on the following questions: Did you have any work-related accident during the last six months? Did you have any work-related disease or sickness during the last six months? Adjusted odds ratios were calculated using the antilogarithm of the regression coefficient found to be statistically significant after adjusting for all of the other variables included in the logistic regression model.

Table 1

Descriptive statistics of selected occupational history characteristics
of maquiladora workers, by gender

Variable	Males			Females		
	n	Mean	SD	n	Mean	SD
Hours worked per	247	51.2	7.7	247	51.0	7.5
week	63	14.5	6.0	54	16.0	7.2
Extra hours worked						
Weekly wages, base salary, pesos	248	108,812	35,106	247	99,627	20,718*
Weekly wages, bonus, pesos	205	27,629	23,147	196	22,895	13,093*
Weekly wages, extra hours, pesos	64	68,042	46,531	48	60,892	34,798
Number of different jobs within plant	63	2.8	1.5	48	2.7	1.1

*Significant t-value $P < .05$.

RESULTS

A total of 248 males and 249 females participated in the study. Of the total sample, 56.6 percent were single, 41.4 percent had children, 26.2 percent were born in Nogales, and 29.5 percent were identified as heads of household. Some attributes of interest from the sample are those related to variables such as education, age, income, and migration. More than 50 percent of both men and women had more than elementary education. More than 45 percent of the sample migrated for reasons associated with better work opportunities. The labor force of the maquiladora industry in Nogales is a relatively young population. The mean age of men and women fluctuates between 22 and 23 years of age. However, 12 percent of the work force consisted of workers over 30 years. Differences in income were found between men and women, even though there were no differences in the number of hours they worked (Table 1).

The average number of hours of work for the sample was 51, with 7.6 percent of the subjects working between 65 and 81 hours per week. The results on the number of different jobs performed within the plant (2.8 percent for men and 2.7 percent for women) show that there is some internal mobility within the plant between different jobs. These numbers are greater than those reported for other border cities.

A careful examination of the occupational history factors reported by the workers sheds light on the type and quality of working environment within the maquiladora plants sampled (Table 2). Among the important factors to consider are changes in standards of production, working relationships with the supervisor, changes in task performance, and satisfaction with the job and/or with the manager. Close to 45 percent of the sample had previously worked in maquiladoras.

A detailed description of work-related health problems and perceptions about health risks is shown in Table 3. In our sample, 12.6 percent (61 cases) reported having an accident within the last six months while working in the maquila, and 18.3 percent (89 cases) reported having an episode of sickness/disease related to work. More than 40 percent of the accidents required at least one day of disability from the IMSS (Mexican Institute of Social Security). The parts of the body most affected were the fingers and the hands. More than 50 percent of the sample reported that working conditions carried some types of health risk. The types of risk mentioned most frequently were damage produced by machines and instruments, damage produced by toxic substances, damage to the eyes, and burns.

From a public health standpoint, it is important to describe the occupational health problems of maquiladora workers in terms of the different factors associated with work-related accidents or diseases. This information is crucial to the design of effective occupational health programs. Thus, health outcomes associated with work-related accidents (Table 4) and work-related disease/sickness (Table 5) were used as dependent variables. Unadjusted odds ratios and their 95 percent confidence intervals were calculated for all the dichotomous variables.

For the outcome variable "having a work-related accident in the last six months" (unadjusted odds from Table 4), four factors were associated with a higher probability of being classified as having a work-related accident at the bivariate level: head of household, changes in production standards, and the two risk perception variables. The greatest odds were associated with the two risk perception variables. The presence of a doctor or nurse at the plant was related to a lower probability of having a work-related accident.

Table 5 describes the factors found statistically significant when tested individually against the variable presence of work-related disease/sickness in the last six months (unadjusted odds). The following factors were associated with the presence of work-related disease/sickness: perceptions of risk, other job just before working in maquiladora, and weekly wages below the mean base salary. Other factors—being a male, being born in Nogales, agreeing on how problems are solved, and the plant offering information about work-related risks—were associated with a lower probability of work-related disease/sickness.

Finally, in order to validate the bivariate analysis, we performed multiple logistic regression analyses for those variables associated with work-related accidents (Table 4) and work-related disease/sickness (Table 5). The adjusted odds

Table 2

Frequency distribution of occupational history variables of
maquiladora workers for the total sample

Variable	N	Percent
Have you worked before in other maquiladora?		
Yes	221	44.7
No	273	55.3
Total	494	100.0
In how many maquiladoras have you worked before?		
1	116	52.5
2	65	29.4
3	22	10.1
>3	18	8.1
Total	221	100.0
Are there production standards in your job?		
Yes	262	53.1
No	231	46.9
Total	493	100.0
Has the production standard changed?		
Yes	78	29.8
No	184	70.2
Total	262	100.0
Have you had the same task at the maquiladora?		
Yes	387	78.4
No	106	21.6
Total	493	100.0
Have you received training for performing each task?		
Yes	74	66.1
No	38	33.9
Total	112	100.0
Has the change in tasks signified any improvement?		
Yes	61	54.5
No	51	45.5
Total	112	100.0
Did you have another job just before working in maquiladora?		
Yes	202	40.9
No	292	59.1
Total	494	100.0

Table 3

Frequency distribution of health-related risks associated with working
conditions of maquiladora workers for the total sample

Variable	N	Percent
Is there a doctor/nurse where you work?		
Yes	414	83.5
No	81	16.5
Total	495	100.0
Do you perceive some risk associated with working conditions?		
Yes	258	52.1
No	237	47.9
Total	495	100.0
Does the plant offer information about work-related risks?		
Yes	341	69.0
No	153	31.0
Total	494	100.0
Have you received safety equipment at the plant?		
Yes	270	54.4
No	224	45.6
Total	494	100.0
Is there a health/safety commission at the plant?		
Yes	311	63.3
No	89	18.1
Don't know	91	18.6
Total	491	100.0
Did you have a work-related accident in the last 6 months?		
Yes	61	12.6
No	425	87.4
Total	486	100.0
What part of your body was injured?		
Eyes	3	4.9
Fingers	28	45.9
Hands	10	16.4
Arms	4	6.6
Feet	1	1.6
Other	15	24.6
Total	61	100.0

Table 3 (Cont'd.)

Variable	N	Percent
Where did you receive medical treatment/care?		
Physician at plant	16	26.2
IMSS	20	32.8
Private doctor	2	3.2
Other	23	37.8
Total	61	100.0
Number of disability days		
1–7	14	22.9
>7	15	24.6
None	32	52.5
Total	61	100.0
Does your work carry a risk for accidents?		
Yes	297	60.0
No	198	40.0
Total	495	100.0
Have you had a work-related disease/sickness in the last 6 months?		
Yes	89	18.3
No	398	81.7
Total	487	100.0
Were you incapacitated?		
Yes	9	10.1
No	80	89.9
Total	89	100.0

ratios and their 95 percent confidence intervals are also included in Tables 4 and 5. For the variable "work-related accidents" (adjusted odds, Table 4) two factors remain statistically significant: the presence of a doctor or nurse at the plant and the risk perception variable. Having a doctor or nurse was associated with a lower probability of work-related accidents; risk perception was highly related with the probability of a work-related risk. Five factors were found to be statistically significant for the variable "work-related disease/sickness" (adjusted odds, Table 5). Interestingly, women had a greater probability of a work-related disease/ sickness. In addition, the variable "plant offers information about work-related risks" was associated with a lower probability of work-related disease/ sickness. As expected, the risk perception factor had the highest adjusted odds ratio.

Table 4

Odds ratios (O.R.) and 95 percent confidence intervals (C.I.) of variables found
statistically significant when tested against variable "Did you have a
work-related accident in the last 6 months?"

Variable	O.R.[a]		95% C.I.	
	Unadj.	Adj.	Unadj.	Adj.
Head of household?				
(Yes)	1.62		1.01–2.60	
Has the production standard changed?				
(Yes)	2.20		1.20–4.04	
Is there a doctor/nurse where you work?				
(Yes)	0.54	0.30	0.32–0.91	0.11–0.93
Do you perceive some risk associated with working conditions?				
(Yes)	4.08		2.17–7.65	
Does your work carry a risk for accidents?				
(Yes)	12.84	52.21	4.08–40.41	5.74–474.40

[a]Unadj., unadjusted odds ratio; Adj., adjusted odds ratio controlling for the other variables in the logistic regression model.

DISCUSSION

The results of this study clearly demonstrate the need to consider the occupational health problems of maquiladora workers in the border region when formulating public health programs and policies at both the governmental and nongovernmental levels. Overall, our results are in accord with some of the occupational health problems reported in previous studies (2, 4). In our sample, more than 60 percent of the subjects perceived health-related risks or reported an accident related to working conditions. These results suggest the need to find specific programs and policies to improve safety conditions in the maquiladora industry.

The identification of risk is necessary to its elimination, reduction, correction, or prevention (9). According to the results of this study, half the accidents

Table 5

Odds ratios (O.R.) and 95 percent confidence intervals (C.I.) of variables found
statistically significant when tested against variable "Have you had a
work-related disease/sickness in the last 6 months?"

	O.R.[a]		95% C.I.	
Variable	Unadj.	Adj.	Unadj.	Adj.
Sex				
(Male)	0.90	0.40	0.83–0.98	0.22–0.74
Born in Nogales				
(Yes)	0.56		0.33–0.94	
Did you have other job just before working in maquiladora?				
(Yes)	1.50	2.09	1.03–2.19	1.17–3.75
Weekly wages (mean base salary)				
(<104,228 pesos)	1.12	2.15	1.03–1.21	1.16–3.97
Do you agree on how problems are solved?				
(Yes)	0.55	0.49	0.37–0.82	0.27–0.89
Do you perceive some risk associated with working conditions?				
(Yes)	2.92	8.97	1.85–4.60	2.71–29.70
Does the plant offer information about work-related risks?				
(Yes)	0.49	0.39	0.34–0.71	0.22–0.68
Does your work carry a risk for accidents?				
(Yes)	1.85		1.19–2.87	

[a]Unadj., unadjusted odds ratio; Adj., adjusted odds ratio controlling for the other variables in the logistic regression model.

reported by the workers were not registered as such by the IMSS. For example, the incidence of work-related accidents reported by the subjects in this study was 12.6 percent, much greater than the incidence rate of 6.4 percent for 1989 reported by IMSS in Nogales. In recent years this rate has decreased even further (9). The 12.6 percent rate in our sample excludes workers who had suffered a sufficiently serious accident to quit work and therefore were not available for interview. This selection bias could have masked a much greater incidence of negative health outcomes (accidents and/or work-related disease conditions) in this study. Furthermore, underreporting clearly depicts a flaw in the registration and monitoring of accidents and diseases associated with the maquiladora industry. Underregistration of accidents by IMSS may be due to several factors. A likely explanation is that IMSS tends to register as work-related accidents only those incidents reported officially by the maquiladora and which require sick leave. It is also highly probable that the increased medical attention offered at the workplace has resulted in the decreased number of work-related accidents reported by IMSS. In our survey, 84 percent of the workers reported the presence of medical services at the maquiladora plants. This is a relatively new phenomenon in the maquilas and requires additional research.

The problem associated with lack of reporting of health problems in the maquiladora industry is augmented by the migration of workers to other maquiladoras. Furthermore, evaluation of the type of maquila industry (textile, electronic, apparel, etc.) is crucial for the identification of specific health problems related to a variety of working conditions. Unfortunately, in this study we could not obtain this type of specificity.

Our results provide valuable subjective information on workers' feelings, attitudes, and perceptions toward health problems associated with the maquiladora industry. This type of information has not been documented in previous studies and needs to be included in any research intended to consider workers' health, including maquiladora workers (5, 6). Although we believe that our results are real in terms of perceptions of risk and of work-related accidents and diseases/sickness reported by the workers interviewed, the possibility of overreporting of risk perception by those who experienced an accident cannot be ruled out. Longitudinal studies are needed to overcome this problem.

In fairness to the maquiladora industry, the negative results on occupational health reported in this research should not be extrapolated to cover the whole gamut of industries in the border cities. A recent study conducted by Guendelman and Silberg (6) points out the possibility that previously reported adverse effects of maquiladoras have been exaggerated. This is not to diminish, however, the need to elucidate more carefully the specific health detriments associated with working conditions regarded as highly risky—namely, exposure to carcinogens, toxins, and other hazardous substances, long and monotonous working conditions, lack of safety procedures in the working environment, dissatisfaction with managerial procedures, etc. In fairness to the workers, it is also imperative that additional resources be allocated to resolving health issues associated with maquiladoras, both at the research level and for the development of intervention programs.

Future studies should incorporate both male and female workers, evaluate gender differences in risk perception and health-related problems, and examine the factors that predict these outcomes. Our study found a lack of availability of medical personnel and a lack of pertinent information about the risks of work-related disease/sickness. These factors have important implications for health policy in Nogales, Sonora, and probably in many other border cities. In this regard, not only should medical personnel be available at the plants, but these personnel should be trained to identify health risks associated with working conditions. A particular concern is that most maquiladora physicians we have interviewed in Nogales are not occupational medicine specialists and are not trained to identify and deal with work-related problems. In addition, it is crucial that new policies be established to incorporate preventive measures within plant operations.

Finally, we must consider the opinions of the workers themselves on improvements to augment work satisfaction and reduce the health risks in the maquiladoras. We have identified several recommendations in our recent publication (9).

REFERENCES

1. EPA-SEDUE. Integrated environmental plan for the Mexico–U.S. border area. First stage, 1992–1994. Working draft. U.S. Environmental Protection Agency and Secretaria De Desarrollo Urbano y Ecologia. August 1991.
2. Instituto Nacional de Estadistica, Geografia e Informatica. Servicios de Informacion Oportuna. No. 45. Aguascalientes, Mexico, 1993.
3. Sanchez, R. Manejo transfronterizo de residuos toxicos y peligrosos: una amenaza para los paises del tercer mundo. *Frontera Norte* 2: 91–114, 1990.
4. Denman, C. Tiempos modernos: trabajar y morir. Toxicos en la maquila. In *Modernizacion y Legislacion Laboral En El Noroeste de Mexico*, pp. 195–220. El Colegio de Sonora, Universidad de Sonora y Fundacion Friedrich Ebert, 1990.
5. Hovell, M., et al. Occupational health risks for Mexican women: The case of the maquiladora along the Mexican–United States border. *Int. J. Health Serv.* 18: 617–627, 1988.
6. Guendelman, S., and Silberg, M. The health consequences of maquiladora work: Women on the US–Mexican border. *Am. J. Public Health* 83: 37–44, 1993.
7. Lemasters, G., et al. Reproductive outcomes of pregnant workers employed at 36 reinforced plastics companies. II. Lowered birth weight. *J. Occup. Med.* 31: 115–120, 1989.
8. Lipscomb, J., et al. Pregnancy outcomes in women potentially exposed to occupational solvents and women working in the electronics industry. *J. Occup. Med.* 33: 597–604, 1991.
9. Denman, C., et al. Reestructuracion productiva y condiciones de trabajo en la maquila en Sonora. In *Sindicalismo, Relaciones Laborales y Libre Comercio*, pp. 135–163. El Colegio de Sonora, 1993.

CHAPTER 17

Sugar and Spice and Everything Nice: Health Effects of the Sexual Division of Labor among Train Cleaners

Karen Messing, Ghislaine Doniol-Shaw,
and Chantal Haëntjens

In many countries, women in the paid labor force work at a small number of jobs (1–5). It has been calculated that in order for North American men and women to be distributed randomly across occupational categories, two-thirds of the total working population would have to change jobs (6). In Canada, for example, 55 percent of women work at only 20 jobs, primarily clerical, health care, teaching, waitressing, hairdressing, or assembly line work such as sewing machine operator. Only five occupations are common to the lists of the top 20 men's and women's jobs (7).

Studies done in several countries have shown that women are further segregated into specific tasks within occupations. In the Québec Ministry of Social Affairs, where 73 percent of workers in 1979 were women, an analysis showed that men and women had separate job titles and separate responsibilities at all levels (8). In factories in France (9), Québec (10), Nova Scotia (11), and Norway (12), women and men are in different parts of the production line.

This sexual division of labor is a major factor determining male–female wage differences (5, pp. 41–46; 13, pp. 15–20; 14). For this reason, women are entering nontraditional jobs in increasing numbers. However, desegregation has often been blocked using arguments based on presumed biological differences between the sexes; women are thought to be assigned to specific jobs because they are too exacting, and women are intrinsically weaker and technically less competent than men (13, pp. 35–39; 15). Others have suggested that the sexual division of labor is

This work was supported by a collaborative fellowship from the Québec and French governments and by the Women and Work program of the Social Sciences and Humanities Research Council of Canada.

based not on women's abilities or job characteristics, but rather on shifting demands of the labor market (1, 16).

The question of whether the sexual division of labor is based on biological differences between the sexes has been approached in two ways. First, the experience of women in nontraditional jobs has been examined. Social barriers to the employment of women in nontraditional jobs have been described (13, 16), but biologically based arguments have also been invoked. Exclusion of women because of their "natural" qualities sometimes appears to be borne out by events in the workplace. In 1982, a group of women brought a case before the Canadian Human Rights Commission asking that women be hired in blue-collar jobs in a railway company. The employer argued that women did not like to do dirty jobs and were unable to do heavy work. The Commission found that the tests used to qualify workers for these jobs were inappropriate, and ordered the company to begin an affirmative action program in order to hire women in nontraditional jobs. However, ten years later, only three of the 20 or so women hired were still employed in this company, whose workforce is over 1,200 (17).

This sequence, in which women attempt to enter nontraditional jobs and are eliminated, may reinforce stereotypes concerning women's strength and aptitudes (18). Addressing this issue, ergonomic analyses of some jobs from which women have been eliminated, including jobs in the railway company mentioned above (17), have revealed that there may be obstacles to women's integration because of the dimensions of working surfaces and tools, resulting in a higher probability of injury for women workers in nontraditional jobs, as well as greater difficulties for women workers in maintaining production (19). Changes in tools and equipment can enable women (and other smaller workers) to perform more safely and efficiently. To some extent at least, difficulties attributed to biological differences may be remedied by job redesign.

A second approach to examining biological differences in job qualifications has been to ask whether women's traditional work is less exacting than men's. Several authors have reviewed the specific physical and technical characteristics of women's work (7, 12, 20). An ergonomic study of data entry work showed that such "unskilled," low-paid work involved a high degree of technical competence whose exercise was not only unrecognized but sometimes had to be hidden from supervisors (21). A study of workers in a cookie factory has shown that technical requirements of women's jobs were unrecognized by both women and men (22).

A fast workspeed is probably the most common characteristic of women's jobs in factories and offices, and a fast overall pace is one of the costs of the "double workday" (19, 23). Women in poultry slaughterhouses make 60 movements per minute; sewing machine operators sew 225 pairs of pants an hour; typists may be controlled by their microcomputers, which scold them if they haven't "produced" a sufficient number of characters in a given time period; hospital workers describe intense time pressures; working mothers rush from job to stores to home (24–26). The physical load resulting from a fast workspeed has been associated with musculoskeletal problems among workers in women's employment "ghettos" (27–29), and the resulting mental load has been associated with stress-related illness (30).

Thus, researchers have suggested that, far from respecting men's and women's biology, the sexual division of labor may have adverse effects on health (31–33). In the course of an ergonomic analysis of train cleaning in France we found a rigid sexual division of labor (34). We present here the results of the analysis and some reflections on the health implications of this sexual division of labor.

The approach that we used, developed by French ergonomists (35), combines observation of work in real-life situations with information obtained from interviews with workers and management. Workers are asked to explain various aspects of their ways of doing their job ("modes opératoires") in the hope that the explanations will reveal technical and physical requirements of their work not apparent in their job descriptions. For example, the data entry clerks mentioned above explained to the research team that they secretly programmed the central computer in order to save time on their jobs (21). Women sewing gloves on an assembly line explained the complexities involved in matching the two halves of a badly cut glove, and researchers were enabled to understand why the physical requirements of this apparently routine undemanding job made it difficult for any but the youngest workers (36). Although such ergonomic studies of a very limited number of workers do not permit generalizations regarding women's work, they can furnish rich detail about the work actually done by some women. We describe here a single job, toilet cleaning, assigned specifically to women. Since we found that there was great resistance to men doing this job, we present it as an example of physical characteristics of a job that can justly be described as "women's work."

MATERIALS AND METHODS

The Cleaning Company

The employer was a cleaning service that had recently signed a contract with the French Société nationale des chemins de fer (SNCF), for a period of three years. The contract requires cleaning of suburban trains according to a schedule determined by the SNCF, which approves the tools and materials used and inspects the trains after cleaning. In France, contracting companies are required to hire the personnel of the previous contractor; thus, the employees' seniority had been acquired with a series of previous employers. During the present study, the employer went bankrupt and its contract was taken over by another branch of the same company.

Access to the site was gained through the recommendation of the occupational health physician. Although the researchers were allowed unlimited observation time, workers were not freed for organized interviews or information gathering. Conversations and interviews with the latter were always conducted on an informal basis and were held either while working or during coffee breaks.

Study Population

Nineteen men and 17 women were employed on a permanent basis; several people were employed occasionally or for short contracts. The mean age of regular male employees (on December 1, 1990) was 47 ± 9.5 years, and the mean age of the women was 39 ± 9.5 years. Four times as many men as women were over 50. The average seniority of men was 16 ± 7 and of women 8 ± 8 years (Figure 1).

Data Collection

Work was done in shifts. The morning shift (12 to 16 workers) was from 7:30 a.m. to 4:18 p.m.; a group of five to six worked from 8:45 a.m. to 5:33 p.m.; the afternoon shift of 12 to 16 workers was between 2:45 p.m. and 11:33 p.m. Numbers of workers per shift varied according to peak days, and an extra shift was added on Fridays. Our observations were concentrated on the morning shift. Work was observed globally during four two-hour periods, three in the morning and one during the afternoon. In addition, toilet cleaning by three workers was observed systematically for a total of ten hours during morning shifts. Observations of the first five of the ten hours were recorded using paper and pencil (three hours noting actions performed plus two hours noting postures), and the

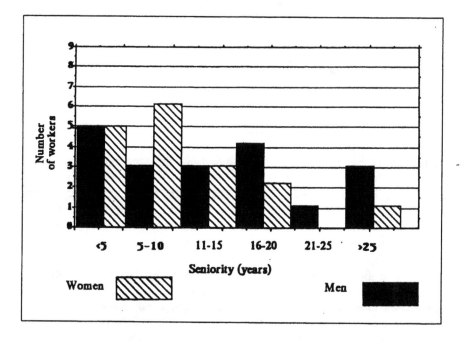

Figure 1.   Distribution of seniority, by sex, among French train cleaners.

rest of the observations were done using the Psion Organiser II programmed with the Kronos program (patented by Alain Kerguelen), which permits simultaneous recording of several categories at a time. We recorded postures, time per toilet, the state of the toilet, and the state of the water supply. Postures were classified as "standing," "slightly bent," (angle between trunk and legs < 135°), "bent" (angle < 90°), and "crouched" (angle < 45°).

Distances were calculated using the K & E "Thermor" pedometer previously calibrated with the stride of the individual worker and against a measured distance.

Interviews were carried out on work content with the company director, the union representative ("délégué du personnel"), the section head ("inspectrice de chantier"), and the foreman ("chef de chantier"). Conversations about work content and health symptoms took place with the three regular toilet cleaners, and informal conversations occurred with many other employees. In addition, depersonalized compilations of health symptoms existing at the time of any medical interview during the previous five years were supplied by the company's occupational health physician.

Absence records were compiled from the registers of the company for the four months starting September 1990, for all permanent employees. Train schedules were compiled for typical workdays.

RESULTS

Work Organization

The cleaning of suburban trains was organized as follows (workers refer to themselves by the names of their tools or the objects cleaned). The "brush" picked up all objects (newspapers, soft drink cans) from the floor under the seats and the seats themselves, leaving them in the aisle. The "broom" swept the aisle and put all rubbish and dirt into a bag. The mechanized "water cart" drove from car to car and filled the reservoirs for the bathrooms, which were cleaned by the "toilet." The "railings" polished railings and chrome surfaces. The "team leader" dusted after all others had passed. The "foreman" worked out of an office, where he planned the work. If numbers permitted, most cleaning tasks were done by two people who cleaned alternate cars. The cleaning of main line trains was organized in a similar way, with the addition of three tasks: emptying ashtrays, cleaning the bar, and polishing the tray tables at each seat.

The sexual division of labor was clear. The positions of "water cart," "railings," "team leader," and "foremen" were always men; "brush" was mixed; and "broom" was usually a woman. "Toilet cleaners," "ashtrays," "tray tables," and "bar" were always a woman. In fact, strikes were threatened on two occasions when the sexual division of labor was questioned, once when men were asked to clean toilets and once when the company offered to train women to drive the water cart. In both cases the company backed down and the changes were never instituted.

Constraints Associated with These Jobs

Time constraints were very heavy. Twenty to 30 trains were cleaned per shift, concentrating during peak periods. Most of these were suburban trains, which were cleaned in four to 12 minutes, depending on the time available. Time available to clean a train began from the arrival of the train and ended when the first passenger was allowed to embark, ten minutes before departure. Trains often arrived late and time for cleaning was thereby reduced. During the study, a work accident ensued when a "broom," in her hurry to begin cleaning the train, positioned herself next to the steps and was hit in the eye with the briefcase of a disembarking passenger.

The complaint voiced first by all workers asked "What is the principal problem on your job?" was, "We run all the time"; this was also the major complaint raised during a five-day strike during the course of the study. Since the trains could arrive on any track and the sequence of tracks was not coordinated with the cleaning schedule, cleaners had to move constantly between different tracks as well as along the 100- to 200-meter long trains. Often, two halves of a train would depart at different times; workers would clean the front half, then clean a train eight or more tracks distant before returning to clean the second half. Pedometer readings for "broom" and "toilet cleaning" gave 22.2 ± 1.6 kilometers per shift.

Health Problems and Absences

In France, the occupational health physician must examine each worker once a year. Table 1 presents the problems reported during the previous five years' examinations of the 19 men and 17 women. Despite the relative age and greater seniority of the men (Figure 1), they reported many fewer health problems, particularly musculoskeletal problems.

Absenteeism was very high among cleaners, averaging 13 percent (number of days absent as percentage of number of days scheduled to work). Absent workers were not replaced, and those present were asked to do the work of those absent. Women's rate of absence was nearly three times that of men (Figure 2), and 76 percent of women were absent at least once during the four month sampling period, compared with 45 percent of men. The reasons for absence were not available from company records.

Absences of women posed a particular problem for toilet cleaning, because men would not be asked to clean toilets. Thus, although three women per shift were usually assigned to this task, all regularly employed women were assigned to this task at least once during the study period. In the afternoon shift, it was difficult to recruit enough women, because when they acquired seniority they transferred to the morning shift (Table 2), which was easier for them because of family responsibilities. In addition, the company doctor forbade several women with back problems to do tasks that required bending and kneeling, such as toilet cleaning. This contributed to the shortage of women for this task. One 40-year-old woman reported that her foreman refused to accept her medical certificate and

Table 1

Pathologies recorded during annual medical
examinations of French train cleaners, 1985–1990

Pathology[a]	Women (N = 17)	Men (N = 19)
Back pain	7	3
Wrist pain	5	2
Joint pain, upper limb	1	0
Ankle pain	2	0
Knee pain	2	0
Stomach pain	2	5
Circulatory problems		
Heavy legs	11	4
Varicose veins	7	0
Phlebitis	2	2
Asthenia at end of workday	12	1

[a]The same worker could have more than one pathology.

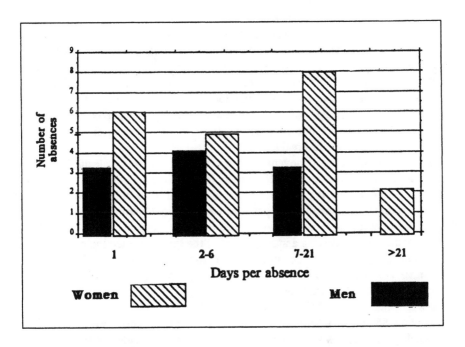

Figure 2.   Distribution of absences from work, by sex, among French train cleaners, September–December 1990.

Table 2

Seniority by shift among French train cleaners

	Morning shift		Afternoon shift	
	Women	Men	Women	Men
Seniority, years	10	15	5	12
Number of workers	12	7	5	11

threatened her with the loss of her job if she would not clean toilets on a Sunday morning when she was the only woman present.

Characteristics of Toilet Cleaning

Between 180 and 240 bathrooms were cleaned per shift. Workers were required to clean taps, sinks, and mirrors, remove stains from walls, wash floors, and clean toilet fixtures in each cubicle. Two women were normally assigned to cleaning toilets, but there were frequent exceptions. The second toilet cleaner often replaced absent or reassigned colleagues. On weekends and during slack periods, only one toilet cleaner was assigned.

Cleaning time varied between 63 and 108 seconds per toilet as a function of the number of cleaners available. If one worker was available she took 63 seconds to clean each toilet (average of 86 toilets); in the presence of a coworker, she took 108 seconds (average of 30 toilets) to clean each of half the number of toilets. Toilet cleaning time also varied as a function of how dirty the toilets were. About three-quarters (72 percent) of the toilet cleaner's time was occupied by cleaning toilets or moving from one to another, 20 percent by waiting for trains, and 8 percent was allowed for breaks.

A number of difficult movements were involved in toilet cleaning. Toilet cleaners carried a bucket with all their tools and cleaning solutions, weighing 2 to 3 kilograms, during their movements between cars and between trains. A large number of uncomfortable postures were required because of space limitations. Observation of 35 toilets showed that the workers spent only 11 percent of their cleaning time standing and 25 percent of the time in a kneeling or crouched position. They changed from one position to another once every 3.0 ± 0.2 seconds. Thirty-eight percent of a sample of 317 postural changes involved a displacement for the trunk over an angle of greater than 90° with the legs (between "standing" and "bent," for example).

Among 86 toilets where the operations were noted, very few toilets were cleaned in the same way. Adjustments were constantly made for the type and location of dirt. Angles of attack, scrubbing motions, and sequences of movement were all modified in response to the specific situation encountered in each toilet.

In addition, some operations were added or eliminated in response to time constraints, changes in water supply, and the state of the toilet (6).

Toilet cleaners reported feeling disgusted in various situations. In one toilet in five (of 86 sampled), human solid waste had been deposited elsewhere than in the bottom of the toilet bowl, requiring a special effort to scrub it off. On one occasion, a dog defecated on one of the train seats and the "brush" normally assigned to clean the seats called on the toilet cleaner to remove it, resulting in a quarrel over jurisdiction. On weekends, vomitus was frequently found on the floors. No special precautions were taken with this material other than the use of gloves.

DISCUSSION

Characteristics of Women's Work in Train Cleaning

Men's and women's jobs in train cleaning were not compared. However, one job that was exclusively assigned to women, toilet cleaning, had characteristics sometimes thought to be associated with stereotypes of male jobs, that is, it was physically demanding, required technical knowledge, and involved considerable exposure to dirt and filth.

Physical Load

Physical strength is the aspect most often mentioned as a justification of differential job assignment, by both employers and employees (18, 37, 38). In fact, jobs that involve lifting of heavy weights all at once with rest intervals between each lift are most frequently assigned to men, with the exception of patient care tasks in the health care professions and lifting children in day care centers (39). However, it has been shown that traditional women's jobs often involve manipulating a large *total* weight per day. Laundry workers in one study lifted 1,800 kg of wet sheets per day, one by one, and they also pushed or pulled 6,000 kg per day (40). In another factory, sewing machine operators manipulated a total of 3,500 kg per day with their arms and 16,000 kg with their legs (41). Although force was not systematically measured in the present study, the task of toilet cleaning shows a similar pattern of exertion. Workers exert themselves constantly during scrubbing tasks and carry a loaded bucket over long distances, although they do not lift single heavy weights.

The sexual division of labor is often justified by the estimate that women average two-thirds of men's physical strength, based on laboratory tests using psychophysiological testing, in which subjects are asked to lift objects whose weight is increased until the subject reports feeling uncomfortable (42); biomechanical testing, in which dynamic strength is measured by exerting a maximal force against a machine; or physiological testing, in which energy consumption is monitored in relation to exertion (43). However, these tests do not measure suppleness, such as the ability to bend and twist constantly at great speed as in the work of the toilet cleaners, or endurance, such as the ability to keep up a fast work speed throughout the day.

Endurance may be an especially important physical component of women's traditional jobs when the domestic workload is taken into account (44). Although no systematic study of the length of the domestic workday was undertaken in this workplace, a contemporary study revealed that women working full-time in French slaughterhouses do an average of 20 hours of domestic tasks weekly (compared to two hours for the average male coworker) (45). Informal conversations with women train cleaners revealed that most women with families lived outside Paris and commuted up to two and a half hours per day. Several married women said they had exclusive responsibility for domestic tasks; greater female responsibility for these tasks was indicated by the male–female differential in the relationship between shift preference and sex (shown in Table 2). One toilet cleaner spoke of a workday that began at 4 a.m. with making the family breakfast and finished at 9 p.m. with helping the children with their homework.

Technical Competence

A requirement for technical competence is often used to justify assigning men to machine maintenance and surveillance, and women often refuse jobs with machines because of the fear of technical inadequacy (46). However, traditional women's work involves its own requirements for technical competence. As mentioned above (21, 36), hidden qualifications may be involved in apparently routine tasks. In toilet cleaning, technical skill is required to clean a toilet adequately in 63 seconds, while adjusting one's techniques for all the possible locations and types of dirt.

Dirt and Filth

In hospitals, women are assigned to many tasks involving exposure to human excretions. In the home, women have traditionally cared for infants, including changing diapers. The assignment of toilet cleaning in trains to women appears to follow a trend in which dirty jobs are preferentially assigned to women. The fact that a woman was called to clean up the dog excrement although its location made it part of the task of a man illustrates the extent to which this activity was sex-typed.

Biological Basis of the Sexual Division of Labor

The suggestion that the sexual division of labor is based on biological differences between the sexes appears to be supported by the association between women's work and certain job characteristics such as fast movements, repetition, and lack of autonomy (9, 19, 47–49). Men's traditional work, on the other hand, is thought to be heavy and dirty and to require technical knowledge (17–19). The present study shows that toilet cleaning, done by women, involves fast movements and repetition, and thus to some degree bears out this association.

It may be that the type of physical expenditure in traditional jobs is better adapted to the characteristics of the average woman than to those of the average man. Men's larger mean muscle mass facilitates lifting heavy weights. Other parameters of the capacity to do physical work have not yet been fully explored in relation to sex differences. For example, it has been suggested that women have more "fast twitch" fibers than men, and thus might be better suited to work at jobs requiring endurance, although this hypothesis has not been confirmed experimentally (50).

However, this study also shows that requirements for heavy physical labor, technical knowledge, and tolerance of dirt do not prevent jobs from being assigned to women, and may indeed be characteristic of certain jobs considered to be "women's work."

Health and Safety Implications

The health problems observed in this study can be attributed to working conditions poorly adapted to human physiology. Toilet cleaning, done at some time during our study by all 17 women workers, requires walking 20 kilometers per day, cleaning 180 to 240 toilets, spending 49 minutes kneeling or crouched, and changing postures about 5,000 times (200 toilets) 25 posture changes per toilet). We think that illness and fatigue caused by these job requirements could explain the high rate of absence among these women. Although women workers' absences were attributed by various members of the administrative staff to women's family responsibilities, this explanation was not borne out by the fact that women's absences were of relatively long duration (Figure 2). Policies dealing with absences appeared to exacerbate the problem; for example, the fact that absent workers were not replaced meant that the second toilet cleaner was often eliminated. The remaining woman had to cope with a sharply increased workload, which was a result but possibly also a further cause of the high level of absenteeism among women. Although the hypothesis that absenteeism was related to occupational illness could not be verified, since reasons for absence were confidential, it is borne out by the relatively high incidence of various health symptoms, particularly musculoskeletal symptoms, among women workers.

The health problems may reflect combined effects of employment in train cleaning and in the home on women workers. Absence could be due to adverse effects of heavy workload on health and to a reluctance to face such heavy work on any days when the workers are feeling even a bit under the weather.

The sexual division of labor based on male–female biological differences is only one type of worker selection. Older or disabled workers, for example, may be unable to perform certain tasks. Genetic screening has been proposed in order to select workers who may be resistant to toxic chemicals in the workplace. Thus, worker selection is used as a method of promoting efficiency and preventing industrial disease (51). However, it has been argued that the health of all workers may be protected more efficiently by adapting workplaces to a wide variety of physical types than by selecting workers in relation to single, rigidly conceived positions (38). Work would thus be rendered less dangerous for all, irrespective of body type.

Unduly heavy work in train cleaning is not limited to women workers. Many of the other jobs are also extremely demanding. The "brush" works bent over most of the time, the "railings" and "water cart" must occasionally carry heavy loads, and "ashtrays" and "tray tables" require rapid wrist movements that have been suspected of giving rise to carpal tunnel syndrome ("wrist pain" in Table 1). The repetitive character of most of these tasks combined with the awkward movements performed may involve a risk of disability in later life, as has been observed for clothing industry workers (27). Although women train cleaners show a larger proportion of health problems at this time, some of the men may eventually suffer long-term effects of their tasks.

The report submitted to the company and to the employee representative recommended several changes, including better tools, improved conditions for breaks, increases in personnel, and redesign of train bathrooms to facilitate cleaning (34). Workers generally agreed with these recommendations. However, there was much greater resistance to our recommendation to rotate all jobs so that difficult tasks would be shared and to avoid repetitive strain injury. This resistance was heard from both women and men. Similar resistance has been noted to sharing of domestic tasks (52–54). Walkerdine (55) and Cockburn (13) have suggested that changes in sex roles and in sex-based task assignments encounter resistance because of their profound roots in identity and fantasy life as well as their relation to issues of power and dominance. It may therefore be difficult to change the sexual division of labor even though it appears to involve a heavy cost for women train cleaners, and may also involve health effects for their male colleagues.

Acknowledgments — This work would not have been possible without the enthusiastic collaboration of the cleaning staff, especially Nina, Patricia, and Michelle. We are grateful to the cleaning company for generous access to the site and to some company records.

REFERENCES

1. Bradley, H. *Men's Work, Women's Work.* University of Minnesota Press, Minneapolis, Minn., 1989.
2. Reskin, B. *Sex Segregation in the Workplace.* National Academy Press, Washington, D.C., 1984.
3. Corvi, N., and Salort, M. *Les Femmes et le Marché du Travail.* Hatier, Paris, 1986.
4. Walby, S. *Sex Discrimination at Work.* Open University Press, Milton Keynes, England, 1988.
5. Armstrong, P., and Armstrong, H. *Theorizing Women's Work.* Garamond Press, Toronto, 1991.

6. David, H. *Femmes et emploi: le défi de l'égalité.* Presses de l'Université du Québec, Montréal, 1986.
7. Messing, K. *Occupational Health and Safety Concerns of Canadian Women.* Labour Canada, Ottawa, 1991.
8. Gaucher, D. L'égalité: Une Lutte à Finir. M.A. thesis, Département de sociologie de la santé, Université de Montréal, 1979.
9. Kergoat, D. *Les Ouvrières.* Sycomore, Paris. 1982.
10. Messing, K., and Reveret, J.-P. Are women in female jobs for their health? A study of working conditions and health effects in the fish-processing industry in Québec. *Int. J. Health Serv.* 13: 635–643, 1983.
11. Lamson, C. On the line: Women and fish plant jobs in Atlantic Canada. *Relations industrielles* 41: 145–157, 1986.
12. Kaul, J., and Lie, M. When paths are vicious circles: How women's working conditions limit influence. *Econ. Industr. Democracy* 3: 465–481, 1982.
13. Cockburn, C. *Machinery of Dominance: Women, Men and Technical Know-how.* Pluto Press, London, 1985.
14. Stathan, A., Miller, E. M., and Mauksch, H. O. *The Worth of Women's Work.* State University of New York Press, Albany, N.Y., 1988.
15. Messing, K. Do men and women have different jobs because of their biological differences? *Int. J. Health Serv.* 12: 43–52, 1982.
16. Reskin, B., and Roos, P. A. *Job Queues, Gender Queues.* Temple University Press, Philadelphia, 1990.
17. Courville, J., Vézina, N., and Messing, K. Analysis of work activity of a job in a machine shop held by ten men and one woman. *Int. J. Industr. Ergon.* 7: 163–174, 1991.
18. Ward, J. S. Sex discrimination is essential in industry. *J. Occup. Med.* 20: 594–596, 1978.
19. Courville, J., Vézina, N., and Messing, K. Analyse des facteurs ergonomiques pouvant entraîner l'exclusion des femmes d'un poste de travail de tri mécanisé de colis postaux. *Le Travail Humain,* 1992, in press.
20. Mergler, D. Rapport-synthèse. Les conditions de travail des femmes. In *Les effets des conditions de travail sur la santé des travailleuses,* edited by J.-A. Bouchard, pp. 215–227. Confédération des syndicats nationaux, Montréal, 1983.
21. Teiger, C., and Bernier, C. Ergonomic analysis of work activity of data entry clerks in the computerized service sector can reveal unrecognized skills. *Women and Health* 18: 67–78, 1992.
22. Dumais, L., et al. Baker's man, baker's woman, make me a cake as fast as you can: The sexual division of labour in an industrial bakery during hard times. Unpublished manuscript. CINBIOSE, Université du Québec à Montréal.
23. Kauppinen-Toropainen, K., Kandolin, I., and Mutanen, P. Job dissatisfaction and work- related exhaustion in male and female work. *J. Occup. Behav.* 4: 193–197, 1983.
24. Mergler, D., et al. The weaker sex? Men in women's jobs report similar health symptoms. *J. Occup. Med.* 29: 417–421, 1987.
25. Leppänen, R. A., and Oikinuora, M. A. Psychological stress experienced by health care personnel. *Scand. J. Work Environ. Health* 13: 1–8, 1987.
26. Billette, A., and Piché, J. Organisation du travail et santé mentale chez les auxiliaires en saisie des données. *Santé mentale au Québec* X: 86–98, 1985.
27. Brisson, C., Vinet, A., and Vézina, M. Disability among female garment workers. *Scand. J. Work Environ. Health* 15: 323–328, 1989.
28. Punnett, L. Soft tissue disorders in the upper limbs of female garment workers. *Scand. J. Work Environ. Health* 11: 417–425, 1985.

29. Hägg, G., and Suurküla, J. Relations between shoulder/neck disorders and myoelectric signs of local muscle fatigue in female assembly workers. *Proceedings of the 1984 International Conference on Occupational Ergonomics* 1: 324–327, 1984.
30. Alexander, R. W., and Fedoruk, M. J. Epidemic psychogenic illness in a telephone operators' building. *J. Occup. Med.* 28: 42–45, 1986.
31. Stellman, J. *Women's Work, Women's Health.* Pantheon, New York, 1977.
32. Hunt, V. *Work and the Health of Women.* CRC Publications, Boca Raton, 1978.
33. Chavkin, W. *Double Exposure.* Monthly Review Press, New York, 1984.
34. Messing, K., Haëntjens, C., and Doniol-Shaw, G. L'invisible nécessaire: l'activité de nettoyage des toilettes sur les trains de voyageurs en gare. *Le travail humain,* 1993, in press.
35. Guérin, F., et al. *Comprendre le travail pour le transformer.* Editions de l'ANACT, Montrouge, France, 1991.
36. Teiger, C. Les contraintes du travail dans les travaux répétitifs de masse et leurs conséquences sur les travailleuses. In *Les effets des conditions de travail sur la santé des travailleuses,* edited by J.-A. Bouchard, pp. 33–68. Confédération des syndicats nationaux, Montréal, 1984.
37. Ward, J. S. Women at work. Ergonomic considerations. *Ergonomics* 27: 475–479, 1984.
38. Messing, K., Courville, J., and Vézina, N. Minimizing health risks for women who enter jobs traditionally assigned to men. *New Solutions: A Journal of Environmental and Occupational Health Policy* 1: 466–471, 1991.
39. Lortie, M. Analyse comparative des accidents déclarés par des préposés hommes et femmes d'un hôpital gériatrique. *J. Occup. Accidents* 9: 59–81, 1987.
40. Brabant, C., Bédard, S., and Mergler, D. Cardiac strain among women laundry workers doing repetitive, sedentary work. *Ergonomics* 32: 615–628, 1989.
41. Vézina, N., and Courville, J. Integrating women into traditionally masculine jobs. *Women and Health* 18: 97–118, 1992.
42. Snook, S. H., and Ciriello, V. Maximum weights and work loads acceptable to female workers. *J. Occup. Med.* 16: 527–534, 1974.
43. Aghazadeh, F., and Dharwadkar, S. R. Effect of gender on physical work capacity and strength. In *Trends in Ergonomics/Human Factors,* II, edited by R. E. Erberts and C. G. Erberts, pp. 551–557. Elsevier Science Publishers, Amsterdam, 1985.
44. Tierney, D., Romito, P., and Messing, K. She ate not the bread of idleness: Exhaustion is related to domestic and salaried work of hospital workers in Québec. *Women and Health* 16: 21–42, 1990.
45. Messing, K., Romito, P., and Saurel-Cubizolles, M.-J. "Moonlighting" as a Mom: Domestic Workload Should Be Considered when Evaluating the Effects of Shiftwork. Paper presented at the Colloque sur le travail posté de l'Association Internationale d'ergonomie, Paris, July 1991.
46. Cockburn, C. Technical Competence, Gender Identity and Women's Autonomy. Paper presented at the World Congress of Sociology, Madrid, July 9–13, 1990.
47. Molinié, A.-F., and Volkoff, S. Les conditions de travail des ouvriers . . . et des ouvrières. *Economie et Statistique* 118: 25–28, 1980.
48. Kauppinen-Toropainen, K., Kandolin, I., and Haavio-Manila, E. Sex segregation of work in Finland and the quality of women's work. *J. Organizational Behav.* 9: 15–27, 1988.
49. Klitzman, S., et al. A women's occupational health agenda for the 1990s. *New Solutions* 1: 1–11, 1990.
50. Courville, J. Différences biologiques entre les hommes et les femmes et activité de travail. M.Sc. thesis, Department of Biological Sciences, Université du Québec à Montréal, 1990.
51. Hubbard, R., and Henifin, M. S. Genetic screening of prospective parents and of workers: Some scientific and social issues. *Int. J. Health Serv.* 15: 231–251, 1985.

52. Vandelac, L. The New Deal des rapports hommes-femmes: Big deal! In *Du travail et de l'amour*, edited by L. Vandelac. Editions St-Martin, Montréal, 1985.
53. Romito, P. *La naissance du premier enfant,* Chapt. 8. Delachaux et Nestlé, Lausanne, Switzerland, 1990.
54. Le Bourdais, C., Hamel, P. J., and Bernard, P. Le travail et l'ouvrage. Charge et partage des tâches domestiques chez les couples québécois. *Sociologie et sociétés* 19: 37–55, 1987.
55. Walkerdine, V. *Schoolgirl Fictions.* Verso Press, London, 1990.

CHAPTER 18

State-Level Clustering of Safety Measures and Its Relationship to Injury Mortality

*Phil Brown, Nicole Bell, Peter Conrad,
Jonathan Howland, and Martha Lang*

Most indicators of overall societal health focus on general mortality, infant mortality, and morbidity and mortality of major disease categories such as cardiovascular disease and cancer. Injury is rarely discussed as a major indicator, despite its importance. Injuries accounted for nearly 150,000 deaths in the United States in 1991, one-fourteenth of the total, ranking third after heart disease and cancer. For ages 1 to 44, injuries were the leading cause of death (1). Injuries are the leading cause of lost years of potential life, accounting for 4.3 million lost years of expected life annually, compared with approximately 3 million each for cancer and heart disease (2).

Injuries also represent a major economic cost. In 1991 unintentional injuries alone cost society $177.2 billion (3). Injuries resulted in 114 million physician visits in 1985, second only to respiratory illness (1).

Injuries are very much a social phenomenon, akin to most elements of health status. Many injuries show strong class, race, and sex gradients, and often appear to be the result, primarily, of "exogenous" factors, such as vehicles, poisons, worksites, and weapons (1). This suggests potential biogenic (e.g., genetic and physiological) causes may be of less importance than social structural causes. This is important in that exogenous variables are more likely to be amenable to change through intervention. However, to date, the role of such social factors has not been incorporated into the study of injury etiology or prevention.

Existing research on injuries in general is limited. It typically focuses on distinctions such as intentional versus unintentional, or merely lists each major category of injury (e.g., falls, drowning, poisoning). Although there is much

This research was supported by grants from the Henry J. Kaiser Family Foundation and from the Small Grants Program of the Brown University Dean of Research.

attention given to motor vehicle injuries, surprisingly little attention has been given to many other categories. As yet, there has been no systematic look at social structural causes and distribution of injuries. We already know that societally developed preventive measures are often quite effective in reducing injuries (e.g., seat belt laws, automobile redesign regulations, smoke detectors). Some of the most effective strategies, such as motor vehicle safety initiatives, have strong social ramifications in pointing to flaws in corporate and governmental policies.

We propose a new social model for investigating injury morbidity and mortality. This approach is guided by the "Society and Health" perspective (4) which incorporates both micro-level features such as normative values, and macro-level features such as social inequality and state regulation. We view the normative values of safety as, first, a set of assumptions about government and citizen roles in creating a safer society, and second, the legislation and regulation that stem from that set of assumptions. Norms are especially important because they are needed to mobilize the production of new safety policies. Changes in norms can arise from a variety of sources, perhaps especially from social movements (e.g., Mothers Against Drunk Drivers (MADD)). The media also provide a source of norm development, as in the designated driver campaign ("Friends don't let friends drive drunk"). Also important are changes in professional views, for example the new epidemiologic knowledge that drunken driving is largely a phenomenon not of chronic alcoholics, but of many ordinary people. In some cases there is a *norm lag*, in which regulation and legislation must catch up to public norms. But when regulation and legislation do occur, they formalize the identification and redefinition of certain social problems. For example, smoking in public becomes labeled a deviant act once there is a sufficient normative basis, combined with a regulatory apparatus.

The macro-level element of state regulation flows in part from the prevailing social norms, as discussed above. But regulation also has a long-standing position in the state apparatus. State action to regulate industry, natural resources, transportation, and communication has long been a large factor in society, frequently the result of struggles between classes or other social groupings. In our view, many of the safety-oriented policies that we are looking at in this analysis are the result of political struggles to make a safer society. Advocates for this direction are motivated by a long history of other state regulation.

This leads to a discussion of the role of inequality in safety policies, as well as social inequality in injury mortality. The above-mentioned legacy of safety advocacy often stems from a desire to make the whole society more equitable. Because the least privileged work at the most dangerous jobs, live in the unhealthiest areas, and have less access to health services, they suffer more injuries and have a greater need for safety policies.

Over the last several decades injury rates have declined (1). Essentially, U.S. society is getting safer over time. One interpretation is that there may be an ongoing process whereby we are consciously working to make the country a safer, hence better place. This leads us to conceptualize a higher level of both humane social organization and socioeconomic development. At the same time, this general advance is uneven and is accompanied by socially structured differences. For example, men continue to have higher injury morbidity and mortality for most categories of injury. This may be due both to different work roles and work settings and to greater risk-taking by men. In addition, income remains important—the living environments of the poor are less safe. Melvin Nelson's evidence from South Carolina is striking here (5). He compared overall childhood mortality (age 28 days to 17 years) between AFDC children (children whose families receive Aid to Families with Dependent Children) and non-AFDC children, and found that AFDC children had 2.7 times the overall mortality. For cause-specific mortality, the ratio of AFDC to non-AFDC mortality is even more telling, as shown in Table 1, listed in descending magnitude of the ratios. The two highest class disparities, fires and poisoning injuries, are 6.9 and 6.1 to 1, respectively. With the addition of homicide and suffocation (both injury categories), four of the six greatest class disparities in mortality were observed for injuries.

Injuries are measurable, describable, and predictable events following fairly well-defined epidemiologic patterns (6). Injury morbidity and mortality is often preventable, and the processes for prevention are very much a feature of political action and social movements. As such, examination of injuries as a social structural phenomenon may be useful. While numerous social units might be used to investigate the influence of social factors on injury, in the United States states may be particularly useful since systematic data are collected for these entities and since states have much leeway in designing safety laws and regulations.

State-level data have been too infrequently analyzed in research on health status. Bird and Baumann (7), noting that state-level data have rarely been used to examine infant mortality, found that political, economic, and social variables had high explanatory power for infant mortality, accounting for more variation than did health services variables. Strauss (8) makes a strong case for using state-level data. He notes that many social scientists have argued against analysis of state-level data on the assumption that state populations are too heterogeneous. But, as Strauss points out, so are cities. State-level data exist for a large array of concerns, and thus should be used. To bolster his argument, Strauss hypothesized that Standard Metropolitan Statistical Areas (SMSAs) and non-SMSA areas in a state would be similar on a large number of social indicators. He computed correlations for all 90 variables in the *County and City Data Book*, finding that 85 were significant, with more than half having $r > 0.70$. Strauss noted that states have major roles in legislation and administration of many areas of social life, and thus are a very appropriate level of analysis. We believe this can be relevant to the public policies that might affect injury mortality.

Table 1

Differences in childhood mortality between children in families receiving
AFDC and other children, aged 28 days to 17 years[a]

Mortality category[b]	AFDC/non-AFDC ratio		
	White	Nonwhite	Total
All causes	2.8	2.3	2.7
Fire	6.8	4.2	6.9
Poison	11.2	—	6.1
Perinatal conditions	6.7	3.7	5.4
Pneumonia and flu	8.9	2.2	4.8
Homicide	4.3	2.7	4.7
Suffocation	—	3.4	4.3
Heart disease	3.1	3.1	3.8
Congenital anomalies	5.1	2.8	3.5
Inhalation/ingestion	7.8	—	3.3
Drowning	—	2.1	2.3
Cancer	2.8	—	1.8
Motor vehicle	—	1.7	1.4

[a]Source: adapted from reference 5, p. 1132.
[b]Specific causes are shown in descending order of AFDC/non-AFDC ratio, based on total population of all races.

There is a lot of evidence that unsafe behaviors cluster (9). For example, people who drive drunk are likely to also speed, drive recklessly, and engage in other dangerous behaviors (10). People who smoke are more likely to drink and drive and are less likely to wear seat belts (11). Risk-taking behaviors in adolescents also cluster (12). If we assume that laws and regulations are a response to unsafe behaviors, then there is reason to believe that state safety laws will cluster. Hence, we hypothesize that state-level laws and regulations concerning safety practices cluster together. Further, we expect that such clustering of safety features may be associated with injury morbidity and mortality. These safety features, we believe, will cluster in a manner allowing us to identify a "safety index" for each individual state.

Because this is the first time researchers have looked at injuries through state-level data in this manner, our study is an explanatory effort to determine if there are clusters of safety measures, if those clusters play any role in injury mortality, and if social structural variables play any role in injury mortality. We are unable in our ecologic approach to make a temporal, causal argument, but we believe this initial attempt can lead to more fruitful work.

METHODS

Three hypotheses are presented and explored through state-level analysis of injury and safety policy data.

- Hypothesis 1: Safety measures cluster together in one or more groupings.
- Hypothesis 2: Groupings of safety measures play a significant role in injury mortality.
- Hypothesis 3: Injury mortality is very highly associated with social structural variables.

To test these hypotheses, we examined laws and regulations concerning motorcycle helmets, seat belts, speed limits, drunken driving, gun control, and smoke detectors. We selected these measures because much health research focuses on them, because some interventions have been successfully targeted at them, and because they seemed logical choices for examining "state safety-ness." We used the most recently available data, which ranged from 1990 to 1993. We employed factor analysis, with varimax rotation, to determine if the selected safety measures cluster in recognizable factors. This technique examines all the cases—in this instance, the 50 states—and identifies patterns of association between the regulations.

We then used ordinary least squares regression with the extracted factors, as well as a variety of social structural variables. We initially entered all the extracted factors, and selected the other independent variables with at least a moderate association with injury mortality, by examining a correlation matrix. When independent variables measuring similar phenomena were highly correlated, we avoided multicollinearity by removing all but the variable most highly correlated to the dependent variable, overall injury mortality. Only the most parsimonious models, showing only significant coefficients, are included here, for ease of presentation. We examined injury mortality in three categories: overall, motor vehicle, and non–motor vehicle. Motor vehicle and non–motor vehicle accidents are moderately associated, correlated at $r = 0.36$, making separate analysis necessary. Despite this moderate correlation, regression analysis produced fairly similar results.

RESULTS

Figure 1 is a plot of motor vehicle versus other unintentional injuries, showing how injury rates correlated by state. Table 2 is a correlation matrix which indicates that state-level mortality rates for various injury categories are moderately to highly correlated. Tables 3 and 4 show results from factor analysis of state safety policies: variance explained (Table 3) and factor loadings (Table 4). There is a clustering of safety policies, as witnessed by the large

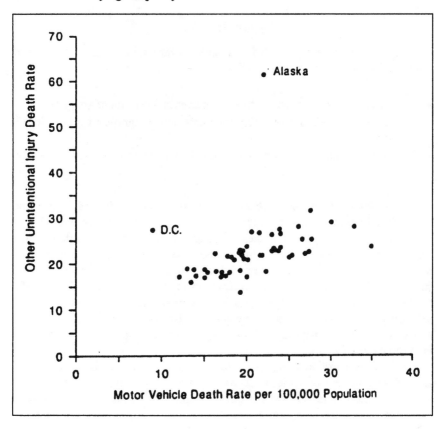

Figure 1. Correlation of motor vehicle injury death rate and other unintentional injury, by state. Source: reference 1, p. 58.

cumulative explained variance of the factors of 67 percent. This analysis does not suggest the presence of a "master" factor, though factor 5 does include helmet laws, minor blood alcohol levels, and smoke detectors, making it the most "global" factor. However, it explains only 7.5 percent of the variance. Factor 1, the strongest factor, includes only two areas: speed limits before 1973 and gun laws (three different laws). Factors 2 and 4 are very specific to two areas: seat belts, and drinking and driving laws. Factor 3 includes gun laws and presence/power of a state cancer registry. Factor 5 includes strength of motorcycle helmet law, low blood alcohol level for children, and strong smoke detector regulations. Factor 6 includes two different, though related, variables: helmet laws and speed limit in 1965. However, the coefficients are smaller than those observed for the other factors.

Table 2

State injury correlation matrix: Age-adjusted rates, 1979–1987[a]

Injury	Guns	Homi-cide	Suicide	Motor vehicle	Burns	Drown-ing	Poison-ing	Falls
Guns	—	—	—	—	—	—	—	—
Homicide	0.69	—	—	—	—	—	—	—
Suicide	0.51	-0.05	—	—	—	—	—	—
Motor vehicle	0.66	0.10	0.70	—	—	—	—	—
Burns	0.51	0.39	-0.19	0.22	—	—	—	—
Drowning	0.41	0.18	0.38	0.48	-0.11	—	—	—
Poisoning	0.46	0.21	0.34	0.22	0.20	0.23	—	—
Falls	0.20	0.31	0.14	-0.10	-0.11	0.11	0.17	—

[a]Source: Derived from data in reference 9.

Table 3

Factor analysis of states' safety regulations: Variance explained

Factor	Eigenvalue	Percent variance	Cumulative percent
1	3.396	21.2	21.2
2	1.843	11.5	32.7
3	1.737	10.9	43.6
4	1.438	9.0	52.6
5	1.208	7.5	60.1
6	1.121	7.0	67.1

Table 5 shows results from regression analyses of safety policy factors, and social structural variables to predict injury mortality. Three models were constructed, predicting overall mortality, motor vehicle mortality, and non–motor vehicle mortality. Two variables are significant in all three analyses: percent metropolitan and factor 2, a factor containing early seat belt laws and seat belt law enforcement. It is not surprising that percent metropolitan provides these large coefficients, since it is well known that rural areas have higher injury mortality. For total accidents, the only significant variables are percent metropolitan and factor 2, the seat belt factor. For non–motor vehicle accidents, percent metropolitan and factor 2 are joined by per capita environmental spending. For

Table 4

Factor analysis of states' safety regulations: Factor loadings

Factor 1		Factor 4	
Maximum speed in 1973	.8052	MADD rating of dwi (driving	
Background check for gun	.5198	while intoxicated) laws	.6615
Ban on juvenile gun possession	.4958	Strength of blood alcohol limit	.5049
Waiting period for gun		Law against open containers	.7177
purchase	.7950		
		Factor 5	
Factor 2		Strength of motorcycle helmet	
Early seat belt law	.8457	law	.4971
Strength of belt enforcement	.8799	Lower blood alcohol for	
		minors	.6637
Factor 3		Smoke detector regulations	.6962
Presence/power of cancer			
registry	−.8023	Factor 6	
Background check for gun	.6126	Current speed limit	−.5288
Child firearm protection law	.6541	Strength of motorcycle helmet	
		law	.3781

Table 5

Regression of safety factors, sociodemographics, and social structural
variables on injury mortality

	Beta coefficients[a]		
	Total mortality	Motor vehicle mortality	Non–motor vehicle mortality
Factor 2 (seat belt law, belt enforcement)	.38**	.33**	.29*
Percent metropolitan	*	*	−.54 (0.8)
Environmental spending per capita	−.61**	−.55**	.35**
Percent Hispanic	*	*	
Percent on AFDC or food stamps		−.21**	
Adjusted R^2		.32**	.45
		−.23*	
	.68	.74	

[a]Statistically significant coefficients are indicated by * <.05   **<.01   ***<.001.
Coefficients approaching significance are in parentheses.

motor vehicle accidents, the above variables are significant, and added to them are percent Hispanic and, negatively, percent on AFDC or food stamps.

DISCUSSION

The factor analysis does provide some provocative evidence for the clustering of safety measures. While we did not find a large master clustering of variables, we did have good explanatory power in the factor model that was developed. Early passage of seat belt laws and enforcement of seat belt laws are clearly important. What is surprising is that this factor is also significant in non–motor vehicle injury mortality. We suggest that there may be a latent safety tendency at the state level which only shows up as the seat belt factor.

The negative relationship between AFDC/food stamps and injury mortality probably reflects the fact that this variable is not a measure of poverty; indeed, it is strongly inversely related to percentage below the poverty level because many states with large poverty populations do not spend a lot on welfare programs. We had included it as a measure of more progressive social policy rather than of poverty. Perhaps states that have better AFDC systems and better food stamp outreach also have better safety policies.

Many variables that predict the likelihood of injury at the individual level do not do so at the state level. On an individual level, poor people do not fare as well as people with higher incomes. However, this does not hold true at the state level. When we look at the states with the lowest injury mortality, we find that five of the top ten are New England states, whose average incomes range from the lowest to the highest in the nation.

On an individual level blacks do worse than whites, but at the state level, the percentage black variable is not significant. Hispanic race is associated with higher motor vehicle mortality. The etiology of this finding is, at present, unclear. However, it may be a reflection of an unassimilated, poor population that is less likely to receive proper medical care and thus to have poorer survival.

We are also puzzled by the environmental spending variable. The more spent on environmental policies, the lower the motor vehicle injury mortality, but the higher the mortality from other injuries. This is difficult to interpret. Perhaps states that spend more money on environmental concerns also make their highways safer, thus reducing accident mortality. Why then the positive relationship between environmental spending and non–motor vehicle mortality? Perhaps states with a history of environmental pollution requiring extensive environmental spending are also states with other unsafe occupations and physical surroundings. These issues require further study.

Implications for Health Policy

In finding that social structural variables were more important than health services variables in predicting infant mortality, Bird and Baumann (7) argued that policy changes are needed that focus more on structural phenomena than health services. Our findings lead us to similar conclusions. While it may seem difficult for health professionals to alter fundamental social structures, we do find it feasible to alter the regulatory environment that reflects social structures. Since we know that injuries are responsive to such changes, we believe it useful to focus more efforts in those directions.

FUTURE RESEARCH

Although the factor analysis of safety policies was only moderately successful, we may expand our array of "social safety" features to include health, social welfare, and environmental policies. With this larger set of potentially clustered elements, we hope to develop a metric "Safety Index" of these measures. We will use this to examine how social structural components of each state affect both safety consciousness/practice and injury morbidity and mortality. For example, how are aggregate income equality and poverty rates associated with scores on the index? We will also investigate the sociodemographic and structural variables to see how they account for mortality differences between states. We also want to look at how different types of injuries cluster together, and see if this suggests an alternative to the traditional injury classifications. In addition, we are interested in the social risk-taking characteristics that lead men to have far higher injury rates and mortality than women.

We also want to understand better the causal direction between state "safety-ness" and mortality. Our analysis here presents a causal link whereby some aspects of "safety-ness" lead to less mortality. But it is conceivable that safety measures are enacted to deal with excess mortality. Therefore it is important to examine injury mortality and safety policy changes over time and to observe when regulations and laws are established.

We cannot yet be as exact as we would like, since this is a new endeavor in a field that has so far had little focus from a broad social health perspective. However, our preliminary findings support a call for a different conceptualization of injuries which incorporates their social nature in the realm of both public policy and social structural features, as well as the social norms related to policy and structure.

Acknowledgments — We are grateful to our colleagues in the Working Group on Society and Health for their support and comments.

Note — This is a revised version of a paper given at the 1994 Annual Meeting of the American Public Health Association, Washington, D.C., October 31, 1994.

REFERENCES

1. Baker, S., et al. *The Injury Fact Book*, Ed. 2. Oxford University Press, New York, 1992.
2. Hall, M., and Owings, M. *Hospitalizations for Injury and Poisoning in the United States, 1991*. Advance Data No. 252, October 7, 1994. National Center for Health Statistics, Hyattsville, Md., 1994.
3. National Safety Council. *Accident Facts*. National Safety Council, Itasca, Ill., 1992.
4. Joint Program in Society and Health. *Mission Statement and Program Description*. Boston, 1994.
5. Nelson, M. Socioeconomic status and childhood mortality in North Carolina. *Am. J. Public Health* 82: 1131–1133, 1992.
6. Robertson, L. *Injury Epidemiology*. Oxford University Press, New York, 1992.
7. Bird, S., and Baumann, K. The relationship between structural and health services variables and state-level infant mortality in the United States. *Am. J. Public Health* 85: 26–29, 1995.
8. Strauss, M. The Validity of U.S. States as Units for Sociological Research. Paper presented at the 1985 Annual Meeting of the American Sociological Association.
9. Centers for Disease Control. *Injury Mortality Atlas*. Atlanta, no date.
10. Fortini, M. Youth, alcohol, and automobiles. In *Drug and Alcohol Use Reviews, Vol. 7: Alcohol, Cocaine, and Accidents*, edited by R. Watson, pp. 25–40. Humana Press, Totowa, N.J., 1995.
11. Cliff, K., Grout, P., and Machin, D. Smoking and attitudes to seat belt usage. *Public Health* 96: 48–52, 1982.
12. Newcomb, M., et al. Substance abuse and psychosocial risk factors among teenagers: Associations with sex, age, ethnicity, and type of school. *Am. J. Drug Alcohol Abuse* 13: 413–433, 1987.

PART 3

Embodied Connections: Cumulative Interplay of Inequalities and Physical and Mental Health

CHAPTER 19

The Social Origin of Cardiovascular Risk:
An Investigation in a Rural Community

Marthe R. Gold and Peter Franks

Despite a 33 percent decline in coronary heart disease (CHD) deaths over the past two decades in the United States (1), cardiovascular disease remains the most common cause of mortality in this country and throughout industrialized nations. Most attention regarding etiology has focused on the individual risk factors of smoking, hypertension, hypercholesterolemia, and obesity. Limited physical activity (2–4) and psychosocial variables such as social isolation (5–7) have also been implicated in the incidence of and survival from CHD.

Over the last 30 years there have been important secular shifts in the social distribution of CHD. For example, recent reports from the United Kingdom (8, 9) and Norway (10) have noted an inverse relationship between occupation and/or social class and ischemic heart disease. This is in contrast to the distribution prior to 1960 when lower social classes had lesser risks of death from CHD in England and Wales (11). The adverse effect of these secular changes on socioeconomically disadvantaged populations has also been observed in the United States. In an ecological study, Wing and associates (12), reported evidence for a secular shift in the burden of ischemic heart disease away from workers in white-collar jobs. The data suggested that this shift primarily reflected changes in the resources and opportunities in communities rather than relating directly to individual workers. In a similar vein, Wing and associates (13) found that populations in metropolitan areas of the United States have experienced an earlier onset of decline in ischemic heart disease deaths than those in nonmetropolitan areas, and that socioeconomic characteristics

This study was supported in part by grants from the Heart and Hypertension Institute, New York State Department of Health, and the O'Connor Foundation.

of these communities could account for most of this variation. Pell and Fayerweather (14), reporting on the incidence and case fatality rate of myocardial infarction from 1957 to 1983 among 100,000 Du Pont employees, noted a decline of 28 percent in disease incidence in male employees. Salaried workers experienced twice the rate of decrease as did hourly blue-collar employees; the curves of these two groups crossed in the mid-1960s as white-collar workers who began with higher rates of disease incidence ended with lower rates.

Risk factors for CHD also show a social distribution. Hypertension is more prevalent among less educated and lower income persons in most (15–18) but not all (19) studies. Cigarette smoking is reportedly more common among less advantaged groups (20–23). Reports of serum cholesterol levels by social class are conflicting. Some investigations report a decreasing level of cholesterol in association with increasing social class (19, 20, 22). Studies in Britain (22, 24) and the Health Examination Survey in the United States (25) found the reverse gradient. Other studies in the United States found essentially no association between cholesterol levels and social class (19, 26, 27). Marmot and coworkers (22) noted a steep inverse association between occupational grade and cardiovascular mortality in their longitudinal study of 17,530 British civil servants. Only 25 percent of this discrepancy was explained by the traditional risk factors of hypertension, age, hypercholesterolemia, family history, obesity, and sedentary life-style. Thus, the etiology of cardiovascular disease is multifactorial and consists of elements that appear to be both individually and socially determined.

The focus in recent U.S. public health and medical literature has been on individually mediated causes of and solutions to cardiovascular disease. Little has been written of late about the interplay of individual and social determinants of cardiovascular risk and disease in U.S. populations. Reported here is the clustering of physiological, behavioral, and psychosocial cardiovascular risk factors in less advantaged members of a cohort of white adults living in two contiguous towns in rural New York State. The literature discussed above suggests the conceptual model illustrated in Figure 1, which was used to inform this study. Sociodemographic factors (age, sex, income, education, and occupation) are posited to have direct effects on psychosocial and behavioral risk factors, on physiological risk factors, and on CHD. Behavioral and psychosocial risk factors, in turn, influence physiological risk and CHD. Thus, psychosocial and behavioral risk factors are viewed as intervening variables, but in addition, sociodemographic factors have an effect on physiological risk independent of measured psychosocial and behavioral factors. It is assumed here that there are also unmeasured external influences on each group of variables, but they do not confound the relationships illustrated in Figure 1. Because the study was cross-sectional in design, the relationships among risk factors and CHD were not examined.

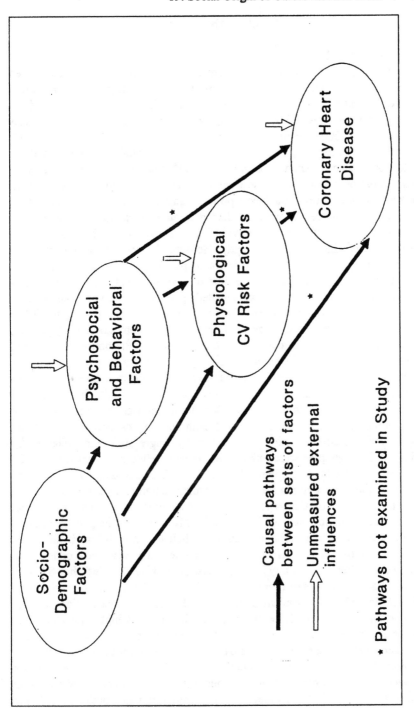

Figure 1. A model for the etiology of coronary heart disease (*CV*, cardiovascular).

MATERIALS AND METHODS

This population-based study was conducted as part of a community-oriented primary care project that sought to define and address the increased burden of cardiovascular death experienced in an economically depressed agricultural region of central New York State. Delaware County is a sparsely populated dairy farming region. In 1980, 20 percent of the population lived at 125 percent or less and 40 percent at 200 percent or less of the poverty level. Between 1984 and 1987, 20 percent of county dairy farms closed. From July through November of 1987, two towns in central Delaware county (Meredith and Kortright) were surveyed and screened on a house-to-house basis by community health workers trained in survey administration and blood pressure and cholesterol measurement. A pilot survey and screening were conducted in an adjacent town to familiarize the workers with techniques and provide field supervision. All houses occupied year-round were included in the study. Households were contacted either by telephone or by leaflets. The program was explained, and an appointment was made (telephone) or an approximate time of revisit indicated (leaflet). Households where no one was at home were visited up to a maximum of three times.

In addition to the measurement of cholesterol and blood pressure, the home visits elicited survey information including standard demographics (age, sex, marital status, family size, occupation, employment status, household income, and education), height and weight, and history of hypertension and hypercholesterolemia. The health workers asked questions about habits relevant to cardiovascular health, including smoking history; dietary intake of salt, cholesterol, and alcohol; and level of leisure exercise. Social support was measured using the social support questions from the COOP Health Status Questionnaire (28). Blood samples for cholesterol testing were drawn by finger stick and collected by capillary tubes. Samples were refrigerated immediately and analyzed within 24 hours using the Kodak Ektachem DT 60 analyzer. Blood pressure was measured twice, with the subject sitting for at least 30 minutes before measurement.

For the purpose of this report, the socioeconomic, behavioral, and social support characteristics were dichotomized. This was done in part to allow a uniform analysis of the variables (described below). In addition, it facilitates comparison of the relative effects of each variable using prevalence odds ratios. Poverty was defined as a family income of less than $10,000, or less than $20,000 for households with five or more members. Manual labor included semi-skilled and unskilled laborers, farmhands, and truck drivers. This occupation variable excluded those not currently working outside the home. A high-cholesterol diet was defined as one including more than two eggs and two dinner meals of red meat each week, and a salty diet as use of a salt shaker at meals either "often" or "always." Increased alcohol consumption was defined as at least seven drinks per week. Persons conducting no vigorous exercise (i.e., exercise to the point of shortness of breath; for example, running, swimming, and basketball) during leisure time were characterized as having low leisure activity. Persons reporting little or no access to social support were considered isolated. Obesity was defined as a body mass index—weight (kg)/height^2 (cm^2)—greater than 26.

The multivariate analyses proceeded in stages corresponding to the previously described model (Figure 1) for cardiovascular risk. First, we examined the age- and sex-adjusted effects of the social class variables (income, education, and occupation) on each of the dichotomous behavioral and psychosocial variables (smoking status, exercise, obesity, cholesterol, alcohol and salt consumption, and social support). Thus age, sex, and social class were treated as independent variables, and the behavioral and psychosocial variables as dependent variables in a series of logistic regressions. Next we examined the effects of the age- and sex-adjusted social class variables on the physiological risk factors (systolic blood pressure and serum cholesterol) using linear regression equations. Finally, the behavioral and psychosocial variables were added (as independent variables) to these linear regression analyses. This allowed us to examine the extent to which the sociodemographic factors acted indirectly through the behavioral and psychosocial pathway to affect physiological risk.

For all variables except the socioeconomic (income, education, and occupation), only main effects were included in the equations. In order to examine more carefully the separate and cumulative effects of the socioeconomic variables, their interaction terms were included if their main effects made a significant ($P < 0.1$) contribution to the equation. For equations where occupation made no significant ($P < 0.1$) contribution, the variable was excluded from the analyses reported here. This allowed inclusion of the whole sample, including those not working outside the home.

RESULTS

Of the 557 households contacted, 508 (91 percent) participated. Of 1063 persons over age 16, 1017 (96 percent) had blood pressures recorded and 973 (92 percent) were screened for cholesterol level.

Table 1 shows the distribution of dichotomous risk factors and their relationships with the social class factors. Manual laborers composed roughly one third of the 776 subjects who worked outside their homes. A quarter of the adult population were not high school graduates, and 30 percent were poor. These three socioeconomic categories did not fully overlap. Of the 776 who worked outside the home, 244 (31.4 percent) had only one of these three risk factors and 356 (46 percent) had none. The prevalence of most risk factors was increased in the presence of each of the three social class risk factors.

Each row of Table 2 summarizes the results of a logistic regression analysis showing the age- and sex-adjusted effect of the social class variables on each behavioral and psychosocial variable. It can be seen that at least one and usually two or three of the markers for socioeconomic disadvantage are associated with

Table 1

Prevalence of dichotomous risk factors[a]

		Social class factors, percent		
Risk factor	Overall risk factor present, percent	Manual labor	<12 years school	Poverty
Manual labor	31.2	100	45	43
<12 years of school	25.6	34	100	36
Poverty	31.0	37	44	100
Male sex	50.3	81	57	48
Smoker	26.1	38	29	29
Low leisure activity	86.5	92	90	89
Obesity	47.5	54	51	45
High-egg/meat diet	32.9	47	36	41
High-salt diet	45.5	55	50	50
High alcohol use	21.0	27	18	18
Social isolation	12.3	9	9	16

[a]The overall percentages were based on the total sample (1063) except for manual labor, which was based on those working outside their home (776). The percentages under "Social class factors" represent the percentage of those with that social class factor who also have the other risk factor.

a statistically significant increased prevalence of each of the behavioral and psychosocial risk factors, except alcohol consumption.

The effects of the social class variables on systolic blood pressure are shown in Table 3. Manual laborers and those without high school graduation had higher systolic blood pressures. After adjustment for age and sex, manual labor and lack of high school graduation retained their independent association with higher systolic blood pressure. Furthermore, the presence of both risk factors was associated with essentially an additive effect on systolic blood pressure. Poverty made no additional statistically significant contribution ($P < 0.6$) to the equation. After also adjusting for the behavioral and psychosocial variables, the parameter estimates for the effects of manual labor and lack of high school graduation on systolic blood pressure were slightly higher.

The effects of the social class variables on cholesterol are shown in Table 4. The unadjusted effect of poverty was to lower serum cholesterol by 8.9 mg/100 ml. After age and sex adjustment, poverty and lack of a high school graduation

Table 2

Age- and sex-adjusted prevalence odds ratios (and 95 percent confidence intervals)
of socioeconomic factors with behavioral and social support risk factors[a]

Risk factor	Socioeconomic factors		
	Manual labor[b]	<12 years school	Poverty
Smoking	1.39 (1.16, 1.66)**	1.21 (1.07, 1.36)*	1.03 (0.85, 1.24)
Obesity	—	1.21 (1.07, 1.36)*	0.88 (0.74, 1.05)
Diet (increased use)			
Salt	1.22 (1.03, 1.45)*	1.28 (1.06, 1.55)**	1.00 (0.84, 1.19)
Eggs/red meat	1.31 (1.1, 1.56)**	1.14 (0.93, 1.39)	1.24 (1.04, 1.48)*
Alcohol	—	0.89 (0.72, 1.10)	0.89 (0.74, 1.07)
Low leisure activity	1.39 (1.04, 1.84)*	1.69 (1.16, 2.48)**	1.18 (0.89, 1.57)
Social isolation	1.67 (1.38, 2.03)**	1.65 (1.35, 2.01)**	1.49 (1.24, 1.8)**

[a]The prevalence odds ratios reported in each row are adjusted for other socioeconomic factors as well as age and sex.
[b]—, no values reported since occupation did not make a significant ($P > 0.1$) contribution and persons not working outside the home were included in the equation.
*$P < 0.05$.
**$P < 0.01$.

independently were associated with lower cholesterol, although these effects were not statistically significant ($P = 0.07$ for poverty, and $P = 0.1$ for lack of high school graduation). The presence of both risk factors had a cumulative decremental effect on cholesterol ($P = 0.01$ for both factors present versus neither). After also adjusting for the behavioral and psychosocial factors, the parameter estimates for the social class variables were little changed, though the confidence intervals were narrower.

DISCUSSION

This study of intermediary risks for cardiovascular disease in a rural, relatively disadvantaged population has corroborated the findings of other population-based studies that have noted clustering of risk factors among members of lower socioeconomic groups (20–24, 29). Less advantaged persons in this community are at higher risk on many counts. We found them to have increased smoking rates, higher intake of salt- and cholesterol-rich diets, higher prevalence of leisure

Table 3

Effects of social class variables on mean systolic blood pressure

Predictor	Parameter estimate, mm Hg[a]	95% confidence interval
Unadjusted		
Manual labor	3.69	0.94, 6.44
<12 years of school	7.99	5.46, 10.51
Poverty	−1.39	−3.8, 1.02
Sociodemographic[b] adjustment		
Manual labor	4.59	1.67, 7.52
<12 years of school	3.64	0.71, 6.57
Poverty	−1.70	−4.39, 0.99
Manual labor and <12 years of school	8.23	4.31, 12.15
Sociodemographic,[b] behavioral, and psychosocial adjustment		
Manual labor	5.20	2.34, 8.46
<12 years of school	6.20	0.38, 12.02
Poverty	−0.88	−3.69, 1.94
Manual labor and <12 years of school	9.50	5.46, 13.54

[a]Parameter estimate represents the effect of predictor on mean systolic blood pressure.
[b]Adjustment for age, sex, and other social class variables.

inactivity, and higher levels of obesity, and they were more socially isolated than the more privileged. In addition, they had significantly higher blood pressures. The adjusted 3.6 to 9.5 mm Hg increase in systolic blood pressure found in lower educational and occupational groups provides evidence for a direct effect of social class variables on the physiological risk of CHD that operates independently of measured behavioral variables.

Social class was measured indirectly by occupation, education, and income. Neither the literature nor our results allow precise specification of the theoretical relationship among these indicator variables or the latent variable, social class. Thus is remains uncertain why the social class indicators found to be predictors of

Table 4

Effect of social class variables on serum cholesterol

Predictor	Parameter estimate,[a] mg/100 ml	95% confidence interval
Unadjusted		
Manual labor	−0.59	−6.94, 5.76
<12 years of school	0.97	−4.99, 6.93
Poverty	−8.90	−14.47, −3.33
Sociodemographic[b] adjustment		
<12 years of school	−5.07	0.90, −11.05
Poverty	−5.52	0.38, −11.42
<12 years of school, and poverty	−10.59	−0.25, −18.68
Sociodemographic,[b] behavioral, and psychosocial adjustment		
<12 years of school	−6.20	−12.02, −0.38
Poverty	−4.80	−10.65, 1.05
<12 years of school, and poverty	−11.00	−18.90, −3.10

[a]Parameter estimate represents the effect of predictor on cholesterol.
[b]Adjustment for age, sex, and other social class variables.

blood pressure (occupation and education) are different from those that predict serum cholesterol (income and education). We view these aspects of the results as exploratory and requiring confirmation. It is also important to note that the marginal statistical significance found in the case of the individual social class predictors of serum cholesterol reflects in part the shared variance of those predictors. For example, when poverty alone was used as the measure of social class, the parameter estimate of its effect adjusted for other predictors on lowering cholesterol was 9.7 ($P = 0.005$, 95 percent confidence interval = 2.9, 16.5), which is only slightly less than the combined adjusted effect of both poverty and lack of high school graduation.

It is possible that some misclassification bias was introduced by the use of dichotomous variables (which were used to facilitate a uniform analysis and to aid clinical interpretation). However, similar results were obtained when more complete categorical, ordinal, or continuous versions of the variables were used.

The significantly lower levels of cholesterol among the poor in this community are congruent with data from the National Health and Nutrition Examination

Survey 1976–80 NHANES II (30). Of note, however, is the changing gradient of serum cholesterol with regard to education between the 1960–62 Health Examination Survey (25) and NHANES II. In the first survey, persons with lower educational levels had consistently lower levels of cholesterol; the second survey revealed almost identical mean levels of cholesterol across educational categories.

The measure of cholesterol consumption used in this study, while lacking precision, does serve as an indicator of the extent to which this population has responded to two well-publicized components of cholesterol-restricting diets. The discrepancy noted between the higher cholesterol intake of these persons of low socioeconomic status and their lower serum cholesterol levels is surprising. Other cross-sectional studies have also been unsuccessful in demonstrating an association between dietary and serum cholesterol (31–35), despite the evidence found in longitudinal trials that a direct relationship exists (36–38). In the early 1970s, dietary patterns of affluent Americans were more likely to include high-fat and high-cholesterol foods than were those of poorer people (39). A similar dietary discrepancy between upper and lower income households was seen in the United Kingdom in those years (40). By the late 1970s a change in dietary habits by economic status is reflected in U.S. data. Persons below the poverty level were eating higher levels of dietary cholesterol and similar levels of dietary fat compared with nonpoverty individuals (41).

Taken together these results suggest that a social transformation of cholesterol-attributable cardiovascular risk has been occurring over the last 20 years. The gradient that has traditionally favored lower socioeconomic persons is shifting. The relative dietary risk of less advantaged people is increasing, and this is becoming visible in measures of serum cholesterol. Parenthetically, it is interesting to note that this effect has lagged behind the social change in CHD distribution. It is probable that this rural, relatively disadvantaged population is being observed at an early stage of this transformation. Most likely, persons of higher socioeconomic status with readier access to health care and more options for "life-style" (i.e., dietary) changes will be the primary beneficiaries of dietary and pharmacological interventions to decrease cholesterol.

This is foreshadowed in two recent reports. Walter and associates (38) conducted a five-year cardiovascular risk reduction program among school-age children in the Bronx and Westchester. At entry, children in the lower income schools of the Bronx had higher mean cholesterol levels than those in the more affluent Westchester system. While intervention groups in both school systems showed a drop in mean cholesterol levels, the Westchester drop was twofold greater and statistically significant. Both populations had similar knowledge of cardiovascular risk both at the beginning and the end of the project. Similarly, findings from the Rand Health Insurance Experiment revealed a significant decrease in cholesterol in the at-risk high-income group when compared with the at-risk low-income group receiving care in a health maintenance organization (42).

Rose (43) has demonstrated a ten-year "incubation period" between exposure to higher serum cholesterol levels and increased mortality from CHD. Accordingly, the adverse social gradient in cardiovascular mortality for poor people may worsen as cholesterol levels begin to drop more in higher socioeconomic populations.

The most recent strategy among the mainstream of preventive cardiovascular policy has been to take an individually focused view of disease causality and treatment. Hence, it is fashionable to focus cardiovascular prevention campaigns on a kind of individual shaping-up ethos. People are admonished to get regular aerobic exercise, eat healthfully, stop smoking, and have regular cholesterol and blood pressure checks. Once case- finding has uncovered physiological risk, medical regimens are tailored to the needs of the individual. The inadequacy of this paradigm stems both from its focus on the relatively small contribution of behavioral risk factors to CHD and the attendant implication that people who do not or cannot follow the rules for healthful living and regular checkups are to blame for the consequences. There is little recognition in such a model for the large role of social forces on the etiology and outcome of this illness.

When the same segments of a population are repeatedly found to exhibit increased risk, it may be more appropriate to widen the approach to the treatment of cardiovascular disease to a sociological perspective that broadens the field for investigation and intervention. Although there is a need to address these social inequalities directly, health services can provide a defense against the consequences of poverty (44, 45). The results of randomized trials also suggest that providing access to medical care to poor (46) and black (47) persons can reduce social inequities in the prevalence of uncontrolled hypertension. One obvious approach within medicine's purview would be to advocate universal access to high-quality health care for all members of the population.

Just as infectious disease deaths were inequitably distributed between poor and nonpoor at the turn of the century, the same pattern appears in the current public health scourge. Improvement in social conditions is widely credited with the major role in curtailing infectious disease deaths, and the most important mechanism for curbing cardiovascular disease may likewise be further advancements in social welfare. While it is important for educators and clinicians to continue to motivate individual behavioral changes, a sound public health policy seems to require action on a wider front.

REFERENCES

1. National Center for Health Statistics. *Health, United States, 1983.* U.S. Department of Health and Human Services, Publication No. (PHS) 84-1232. Public Health Service. U.S. Government Printing Office, Washington, D.C., 1983.
2. Salonen, J., Slater, J., and Tuomilehto, J. Leisure time and occupational physical activity: Risk of death from ischemic heart disease. *Am. J. Epidemiol.* 127: 87–94, 1988.

3. Kannel, W., Wilson, P., and Blair, S. Epidemiological assessment of the role of physical activity and fitness in development of cardiovascular disease. *Am. Heart J.* 109: 876–885, 1985.

4. Folsom, A., et al. Leisure time physical activity and its relationship to coronary risk factors in a population based sample: The Minnesota Heart Survey. *Am. J. Epidemiol.* 121: 570–579, 1985.

5. Ruberman, W., et al. Psychosocial influences on mortality after myocardial infarction. *N. Engl. J. Med.* 311: 552–559, 1984.

6. Kaplan, G., et al. Social connections and mortality from all causes and from cardiovascular disease: Prospective evidence from Eastern Finland. *Am. J. Epidemiol.* 128: 370–380, 1988.

7. Berkman, L. F., and Syme, S. L. Social networks, host resistance, and mortality: A nine-year follow-up study of Alameda County residents. *Am. J. Epidemiol.* 109: 186–204, 1979.

8. Popcock, S. J., et al. Social class differences in ischaemic heart disease in British men. *Lancet* 2: 197–201, 1987.

9. Marmot, M. G., Shipley, M. J., and Rose, G. Inequalities in death—specific explanations of a general pattern? *Lancet* 1: 1003–1006, 1984.

10. Holme, I., et al. Four-year mortality by some socioeconomic indicators: The Oslo study. *J. Epidemiol. Community Health* 34: 48–52, 1980.

11. Rose, G., and Marmot, M. G. Social class and coronary heart disease. *Br. Heart J.* 45: 13–19, 1981.

12. Wing, S., et al. Changing association between community occupational structure and ischemic heart disease mortality in the United States. *Lancet* 2: 1067–1070, 1987.

13. Wing, S., et al. Socioenvironmental characteristics associated with the onset of decline of ischemic heart disease mortality in the United States. *Am. J. Public Health* 78: 923–926, 1988.

14. Pell, S., and Fayerweather, W. Trends in the incidence of myocardial infarction and in associated mortality and morbidity in a large employed population 1957–1983. *N. Engl. J. Med.* 312: 1005–1011, 1985.

15. National Center for Health Statistics. Hypertension in adults 25–75 years of age, United States 1971–75. *National Health Survey*, Series 11, No. 221. U.S. Department of Health and Human Services, Public Health Service. U.S. Government Printing Office, Washington, D.C., 1981.

16. Dyer, A. R., et al. The relationship of education to blood pressure. Findings on 40,000 employed Chicagoans. *Circulations* 54: 987–992, 1976.

17. Hypertension Detection and Follow-up Program. Race, education and prevalence of hypertension. Co-operative Group. *Am. J. Epidemiol.* 106: 351–361, 1977.

18. Wadsworth, M. E. J., et al. Blood pressure in a national birth cohort at the age of 36 related to social and familial factors, smoking, and body mass. *Br. Med. J.* 291: 1534–1538, 1985.

19. Haynes, S. G., et al. The relationship of psychosocial factors to coronary heart disease in the Framingham Study. I. Methods and risk factors. *Am. J. Epidemiol.* 107: 362–383, 1978.

20. Holme, I., et al. Coronary risk factors and socioeconomic status. Lancet 2: 1396–1398, 1976.

21. Kraus, J. F., Borhani, N. O., and Franti, C. E. Socioeconomic status, ethnicity and risk of coronary heart disease. *Am. J. Epidemiol.* 111: 407–414, 1980.

22. Marmot, M. G., et al. Employment grade and coronary heart disease in British civil servants. *J. Epidemiol. Community Health* 32: 244–249, 1978.

23. Jacobsen, R. K., and Thelle, D. S. Risk factors for coronary heart disease and level of education. The Tromso Heart Study. *Am. J. Epidemiol.* 127: 923–931, 1988.
24. Thelle, D. S., et al. Blood lipids in middle-aged British men. *Br. Heart J.* 49: 205–213, 1983.
25. National Center for Health Statistics. Serum cholesterol levels of adults. U.S. 1960–1962. *Vital and Health Statistics*, Series 11, No. 22. U.S. Department of Health, Education and Welfare. U.S. Government Printing Office, Washington, D.C., 1967.
26. Liu, K., et al. Relationship of education to major risk factors and death from coronary heart disease, cardiovascular diseases and all causes; findings of three Chicago epidemiologic studies. *Circulation* 66: 1308–1314, 1982.
27. Khoury, P. R., et al. Relationships of education and occupation to coronary heart disease risk factors in school children and adults; the Princeton School District Study. *Am. J. Epidemiol.* 113: 378–395, 1981.
28. Nelson, E., et al. Assessment of function in routine clinical practice: Description of the COOP chart method and preliminary findings. *J. Chronic Dis.* 40(Suppl. 1): 55S–63S, 1987.
29. Millar, W. J., and Wigle, D. T. Socioeconomic disparities in risk factors for cardiovascular disease. *Can. Med. Assoc. J.* 134: 127–132, 1986.
30. National Center for Health Statistics. Total serum cholesterol levels of adults 20–74 years of age. U.S. 1976–80. *Vital and Health Statistics*, Series 11, No. 236. Public Health Service. U.S. Government Printing Office, Washington, D.C., 1986.
31. Nichols, A. B., et al. Daily nutritional intake and serum lipid levels. The Tecumseh Study. *Am. J. Clin. Nutr.* 29: 1384–1392, 1976.
32. Stulb, S., et al. The relationship of nutrient intake and exercise to serum cholesterol in white males in Evans County, GA. *Am. J. Clin. Nutr.* 16: 238–242, 1965.
33. Kahn, H., et al. Serum cholesterol: Its distribution and association with dietary and other variables in a survey of 10,000 men. *Isr. J. Med. Sci.* 5: 1117–1127, 1969.
34. Kannell, W. B., and Gordon, T. (eds.). The Framingham Study—an epidemiologic investigation of cardiovascular disease. Section 24: The Framingham diet study; diet and the regulation of serum cholesterol. U.S. Department of Health, Education and Welfare, Public Health Service, National Institutes of Health. U.S. Government Printing Office, Washington, D.C., 1970.
35. Jacobs, D. R., Jr., Anderson, J. T., and Blackburn, H. Diet and serum cholesterol: Do zero correlations negate the relationship? *Am. J. Epidemiol.* 110: 77–87, 1979.
36. Shekelle, R. B., et al. Diet, serum cholesterol and death from coronary heart disease. *N. Engl. J. Med.* 304: 65–70, 1981.
37. Turpeinen, O., et al. Dietary prevention of coronary heart disease: The Finnish Mental Health Study. *Int. J. Epidemiol.* 8: 99–118, 1979.
38. Walter, H. J., et al. Modification of risk factors for coronary heart disease: Five year results of a school-based intervention trial. *N. Engl. J. Med.* 318: 1093–1100, 1988.
39. National Center for Health Statistics. Food consumption profiles of white and black persons aged 1–74 years: United States 1971–74. *National Health Survey*, Series 11, No. 210. U.S. Department of Health, Education and Welfare Publication No. (PHS) 79-1658. Hyattsville, Md., 1979.
40. National Food Survey Committee, Ministry of Agriculture, Fisheries and Food. *Household Food Consumption and Expenditure 1970 and 1971.* Her Majesty's Stationery Office, London, 1973.
41. National Center for Health Statistics. Dietary intake source data: United States 1976–80. U.S. Department of Health and Human Services, Publication No. 83-1681, Series 11, No. 231. U.S. Government Printing Office, Washington, D.C., 1981.

42. Ware, J. E., et al. Comparison of health outcomes at a health maintenance organisation with those of fee-for-service care. *Lancet* 2: 1017–1022, 1986.
43. Rose, G. Incubation period of coronary heart disease. *Br. Med. J.* 284: 1600–1611, 1982.
44. Blaxter, M. Health services as a defence against the consequences of poverty in industrialised societies. *Soc. Sci. Med.* 17: 1139–1148, 1983.
45. Mundinger, M. O. Health service funding cuts and the declining health of the poor. *N. Engl. J. Med.* 313: 44–47, 1985.
46. Keeler, E. B., et al. How free care reduced hypertension in the health insurance experiment. *JAMA* 254: 1926–1931, 1985.
47. Hypertension Detection and Follow-up Program Cooperative Group. Five-year findings of the hypertension detection and follow-up program. II. Mortality by race-sex and age. *JAMA* 242: 2572–2577, 1979.

Latina and African American Women: Continuing Disparities in Health

Marsha Lillie-Blanton, Rose Marie Martinez, Andrea Kidd Taylor, and Betty Garman Robinson

Race and gender are powerful determinants of life experiences in the United States. A legacy of racial discrimination and segregation continues to affect the quality of life of U.S. racial and ethnic minority populations. Similarly, discrimination based on gender has affected the life experiences of women. As members of both population subgroups, Latina and African American women have encountered discrimination based on their gender and race. Blatant and subtle barriers have affected minority women's access to educational and employment opportunities. Moreover, racism affects where individuals live and the quality of resources available within those neighborhoods. Both gender and race have historically triggered social relations (i.e., in the family and work environment) which are risk factors for diminished health.

Social class stratification in the United States also shapes the life experiences of women of color. Social class status, sometimes referred to as socioeconomic status (SES), is generally measured by an individual's family resources and/or the occupation and educational attainment of the head of household (1). These indices, however, are affected by discriminatory policies and practices that persist despite legislation and judicial decisions prohibiting discrimination based on race and gender. Thus, social class status is socially determined and inseparably linked to this nation's history of social inequities. As such, the burden of illness and injury facing minority women reflects the common life experiences they share as a consequence of their race, gender, and social class.

Women represent about half of the 30.8 million African Americans and 21.4 million Latino Americans identified in the 1990 Census. Although stereotypically portrayed by contrasting profiles, Latina and African American women represent a diversity of socioeconomic and psychosocial backgrounds. For example, African American women often are described as disproportionately poor, single heads of household who are dependent on public welfare programs such as AFDC (Aid to Families with Dependent Children). The profile is one of women who are irresponsible and a financial burden on society. In contrast, there is an abundance of research—some disputed—on the "black matriarchy" (2). Sociologists have portrayed African American women as the "rocks of Gibraltar" who provide the stabilizing and nurturing foundation for the black family (3, 4). Latina women are often characterized as submissive, self-denying, and self-sacrificing (5). Within the family environment, the profile is one of women who place the needs of children and husband first and ask little for themselves in return. Their submissiveness and self-denial is said to contribute to their general lack of power and influence within American society.

As with most women, Latina and African American women have had what paradoxically could be considered both the good fortune and ill-fortune of being the primary caretaker of the family's children and elderly. While caretaking roles expand the depth of compassion women feel for others, they also compromise women's ability to compete in a rapidly evolving market economy. While there is substantial evidence for their portrayal as pillars of strength, the health consequences of being a primary caretaker in a frequently hostile social environment deserve investigation.

The meaning of racial/ethnic classifications is a subject of intense debate and controversy. In U.S. census and survey data, respondents are generally asked to report their racial group as: white; black; Asian or Pacific Islander; Aleut, Eskimo, American Indian; or other. In another question, information about Hispanic national origin is asked and persons of Hispanic origin may be of any of the racial categories. When individuals have an opportunity to self-define their race, a small but sizable percentage report their race as "other" rather than one of the four major racial groups. We recognize that these categories oversimplify race/ethnic origin, but they are the social designations used for U.S. census and survey purposes.

Racial/ethnic classifications denote group membership in which there is some assumed commonality of inheritance and contemporary life experiences. Nonetheless, women classified by U.S. census or survey data as of Hispanic origin are a tremendously heterogeneous group ethnically, consisting primarily of individuals with Mexican, Puerto Rican, Cuban, and South and Central American ancestry. These ethnic groups share a common bond of language and culture, but there are major subgroup differences in terms of their inclusion in society and access to resources. African American women are a more homogeneous group but are also ethnically diverse, including individuals with African, Caribbean, Indian, and European ancestry. Latina and African American women, as evidenced by their varying shades of color, have experienced considerable cross-generational mixing of racial/ethnic groups. As a consequence, racial/ ethnic classifications are more a measure of the sociocultural experience of being a member of a particular racial/ethnic group than a marker of biological inheritance. Although a number of biological explanations for racial differences in health have been advanced, there is little scientific evidence to support these theories (6, 7).

SCOPE OF THE INVESTIGATION

In an effort to assess the quality of life experienced by Latina and African American women, this chapter provides descriptive information on racial/ethnic differences in women's social conditions, health status, exposure to occupational and environmental risks, and use of health services. We examine indices of the quality of life using a framework that considers life experiences associated with being female, a racial/ethnic minority, and a member of a particular social class. This assessment attempts to address some of the limitations of past research but, at most, represents an initial exploration into an issue that deserves more in-depth review.

Framework for the Study of Minority Women's Health

Several articles assisted us in establishing a framework for examining the health of minority women (8–10). Zambrana (8) provides a thoughtful and poignant critique of the research on the health of minority women, noting that even authors sensitive to women's issues have failed to address social class and racial/ethnic differences among women. She proposes a conceptual model for studying the health of minority women that considers health status as an interactive relationship among socioeconomic, behavioral, and environmental factors. Focusing on reproductive health issues, Zambrana applies this conceptual model while illustrating the limitations of existing research. Asserting that adolescent sexuality and childbearing are influenced by sociocultural background and SES, Zambrana also sees their consequences for the mother's education and employment opportunities and the child's health. In reviewing data on pregnancy outcomes, she notes that Mexican American women have high childbirth mortality rates and African American women have high rates of low birthweight infants. Zambrana advances the premise that poorer outcomes are due to differences in use of prenatal care, social class, and psychosocial factors such as chronic stress and social support.

Bennett (9) and Bassett and Krieger (10) have examined minority women's health from a perspective that acknowledges the impact of social class on health. Bennett explores the premise that life stressors associated with poverty are risk factors for emotional distress and even mental illness. The relation between social class and mental health has been well documented (11); research, however, is limited regarding the impact of race, gender, and SES on mental health (12, 13). Bennett asserts that social strata are not necessarily comparable across racial/ethnic groups because who is considered poor is relative, depending on the wealth among one's peers. Using clinical case studies, Bennett describes some of the economic circumstances of African American single women that potentially exacerbate life stressors associated with loneliness or parenting. The author argues that, depending on a woman's problem-solving skills, poor resolution of problems could lead to diagnosable emotional distress. Bassett and Krieger (10) examine the impact of race and social class on breast cancer survival in a population-based sample. After adjusting for social class, in addition to age and other medical predictors of survival, the authors found that black-white differences in breast cancer survival rates diminished greatly. The results provide strong evidence that racial differences in today's breast cancer survival rates are largely attributable to the poorer social class standing of black women.

Data Sources and Key Measures

Data on health indices of minority women are presented from a number of sources, including the 1990 U.S Census, the National Health and Nutrition Examination Survey II (NHANES; 1976–1980), and the Hispanic Health and Nutrition Examination Study (HHANES; 1982–1984). We also analyze and present original data on women aged 18 to 64 from the 1988 Health Interview Survey (HIS).

When possible, this chapter presents data on mutually exclusive racial/ethnic categories. In most of the analyses, women are classified as: white American, not of Hispanic origin; African American, not of Hispanic origin; or Latina.[1] Although these categories inadequately capture the racial/ethnic diversity within a population subgroup, they are used to yield a more accurate comparison of the indices of racial/ethnic minority women with those of nonminority women. Since most Latinos are classified racially as white (in the 1990 census, 96 percent of the 21.4 million persons of Hispanic origin are identified as white), analyses in which they are not examined as a distinct population group could diminish the magnitude of the race/ethnicity differentials.

Additionally, health and access indices from the HIS are stratified by family income categories of: below $10,000; $10,000 to $19,999; $20,000 to $34,999; and $35,000 and above. Stratifying by income is intended to limit the confounding effects of social class on the comparison of racial differences and also to gain some insight into the impact of income differences on the health indices of racial/ethnic minority women. When racial differences in health are presented, questions inevitably arise about the extent to which disparities can be attributed to racial differences in poverty, or more broadly, to differences in social class. Despite the imprecision of family income as a measure of social class, we considered it the best of the readily available indicators.

---

[1] Women of other racial groups (i.e., Asian and Pacific Islanders, Native Americans, etc.) were excluded from the analysis of the HIS data.

SOCIAL CONDITIONS OF LATINA AND
AFRICAN AMERICAN WOMEN

Social environmental conditions are recognized as one of several determinants of a population's health. The term "social condition" is used to refer to sociodemographic factors (e.g., employment) and to physical surroundings (e.g., neighborhood of residence). Factors such as these, individually and in combination with more personal factors, are determinants of health status. Employment, for example, is not only a source of income, it is often important to an individual's sense of self-worth and is a potential source of life stress. Additionally, it is the means by which most Americans obtain health insurance. Social conditions also affect other determinants of health such as physiological factors, lifestyle behaviors, and access to and use of health services.

For racial/ethnic minority women, the social environment has undergone tremendous change during the last three decades (1960s through 1980s). Progress has been achieved in legally and socially challenging traditional male-female gender roles. Minority women have benefited from policies that foster greater inclusion of women in all sectors of society. Enforcement of antidiscrimination laws helped to assure minority women greater equity in access to educational and employment opportunities. Nonetheless, data on indicators of life conditions continue to suggest that minority women encounter barriers that prevent full participation in the opportunities available in society.

Income, Poverty, and Family Structure

A disproportionate share of racial/ethnic minority women face circumstances of low-wage jobs and/or poverty. After a sharp decline in poverty rates between 1960 and 1970, the percentage of the population with incomes below the federal poverty level has remained relatively unchanged in the last two decades (Figure 1).[2] In 1990, about three times as many African Americans (32 percent) and Latino Americans (28 percent) as white Americans (11 percent, including whites of Hispanic origin), had family incomes below poverty (14). (The rate for whites not of Hispanic origin was 8.8 percent). While the poverty rate is similar for Latino and African Americans, families headed by women represent 75 percent of all poor African American families, as compared with 46 percent of all poor Latino families.

Family composition has major implications for the economic resources and social support available to a family. Nearly one-third (31 percent) of African American and 19 percent of Latino American families were headed by women in 1990. In contrast, only 9 percent of white American families were headed by

---

[2] The average poverty threshold for a family of four was $13,359 in 1990.

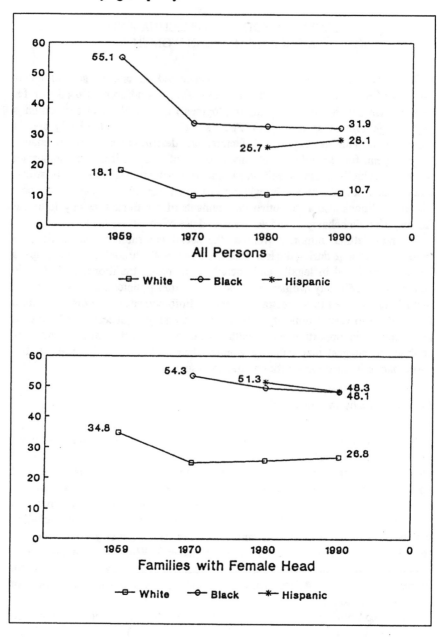

Figure 1. Poverty rates in the United States, by race/ethnicity, for all persons and for families with a female head of household, 1959–1990. Persons of Hispanic origin may be of any race. Source: reference 14.

women. As shown in Figure 1, about half of Latino and African American families headed by women had incomes below poverty. High rates of poverty among minority populations have been attributed to the shift in the number of families with a female head of household.[3] However, the National Research Council's report on the Status of Black Americans (16) found that if family structure in 1984 were the same as in 1973, the percentage of children and/or persons in poverty would have changed only modestly. The report concluded that the decline in wages, not an increase in female-headed households, accounts for persistently high poverty rates.

Median income, another measure of a person's economic condition, shows continuing disparity between men and women, as well as racial/ethnic differences among women. Table 1 shows that despite greater opportunities, the 1988 median income for households headed by women barely approached two-thirds of the median income for households headed by men. For Latina and African American families headed by women, the median income was slightly more than half that reported for white American families headed by women. Findings are somewhat better for single women (i.e., nonfamily households headed by women), with median incomes for African American and Latina American women being about three-quarters of the income for white American women. Thus, even with considerable growth in employment opportunities, the earnings of women of color are still lower than those of whites.

The increasing number of African American families headed by women is a recurring subject of policy debate. A number of factors, such as increasing rates of divorce and separation among all racial/ethnic groups, contribute to the rise in families headed by women; however, the small and declining pool of marriageable black males is one factor that cannot be overlooked. In 1989, the ratio of males to females aged 25 to 44 years was 87 per 100 for blacks, compared with 101 and 107 per 100 for whites and Latinos, respectively (17). These statistics reflect, in part, the high rates of incarceration and premature mortality among young African American males.[4] The difficulties facing minority males are directly linked to the options and resources of minority families.

Demographic and Housing Patterns

Racial and ethnic minority populations are primarily concentrated in densely populated large urban areas. In 1988, over half (57 percent) of African Americans

---

[3] The percentage of Latino and African American families headed by women increased by about 40 percent between 1970 and 1990, from 21.8 to 31.2 percent among African American families and from 13.3 to 18.8 percent among Latino American families (15).

[4] There was a twofold increase in the prison population during the 1980s, with young black males comprising almost half of that population in 1986 (15). Moreover, African American males aged 25 to 44 years have the highest mortality rates, 2.5 times the rate for white males in 1988 (10).

Table 1

Sociodemographic characteristics of the U.S. population
by race and ethnicity, 1990[a]

Characteristic	White	Black	Hispanic[b]	Ratio B:W	Ratio H:W
Household composition (1990), %					
Married couple	58.6	35.8	57.2	0.61	0.98
Male householder	2.9	4.3	5.5	0.48	1.90
Female householder	9.1	31.2	18.8	3.43	2.07
Nonfamily households	29.4	28.8	18.4	0.98	0.63
Years of school completed (1989), %					
<12 yrs	21.7	35.0	49.3	1.60	2.27
12 yrs	42.3	36.7	29.6	0.87	0.70
12+ yrs	35.9	28.4	21.2	0.79	0.59
Median income (1988), thousands of dollars					
Family					
Male householder	$30.7	$19.5	$23.7	0.64	0.77
Female householder	18.7	11.0	11.3	0.59	0.60
Nonfamily					
Male householder	19.6	10.9	12.7	0.56	0.65
Female householder	12.1	7.1	7.5	0.59	0.62
Occupation of employed females (1989), %[c]					
Managerial/professional	30.1	20.0		0.66	
Technical/sales administrative	43.4	35.5		0.82	
Service	14.6	28.0		1.92	
Precision production	2.4	2.6		1.08	
Operators/fabricators	8.4	13.6		1.62	
Farming/forestry	1.2	0.4		0.33	

[a]Source: reference 17, Tables 58, 224, 725, and 656, respectively, for the listed characteristics.
[b]Persons of Hispanic origin may be of either race.
[c]Data not available for Hispanic women.

resided in central cities of metropolitan areas, compared with 27 percent of whites. Similarly, 90 percent of Latinos reside in urban areas, with the largest concentration living in four cities: New York, Los Angeles, Chicago, and San Antonio. African Americans and white Americans live primarily in racially segregated neighborhoods. Using an index in which 100 means a racially homogeneous neighborhood, Jaynes and Williams (16) found that although residential segregation declined during the 1970s, the average index for black-white neighborhoods in 1980 was about 80 points. Indices for Latino and Asian American neighborhoods, however, averaged about 45 points. It is likely that the impact of residential segregation varies depending on the quality of life in a particular neighborhood. However, the life experiences of minority women living in urban ghettos and barrios or in rural slums differ considerably from those of minority women living in more affluent, although segregated, neighborhoods.

Education and Employment

Educational achievement, as measured by years of completed school, provides some of the explanation for income differentials by race/ethnicity. Table 1 shows that in 1989, twice as many Latina American as white American women aged 25 and older had not completed high school (49 versus 22 percent). For African American women, the percentage not completing high school (35 percent) was somewhat less than the percentage for Latina American women but was still about 60 percent more than that for white American women. Women without a high school degree, or its equivalent, are more likely to enter the work force in low-wage, dead-end positions.

Employment patterns also help to explain the lower income of minority women. Over half of African American (58.7 percent), Latina American (53.5 percent), and white American (57.2 percent) women were in the labor force in 1989. Government enforcement of antidiscriminatory policies, however, has occurred in an era when there are fewer employment and business opportunities for those with less technically sophisticated skills. Data from the Bureau of Labor Statistics presented in Table 1 show that in 1989, African American women were less likely than white American women to work in managerial, professional, and technical positions and more likely to be employed in service occupations (17). Almost twice as many African American as white American women were employed in service positions such as food service, health service, and private household work (28 versus 15 percent). Additionally, 60 percent more African American women than nonminority women were employed in positions classified by the U.S. census as operators or fabricators (e.g., machine operators and assemblers). Current statistics are not stratified by gender for Latino Americans, although statistics similar to those of African American women probably hold true.

Due to long-standing inequities in education and training, minority women face difficulty taking advantage of new opportunities. As a consequence, the economic benefits of the transitions occurring in society have been shared unevenly across racial/ethnic groups.

Linking Health and Social Conditions

Latina and African American women have lower median incomes than white American women, and nearly half of Latino and American families headed by women have faced conditions of poverty for the last two decades. Also, minority populations live primarily in inner cities that lack the economic resources to address the varied problems associated with high rates of poverty. Many factors contribute to disparities in health; however, inadequate financial resources, limited education, and the stress of life in densely populated inner cities are important contributing factors that cannot be discounted. Furthermore, when illness or injury occurs, it not only raises a family's health care costs but can compromise an income earner's ability to work. Our society recognizes airline pilots, combat soldiers, and police officers, for example, as individuals who face life circumstances that place them at risk for stress-related illnesses and premature mortality. Yet we fail to recognize the similar impact of having inadequate resources to live, being perceived as inferior, or being part of a marginal, expendable workforce. Many racial/ethnic minority women, irrespective of their status as parents, experience life conditions that place them at risk for ill-health and injury. Measurement tools for the impact of these factors are not yet well developed, but statistics capturing the social environments of minority women are objective indications of the risks.

MINORITY HEALTH: A DEARTH OF RESEARCH

In our review of the literature, we found that most reports addressing the health status of racial/ethnic minority population groups did not provide data by gender and race or were limited in the ethnic groups included (18–24). Also, research involving the health of women in general, and of minority women in particular, is limited (15, 25), and few studies have explored the effects of race and social class on health (24, 26–29). The Secretary's Task Force on Black and Minority Health (18), reporting in 1985, was a first attempt at providing a national perspective on the health of racial/ethnic minority groups. In many cases, data were disaggregated by gender. However, information on the health of Latinos was not included in this report due to the lack of data specifically identifying ethnic origin.

Since 1960, U.S. racial/ethnic minority population groups have experienced considerable gains in health status (18–21). The magnitude of racial disparities, however, has changed little in the last two decades. In some cases, the gap has widened. Mortality statistics, one of the most dramatic and reliable indicators of a population's health, are evidence of continuing racial disparities.

The Secretary's Task Force contributed significantly to our understanding of the differences in mortality between African Americans and white Americans. As an indicator of the severity of racial disparities in health, the Task Force computed the number of "excess deaths" that occur among racial/ethnic minority women and men. Excess deaths reflect the number of deaths that would not have occurred if racial/ethnic minority populations experienced the same death rates, by age and sex, as whites. The measure reflects a standard of health that presumably could be achieved given the current state of knowledge and use of comparable resources. Using this approach, six health problems were identified as accounting for most of the excess deaths among African Americans of both genders.[5] The health problems that contributed most to the average annual excess deaths among female African Americans under the age of 70 were: cardiovascular disease (41 percent), infant mortality (12 percent), cancer (10 percent), homicide (6 percent), diabetes (5 percent), cirrhosis (3 percent), and accidents (1 percent). All other deaths continued to account for the remaining 22 percent of excess deaths for females in this age group.

More current information on the mortality experience of African American and Latino Americans as compared to white Americans is presented in Table 2 (22). Although the data are not gender specific, they provide an indication of the causes of death experienced more frequently among racial/ethnic minority groups than among white Americans. In 1990, African Americans of all age groups showed higher rates of mortality than white Americans for almost all causes of death examined. However, death rates for homicide, cerebrovascular disease (ages 45 to 64), HIV Infection, and diseases of the heart (ages 25 to 44) were substantially higher for African Americans than for white Americans.

The mortality experience of Latino Americans differs greatly from that of African Americans. For the majority of causes, Latino American mortality rates are similar to or lower than those of white Americans. Two exceptions are the higher death rates for homicide and HIV infection. It should also be noted that death rates for malignant neoplasms, diseases of the heart, and cerebrovascular disease were lower for Latinos than for white Americans.

Several recent articles have examined the effects of race and social class on health (26–29). Navarro (26) estimated mortality rates for heart disease using data from the 1986 National Mortality Followback Survey and the 1986 U.S. Occupational Census. Blue-collar workers such as operators, fabricators, and laborers had mortality rates for heart disease that were 2.3 times higher than those of managers and professionals. Navarro found that class differentials in mortality were larger than race differentials. Lerner and Henderson (27, 28), using Baltimore, Maryland, census tract data on neighborhood character-istics, found that both race and income were significant factors in mortality due to cerebrovascular disease and cancer, but race was not independently associated with mortality due to heart disease. Since both of these studies analyzed aggregate population-based indicators (e.g., occupational group and census tract median income) rather than person-specific data, relations among variables must be interpreted with caution. Using multivariate analytic techniques

---

[5] These health problems were heart disease and stroke, cancer, cirrhosis and other liver disease, diabetes, homicide and unintentional injuries, and infant mortality.

Table 2

Ratio of African American and Latino American to white American
death rates for selected causes and age groups, 1988[a]

Age group/selected causes	African Americans	Latino Americans
Age group 1–14		
Total	1.6	1.0
Injuries	1.5	0.9
Homicide	5.0	2.0
Malignant tumors	1.0	1.0
Other	1.6	1.1
Age group 15–24		
Total	1.5	1.2
Injuries	0.7	0.9
Homicide	7.4	3.5
Suicide	0.6	0.7
Other	2.0	1.2
Age group 25–44		
Total	2.5	1.2
Injuries	1.4	1.2
Homicide	7.0	3.1
Diseases of the heart	2.6	0.7
HIV infection	3.6	2.3
Other	2.3	1.1
Age group 45–64		
Total	1.7	0.8
Injuries	1.7	1.2
Diseases of the heart	1.7	0.7
Malignant neoplasms	1.4	0.5
Cerebrovascular disease	3.0	1.1
Other	2.1	1.1
Age group 65+		
Total	1.1	0.7
Diseases of the heart	1.1	0.6
Malignant neoplasms	1.2	0.6
Cerebrovascular disease	1.2	0.6
Other	1.1	0.8

[a]Source: reference 22.

and person-specific data, Otten and associates (29) found that about one-third
(31 percent) of the mortality differential by race could be explained by six
well-established risk factors and that 38 percent could be accounted for by family
income. This left 31 percent of the mortality differential by race unexplained.

HEALTH INDICES OF LATINA AND
AFRICAN AMERICAN WOMEN

It is generally known that women have a longer life expectancy, report more symptoms of acute illness, and are more likely to make a physician visit than men; very little is known, however, about the extent to which women vary by race/ ethnicity in patterns of illness and risk factors for ill-health. In this section, we provide descriptive information on several health indicators and risk factors for ill-health. The health measures (perceived health status, percentage with activity limitations due to chronic conditions, and percentage unable to work due to activity limitations) are indicators of the quality of life experienced by Latina and African American as compared with white American women. Data on risk factors (e.g., smoking, being overweight) reflect lifestyle behaviors that, while generally described as personal choices, also reflect sociocultural patterns, historic dietary practices, and financial resources.

Perceived Health Status

Self-assessment of health status has been found to correlate reasonably well with objective measures of health, including mortality and physician ratings of health (30). As such, it is a good indicator of the extent of health problems in a population. About one in ten women assess their health as fair or poor. As expected this finding varies by race and by income (Table 3). Twice as many African American (17.2 percent) as white American women (8.5 percent) reported their health as fair or poor in the 1988 HIS, and 1.5 times as many Latina American (13.0 percent) as white American women reported their health as fair or poor.

The proportion reporting their health as fair or poor is inversely related to income, with nearly one in four women with incomes under $10,000 feeling that their health was fair or poor, compared with one in 25 women with incomes of $35,000 or more. When examining self-reports of health by race and income, some racial differences persist but they are modest. For example, among women with incomes under $10,000, there are small differences by race/ethnicity in the percentage reporting fair or poor health (21 percent of white Americans, 24 percent of Latina Americans, 30 percent of African Americans). Similarly, among women with incomes of $35,000 or more, the percentage in fair or poor health is less than 10 percent irrespective of race/ethnicity, even though there is an almost twofold difference in the percentage of African Americans and white Americans reporting their health as fair or poor. In each income category, a larger percentage of Latina and African American women than white American women reported their health as fair or poor. Differences across racial groups, however, are smaller than the differences by income within a racial group.

Table 3

Health status measures by race/ethnicity and family incomes,
women aged 18 to 64 (weighted), 1988[a]

Health status measure/ family income	African Americans	Latina Americans	White Americans	Ratio	
				AA:WA	LA:WA
Fair or poor health, %					
All income groups	17.2	13.0	8.5	2.02	1.53
Under $10,000	29.5	24.4	21.0	1.40	1.16
$10,000–19,999	18.0	16.7	12.7	1.42	1.31
$20,000–34,999	9.2	9.6	7.5	1.23	1.28
$35,000+	7.8	5.0	4.2	1.86	1.19
Any activity limitation, %					
All income groups	15.6	10.3	12.9	1.21	0.80
Under $10,000	24.6	20.2	27.6	0.89	0.73
$10,000–19,999	17.8	9.7	18.0	0.99	0.54
$20,000–34,999	8.4	7.7	12.1	0.69	0.64
$35,000+	8.9	5.0	8.2	1.09	0.61
Unable to work due to activity limitations, %					
All income groups	8.2	5.3	4.8	1.71	1.10
Under $10,000	14.4	12.1	14.5	0.99	0.83
$10,000–19,999	9.3	4.9	7.1	1.31	0.69
$20,000–34,999	3.4	3.6	3.8	0.89	0.95
$35,000+	3.6	1.1	2.2	1.64	0.50

[a]Source: Analysis of data from the 1988 HIS.

Limitation of Activity

One frequently used indicator of a population's health is the percentage with limitation of major activity due to a chronic condition. The prevalence of reported chronic conditions is higher among older (aged 45 to 64) than younger (under age 45) women; however, heart disease, high blood pressure, orthopedic impairments, arthritis, sinusitis, and migraine headaches ranked among the leading chronic conditions for women of both age groups (31). Table 3 includes information on the percentage of women that reported limitation of the major activity associated with their age group in the 1988 HIS. For persons aged 18 to 64, the major activity is considered working or keeping house. As noted earlier, over half of women in each racial/ethnic group work outside the home.

Of women aged 18 to 64, 13 percent reported limitation of activity due to chronic conditions. This estimate includes individuals reporting they were (a) unable to perform the major activity, (b) able to perform the major activity but limited in the kind or amount of this activity, or (c) not limited in the major activity but limited in the kind or amount or other activities. Small differences by race/ethnicity are observed, with about 20 percent more African Americans (15.6 percent) and about 20 percent fewer Latinas (10.3 percent) than white Americans (12.9 percent) reporting limitation of activity. Differences by income are striking. Three times as many low-income women (25.7 percent) as upper-income women (7.9 percent) reported limitation of activity. When stratified by income and race, the effects of race observed among all women persist only for women in the highest income category. Data suggest that lower-income and middle-income racial minority women are as likely as or less likely than their white counterparts to report activity limitations. For example, in the $20,000 to $34,999 income group, about 30 percent fewer Latinas (7.7 percent) and African Americans (8.4 percent) reported limitation of activity than did white Americans (12.1 percent).

Inability to Work Due to Activity Limitations

Another measure used to assess health status is the degree to which health problems limit one's ability to work. Table 3 shows the percentage of women who reported they were unable to work due to activity limitations, a subset of those reporting any activity limitation. Health problems limited the working capacity of more African American women than Latinas or white Americans. The percentage of African Americans who were unable to work is 1.7 times greater than that for white Americans and 1.5 times greater than that for Latinas. The proportion of women unable to work is inversely related to income levels, with nearly one of every seven women (13.9 percent) with incomes below $10,000 unable to work because of their health problems. At the higher spectrum of the income level (more than $35,000), one of every 45 women was unable to work (2.2 percent) due to health problems.

When income and race/ethnic group are considered, there are some differences across racial groups within each income level, but these are modest compared with the differences within a racial/ethnic group by income. For example, among women with incomes below $10,000, a similar percentage of African Americans and white Americans were unable to work (14.4 and 14.5 percent, respectively). When considering African American women by income, those with incomes under $10,000 were four times more likely to be unable to work than those with incomes above $35,000. Among white American women, those in the lowest income group were close to seven times more likely to be unable to work due to health problems than women in the highest income group. In general, a lower percentage of Latina women than both African American and white American women were unable to work. However, differences by income are more striking. Latinas in the lowest income level were 11 times more likely to be unable to work than were those in the highest income level.

Lifestyle Behaviors

The health profiles of racial/ethnic minority women often include characteristics of risk factors that are known to be associated with specific states of ill-health and are modifiable. Four common risk factors—overweight, hypertension, high cholesterol, and smoking—are noted in Table 4 for racial/ethnic minority women, with Latina women grouped according to their country of origin.

Being overweight is one of the most common nutritional problems among racial/ethnic minority women. It is an indicator of dietary practices and often signals a diet poor in quality and variety. In the NHANES, almost twice as many African American (44.4 percent) as white American women (23.9 percent) were overweight. A sizable percentage of Latina women in the HHANES were also overweight. The rate varies, however, by ethnic group. Cuban Americans had the lowest percentage of overweight women, and Mexican Americans the highest. The disproportionate number of overweight racial/ethnic minority women is disturbing given the strong associations between obesity and such diseases as diabetes, hypertension, and breast and uterine cancer.

The prevalence of hypertension, an important risk factor for cardiovascular disease, differs considerably among the various racial/ethnic minority groups. Cuban American women, for example, had the lowest rate of hypertension (14.4 percent), compared with 25.1 percent for white women. African American

Table 4

Age-adjusted prevalence rates for specific health risk factors for women, by race/ethnic group, percentages[a]

Health risk factor	Mexican American	Puerto Rican	Cuban	Non-Hispanic black	Non-Hispanic white
Overweight	41.6	40.2	31.6	44.4	23.9
Hypertension	20.3	19.2	14.4	43.8	25.1
High cholesterol	20.0	22.7	16.9	25.0	28.3
Smoking	15.5	23.4	20.2	29.1	28.6

[a]Sources: For all factors except smoking, data for Hispanics are from the 1982–84 Hispanic HANES; data for non-Hispanic blacks and whites from the 1976–80 National HANES. For smoking, data are from the 1988 HIS.

women had the highest rate, 1.7 times that of white American women. Hypertension rates for Latina women of Puerto Rican and Mexican ancestry were about 20 percent lower than that of white women. Higher rates of hypertension among African Americans are believed to be related to environmental factors (e.g., diet and stress) and genetic predisposition (21, 32).

High serum cholesterol level and cigarette smoking are important risk factors for several chronic diseases including heart disease, stroke, and lung cancer. Data from the HIS (Table 4) show Latinas as having a lower prevalence of high serum cholesterol levels and fewer smokers than white American women. Data from the HHANES provide estimates of smoking rates among subgroups of Latinas that are higher than the HIS estimates but are still lower than the rates for white American women. Prevalence rates for high serum cholesterol level and cigarette smoking do not differ substantially for African American and white American women. This finding suggests that these risk factors, although very important to healthy living, are unlikely to be major contributors to the excess heart disease and lung cancer mortality of African American women when compared with white American women.

Another behavior pattern that affects the health of racial/ethnic minority women is drug abuse. In addition to the adverse physiological effects of the drugs used, users today are at higher risk of ill-health due to behaviors related to drug acquisition and use. For example, women who engage in sexual activity in exchange for cocaine are at a higher risk of exposure to sexually transmitted diseases, including HIV infection. Data from the Centers for Disease Control (33) indicate that African American and Latina women represent 86 percent of the AIDS cases among women (13 years and older) reported in 1991. Annual AIDS case rates were 14.5 times higher among African American women and 7.4 times higher among Latinas than among white American women. The high risk of AIDS among minority women is also reflected in the rising number of pediatric AIDS cases among minority children. Children born to minority women make up 81 percent of the cumulative pediatric AIDS cases reported through December 1991.

The risks of HIV infection are enormous for racial/ethnic minority populations because drug use, which can compromise one's judgment, is one of the major modes of transmission. Intravenous drug use was the mode of transmission in 48 percent of the AIDS cases among women in 1991, and having sex with an intravenous drug user exposed another 22 percent of the women to the virus. The high rates of transmission related to intravenous drugs could be an indicator of the prevalence of such drug use in minority communities or reflect racial/ethnic differences in the use of clean needles. For either case, changing the behavior of persons addicted to drugs is one of the greatest challenges facing society. Efforts to reduce HIV infection in racial/ethnic minority women will depend, in part, on the effectiveness of drug abuse prevention and treatment programs.

OCCUPATIONAL AND ENVIRONMENTAL RISKS

The work and home environments, where individuals spend most of their waking hours, often contribute to the experience of ill-health. Hazards in the work place such as exposures to noxious agents, the pace of work, and general safety concerns, among others, have been found to be associated with higher rates of injury, disease, and death. Additionally, some ill-health experiences are localized within a geographic area. In such cases, surrounding environmental conditions may be suspect in contributing to ill-health. Combining information on occupational and environmental hazards with information on health indicators helps us to construct a profile of the health of Latina and African American women.

Occupational Safety and Health

One legacy of discrimination in the United States has been the percentage of Latino Americans and African Americans employed in the lowest paid and least desirable jobs. When racial minorities gained entrance into many industries and skilled trades, they often were assigned the most dangerous jobs (34). Even after controlling for racial differences in years of education and work experience, the disproportionate representation of African American workers in more hazardous jobs and occupations remains strong (35).

The devastating fire that occurred in 1991 in a Hamlet, North Carolina, poultry plant is one example of the dangerous working conditions of minority women. Twenty-five workers (men and women) were killed in the fire because locked safety doors kept them from escaping. Although the majority of the persons fatally injured were white, two-thirds of the plant workforce were African Americans. This tragedy increased the public's awareness of the magnitude of the problems in the workplace and the lax enforcement of Occupational Safety and Health Act (OSHA) guidelines. Over 240 such poultry plants exist today, employing 150,000 workers, the majority of whom are women. Nearly 75 percent of these industries are located in the south, in predominantly poor and African American neighborhoods. The health and safety conditions within these plants are abhorrent. Each year, almost 28,000 workers in poultry plants lose their jobs or become disabled due to work-related accidents or injuries. Icy temperatures, dull knives and scissors, fat and grease build-up, line speed-up, and hand and wrist injuries are only a few of the health and safety problems (36). The majority of these plants are nonunionized, pay minimum wages, and offer no health care benefits to their employees.

A large proportion of Latina American women are employed in the semiconductor and agricultural industries. Studies show that workers in the semiconductor industry experience occupational illness at three times the rate of workers in the general manufacturing industries (37). Farmworkers and their families are exposed to dangerous pesticides, and occupational injuries occur at an alarming rate as the result of using faulty equipment.

The garment industry is another industry in which women of color constitute the majority of workers. Although conditions have improved somewhat with the passage of the OSHA standards regulating exposure to cotton dust, many hazards, similar to the sweatshop conditions of the 19th century, remain. Many garment shops are poorly lit working areas with inadequate ventilation. These conditions are similar to those that existed in New York's Triangle Shirtwaist Factory, where in 1911, a tragic fire killed 146 immigrant women (36). Workers suffer from formaldehyde exposure, carpal tunnel syndrome, and other ergonomic problems.

The majority of office employees are women. For minority women, many of whom are employed in lower level clerical positions, the health risks are substantial (38). The occupational hazards of office work are well known; however, current OSHA standards apply poorly to these hazards. The production line pace of most office settings and the modernization of offices with video display terminals, along with poor office design and inadequate ventilation, have increased employees' risk of developing job-related health problems. Ergonomic problems related to the hands and back (i.e., carpal tunnel syndrome, tendinitis, and back strain), vision problems, headaches, fatigue, colds and allergies due to poor indoor air quality, and job stress are among the most frequently reported health problems of office workers (39).

Environmental Exposures

Three of every five Latino Americans and African Americans live in areas with uncontrolled toxic waste sites (40). The most infamous dumping groups are to be found in rural areas in the South. "Cancer Alley" located in Louisiana, along the Mississippi River between Baton Rouge and New Orleans, is among the worst. The area is lined with oil refineries and petrochemical plants, and its residents are predominantly African American and poor. The abnormally high cancer rates of the alley's residents have prompted one health official to call the alley a "massive human experiment" (41).

From the landfills of rural America to the "fly dumpsites" and toxic incinerators of urban America, the lives and health of racial minority populations are threatened. For example, excess cancer rates, respiratory problems, and birth deformities have been identified in Altgeld Gardens of Chicago, Illinois, and in East Los Angeles, California. These predominantly African American and Latino American communities have toxic dumpsites and incinerators located literally in residents' backyards (42). In Warren County, North Carolina, residents of a predominantly African American community protested against the proposed site of a polychlorinated biphenyl (PCB) landfill (43). In spite of their protest, however, the community became a dumping site for these cancer-causing agents. PCBs not only cause cancer, but also can affect the reproductive system of adults and may pass to a child through the mother's breast milk. Repeated and high exposure to PCBs can also cause liver and nervous system damage.

In a study conducted by the Commission for Racial Justice (40), investigators analyzed a cross section of U.S. commercial hazardous waste facilities and uncontrolled toxic waste sites, and correlated them with the ethnicity of the communities in which they were located. The study found that race/ethnicity is the most significant variable associated with the location of hazardous waste facilities and that African Americans are overrepresented in the populations of metropolitan areas with the largest number of uncontrolled toxic waste sites. The study also found that even though socioeconomic status plays an important role in the location of hazardous waste sites, race is more significant. Bullard and Wright (44) explain that because of housing patterns and limited mobility, middle-income and lower-income blacks, unlike whites, often cannot "vote with their feet" and move when a polluting facility arrives.

ACCESS TO HEALTH SERVICES

Dramatic changes have occurred in the U.S. system of financing and delivery of health services during the last three decades. New initiatives improved the availability of health resources (providers and facilities) within inner city and rural communities. Additionally, with enactment of Medicaid and Medicare in 1965 and federal enforcement of antidiscrimination laws, health care services have become more financially accessible for low-income, elderly, and ethnic minority populations. Yet inequities in access to health care persist, and there are indications that barriers to care have increased for some populations (45, 46). In the last decade, access to care has been threatened by rising uncompensated care (i.e., bad debt and charity care) as well as the increasing costs of medical care.

Blendon (45) and Freeman (46) and their colleagues, analyzing data from a 1986 national survey on access, provide evidence of continuing disparities for racial/ethnic minority populations. Blendon and associates (45) found that the proportion making a physician visit and the average number of visits are significantly lower for African Americans than white Americans. The gap is experienced by all income levels. Racial differences persisted even after using multiple regression analysis to take into account respondent differences in age, gender, health status, and income. In addition to lower rates of use, African Americans reported greater dissatisfaction than white Americans with the care received. Freeman and associates (46) compared access indicators of Latino Americans with those of African Americans and white Americans. This study found that Latino Americans, on average, saw physicians at about the same rate as white Americans, but were less likely to receive hospital care, despite a larger proportion reporting poorer health.

With approximately 38 million people uninsured for their medical costs (47), access to care is problematic for many Americans. Problems are particularly acute for racial/ethnic minority populations. Barriers of language, cultural insensitivity, and the lack of health providers in minority communities compound problems in financial access for the uninsured and underinsured. Moreover, national policy emphasis during the 1980s shifted from expanding access to containing costs.

Table 5 presents information on racial/ethnic differences in indicators of women's access to ambulatory and hospital care (i.e., percentage without a physician visit, average number of physician visits, and hospital discharges per 100 persons), derived from HIS data. Health services utilization is an indicator of a population's health status as well as its access to health services. In general, individuals in poorer health may require more medical care and use services at higher levels than those who are healthier. However, financial and physical barriers to care could reduce utilization. Since many factors determine use of services, the most important of which is health status, measures of utilization, at most, provide suggestive evidence of barriers to care.

Ambulatory Care

The percentages of African American and white American women not visiting a physician in the last year do not differ (Table 5), with about one in five reporting no contact with a physician. Among Latina women, on the other hand, a larger percentage were without a physician visit (24.8 percent). When income is considered, women with incomes between $10,000 and $19,999 were the least likely to visit a physician among all racial/ethnic groups. This finding could reflect gaps in health coverage that are particularly severe for the working poor. Regardless of the reason, it is a disturbing finding that the population group with the largest percentage in fair or poor health has the smallest percentage making contact with our health care system.

Latina American women in all income groups were less likely than either white American or African American women to report contact with a physician. For example, 23.3 percent of Latinas were without a physician visit in 1988, compared with 19 percent of African American and 18.4 percent of white American women with incomes under $10,000. At the higher end of the income spectrum, more Latina American (22.4 percent) than African American (14.6 percent) or white American (17.2 percent) women were without a physician visit. The data suggest that factors other than income may be important determinants of whether Latina women obtain health care services.

The average number of physician visits per person per year also varies by race/ethnicity and income (Table 5). Low-income women in each racial/ethnic group reported more physician contacts than women in higher income groups. This is likely a consequence of their poorer health status. However, when comparing women of similar income, Latina and African American women made fewer physician visits than white American women. Racial/ethnic differences are greatest between Latinas and white American women. The finding provides some

Table 5

Utilization measures by race/ethnicity and family incomes,
women aged 18 to 64 (weighted), 1988[a]

Utilization measure/ family income	African Americans	Latina Americans	White Americans	Ratio AA:WA	Ratio LA:WA
No physician visit in last year, %					
All income groups	19.8	24.8	19.2	1.03	1.29
Under $10,000	19.0	23.3	18.4	1.03	1.27
$10,000–19,999	21.3	27.8	21.0	1.01	1.32
$20,000–34,999	19.9	23.7	19.3	1.03	1.23
$35,000+	14.6	22.4	17.2	0.85	1.30
Physician contacts, per person per year					
All income groups	4.8	4.1	4.8	1.00	0.85
Under $10,000	6.0	5.3	6.9	0.87	0.77
$10,000–19,999	5.1	4.3	5.2	0.98	0.83
$20,000–34,999	4.3	3.8	4.7	0.91	0.81
$35,000+	4.0	3.7	4.6	0.87	0.80
Short-stay hospital discharges, per 100 persons per year[b]					
All income groups	10.7	7.2	9.6	1.11	0.75
Under $10,000	14.9	11.4	17.9	0.83	0.64
$10,000–19,999	12.4	8.3	10.8	1.15	0.77
$20,000–34,999	7.5	5.3	9.3	0.81	0.57
$35,000+	7.4	4.4	7.1	1.04	0.62

[a]Source: Analysis of data from the 1988 HIS.
[b]Excluding childbirth.

evidence that minority women use health services less frequently than non-minority women of comparable income.

Hospital Care

Short-stay hospital discharge rates, unadjusted for health status, show higher annual rates of hospitalization for African American women (10.7 per 100 persons) and lower rates for Latinas (7.2 per 100) than for white American women (9.6 per 100) (Table 5). When hospital discharges are examined by family income, an inverse relation is observed for all racial/ethnic groups. Women in the lowest income groups had close to double the number of hospital discharges compared with women in the highest income category. Given the larger percentage of African American and low-income women in fair or poor health, higher rates may reflect their greater need for care.

Hospitalization rates also were found to vary by race and income. Among women with incomes below $10,000, fewer Latinas (11.4 per 100 persons) and African Americans (14.9 per 100) than white Americans (17.9 per 100) were hospitalized, even though a larger percentage of minority women reported being in poorer health. Also, fewer African American than white American women with incomes of $20,000 to $34,999 received hospital care. Latina women, on the other hand, had lower overall hospitalization rates than white American women and lower rates of hospital care in each income group. The data suggest that racial/ethnic barriers to hospital care exist for Latina women regardless of income; whereas for African American women, possible racial barriers are evident in only two of the four income groups.

DISCUSSION

Latina and African American women, when compared with nonminority women, are more likely to face social environments (e.g., poverty and hazardous work conditions) that place them at risk for illness and injury. Although persistent racial disparities in health are often attributed to the lifestyle behaviors of racial minority populations, they are also a consequence of poorer social conditions as well as barriers in access to quality health services. The complex interplay of racial, economic, and gender-specific barriers has resulted in many minority and poor women experiencing social conditions that adversely affect their health. The health effects of these barriers may be cumulative across generations, with cause and effect difficult to disentangle.

This chapter provides evidence that low-income women, regardless of race/ethnicity, have poorer health indices than their higher income racial/ethnic peers. Moreover, racial disparities in health are reduced when considering a measure of social class such as family income. Nonetheless, within most income categories, African American women have poorer health indices than whites. The unexpected finding, however, is that Latina and African American women experience similar social environments, yet Latinas have health indicators that more closely resemble those of white American women. Many studies have documented a positive relation between socioeconomic conditions and health status, an association that generally holds true for U.S. racial groups. White Americans and Asian Americans, as a group, complete more years of school and have higher incomes and better health indices. In contrast, African Americans and Native Americans, as a group, complete fewer years of school and have lower incomes and poorer health indices. Latinas, for some reason, may be the exception.

Health indicators of Latina women must be considered with caution given the difficulties in accurately identifying ethnic origin. Mortality ratios showing lower or modest differences in death rates between Latinos and whites, for example, may reflect a problem of misclassification of ethnicity. As late as 1988, only 30 states included a Hispanic identifier on their death certificate. Misclassification has been found to be a significant problem plaguing infant mortality statistics. A recent study showed that 30 percent of infants assigned a specific Hispanic origin at birth were assigned a different origin of death (48). Another hypothesis is that the indicators we analyzed do not truly capture the health experiences of Latinas. It is also possible that the indicators are not sufficiently sensitive to detect racial/ ethnic health differences for Latinas in aggregate. The inability to disaggregate Latinas into subgroups based on their country of origin or ancestry (due to the small number of cases) is one of the limitations of the HIS data and thus a limitation of this effort. For example, HHANES health indicators for Cuban-American women differed from those for Puerto Rican women. One must consider whether these differences are related to culture or to the social histories of the population subgroups. Cuban women living in the United States may disproportionately represent white Cubans (of Spanish origin), while Puerto Ricans and Mexican Americans may disproportionately represent black Puerto Ricans (of African descent) and Mexican Indians, respectively. Thus, efforts to understand Latina health will require sample populations of sufficient size and clarity of definition to examine differences in population subgroups.

Utilization indicators suggest that racial/ethnic barriers to care persist, particularly for low-income women. The finding that Latinas are less likely to visit a physician, make fewer visits per person, and receive less hospital care than white women across income groups is an indication of possible barriers in access to care. Latinas who are primarily Spanish-speaking, for example, may prefer to use alternative healers than face the language barriers encountered in the general health care system. For African American women, data suggest that while entry into the health care system may be approaching levels that are somewhat comparable to those for nonminority women, some differences persist in the amount of care women receive. However, an assessment of whether levels of use are appropriate cannot be made unless considering health needs. This analysis shows that low-income (under $10,000) and middle-income ($20,000 to $34,999) African American women receive less hospital care than nonminority women, but overall racial differences in receipt of hospital care as reported by Blendon and associates (45) are not evident from this analysis. One possible explanation for the varying findings is the effect of gender on insurance coverage and thus access to care. Since a larger percentage of minority women than men have health coverage (because of their eligibility for Medicaid through AFDC), they may experience fewer barriers to care than minority men even if problems persist in the quality of care received.

Gaps in Knowledge Hinder Policy and Interventions

Knowledge about the relative impact of race/ethnicity and social class on women's health and use of services is limited. Given the interrelated nature of economic, racial/ethnic, and gender-specific barriers, debate on the primary nature of one factor over the other is, to some extent, an academic exercise. Future research, however, should strive to improve our knowledge about the health effects of all three factors so as to develop interventions that will more precisely target causal factors. Disentangling the interrelated factors is complicated methodologically, but the limited progress to date is more a function of the lack of effort than the complexity of the task.

Much of the published research on the health of minority populations has been descriptive, with few studies exploring causal or contributing factors for ill-health. There are many reasons that could account for the lack of etiologic research, including a dearth of researchers interested in exploring such issues. Also, many epidemiologic studies exclude nonwhites from study populations because of concern about the confounding effects of race, even though there is little scientific evidence to support biological differences among racial/ethnic groups (6, 49). However, the lack of data by race/ethnicity is undoubtedly one major factor accounting for the lack of research. Although vital statistics and national surveys now routinely collect and report data by race/ethnicity, a paucity of national data persists for Latino, Asian, and Native Americans. Vital statistics are collected by state agencies, which vary considerably in definition and data quality. Several national surveys have oversampled racial/ethnic minority populations in the last decade, but the number of observations is generally too small for analyses of specific ethnic groups (e.g., Mexican Americans, Puerto Ricans) or for analyses of nonwhite/nonblack racial groups (e.g., Native Americans and Asian Pacific Islanders) with any confidence.[6]

Moreover, health and safety hazards that largely affect women on the job, including women of color, have not been thoroughly investigated even by the Occupational Safety and Health Administration. Since OSHA's passage in 1970, considerable improvements have been made in occupational safety and health. However, regulating exposures to occupational hazards in jobs traditionally held by women has been slow. As a result of a recent Congressional mandate, in 1991 the Occupational Safety and Health Administration issued a standard covering occupational exposure to bloodborne pathogens. The issuance of this standard is a major step forward and should improve protections available to health care employees, the majority of whom are women.

Limited knowledge about the factors associated with racial disparities in health has hindered the development of policies and programs that could seek to reduce

---

[6] Two notable exceptions are the Hispanic Health and Nutrition Examination Study (HHANES) and the Survey of American Indians and Alaskan Natives (SAIN).

these disparities. In the absence of more precise knowledge, public health interventions can only vaguely address rather than specifically target factors contributing to the greater burden of illness and injury among racial minority women. Future research must move beyond descriptive analyses and investigate causal and contributing factors to ill-health, particularly those associated with modifiable social environmental conditions. Such investigations are critical for identifying risk factors and developing more effective preventive interventions.

The recent National Institutes of Health policy (50) requiring inclusion of "women and minorities in study populations for clinical research, unless compelling scientific or other justification for not including them is provided" is important if this nation is to advance its knowledge of the nature of health problems and the most effective interventions for reducing the health problems of racial/ethnic minority populations. Navarro's (26) urging federal research agencies to collect and analyze information on indicators of social class, such as occupation and income, is also critically important. In order to help us in moving toward a more egalitarian society, our data collection systems and analytic methods should have the capability of monitoring progress in reducing differentials by race/ethnicity and by social class.

Improving Minority Women's Health
Provides Challenge and Opportunity

Further gains in the health of minority women will require a recognition of the role of the socioeconomic environment in facilitating or hindering improvements in health. From generation to generation, minority women's worth has been devalued because of their race/ethnicity and their gender. This has resulted in conditions of poverty and powerlessness. With limited financial resources and minimal political influence, minority women have faced conditions of life defined by others. As is apparent from this study, poorer health indices of minority women are due in part to the disproportionate share of minority women living in poverty, but a disproportionate share live in poverty because of racial and gender-specific barriers that persist in this country.

The major health problems facing minority and nonminority women (e.g., lung cancer, breast cancer, heart disease, AIDS, substance abuse, violence) have behavioral and psychosocial etiologic components that affect their prevention and treatment. Having an impact on these conditions will require multidisciplinary, community-based programmatic efforts. This perspective may result in fewer expenditures on health or shared funding for health and social programs. The challenge confronting public health researchers and practitioners is to deepen the level of understanding of the link between health and social conditions. Social factors theoretically are recognized as important determinants of health, but they are generally considered outside the domain of public health practice. One consequence of our failure to make practical linkages between health and social conditions has been a fragmentation of related interventions, with programmatic efforts addressing different dimensions of the same problem viewed as competing rather than complimentary. In some cases, barriers to improved linkages are organizational as well as conceptual. For example, human service delivery systems that address poverty are organizationally independent of those that seek to prevent injury and illness. Also, service efforts are often organized by bureaucracies that are only modestly informed about the population groups they serve.

To achieve further gains in the health of minority women, public policies must reduce social inequalities and assure greater equity in access to resources that facilitate healthier environments and lifestyles. Minority communities in general, and minority women in particular, must be active participants in efforts that seek to improve their health and well-being. Public health initiatives should be community-based, that is, they should reflect a shared partnership that actively engages minority women in decision-making about their lives and is responsive to the *health* and *social* needs of minority women. Efforts that improve social conditions objectively provide opportunities for healthier lives and lifestyles. However, the need to continue to improve the quality of life of minority women should not overshadow the successes that have been made. The vast majority of Latina and African American women have survived the degrading experiences of second-class citizenship and are productive members of society. The gains achieved by minority women were, in large part, a consequence of public policies that reduced racial and gender-specific barriers to the economic opportunities available in this society. If we seek further progress, we should work to implement public policies that help overcome continuing discrimination and thus serve the goal of social equity and improved health status for all.

Note — This chapter does not reflect the views of the U.S. General Accounting Office.

REFERENCES

1. Hollingshead, A., and Redlich, F. *Social Class and Mental Illness.* John Wiley and Sons, New York, 1958.
2. Jackson, J. J. Black women in a racist society. In *Racism and Mental Health.* University of Pittsburgh, Pittsburgh, 1973.
3. Frazier, F. E. *The Negro Family in the United States.* University of Chicago Press, Chicago, 1939.
4. Clark, K. *Dark Ghetto.* Harper & Row, New York, 1965.
5. Texidor del Portillo, C. Poverty, self-concept, and health: Experience of Latinas. *Women Health* 12(3/4): 229–242, 1987.
6. Cooper, R., and David, R. The biological concept of race and its application to public health and epidemiology. *J. Health Polit. Policy Law* 11: 97–115, 1986.
7. Krieger, N. Shades of difference: Theoretical underpinnings of the medical controversy on black/white differences in the United States, 1830–1870. *Int. J. Health Serv.* 17: 259–278, 1987.

8. Zambrana, R. E. A research agenda on issues affecting poor and minority women: A model for understanding their health needs. *Women Health* 12(3/4): 137–160, 1987.
9. Bennett, M. B. Afro-American women, poverty and mental health: A social essay. *Women Health* 12(3/4): 213–228, 1987.
10. Bassett, M. T., and Krieger, N. Social class and black-white differences in breast cancer survival. *Am. J. Public Health* 76: 1400–1403, 1986.
11. Dohrenwend, B. P., and Dohrenwend, B. S. *Social Status and Psychological Disorder: A Casual Inquiry.* Wiley Interscience, New York, 1969.
12. Neighbors, H. The distribution of psychiatric morbidity in black Americans: A review and suggestions for research. *Community Mental Health J.* 20(3): 5–18, 1984.
13. Neff, J. Race differences in psychological distress: The effect of SES, urbanicity, and management strategy. *Am. J. Community Psychol.* 12(3): 337–351, 1985.
14. U.S. Bureau of the Census. *Poverty in the United States: 1990.* Series P-60, No. 175. Washington, D.C., 1991.
15. U.S. Department of Health and Human Services. *Women's Health.* Report of the Public Health Service Task Force on Women's Health Issues, Vol. II. Washington, D.C., 1985.
16. Jaynes, G. D., and Williams, R. M., Jr. (eds.). *A Common Destiny: Blacks and American Society.* National Academy Press, Washington, D.C., 1989.
17. U.S. Bureau of the Census. *Statistical Abstract of the United States: 1991,* Ed. II. Washington, D.C., 1991.
18. U.S. department of Health and Human Services. *Report of the Secretary's Task Force on Black and Minority Health,* 1: Executive Summary. Washington, D.C., 1985.
19. Trevino, F. M., and Moss, A. J. *Health Indicators for Hispanic, Black, and White Americans.* Vital and Health Statistics, Series 10, No. 148. DHHS Publication No. (PHS) 84-1576. National Center for Health Statistics, Washington, D.C., 1984.
20. Davis, K., et al. Health care for black Americans: The public sector role. In *Health Policies and Black Americans,* pp. 213–247. Transaction Publishers, New Jersey, 1989.
21. U.S. Department of Health and Human Services. *Health Status of Minorities and Low-Income Groups: Third Edition.* GPO:1991 271-848/40085. Washington, D.C., 1991.
22. U.S. Department of Health and Human Services. *Health, United States, 1990.* DHHS Publication No. (PHS) 91-1232. Washington, D.C., 1991.
23. Trevino, F. M., Falcon, A. P., and Stroup-Benham, C. A. (eds.). Hispanic Health and Nutrition Examination Survey, 1982–84: Findings on health status and health care needs. *Am. J. Public Health* 80(Suppl.): 1–72, 1990.
24. Miller, W. J., and Cooper, R. Rising lung cancer death rates among black men: The importance of occupation and social class. *J. Natl. Med. Assoc.* 74: 253–258, 1982.
25. Muller, C. F. *Health Care and Gender.* Russell Sage Foundation, New York, 1990.
26. Navarro, V. Race or class or race and class? Growing mortality differentials in the United States. *Lancet* 336: 1238–1240, 1990.
27. Lerner, M., and Henderson, L. A. Income and race differentials in heart disease mortality in Baltimore City, 1979–81 to 1984–86. In *Health Status of Minorities and Low-Income Groups: Third Edition.* GPO:1991 271-848/40085. U.S. DHHS, Washington, D.C., 1991.
28. Lerner, M., and Henderson, L. A. Cancer mortality among the disadvantaged in Baltimore City by income and race: Update from 1979–81 to 1984–86. In *Health Status of Minorities and Low-Income Groups: Third Edition.* GPO:1991 271-848/40085. U.S. DHHS, Washington, D.C., 1991.

29. Otten, M. W., Jr., et al. The effect of known risk factors on the excess mortality of black adults in the United States. *JAMA* 263: 848–850, 1990.
30. Yergan, J., et al. Health status as a measure of need for medical care: A critique. *Med. Care* 19(Suppl. 12): 57–68, 1981.
31. U.S. Department of Health and Human Services. *Current Estimates from the National Health Interview Survey, 1988.* Vital and Health Statistics, Series 10, No. 173, DHHS Publication No. (PHS)89-1501. Washington, D.C., 1989.
32. Klag, M. J., et al. The association of skin color with blood pressure in US blacks with low socioeconomic status. *JAMA* 265: 599–602, 1991.
33. Centers for Disease Control (National Center for Infectious Diseases, Division of HIV/AIDS). *HIV/AIDS Surveillance.* Atlanta, 1992.
34. Michaels, D. Occupational cancer in the black population: The health effects of job discrimination. *J. Natl. Med. Assoc.* 75: 1014–1017, 1983.
35. Robinson, J. Racial inequality and occupational health in the United States: The effects on white workers. *Int. J. Health Serv.* 15: 23–34, 1985.
36. Cromer, L. Plucking Cargill: The RWDSU in Georgia. *Labor Res. Rev.* 16: 15–23, 1991.
37. Lee, P. T. An overview: Workers of color and the occupational health crisis. Labor Occupational Health Program. U.C. Berkeley, California. In *The First National People of Color Environmental Leadership Summit*, pp. 76–79. Washington, D.C., October 1991.
38. Haynes, S. G., and Feinlieb, M. Women, work, and coronary heart disease. *Am. J. Public Health* 70: 133–141, 1980.
39. Rabinowitz, R. *Is Your Job Making You Sick?* Coalition of Labor Union Women, New York, 1991.
40. Commission for Racial Justice, United Church of Christ. *Toxic Wastes and Race in the United States.* Public Data Access, Inc., 1987.
41. Elson, J. Dumping on the poor. *Time Magazine*, August 1990, pp. 46–47.
42. Grossman, K. Environmental racism. *Crisis* 98(4): 14–17, 31–32, 1991.
43. Lee, C. The integrity of justice: Evidence of environmental racism. *Sojourners*, 1990, pp. 23–25.
44. Bullard, R., and Wright, B. H. Environmentalism and the politics of equity: Emergent trends in the black community. *Mid-Am. Rev. Sociol.* 12: 21–38, 1987.
45. Blendon, R. J., et al. Access to medical care for black and white Americans: A matter of continuing concern. *JAMA* 261: 278–281, 1989.
46. Freeman, H. E., et al. Americans report on their access to health care. *Health Aff.* 6(1): 6–18, 1987.
47. Short, P. F., Cornelius, L. J., and Goldstone, D. E. Health insurance of minorities in the United States. *J. Health Care Poor Underserved* 1(1): 9–24, 1990.
48. Hahn, R., Mulinare, J., and Teutsch, S. Inconsistencies in coding of race and ethnicity between birth and death in U.S. infants: A new look at infant mortality, 1983 through 1985. *JAMA* 267(2): 259–263, 1992.
49. Jones, C. P., LaVeist, T. A., and Lillie-Blanton, M. Race in the epidemiologic literature: An examination of the *American Journal of Epidemiology*, 1921–1990. *Am. J. Epidemiol.* 134: 1079–1084, 1991.
50. National Institute on Drug Abuse. *Research Grants Program Catalog of Federal Domestic Assistance*, No. 93.279: Announcements and Guidelines. U.S. DHHS, Rockville, Md., 1990.

CHAPTER 21

Risks Associated with Long-Term Homelessness among Women: Battery, Rape, and HIV Infection

Barbara Fisher, Mel Hovell,
C. Richard Hofstetter, and Richard Hough

Women comprise an increasing proportion of the homeless population; approximately one-third of the homeless are now women and their children, and approximately 12 percent of the homeless are single women (1–3). These figures raise serious questions about the effectiveness of safety-net programs for families and underline the need to understand more about these women and their needs, the causes of their homelessness, and the risks they face while they are homeless.

The major support program for poor single women and their children, Aid to Families with Dependent Children (AFDC), has failed to protect large numbers of women from the debilitating effects of homelessness. More severe restrictions on eligibility enacted in the early 1980s and decreases in benefit level later in the decade—a 39 percent decrease between 1970 and 1990 (4)—have had a devastating effect. Family breakdown and limited job opportunities for women may also play a role in the "feminization of poverty" and the decline into homelessness among women (5, 6). Forty-six percent of female-headed families with children under 18 years of age are poor, three times the rate among two-parent families with children (5). As with most poor people, homeless women lack some of the basic essentials to maintain health and have a high prevalence of physical and mental diseases (7, 8). Comparisons of poor homeless and nonhomeless clinic users have found that the homeless are at greater risk than the domiciled poor for chronic obstructive pulmonary disease, weight loss, and substance abuse (9, 10). In addition, homeless clinic users were twice as likely as domiciled clinic users to have been attacked and four times more likely to have been raped in the last year (10). One retrospective study found significant drug abuse and psychiatric hospitalization with increasing period of homelessness among those with no impairment at onset of homelessness (57 percent of women) (11).

The use of drugs, the risk of rape, and mental health problems may place homeless women at high risk for AIDS as well. Drug abuse increases risk of HIV infection through use of contaminated needles and having sex with an intravenous drug user or other HIV-infected partner (12, 13). Alcohol abuse can decrease judgment and interfere with safe sex practices (14). Crack use also has been associated with an increased risk of HIV infection (15, 16). A sample of chronic mentally ill at a community clinic were found to have a high level of risky behavior as well as encountering HIV risk situations (17). Mental health symptoms during adolescence have been found to be associated with higher numbers of HIV risk behaviors during young adulthood (18).

Homeless women may be at further risk of HIV infection from behaviors that are important to their survival on the streets. They may engage in prostitution as one of their few sources of money. They may associate with one man for protection from violence; that man may be an intravenous drug user. Those who are in a dependent relationship may be unable to negotiate safe sex practices (19).

As a group, women who are homeless may be at greater risk of HIV infection because of the higher prevalence of abuse history in homeless than in domiciled women (3, 20). Women with a history of childhood sexual abuse exhibit high risk behaviors for HIV infection (21), and this may be true of victims of abuse later in life as well. In surveys, 22 percent (22) to 85 percent (23) of homeless women cited domestic conflict as the reason for their homelessness. Researchers agree that domestic violence is a major cause of homelessness (24–26).

The length of the homeless experience may also affect behavior. Women who are homeless for a brief period may have less need to trade sex for money and protect themselves through relationships with men, particularly if they are sheltered for most of that time.

There have been few reported epidemiological studies of the HIV risk behavior of homeless women (27, 28) and none requiring a certain length of homelessness. Studies of health risks among the homeless are frequently based on convenience sampling and contain few women (ranging from 6 percent (29) to 12 percent (11) to 27 percent (30)). Women often avoid congregation areas (7, 31, 32), making it difficult to locate and recruit women to studies of homelessness.

The following is an exploratory study of a sample of women who were homeless for at least three months. The purpose was to explore the risks for chronically homeless women and compare those risks with those reported in other studies. This report focuses on battery, rape, and HIV infection risks among homeless women.

METHODS

Sample

To be eligible for inclusion in the study, women had to be: (*a*) homeless for at least three months in the past 12; (*b*) English speaking; (*c*) living independently of their parents; (d) nonviolent; and (e) mentally competent. If the woman had lived at an emergency shelter, outdoors, in a space not designed for shelter or in a home, motel, or institution for less than 60 days and with no home available in the future, she was considered "homeless" (33).

Cluster sampling was used to obtain 53 homeless women almost equally distributed between night and day shelters. Women from shelters specifically serving battered women were excluded from the study so that the sample would not be artificially weighted toward women who had been battered prior to becoming homeless.

Women volunteers from five of the ten night shelters serving women in San Diego and all the women at the one women's day shelter who met the criteria for the study were interviewed between June and October, 1991. Two respondents were in a class for homeless teens, and one was a referral from an outreach project. A total of 53 women provided informed consent and were given five dollar for participation.

Four women were given a mini mental status exam adapted from Paveza and colleagues (34) because their ability to recall events accurately was questioned. One was excluded because she was unable to provide the current date or her date of birth. The remaining three passed the test and were included in the study. No women had to be excluded because they appeared to be threatening or violent.

Data Collection

Trained senior undergraduates in psychology or graduate students in public health conducted the 90- to 120-minute structured interview. Interviews were conducted in a closed room or, in one case, a private area of a park.

Measures

In addition to demographic information, the interview protocol included measures of the women's mental health, sexual relationships, assertiveness, risks of sexually transmitted diseases (STDs), and the occurrence of battery, rape, threats, and robbery.

Mental Health Status. Mental distress was measured on a five-item, six-point psychological distress scale developed by Ware and colleagues (35). A Cronbach's alpha reliability coefficient of .83 was achieved with this sample for this scale.

Social Support/Social Demands. The measure of social support was adapted from a questionnaire used in Solarz and Bogat's (36) study of the homeless. While the formal reliability and validity was not tested, the measure was successfully used to identify significant relationships in Solarz and Bogat's 1990 study, providing some evidence of validity. The protocol also included three questions that delineated people who placed demands on the participant (37) and two questions about the people who made life difficult for the participant.

Assertiveness. A measure of assertiveness was obtained by summing assertive responses to the seven questions in Table 1. Responses were coded as assertive if the woman was watchful and alert, talked her way out of a situation or tried to defuse it, or said that she held her ground. Four questions were open-ended and the remaining three offered five options as well as the opportunity to express an alternative response. The latter questions are typical of those used to measure assertion in violation of rights situations (38) adapted to situations common to homeless women.

Alcohol and Drug Use. A participant was identified as having alcohol problems if she responded affirmatively to two or more of the four questions that comprise the CAGE questionnaire (39). The measure has been used by other researchers studying homeless populations (33). The women were asked if they had used eight specific drugs in the past year.

STD Risks. The interview included questions from the Project STARRT Evaluation Questionnaire (PSEQ) (40) to assess AIDS risk-related behaviors and the prevalence of eight STDs. Responses to questions on sexual behavior used to assess HIV risk correlated with other measures as expected. Those who had sexual intercourse in the last year were younger ($r = -.41; P < .002$) and less assertive ($r = -.38; P < .003$) than those who had not had intercourse in the past year, and were more likely to respond in the affirmative to the CAGE

Table 1

Questions for measure of assertiveness

Open-ended
1. What do you do when someone threatens you verbally?
2. What do you do when someone threatens you with a weapon?
3. What do you do to protect yourself when you're walking on the streets during the day?
4. What do you do to protect yourself when you're walking on the streets at night?

Five-point questions with option for "other" responses
1. If someone pushed ahead of me at a food line, I would . . .
2. If another woman tried to steal my jacket, I would . . .
3. If someone near me was continuing to annoy me, I would . . .

---

questionnaire assessing alcoholism ($r = .28$; $P < .020$). Those who had had intercourse for drugs, money, or other financial benefit were more likely to have a sexual partner who used intravenous drugs ($r = .59$; $P < .001$) and to respond affirmatively to the CAGE questionnaire. Those who had had intercourse with someone who used intravenous drugs were more likely to use heroin themselves ($r = .44$; $P < .001$) and to respond affirmatively to the CAGE questionnaire ($r = .32$, $P < .011$).

Victimization. A number of questions measured the participants' exposure to rape, battery, and threats with a weapon. The 15-item checkoff list of injuries following rape or battery was taken from the common injuries list (41).

Reliability and Validity. Several internal checks were built into the interview to check the reliability of responses since some questions were sensitive and since women who were transient may have had difficulty recalling events reliably. The correlation between the number of months the participant was homeless in the last two years (asked at the beginning and end of the interview) was .99 ($P < .001$). In examining two related questions on partners' drinking history, 100 percent agreement was obtained. Six women were interviewed a second time to test reliability of certain measures. Since the women were highly mobile, retesting took place between 4 and 35 days later, and most were done by a different interviewer. There was 100 percent agreement in the women's retest response to whether they had been beaten or raped while homeless and while domiciled, but only 83 percent agreement concerning robberies. There was 100 percent agreement in response to crack and crystal use, but only 60 percent agreement in response to marijuana use.

Since the assertive measure was developed specifically for this study, we tested this measure's validity. The assertive measure was negatively correlated with having a protector ($r = -.23$; $P < .048$) and marijuana use ($r = -.26$; $P < .031$) but not with crystal use. The measure was positively associated with age ($r = .36$; $P < .005$) and with positive responses to the question "when walking outside, I look to see who is a danger to me" ($r = .34$; $P < .006$). Based on these analyses, these measures were assumed to be satisfactorily reliable; associations among variables suggest moderate levels of divergent and convergent validity (42).

RESULTS

Sample Characteristics

This study departs from the majority of studies on homeless women because it excludes those women who have been homeless for only short periods. The median length of homelessness was 24 months.

Despite differences in the length of homelessness, the sample's demographic characteristics (Table 2) were similar to a sample of homeless men and women. The average age was 35 ± 8.5 years (range, 18 to 56 years). Fifty-seven percent of the women were white, 24 percent African-American, 8 percent Latina, and 11 percent other, most of whom were Native American. Mean length of education was 12 ± 2.5 years. Thirteen percent of the women were married, 21 percent were in a long-term relationship, and 65 percent were single.

Table 2

Sociodemographic characteristics of long-term homeless
women and homeless clinic-users

Characteristic	Homeless women	Homeless clinic-users[a]
Age (n = 53)		
17-20	6%	
21-30	28%	
31-40	45%	
41-56	21%	
Mean ∫ S.D. (age in years)	35 ± 8.5	33 ± 9.7
Ethnicity (n = 52)		
White	57%	50%
African-American	24%	23%
Latina	8%	8%
Other	11%	6%
Education (n = 51)		
<12 years and no G.E.D.	27%	
High-school graduate only	16%	
G.E.D. and no further education	16%	
High-school graduate and further education	37%	
G.E.D. and further education	4%	
Mean ∫ S.D. (years of education)	12 ± 2.5	12 ± 2.4
Marital status (n = 52)		
Married	13%	9%
Long-term relationship	21%	
Single	65%	
Ever married	67%	
Ever divorced	42%	
Ever separated	25%	

[a]Source: reference 10.

Alcohol and Drug Use

Seventeen percent of the sample had been hospitalized or institutionalized for drug and alcohol problems at some time in their lives. Thirty percent of those hospitalized had been treated within the last 18 months. Although 30 percent were alcoholics according to the CAGE questionnaire, only 8 percent reported drinking more than eight times a month. The discrepancy may be due to the retrospective nature of the CAGE questionnaire, the strict rules against drinking at the day shelter, or underreporting (43).

Mental Health Status

The mean score on the six-point psychological distress scale was 3.49, compared with a mean of 2.10 in a general population (44) and 3.10 in Gelberg and Linn's (45) community-based study of homeless men and women (Table 3). Forty-three percent reported being afraid of being attacked or hurt for at least one hour each night. Fear of attack correlated with the frequency of nervousness ($r = .29$; $P < .017$).

Twenty-six percent of the women had required psychiatric hospitalization. Of those hospitalized, 43 percent (n = 6) had been hospitalized within a year prior to their interview. However, there was no significant difference in mental

Table 3

Psychological distress scale statistics for sample, comparable sample of homeless adults, and general population[a,b]

	Descriptive statistics ($X +$ S.D.)		
	Sample population (n = 53)	Gelberg and Linn (n = 529)	General population (n = 2,008)
Nervous person[c]	4.04 ± 1.37	3.01	2.14
Calm and peaceful	4.19 ± 1.27	3.57	2.64
Downhearted and blue[c]	3.30 ± 1.37	3.20	1.97
Happy	3.58 ± 1.29	3.47	2.36
Nothing could cheer[c]	2.32 ± 1.41	2.22	1.41
Total scale	3.49 ± 1.04	3.10	2.10

[a]Sources: Gelberg and Linn, reference 45, p. 293; general population, reference 44.
[b]Scores: 1 = all of the time; 2 = most of the time; 3 = a good bit of the time; 4 = some of the time; 5 = a little of the time; 6 = none of the time.
[c]These items were recorded so that a higher score represents more nervousness and depression.

distress between those ever hospitalized and those never hospitalized or between those hospitalized in the last year and those not hospitalized in the last year for mental health problems.

Family Relationships and Social Support

The women had an average social support network of three people. Only 35 percent of the women were married or in a long-term relationship at the time of the interview. Of the 35 women who had been married, only 20 percent were still married. Almost one-third of the women had children with them. These families had been homeless an average of seven months in the last year, and 56 percent had slept outside. Over half of those women with children were separated from them.

Battery and Rape

For the purposes of this study "battered" was defined as an affirmative response to the question "Have you ever been beaten or battered?" Ninety-one percent of the homeless women stated that they had been battered at some time in their lives. Thirty-eight percent had been battered only when domiciled, 48 percent both while domiciled and homeless, and 4 percent only when homeless. Fifteen percent reported that their most recent partner hit them an average of eight times a month or more.

Twenty-nine women (56 percent) in this study had been raped at some time in their lives, and 15 percent had been raped in the last year.

Sexual Relationships and Drug Use

Of those who were presently in a sexual relationship (45 percent), 42 percent had partners who used some form of drug, though not necessarily injectable. Of all women, 19 percent reported that their most recent sexual partner drank daily, and 49 percent that their most recent sexual partner used other drugs.

Risks of HIV

Women were divided into four groups according to their risk for HIV infection in the last year. The following is the authors' best judgment as to the probability of exposure, although we recognize that such an assessment is subject to argument.

Twelve women (23 percent) were in the "high-risk" group, characterized by one or more of the following behaviors within the past year: (a) heroin use, (b) intercourse with an intravenous drug user, or (c) intercourse for drugs, money, or other benefit. Half of the high-risk group engaged in two or more of these high-risk behaviors. Over 83 percent of the high-risk group did not use condoms all the time.

Of the total sample, four (8 percent) reported heroin use in the past year, nine (17 percent) had partners who used intravenous drugs, and six (11 percent) had intercourse in return for drugs, money, or other benefit (half of these with three or more men in the last year).

Those who had not had intercourse and had not used heroin within the past year were placed in a "no-risk" group. Although this group, comprising 32 percent of the total sample, still had some risk of HIV infection, that risk was very low. According to this definition, one lesbian was included in the no-risk group. While female to female transmission is possible, the risk is admittedly very low, and some might place this individual in a zero-risk group. However, placement of this individual in a different group would make no material difference in the analyses or overall results.

The remaining women were placed in two intermediate risk groups. Thirty percent were in the "low-risk" group because they were either monogamous or always used a condom during intercourse and had no other reported high-risk practice. The remaining 15 percent were in the "medium-risk" group, those who had more than one sexual partner in the last year and did not always use condoms.

Of the 85 percent who responded to a question about condom use, 60 percent never used a condom during the last ten times they had had intercourse and 22 percent always used a condom.

AIDS Risk Correlates

An AIDS risk variable was created by assigning the four risk groups an ordinal scale from one to four. An analysis was performed using Pearson's r correlations for bivariate associations between AIDS risk and selected variables. A Pearson's r value of greater than $\pm.20$ was systematically selected as a minimum standard for assuming an important relationship (Table 4).

In addition, two logistic regression analyses were performed to determine variables that distinguished those in the no-risk group from those not in the no-risk group, and those in the high-risk group from those not in the high-risk group. The results of these regression analyses are shown in Table 5. In view of the small sample size, we considered an odds ratio of 1.9 or more as a potentially real relationship worthy of comment and confirmation research.

The number of affirmative responses to the four questions in the CAGE questionnaire, a measure of alcoholism, was a significant factor in distinguishing the high-risk group ($P < .020$) and close to significant in distinguishing the no-risk group ($P < .103$). For each additional affirmative response to these four questions, homeless women were nearly twice as likely to be in the high-risk group as to not be in the high-risk group, controlling for other terms in the model. Those who

Table 4

HIV risk correlates with Pearson's r values
greater than $\lceil.20$

Variables	r	P
Alcohol use	.42	<.002
Crystal use	.24	<.042
Marijuana use	.32	<.011
Assertiveness	−.25	<.051
Protector	.25	<.036
Sleeping outside	.29	<.019
Mental distress	.20	<.072

Table 5

Logistic regression analyses of HIV risks on several behavioral variables

HIV risks/variable	β	Partial S.E. β	P	Odds ratio
"High HIV risk" vs "not high HIV risk"				
Alcoholism	.646	.276	<.020	1.907
Use of crystal and/or marijuana	.892	.554	<.108	2.441
Assertiveness	.110	.323	<.733	1.117
No protector	−.085	.426	<.842	.918
Sleeping outside	.547	.553	<.323	1.728
Psychological distress	.308	.467	<.511	1.360
"No HIV risk" vs "some risk"				
Alcoholism x (−1)	.654	.401	<.103	1.923
Use of crystal and/or marijuana x (−1)	.481	.587	<.413	1.618
Assertiveness	.500	.308	<.105	1.649
No protector	.904	.469	<.055	2.469
Sleeping outside	−.230	.489	<.639	.795
Psychological distress x (−1)	.315	.362	<.384	1.371

used crystal or marijuana were 2.4 times as likely to be in the high-risk group as those who did not use either ($P < .108$).

Those who did *not* have a "protector" (were *not* able to name a particular person whom they could count on to protect them if someone were trying to hurt them) were 2.5 times more likely to be in the no-risk group than those who did have a protector ($P < .055$).

Assertiveness was negatively associated with increased risk of HIV infection ($r = -.23$; $P < .051$) and was close to significant in distinguishing the "no-risk" group from those with some risk (odds ratio = 1.6; $P < .105$).

Although in this small sample, greater frequency of sleeping outside and greater mental distress were not significant variables for distinguishing the no-risk or high-risk groups. Pearson's r correlations indicated that these variables may have some affect on risk (no-risk: $r = .20$; $P < .019$; high-risk: $r = .20$; $P < .072$). There was very little improvement in predicting the high-risk group. There was an 11 percent improvement over chance in predicting who would be in the no-risk group when the following variables were used: alcohol use, marijuana and/or crystal use, assertiveness, having a protector, mental distress, and frequency of sleeping outside.

DISCUSSION

Our results should be considered cautiously in the light of sampling procedures, the modest sample size, and the cross-sectional design. We cannot determine from this study whether associations are causal, the direction of causality, or whether other factors affect possible causal relationships. Our conclusions are tempered by other design limitations including self-report bias, recall bias, and possible selection bias. The interview did not include a direct measure of intravenous drug use or the frequency of anal intercourse, which may lead to underestimates of HIV infection risk.

On the other hand, the study had many strengths compared with available information concerning homeless women. The use of fully trained, empathetic, same-sex interviewers, the guarantee of anonymity, and specific language giving permission for socially unacceptable behavior increased the face validity of responses to sensitive questions. Most measures were taken from prior studies that had established reliability or validity. Women were selected who were known to have been homeless for at least three months, resulting in a median length of homelessness of 24 months.

The demographic characteristics and drug use patterns of this group of women appear to be similar to those of other samples of homeless people reported in the literature. Comparisons are difficult to make since there are few studies that exclusively study homeless women or report results from their sample of women separately. Studies of homeless women with children are not an appropriate comparison since these women are different from those without children (2). Our sample of women was within 1 to 3 percentage points of the proportion of blacks and had fewer Hispanics than two other studies reporting statistics on homeless women in California (46, 47). Women in our sample appeared to be slightly better educated, although this may have been due to considering a G.E.D. equivalent to high-school graduation. Compared with male and female homeless clinic users in Los Angeles, the homeless women in our sample had the same mean years of education, consisted of approximately the same proportion of African-Americans and Latinas, were two years older on average, and had similar drug use patterns (10). Reported drug use in the last year and the last month for our sample and the clinic sample were, respectively: marijuana, 38 vs 41 percent; crack or cocaine, 21 vs 18 percent; uppers, 9 vs 8 percent; and heroin, 7 vs 4 percent. Our study found that 30 percent of the women were alcoholics, comparable to the 32 percent of women found by another study (48). These findings imply that our sample may be similar to other samples of homeless women and that our results are generalizable and sufficiently reliable as a basis for further exploration.

Although the sample was similar in demographics and drug use, the proportions of certain risks were much higher than in other samples of homeless women. The differences may be due to differences between women who were episodically homeless and the women in this study who were homeless for a median of 24 months (49). The higher proportions found in this study may be more representative of the true risks among long-term homeless women and may be a better indication of the public health problems among women who are chronically homeless.

One of the most disturbing findings is the extremely high proportion of women (91 percent) who have been battered over their lifetime. The proportion is much higher than the 63 percent found in another study of homeless women (20). Most of the women in our study suffered severe injury during episodes that they considered to be battery. Ninety percent of the women who had been battered suffered at least one injury more serious than bruises during their worst beating.

Recent exposure to battery was high as well. Forty-two percent of these long-term homeless women reported a battery incident within the last 12 months. By comparison, Maurin, Russell, and Memmott (50) found that only 20 percent of homeless women in their samples had been abused during the same time period, and a nationwide survey of women found that 16 percent had been physically assaulted (51).

The prevalence of rape is also very high. Fifty-six percent of these homeless women had been raped at some time in their life, compared with 58 percent of women in a shelter (20) and 12 percent of adult women in a nationwide survey (52). Padgett and Struening (53) found that 10 percent of the women in their shelter sample had been raped in the last year, compared with 15 percent in our sample.

The high prevalence of battery and rape may be due to greater exposure to such attacks during longer periods of homelessness. In one of the studies noted for comparison, 43 percent of the women had been homeless for less than a month (50). The high proportion also could be due to the fact that women who have been raped or battered have more severe coping problems (54) and thus have more problems taking the difficult steps needed to escape from homelessness. Winkleby and coworkers (46) found that length of homelessness was associated with physical abuse as a child. Abuse as an adult may be a predictor for subsequent homelessness as well. It should be noted, however, that no comparisons were made with domiciled poor women in the same area. Although several studies have shown homeless women to have higher rates of abuse (3, 55), one study found similar rates of abuse among domiciled and homeless poor women (56).

The homeless women in this study reported that 73 percent of the offenders during their most recent battery were present or former sexual partners, a figure similar to the 76 percent of offenders who were known to the victim in the National Crime Survey data (57). This suggests that relationships are a source of battery risk to all women, no matter what their living situation.

A constant, even chronic, state of alertness and anxiety is a consistent response to the dangers that homeless women confront (58). The study found a full point scale difference in the level of nervousness compared to Gelberg and Linn's (45) sample of homeless men and women. Forty percent reported being nervous most or all of the time. The exceptionally high distress level found among these long-term homeless women may be a gender-related response or related to a higher exposure to anxiety-producing events. The distress level correlated with exposure to rape ($r = .23$; $P < .06$).

Women in our study reported a support network of three, whereas a study of homeless-shelter men and women that used a similar support measure found an average of six in the support network (36). The relative lack of social support may be due to the inability to maintain former relationships during longer periods of homelessness (59) or a higher prevalence of long-term homelessness among those who suffer from severe family discord or greater distrust. Distrust is associated with assaults by partners or acquaintances (60), and the homeless women in our study had a high prevalence of such assaults.

Some women associated with men as one of the few means of protecting themselves from violence on the streets (61). Tragically, this action may have placed these homeless women at serious potential risk of HIV infection because of the behaviors of the men they acquired as their protectors and sexual partners. Forty-nine percent said that their most recent sexual partner used drugs, and 70 percent said their most recent sexual partner hit them. These partnerships may not have been during their period of homelessness, however. In such relationships, condom negotiation may be particularly difficult due to physical abuse and dependency for physical protection (19). Thirty-two percent of the women had sex with more than one sexual partner in the last year, compared with 3 percent having sex with more than one partner in 3 months in a national sample (62) and 9 percent in a methadone-clinic study (63). Exchange of sex for protection, money, or drugs may be reasons for the high number of sexual partners in this group of long-term homeless women. Although a greater proportion of the partners of these homeless women always used condoms (22 percent) than the proportion found in a study of heterosexual women in San Francisco (9 percent) (64), the large majority of the women are not protecting themselves from sexual disease risks. Even those homeless women who were celibate were at risk due to forced sexual intercourse, which is prevalent in this group. Sexual assault is associated with alcohol use by the victim (43, 53), a behavior that was prevalent in our sample.

The relationships between HIV risk and other variables found in this small study, while not always clearly significant, reveal important trends that warrant further study to determine significant factors and effective interventions to prevent the spread of AIDS. As in other studies, we found an association between high-risk behavior and alcohol use (14) and found that for every additional affirmative response in the CAGE questionnaire, the subject was twice as likely to be in the highest risk group.

The association with drug use was not as strong, although there was a trend in higher likelihood of being in the highest risk group with marijuana and crystal use. This finding is consistent with studies showing an association between high-risk behavior and crack use (15, 16) as well as with the use among the poor of prostitution to obtain drugs (16, 65). Women who use marijuana and crystal may be more likely to have partners who also use drugs. Studies have found that women who are intravenous drug users have difficulty finding partners who are not also intravenous drug users (66).

Another trend found by logistic regression was an increased likelihood of being in the "no risk" group with increased assertiveness and not having a protector. An association with assertiveness is consistent with other studies (67). These trends suggests that social skills training to increase assertiveness and to teach homeless women effective means of providing their own protection may reduce their need to find a partner for protection and reduce their risk of HIV infection.

Clearly, however, the most effective means of reducing these women's risk of serious injury is to offer a safer environment than inner city streets. The association between high-risk HIV behaviors and sleeping outdoors ($r = .29$; $P < .019$), while not supported by the logistic regression in this small sample, suggests a connection between homelessness and HIV risk.

Our study underlines other acute and chronic risks also associated with long-term homelessness, creating a picture of the long-term homeless woman as an extremely vulnerable person exposed to the serious risks of HIV infection, battery, rape, anxiety, and social isolation. The most effective way to confront these problems is to address the needs of the poor and the causes of homelessness.

Perhaps one measure of the degree of civility in a society is whether it offers the basic necessities of food and shelter to its vulnerable citizens. We cannot hope to change risky behaviors associated with HIV infection for this population without getting women off the streets and away from the dangers the street life imposes, as well as addressing the alcohol and drug abuse problems associated with these high-risk behaviors. A health education program for homeless women on AIDS risks can have little effect on changing behaviors when those behaviors appear necessary for survival on the streets and when the basic needs of clothing and shelter have not been addressed. Even in a domiciled population, knowledge of risks have been shown to be a poor predictor of safe sexual behavior (68).

Some of the solutions to homelessness involve major changes in our laws and social systems. AFDC laws should be changed to provide financial incentives for work while maintaining access to health care. Existing low-income housing should be preserved and public/private partnerships encouraged to build more. We should improve or develop programs for eviction prevention, work training, and discharge planning. Violence prevention, an important public health goal in its own right, may be another important tool to lower the incidence of homelessness and possible consequential HIV infection. A high proportion of these long-term homeless women (86 percent) experienced violence prior to becoming homeless. Other researchers have suggested a causal relationship between abuse and homelessness (58). For some women, homelessness may have seemed a safer alternative than the violence in their homes. One respondent noted that she felt safer on the streets where she could yell or run than when she was confined in an apartment. Lowering the rate of exposure to adult abuse may lower high-risk sexual behaviors. One study found that childhood sexual abuse is associated with high-risk sexual behavior (21).

For those who are homeless, other approaches must be explored. Research is needed to find the best approaches for changing behaviors in the context of a history of rape, abuse, and continued threats. To decrease women's anxiety, programs must offer a secure and safe haven. Day shelters should provide a place where women can learn to let go of protective street behaviors in a safer environment and develop trust. Social skills training should be offered to teach refusal skills for drugs, alcohol, and unprotected sex and alternative coping skills for protection. A small pilot study of a social skills program with women in a drug treatment program found changes in condom use and communication (63).

Studies that include HIV testing would be helpful to more clearly identify behaviors associated with risk in this population. A study of homeless black women in Los Angeles (28) found the same seropositivity rate (1.2 percent) among intravenous drug users as among those who had sex with an intravenous drug user, used nonintravenous drugs, or had unprotected sex with two or more partners. The study found that high-risk homeless women were more depressed and had less self-esteem and greater environmental concerns.

Our study makes clear that long-term homeless women are at high risk for disease and trauma and that the risks may be interactive with one another. These relationships and other possible "determinants" of risk require further study. In the interim, all efforts must be made to prevent homelessness, especially among women, and to provide shelter for those who have become homeless.

REFERENCES

1. The U.S. Conference of Mayors. *A Status Report on Hunger and Homelessness in America's Cities: 1991*, p. 2. Washington, D.C., 1991.
2. Johnson, A. K., and Kreuger, L. W. Toward a better understanding of homeless women. *Soc. Work* 34: 537–540, 1989.
3. Bassuk, E. L., and Rosenberg, L. Why does family homelessness occur? A case control study. *Am. J. Public Health* 78: 783–787, 1988.
4. Weill, J. D. Child poverty in America. *Clearinghouse Rev.* 25: 337–348, 1991.
5. Besharov, D. J. The feminization of poverty: Has legal services failed to respond? *Clearinghouse Rev.* 24: 210–218, 1990.
6. Bassuk, E. L., Rubin, L., and Lauriat, A. S. Characteristics of sheltered homeless families. *Am. J. Public Health* 76: 1097–1101, 1986.
7. Ritchey, F. J., La Gory, M., and Mullis, J. Gender differences in health risk and physical symptoms among the homeless. *J. Health Soc. Behav.* 32: 33–48, 1991.
8. Wright, J. D. Poor people, poor health: The health status of the homeless. *J. Soc. Issues* 46: 49–64, 1990.
9. Ferenchick, G. S. Medical problems of homeless and nonhomeless persons attending an inner-city clinic: A comparative study. *Am. J. Med. Sci.* 301: 379–382, 1991.
10. Linn, L. S., Gelberg, L., and Leake, B. Substance abuse and mental health status of homeless and domiciled low-income users of a medical clinic. *Hosp. Community Psychiatry* 41: 306–310, 1990.
11. Winkleby, M. A., and White, R. Homeless adults without apparent medical and psychiatric impairment: Onset of morbidity over time. *Hosp. Community Psychiatry* 43: 1017–1023, 1992.
12. Lane, S. R., and Levine, R. N. Caring for homeless people with HIV disease. *Focus* 5: 1–2, 1990.
13. Schoenbaum, E. E., et al. Risk factors for human immunodeficiency virus infection in intravenous drug users. *N. Engl. J. Med.* 321: 874–879, 1989.
14. Hingson, R. W. Use of alcohol, drugs and unprotected sex among adolescents. *Am. J. Public Health* 80: 295–301, 1990.
15. Chiasson, M. A., et al. Heterosexual transmission of HIV-1 associated with the use of smokable freebase cocaine (crack). *AIDS* 5: 1121–1126, 1991.
16. Fullilove, R. E., et al. Risk of sexually transmitted disease among black adolescent crack users in Oakland and San Francisco, Calif. *JAMA* 263: 851–855, 1990.
17. Kelly, J. A., et al. AIDS/HIV risk behavior among the chronic mentally ill. *Am. J. Psychiatry* 149: 886–889, 1992.
18. Stiffman, A. R., et al. The influence of mental health problems on AIDS-related risk behaviors in young adults. *J. Nerv. Ment. Dis.* 180: 314–320, 1992.
19. Campbell, C. A. Women and AIDS. *Soc. Sci. Med.* 30: 407–415, 1990.

20. D'Ercole, A., and Struening, E. Victimization among homeless women: Implications for service delivery. *J. Community Psychol.* 18: 141–152, 1990.
21. Zierler, S., et al. Adult survivors of childhood sexual abuse and subsequent risk of HIV infection. *Am. J. Public Health* 81: 572–575, 1991.
22. Mills, C., and Ota, H. Homeless women with minor children in the Detroit metropolitan area. *Soc. Work* 34: 185–189, 1989.
23. Mitchell, J. C. The components of strong ties among homeless women. *Soc. Networks* 9: 37–47, 1987.
24. Seltser, B. J., and Miller, D. E. *Homeless Families: The Struggle for Dignity,* pp. 7–15. University of Illinois Press, Champaign, 1993.
25. Zorza, J. Women battering: A major cause of homelessness. *Clearinghouse Rev.* 25: 420–429, 1991.
26. Ropers, R. H., and Boyer, R. Perceived health status among the new urban homeless. *Soc. Sci. Med.* 24: 669–678, 1987.
27. Christiano, A., and Susser, I. Knowledge and perceptions of HIV infection among homeless pregnant women. *J. Nurse Midwifery* 34: 318–322, 1989.
28. Nyamathi, A. Comparative study of factors relating to HIV risk level of black homeless women. *J. Acquir. Immune Defic. Syndr.* 5: 222–228, 1992.
29. Fischer, P. J., et al. Mental health and social characteristics of the homeless: A survey of mission users. *Am. J. Public Health* 76: 519–524, 1986.
30. Gelberg, L., Linn, L. S., and Mayer-Oakes, S. A. Differences in health status between older and younger homeless adults. *J. Am. Geriatr. Soc.* 38: 1220–1229, 1990.
31. Bachrach, L. L. Homeless women: A context for health planning. *Milbank Q.* 65: 371–396, 1987.
32. Harris, M. *Sisters of the Shadow,* pp. 98–126. University of Oklahoma Press, Norman, 1991.
33. Gelberg, L., and Linn, L. S. Assessing the physical health of homeless adults. *JAMA* 262: 1973–1979, 1989.
34. Paveza, G. J., et al. A brief form of the mini-mental status examination for use in community care settings. *Behav. Health Aging* 1: 133–139, 1990.
35. Ware, J. E., Sherbourne, C. D., and Davies, A. R. *A Short-Form General Health Survey.* Rand Corporation, Santa Monica, Calif., 1986.
36. Solarz, A., and Bogat, G. A. When social support fails: The homeless. *J. Community Psychol.* 18: 79–96, 1990.
37. Hough, R. L., and Timbers, D. M. Social network support and demand: Implications for prevention. In *Psychiatric Epidemiology and Prevention: The Possibilities,* edited by R. L. Hough, et al., pp. 191–206. Neuropsychiatric Institute, Los Angeles, 1985.
38. Kern, J. M. An evaluation of a novel role-play methodology: The standardized idiographic approach. *Behav. Ther.* 22: 13–29, 1991.
39. Ewing, J. A. Detecting alcoholism: The CAGE questionnaire. *J. Am. Med. Soc.* 252: 1905–1907, 1984.
40. Hovell, M. F., et al. *Project STARRT Evaluation Questionnaire (PSEQ).* San Diego State University, San Diego, 1989.
41. Sheridan, D. J., et al. *Guidelines for the Treatment of Battered Women Victims in Emergency Room Settings.* Chicago Hospital Council, Chicago, 1985.
42. Campbell, D. T., and Fiske, D. W. Convergent and discriminant validation by the multitrait-multimethod matrix. *Psychol. Bull.* 56: 81–104, 1959.
43. Fischer, P. J., and Breakey, W. R. The epidemiology of alcohol, drug, and mental disorders among homeless persons. *Am. Psychol.* 46: 1115–1128, 1991.

44. Ware, J. E., and Sherbourne, C. D. Developing and testing the MOS 20-item short form health survey: A general population application. In *Measuring Functioning and Well-Being: The Medical Outcomes Study*, edited by A. Stewart and J. Ware. Duke University Press, Durham, N.C., 1992.

45. Gelberg, L., and Linn, L. S. Psychological distress among homeless adults. *J. Nerv. Ment. Dis.* 177: 291–295, 1989.

46. Winkleby, M. A., et al. The medical origins of homelessness. *Am. J. Public Health* 82: 1395–1398, 1991.

47. Robertson, M. J., and Cousineau, M. R. Health status and access to health services among the urban homeless. *Am. J. Public Health* 76: 561–563, 1986.

48. Breakey, W. R., et al. Health and mental health problems of homeless men and women in Baltimore. *JAMA* 262(10): 1352–1357, 1989.

49. Belcher, J. R., Scholler-Jaquish, A., and Drummond, M. Three stages of homelessness: A conceptual model for social workers in health care. *Health Soc. Work* 16: 87–93, 1991.

50. Maurin, J. T., Russell, L., and Memmott, R. J. An exploration of gender differences among the homeless. *Res. Nurs. Health* 12: 315–321, 1989.

51. Straus, M. A., and Gelles, R. J. (eds.). How violent are American families? Estimates from the national violence resurvey and other studies. In *Physical Violence in American Families*, pp. 95–112. Transaction Publisher, New Brunswick, 1990.

52. National Victim Center. *Rape in America: A Report to the Nation.* Arlington, Va., 1992.

53. Padgett, D. K., and Struening, E. L. Victimization and traumatic injuries among the homeless: Associations with alcohol, drug, and mental problems. *Am. J. Orthopsychiatry* 62: 525–534, 1992.

54. Hilberman, E., and Munson, K. Sixty battered women. *Victimol. Int. J.* 2: 460–470, 1978.

55. Wood, D. L., et al. Health of homeless children and housed, poor children. *Pediatrics* 86: 858–866, 1990.

56. Goodman, L. A. The prevalence of abuse among homeless and housed poor mothers: A comparison study. *Am. J. Orthopsychiatry* 61: 489–500, 1991.

57. Harlow, C. W. *Female Victims of Violent Crime.* U.S. Department of Justice, Washington, D.C., 1991.

58. Milburn, N., and D'Ercole, A. Homeless women: Moving toward a comprehensive model. *Am. Psychol.* 46: 1161–1169, 1991.

59. Goodman, L. A., Saxe, L., and Harvey, H. Homelessness as psychological drama: Broadening perspectives. *Am. Psychol.* 46: 1219–1225, 1991.

60. Carmen, E. H., Rieker, P. P., and Mills, T. Victims of violence and psychiatric illness. *Am. J. Psychiatry* 141: 378–383, 1984.

61. Ranson, M. Personal communication, 1992.

62. Seidman, S. N., Mosher, W. D., and Aral, S. O. Women with multiple sexual partners: United States, 1988. *Am. J. Public Health* 82: 1388–1394, 1992.

63. Schilling, R. F., et al. Building skills of recovering women drug users to reduce heterosexual AIDS transmission. *Public Health Rep.* 106: 297–301, 1991.

64. Catania, J. A., et al. Condom use in multi-ethnic neighborhoods of San Francisco: The population-based AMEN (AIDS in Multi-Ethnic Neighborhoods) study. *Am. J. Public Health* 82: 284–287, 1992.

65. Minkoff, H. L., et al. The relationship of cocaine use to syphilis and human immunodeficiency virus infections among inner city parturient women. *Am. J. Obstet. Gynecol.* 163: 521–526, 1990.

66. Murphy, D. L., Harrison, B., and Hosang, D. Sex Roles and Partnership Acquisition Patterns: Ethnographic, Sociocultural and Epidemiological Perspectives on the Heterosexual Transmission of HIV. Paper presented at VII International Conference on AIDS, Amsterdam, July 19–24, 1992.
67. Rotherman-Borus, M. J., Koopman, C., and Ehrhardt, A. A. Homeless youths and HIV infection. *Am. Psychol.* 46: 1188–1197, 1991.
68. Harrison, J., Mullen, P., and Green, L. A meta-analysis of the studies of the Health Belief Model with adults. *Health Ed. Res.* 7: 107–116, 1992.

CHAPTER 22

Prevalence and Health Implications of Anti-Gay Discrimination: A Study of Black and White Women and Men in the CARDIA Cohort

Nancy Krieger and Stephen Sidney

Little empirical research documents the prevalence of self-reported experiences of discrimination based on sexual orientation among lesbians, gay men, and bisexual women and men in the United States, and even less has examined relationships between exposure to this type of discrimination and somatic health (1–4). Several studies, however, have linked risk of depression and suicide among lesbian and gay adolescents and adults to anti-gay discrimination (3, 5–8); others have documented how such discrimination can impede access to appropriate health care (1, 2, 9–11). Data on hate crimes further underscore how anti-gay harassment, in the form of gay-bashing, can produce injury and death (1, 4, 12, 13). To date, however, the few studies regarding public health implications of anti-gay discrimination have chiefly involved only one portion of the population at risk: namely, white lesbians and gay men, recruited by either announcements directed to, or snowball sampling conducted among, self-defined lesbian and gay communities (2, 7, 10).

To address gaps in current knowledge, the purpose of our study was thus to (*a*) describe the prevalence of discrimination based on sexual orientation reported by black and white women and men with same-sex sexual partners, among members of a cohort not recruited with reference to sexual orientation, and (*b*) explore health-related consequences of this discrimination, in

This investigation was supported by FIRST investigator award 1-R29-HL51151-01, issued by the National Heart, Lung, and Blood Institute. The CARDIA study, overall, is supported by contracts N01-HC-84047, N01-HC-84048, N01-HC-84049, and N01-HC-84050, also issued by the National Heart, Lung, and Blood Institute.

conjunction with self-reported experiences of racial and gender discrimination. We focused on blood pressure because a small but provocative body of literature suggests that experiences of, and internalized responses to, racial discrimination may contribute to elevated blood pressure and excess rates of hypertension among the U.S. black population (14–22). To our knowledge, no study has assessed whether comparable relationships exist for blood pressure and discrimination based on sexual orientation.

METHODS

Study Population

Our study population consisted of a subset of participants enrolled in the Coronary Artery Risk Development in Young Adults (CARDIA) study, a prospective epidemiologic investigation examining evolution of cardiovascular risk factors among young black and white men and women in the United States (23, 24). The CARDIA study design and characteristics of its black and white participants have been described in previous publications (23, 24). At baseline (1985–1986), the study enrolled 5,115 young adults, 18 to 30 years old, representing 51 percent of eligible persons contacted. Participants were recruited by community-based random sampling from three U.S. cities (Birmingham, Alabama; Chicago, Illinois; Minneapolis, Minnesota), and from the membership of a large prepaid health plan in Oakland, California. The study targeted recruitment to 16 groups, defined by race/ethnicity, gender, age (18 to 24 years old, 25 to 30 years old), and education (completed 12 or less, or more than 12, years of education). Recruitment criteria did not address sexual orientation.

The initial CARDIA cohort included 1,480 black women, 1,157 black men, 1,307 white women, and 1,171 white men, of whom 48, 56, 27, and 28 percent, respectively, had completed at most a high school education. Participants subsequently returned for examinations conducted in Year 2 (1987–1988; 90 percent retention), Year 5 (1990–1991; 84 percent cumulative retention), and Year 7 (1992–1993; 79 percent cumulative retention). None of these exams included questions about sexual identity (e.g., lesbian, gay, bisexual, heterosexual). The Year 7 examination included questions on participants' self-reported experiences of discrimination and responses to unfair treatment. All examinations were conducted with the approval of institutional review boards at each institution, and informed consent was obtained at each examination from each study participant.

In 1989, a self-administered HIV-related questionnaire was mailed to a subset of the CARDIA cohort (25). This subset included all participants residing in Minneapolis and a 50 percent random sample of participants living in the other three cities. Response rates ranged from 48 percent among black men and 64 percent among black women to 79 percent among white men and 90 percent among white women; in all four groups, response rates increased with educational level. The present study includes the 412 black women, 221 black men, 619 white women, and 472 white men (N = 1,724) who (*a*) responded to the 1989 HIV questionnaire and (*b*) participated in the Year 7 examination.

Data Collection Methods

At baseline, CARDIA participants provided interviewers with data on their race/ethnicity, gender, and date of birth. These data were verified at each subsequent examination. Participants responding to the self-administered 1989 HIV-related questionnaire provided data on lifetime number of same- and other-sex sexual partners. The questionnaire, however, did not include questions on: sexual identity; age at which respondents, if ever, first, and also most recently, had sex with a same-sex sexual partner; or age at or situations in which, if any, individuals with same-sex partners had "come out" to themselves or to others.

The question about discrimination based on sexual orientation asked at the Year 7 exam, using a self-administered questionnaire, read as follows:

> Have you experienced discrimination, been prevented from doing something, or been hassled or made to feel inferior in any of the following situations because of your sexual preference (heterosexual, bisexual, homosexual)? (yes or no)
> a. In your family
> b. At school
> c. Getting a job
> d. At work
> e. At home
> f. Getting medical care
> g. On the street or in a public setting

The questionnaire, which also included questions about responses to unfair treatment and other kinds of discrimination, was based on an instrument previously developed for a study on hypertension in relation to racial and gender discrimination (14). The first question asked participants how they usually responded if they felt they had been treated unfairly: "accept it as a fact of life" versus "try to do something about it"; and "talk to other people about it" versus "keep it to yourself." Five sets of comparable questions then asked, in the following order, about experiences of discrimination based on "gender," "race or color," "socioeconomic position or social class," "sexual preference," and "religion." Questions about discrimination based on race/ethnicity, social class, and religion each included one situation not listed in the question about discrimination based on sexual orientation ("from the police or in the courts"), omitted "in your family," and substituted "getting housing" for "at home." The question about discrimination based on gender was the same as that about discrimination based on sexual orientation, except for omitting "in your family." For each type of discrimination, the specified situations reflect circumstances in which people have typically reported encountering discrimination (22, 26–38). In this chapter, we present only data pertaining to discrimination based on sexual orientation, race/ethnicity, and gender, since virtually none of the respondents reported experiencing discrimination based on religion and there was little variation in responses to questions about discrimination based on social class.

Additional sociodemographic and anthropometric data were provided by CARDIA participants at the Year 7 exam, as gathered by self- and interviewer-administered questionnaires and physical examination, following standardized protocols (23, 39–41). To measure blood pressure, trained and certified techni-cians used a random zero sphygmomanometer to record participants' resting 30-second pulse, followed by three systolic and fifth-phase diastolic blood pres-sures (measured at 1-minute intervals); we used the average of the second and third blood pressure measurements in our analyses. Participants provided inter-viewers with data on alcohol consumption (ml/day) and reported their cigarette smoking status via a self-administered questionnaire (40, 41). We classified their occupations (social class) as either "working class" (nonsupervisory, nonpro-fessional employees) or "executive, professional, or managerial" (14, 42, 43).

Statistical Analyses

Our analyses sought to describe (*a*) the number and proportion of black and white women and men who had same-sex sexual partners; (*b*) their socio-demographic characteristics; (*c*) their self-reported responses to unfair treat-ment and experiences of discrimination based on sexual orientation, gender, and race/ethnicity; and (*d*) associations of these characteristics with systolic and dia-stolic blood pressure. We examined the discrimination data in terms of each of the three kinds and also in their combinations, and for the blood pressure analyses we focused on comparisons of persons reporting no discrimination, only discrimination based on sexual orientation, and other combinations or types of discrimination.

We analyzed the blood pressure data in two ways: as a continuous variable and as a gender-specific dichotomous variable. For the latter analyses, we set the cut-point at the top 20th percentile of the blood pressure distribution (equal to 120 mm Hg for systolic and 79 mm Hg for diastolic among men, and 113 mm Hg and 74 mm Hg, respectively, among the women). Because both approaches yielded comparable results, and because findings pertaining to systolic and diastolic blood pressure were similar, we present only results regarding systolic blood pressure treated as a continuous variable. To describe and compare distribution of participants' characteristics, we used SAS Version 6.04 for per-sonal computers (44). Given the exploratory nature of our study and constraints imposed by small numbers, we chiefly present descriptive statistics. Where appropriate, however, we calculated mean differences and their 90 percent confidence intervals (C.I.) (equivalent to a one-sided test with $\alpha = 0.05$) for comparisons involving continuous variables, and odds ratios and their 90 percent C.I. for comparisons involving dichotomous variables.

RESULTS

Among the 1,724 study participants, 42 (2.4 percent) reported having only same-sex sexual partners and 162 (9.4 percent) reported sexual partners of both sexes (Table 1). On average, these women and men were in their late 20s when they provided data on lifetime number of sexual partners, and in their early 30s when they participated in the Year 7 exam and answered questions about responses to unfair treatment and experiences of discrimination (Tables 2 and 3). Among each of the four racial/ethnic–gender groups, those reporting exclusively same-sex and those reporting both-sex sexual partners were comparable for most of the sociodemographic and anthropometric characteristics analyzed, and also in their reported responses to unfair treatment and reported experiences of discrimination (data available upon request). In the light of these similarities, and of constraints imposed by small numbers, we combined these two groups into one, defined as persons with at least one same-sex sexual partner. Percentages of respondents belonging to this group ranged from 6 percent among the black women and men to 14 percent and 16 percent among the white women and men.

Among participants with same-sex sexual partners, women and men within each racial/ethnic group had similar socioeconomic profiles, but racial/ethnic disparities were evident (Table 2). Thus, over 60 percent of the black women and men, but only 40 percent of their white counterparts, were employed in working-class occupations; nearly one-quarter, compared with one-tenth, had an

Table 1

CARDIA participants reporting ever having a same-sex sexual partner, by race/ethnicity and gender, among participants with data on lifetime number of sexual partners, Year 7 exam, 1992–1993

Sex of sexual partners	Total, no. (%) (n = 1,724)	Black, no. (%) Women (n = 412)	Men (n = 221)	White, no. (%) Women (n = 619)	Men (n = 472)
Only same-sex	42 (2.4)	3 (0.7)	1 (0.5)	11 (1.8)	27 (5.7)
Both sexes	162 (9.4)	24 (5.8)	12 (5.4)	76 (12.3)	50 (10.6)
Total	204 (11.8)	27 (6.6)	13 (6.0)	87 (14.1)	77 (16.3)

Table 2

Selected sociodemographic and anthropometric characteristics of CARDIA participants with same-sex and only other-sex sexual partners, by race/ethnicity and gender, among participants with data on lifetime number of sexual partners, Year 7 exam, 1992–1993

Characteristic	At least one same-sex sexual partner[a]				Only other-sex sexual partners[a]			
	Black		White		Black		White	
	Women (n = 27)	Men (n = 13)	Women (n = 87)	Men (n = 77)	Women (n = 368)	Men (n = 196)	Women (n = 509)	Men (n = 375)
Age (yrs)								
25–29	15%	8%	13%	20%	36%	29%	19%	18%
30–34	41	62	49	44	38	37	48	47
35–37	44	31	38	36	26	34	33	35
Study center								
Birmingham, AL	22	15	6	10	20	24	13	16
Chicago, IL	7	8	9	10	19	18	16	17
Minneapolis, MN	37	46	61	65	27	33	50	50
Oakland, CA	33	31	24	14	33	26	21	17
Social class								
Working class	62	64	41	43	68	61	43	34
Executive, professional, managerial	38	36	59	57	32	39	57	66
Annual family income								
<$12,000	26	23	13	9	20	15	6	5
$12,000–$24,999	33	31	16	21	25	23	17	15
$25,000–$49,999	22	38	40	40	37	46	40	38
≥$50,000	19	8	31	30	19	15	37	42

	4%	0%	1%	3%	5%	7%	2%	2%
Educational level								
<High school	65	69	40	41	71	73	40	44
≥High school, <4 yrs college	31	31	59	56	24	20	57	55
≥4 yrs college								
Home ownership								
Rents	59	69	41	51	58	57	37	32
Owns	41	31	59	49	42	43	63	68
Health insurance status								
No	30	31	26	30	15	29	15	21
Yes	70	69	74	70	85	71	85	79
Marital/partner status (married/living as married)								
Currently	48	46	67	54	49	58	71	69
Previously	19	8	5	4	18	16	9	6
Never	33	46	29	42	32	27	20	24
Cigarette smoking status								
Never smoked	52	69	45	43	62	54	50	62
Ex-smoker	15	8	31	23	7	11	27	15
Current smoker	33	23	24	34	30	36	23	23
Alcohol consumption								
Non-drinker	11	8	18	1	28	18	13	12
Drinks alcohol	89	92	82	99	72	82	87	88
Alcohol (drinkers only; average ml/day)								
≤2.4	33	33	51	25	49	24	43	27
2.4–11.9	38	17	28	29	32	26	31	28
≥12.0	29	50	21	46	19	50	25	45

Table 2

(Cont'd.)

| Characteristic | At least one same-sex sexual partner[a] | | | | Only other-sex sexual partners[a] | | | |
| | Black | | White | | Black | | White | |
	Women (n = 27)	Men (n = 13)	Women (n = 87)	Men (n = 77)	Women (n = 368)	Men (n = 196)	Women (n = 509)	Men (n = 375)
Body mass index								
<24	22%	31%	52%	47%	31%	28%	58%	32%
24–28	37	38	24	43	29	44	25	48
≥28	41	31	23	10	40	28	17	20

[a] A small number of participants were missing data for the selected characteristics. The distribution of missing data was:

At least one same-sex sexual partner
  Black women: social class = 3, education = 1
  Black men: social class = 2
  White women: social class = 1, body mass index = 1
  White men: social class = 2

Only other-sex sexual partners
  Black women: social class = 26, annual family income = 10, home ownership = 2, education = 3, marital/partner status = 4, health insurance = 2, smoking status = 1, alcohol consumption = 2, body mass index = 12
  Black men: social class = 8, annual family income = 8, home ownership = 3, education = 2, marital/partner status = 3, health insurance = 3, body mass index = 3
  White women: social class = 30, annual family income = 9, home ownership = 3, education = 9, marital/partner status = 3, health insurance = 3, smoking status = 3, alcohol consumption = 2, body mass index = 23
  White men: social class = 3, annual family income = 1, home ownership = 1, education = 3, marital/partner status = 1, health insurance = 1, alcohol consumption = 2, body mass index = 1

annual family income under $12,000; under one-third, compared with nearly two-thirds, completed four or more years of college education; and about two-thirds, compared with under one-half, rented, rather than owned, their homes. Nearly a third in all four groups, however, lacked health insurance, and nearly half or more described their marital/partner status as "living as married." Between 40 and 50 percent of the black and white women and the white men and nearly 70 percent of the black men had never smoked cigarettes. Additionally, virtually all of the white men and 80 to 90 percent of the black and white women and black men reported ever having consumed alcohol. Among drinkers, average daily consumption was notably lowest among the white women and highest among the white and black men. Body mass index was likewise lowest among the white women. To provide context, Table 2 presents these same data for the 1,448 respondents reporting only other-sex sexual partners.

Self-reports of experiences of discrimination varied by race/ethnicity and gender (Table 3). Overall, about one-third of the black men, white women, and white men reported experiencing discrimination based on sexual orientation in three or more of the seven specified situations. The odds of black women reporting this experience, however, was 0.3 times that in the other three groups (90 percent C.I. = 0.1, 0.9). In all four groups, "in public" ranked among the top three selected sites. Other most commonly reported situations were, for both the black women and black men: "in the family," "getting a job," and "at work." For the white women, they were "in the family" and "at work"; and for the white men, "at work" and "at school." Self-reported responses to unfair treatment were comparable among all four groups (Table 3).

Discrimination based on sexual orientation was only one of several types reported by these women and men with same-sex sexual partners (Table 3). About half the women, whether black or white, reported experiencing gender discrimination in three or more of the six selected situations. Approximately 60 percent of the black women and men, moreover, reported experiencing racial discrimination in three or more of the seven specified situations.

To capture more fully experiences of multiple types of discrimination, Table 3 also presents data on whether participants reported having ever experienced any versus none of the three kinds of discrimination, in all eight possible permutations. Nearly all of the women, black and white, reported experiencing some form of discrimination. Almost half the black women reported a combination of racial and gender discrimination, and a third reported all three types of discrimination. A quarter of the black men reported, respectively, racial discrimination only, racial and gender discrimination only, and all three. Similar proportions of the white women reported gender discrimination only, sexual orientation and gender discrimination only, and all three. Among the white men, one-fifth reported experiencing discrimination based only on sexual orientation, an experience reported by very few white women and by none of the black women or men.

Table 3

Self-reported response to unfair treatment and experiences of discrimination based
on sexual orientation, gender, and race/ethnicity, by race/ethnicity and gender,
among CARDIA participants with at least one same-sex sexual partner,
Year 7 exam, 1992–1993

	Black		White	
Characteristic	Women (n = 27)[a]	Men (n = 13)	Women (n = 87)[a]	Men (n = 77)
Response to unfair treatment				
Take action + talk to others	74%	85%	85%	74%
Take action + keep to self	4	0	2	0
Accept + talk to others	22	15	12	21
Accept + keep to self	0	0	1	5
Reported experiences of discrimination based on:				
Sexual orientation ("yes")				
In family	22	23	38	29
At home	7	15	14	4
At school	7	38	24	32
Getting a job	15	23	17	21
At work	15	23	28	36
Getting medical care	0	15	16	14
In public	18	38	48	51
No. of "yes" responses				
0	67	61	48	44
1 or 2	18	8	20	20
3 or more	15	31	33	36
Gender ("yes")				
At home	23	23	36	4
At school	44	23	38	13
Getting a job	48	15	44	23
At work	56	31	58	17
Getting medical care	26	23	22	3
In public	63	38	83	22
No. of "yes" responses				
0	11	46	12	58
1 or 2	41	39	35	30
3 or more	48	15	54	12

Table 3

(Cont'd.)

Characteristic	Black		White	
	Women (n = 27)[a]	Men (n = 13)	Women (n = 87)[a]	Men (n = 77)
Reported experiences of discrimination based on:				
Race/ethnicity ("yes")				
At school	48%	38%	14%	3%
Getting a job	52	62	6	3
At work	59	54	13	4
Getting housing	44	46	0	3
Getting medical care	15	15	2	1
From police or in courts	38	54	4	0
In public	63	69	36	25
No. of "yes" responses				
0	15	23	61	69
1 or 2	30	15	31	30
3 or more	56	62	8	1
Multiple types of discrimination (one or more "yes" responses)				
None	7	15	8	25
Sexual orientation only	0	0	4	20
Sexual orientation + race/ ethnicity only	0	8	0	6
Sexual orientation + gender only	0	8	23	17
Race/ethnicity only	4	23	0	8
Gender only	8	0	26	8
Race/ethnicity + gender only	48	23	14	4
All three (sexual orientation, race/ethnicity, gender)	33	23	26	13

[a]Data on response to unfair treatment were missing for only one white woman, and data on reported experiences of discrimination were missing for only one black woman and one white woman.

Analyses of systolic blood pressure in relation to reported experiences of multiple types of discrimination were limited by small numbers (data available upon request). Among the white men, however, systolic blood pressure was 3.3 mm Hg higher (90 percent C.I. = −0.3, 7.0) and 5.4 mm lower (90 percent C.I. = −9.4, −1.4), respectively, among the 19 men reporting no discrimination and among the 15 men reporting discrimination based only on sexual orientation than among the remaining 43 men. Systolic blood pressure among these white men was thus 9 mm Hg lower among those reporting only discrimination based on sexual orientation than among those reporting no discrimination. Among the white women, blood pressure was also lowest among the three women reporting only discrimination based on sexual orientation. Small numbers, however, preclude meaningful analyses of these data and the data for the black women and men.

DISCUSSION

Our study found that, in a community-based cohort of urban adults, 25 to 37 years old, not selected on the basis of sexual orientation, more than one-third of the black women and men and one-half of the white women and men with same-sex sexual partners reported experiencing discrimination based on sexual orientation. Depending upon participants' race/ethnicity and gender, reports of discrimination based on sexual orientation often—but not always—overlapped with reports of racial and gender discrimination. Additionally, among white men with same-sex partners, systolic blood pressure tended to be highest among those reporting no experiences of discrimination based on sexual orientation.

Before considering the plausibility of our findings, we note several caveats regarding interpretation of our data. These concern classification of who was at risk of experiencing anti-gay discrimination and, among those experiencing such discrimination, who reports this experience.

First, we lacked data on how participants identified their own sexual orientation. Our limited data on sexual behavior do not necessarily match data on self-identified sexual orientation, since individuals who have same-sex sexual partners may not identify as lesbian, gay, or bisexual (45–51). Results of a recent national probability survey on sexual behavior among 3,432 U.S. adults found, for example, that whereas 7.6 percent of white men reported ever having same-sex sexual partners, only 3.0 percent identified as "homosexual" or "bisexual"; the corresponding proportions for white women were 4.0 and 1.7 percent; for black men, 5.8 and 1.5 percent; and for black women, 3.5 and 0.6 percent (45, p. 305). The slightly higher proportions for lifetime history of same-sex sexual partners observed in our study for black CARDIA participants, and notably higher proportions among white participants, may be artifactual, reflecting error due to response bias (since likelihood of having a same-sex sexual partner increases with education (45, pp. 302–310), and nonresponse to the CARDIA HIV questionnaire was inversely related to educational level) and also chance, related to our relatively small sample size. To our knowledge, except for the one national survey mentioned above (45), no other contemporary data are available on proportions of U.S. adults reporting same-sex sexual partners stratified by race/ethnicity and gender (46, 47), thus limiting possibilities for comparing results across studies.

Our data on sexual partners also did not permit us to distinguish between participants with markedly different lifetime patterns of same-sex sexual partners. Individuals who had several same-sex sexual partners when in their teens, and thereafter had only other-sex partners, for example, could not be differentiated from those who had several other-sex sexual partners in their teens and thereafter had only same-sex partners. Thus, our group of persons with same-sex sexual partners (most of whom had partners of both sexes) most likely included individuals with limited as well as extensive histories of same-sex sexual partners. This type of misclassification would dilute estimates of both prevalence of anti-gay discrimination and associations between blood pressure and anti-gay discrimination, compared with what would be observed among individuals who identify as lesbian or gay.

Second, we lacked data on the age at which participants first and also most recently, if ever, had sex with a same-sex sexual partner, and also on the age at which and contexts in which individuals identifying as lesbian, gay, or bisexual had "come out" (to themselves or others). In contrast to persons experiencing discrimination based on race/ethnicity or gender (traits typically ascribed by external observers from birth onwards), many people who identify as lesbian, gay, or bisexual often do not articulate this identity until or after adolescence and can, to protect themselves, more readily "pass" as heterosexual (by remaining "in the closet") than can people of color "pass" as white or women "pass" as men (11, 34–36, 48, 52–54). An in-depth study of eight black lesbians on the impact of perceived discrimination upon their intimate relationships (54), for example, found that five of these women reported experiencing both racial and gender discrimination whereas only one reported experiencing discrimination based on sexual orientation. The other seven reported they had not experienced this type of discrimination because they were not "out" in their work settings and had disclosed their sexual identity only to "select friends," a decision reflecting awareness of anti-gay discrimination and thus motivation for being "in the closet." Lacking data on the relevant etiologic period and contexts for exposure to anti-gay discrimination would likewise dilute estimates of the occurrence and health effects of anti-gay discrimination.

A third concern is that some people who experience discrimination may not acknowledge or report it as such. Research indicates that individuals belonging to groups that experience discrimination are more likely to state that members of their group, rather than they themselves, have experienced discrimination (6, 22, 26–31, 55). This phenomenon may reflect what some have termed "internalized oppression" (including "internalized homophobia") (5, 7, 22, 56), whereby unfair treatment is perceived by members of stigmatized groups as "deserved" and nondiscriminatory. By contrast, individuals belonging to stigmatized groups but who refuse to accept a stigmatized status may be more able and willing to name discriminatory treatment. Additional theoretical and empirical work, primarily concerning racial discrimination, suggests that individuals who have been discriminated against—and who feel relatively powerless to challenge this discrimination—may find it painful, and thus difficult, to admit, either to themselves or to another person, that they have experienced discrimination (14; 22; 26, pp. 25, 276; 27, pp. 96, 112, 168; 28, pp. 77–79; 55). Supporting this interpretation, some preliminary research on internalized oppression and racial discrimination among black women and men in the United Kingdom has found that individuals who initially report not having experienced racial discrimination, upon being asked more probing questions, acknowledge having experienced discrimination and find it hard to talk about (55). The net effect, again, would be to underestimate the prevalence of anti-gay discrimination and bias estimates of its effects upon health status.

Absent data on the likelihood and extent of exposure to anti-gay discrimination, and on participants' ability and willingness to report such discrimination, our findings on reported prevalence of anti-gay discrimination and its association with blood pressure are provisional at best. Even so, because our data raise important questions about studying patterns and possible health consequences of anti-gay discrimination, topics which have received little attention in public health literature, we consider three implications of our data, bearing these caveats in mind.

First, our view that our findings most likely underestimate, rather than exaggerate, prevalence of anti-gay discrimination is supported by results of the handful of other empirical studies on this topic. A 1986 study of 166 lesbian/gay/bisexual respondents recruited at lesbian and gay events and through friendship networks at Yale University found that even though approximately half hid their sexual identity from their classmates, teachers, and colleagues, 65 percent reported having experienced verbal insults, 50 percent had been threatened with physical violence or chased or followed, and 10 percent had personal property damaged on account of their sexual orientation (4). Similar results were found in a 1989 study of 125 lesbian/gay/bisexual respondents at Pennsylvania State University (57). Anti-gay violence and discrimination were also reported, respectively, by 12 and 16 percent of 741 primarily white, college-educated, and "out" gay men in New York City, in a 1987 study that enrolled participants through personal friendship networks and mailing lists of gay organizations (7). Moreover, among 1,925 primarily white, college-educated U.S. lesbians who filled out a survey distributed between 1984 and 1985 among lesbian friendship networks and through lesbian, gay, and women's organizations and bookstores, even though fewer than one-third were "out" to their heterosexual colleagues, friends, and families, 52 percent reported having been verbally attacked, 8 percent had lost their jobs, and 6 percent had been physically attacked on account of being lesbian (3).

Studies on anti-gay discrimination in medical settings provide less consistent data. A 1992 study noted that fewer than 5 percent of the gay/bisexual men enrolled in the Multicenter AIDS Cohort Study said they had been refused medical or dental treatment because of their sexual orientation (58). By contrast, half of the 711 lesbian/gay/bisexual physicians and medical students responding to a 1994 national survey reported "actually observing colleagues providing reduced care or denying care to patients because of their sexual orientation"; 88 percent recalled "hearing colleagues making disparaging remarks about lesbian, gay, and bisexual patients"; and 67 percent knew of "lesbian, gay, or bisexual patients who had received substandard care or been denied care because of their sexual orientation" (9). One-third of the respondents also said they had either been refused medical privileges, fired, denied employment or a promotion or a loan, or had been denied referrals from other physicians because of their sexual orientation, and the same proportion, along with half of the medical students, reported they had been "subjected to verbal harassment or insulted by their medical colleagues" (9).

The higher levels of anti-gay discrimination reported in these studies may reflect, in part, differences in study population and study design. Most of these prior investigations focused chiefly on experience of college-educated white lesbians and gay men recruited either by announcement directed to, or snowball sampling conducted among, self-defined lesbian and gay communities (2, 4, 7, 9, 57). Because these studies document experiences of individuals most likely to be at risk of, conscious of, and able to name anti-gay discrimination, it is not surprising that our study yielded somewhat lower, but still disturbing, estimates of self-reported experiences of discrimination based on sexual orientation—estimates which, to the best of our knowledge, are the first to be derived from a community-based cohort selected without reference to sexual orientation.

A second implication of our findings is that studies of anti-gay discrimination and health should consider diverse, not single, types of discrimination. Notably, only the white men and women reported experiencing discrimination based only on sexual orientation, whereas the black men and women were far more likely to report experiencing racial discrimination, and both the black and white women reported substantial levels of gender discrimination. Analyzing how discrimination affects the health of people who, among other things, identify as lesbian or gay may thus require considering other kinds of discrimination to which they may be exposed. Along these lines, a 1994 study of 603 and 829 African American women and men with at least one previous homosexual experience found that both the women and men reported higher levels of depressive distress than would have been expected based on their race/ethnicity, gender, or sexual orientation alone (5). The authors interpreted these findings as being indicative of cumulative effects of multiple types of discrimination. Thus, rather than assume there is some "universal" lesbian/gay/bisexual experience, our study likewise indicates that analyses of lesbian/gay/bisexual health should be conducted among diverse sectors of this population. Another implication is that our estimates of the prevalence of anti-gay discrimination may not be generalizable to populations *not* represented in the CARDIA cohort, that is, teens and older or rural women and men, whether black or white, or who are impoverished or belong to other racial/ethnic groups.

Finally, our tentative findings of an inverse relationship between self-reported experiences of anti-gay discrimination and elevated blood pressure among only the white men with at least one same-sex sexual partner resemble results of two prior studies on racial discrimination and blood pressure (14, 15). In these studies, blood pressure was highest, especially for working-class black study participants, among those reporting *not* having experienced racial discrimination. One possible explanation is that transient increases in blood pressure associated with not expressing anger, and possibly denial or repression of adverse experiences, may, over time, result in permanently elevated blood pressure (14–21, 59, 60). Thus, among groups defined, in part, by discrimination, those most able and willing to name experiencing this discrimination may be at lower risk of elevated blood pressure than those stating they have not experienced discrimination. That such a pattern in relation to anti-gay discrimination was apparent only among the white men most likely reflects their not being subject to racial and gender discrimination, thus increasing the likelihood of detecting health-related consequences of solely anti-gay discrimination. The cross-sectional nature of our study design, however, along with the small numbers, sharply limits causal inference (61) linking reported experiences of anti-gay discrimination to elevated blood pressure.

In summary, our study indicates that self-reported experiences of discrimination based on sexual orientation are sufficiently common to warrant consideration as an important obstacle to good health among lesbian, gay, and bisexual populations. At issue are not only overt ways in which people can be directly harmed on account of their sexual orientation, such as by queer-bashing, but also other ways that discrimination can hurt: by impeding access to health care, by harming people's chances to succeed at school and in the workforce, and by devaluing one's sense of oneself.

To better assess the hypothesis that anti-gay discrimination adversely affects health (in addition to being morally and politically unacceptable), we thus recommend that future studies (*a*) incorporate better, longitudinal data on sexual identity and sexual partners, and on duration, frequency, and intensity of exposure to discrimination and responses to this discrimination; (*b*) consider a wider variety of health outcomes; and (*c*) be conducted among larger, more diverse populations more varied with regard to race/ethnicity, social class, age, and geographic locale. Only in this way will public health realities and needs of complex yet understudied populations of lesbians, gay men, and bisexuals be better understood.

Acknowledgments — We would like to thank Heather McCreath for assistance with computer programming, and Dr. Sally Zierler for helpful suggestions on analysis and interpretation of the data.

Note — A talk entitled "Prevalence and Health Implications of Discrimination Based on Sexual Orientation: A Study of Black and White Women and Men with Same-Sex Sexual Partners in the CARDIA Cohort," based upon the results of this investigation, was presented by Dr. Nancy Krieger at the 123rd annual meeting of the American Public Health Association, San Diego, October 30 to November 2, 1995.

REFERENCES

1. Council on Scientific Affairs, American Medical Association. *Health Care Needs of Gay Men and Lesbians in the U.S.* CSA Report 8-I-94. December 1994.
2. Stevens, P. E. Lesbian health care research: A review of the literature from 1970 to 1990. *Health Care Women Int.* 13: 91–120, 1992.
3. Bradford, J., Ryan, C., and Rothblum, E. D. National lesbian health care survey: Implications for mental health care. *J. Consult. Clin. Psychol.* 62: 228–242, 1994.
4. Herek, G. M. Documenting prejudice against lesbians and gay men on campus: The Yale Sexual Orientation Survey. *J. Homosex.* 25: 15–30, 1993.
5. Cochran, S. D., and Mays, V. M. Depressive distress among homosexually active African American men and women. *Am. J. Psychol.* 151: 524–529, 1994.
6. Mays, V. The Impact of Perceived Discrimination on the Health and Well-being of African Americans. Paper presented at the 122nd annual meeting of the American Public Health Association, Washington, D.C., October 29–November 4, 1994.
7. Meyer, I. H. Minority stress and mental health in gay men. *J. Health Soc. Behav.* 36: 38–56, 1995.
8. Erwin, K. Interpreting the evidence: Competing paradigms and the emergence of lesbian and gay suicide as a "social fact." *Int. J. Health Serv.* 23: 437–453, 1993.
9. Schatz, B., and O'Hanlan, K. *Anti-gay Discrimination in Medicine: Results of a National Survey of Lesbian, Gay, and Bisexual Physicians.* American Association of Physicians for Human Rights, San Francisco, May 1994.
10. Taylor, I., and Robertson, A. The health needs of gay men: A discussion of the literature and implications for nursing. *J. Adv. Nurs.* 20: 560–586, 1994.
11. Cochran, S. D., and Mays, V. M. Disclosure of sexual preference to physicians by black lesbians and bisexual women. *West. J. Med.* 149: 616–619, 1988.
12. Cotton, P. Attacks on homosexual persons may be increasing, but many 'bashings' still aren't reported to police. *JAMA* 267: 2999–3000, 1992.
13. Dunlap, D. W. Survey on slayings of homosexuals finds high violence and low arrest rate. *New York Times*, December 21, 1994, p. A10.
14. Krieger, N. Racial and gender discrimination: Risk factors for high blood pressure? *Soc. Sci. Med.* 30: 1273–1281, 1990.
15. Krieger, N., and Sidney, S. Racial discrimination and blood pressure: The CARDIA study of young black and white women and men. *Am. J. Public Health* 86: 1370–1378, 1996.

16. Armstead, C. A., et al. Relationship of racial stressors to blood pressure and anger expression in black college students. *Health Psychol.* 8: 541–556, 1989.
17. James, S. A., et al. John Henryism and blood pressure differences among black men. II. The role of occupational stressors. *J. Behav. Med.* 7: 259–274, 1984.
18. Dressler, W. W. Lifestyles, stress, and blood pressure in a southern black community. *Psychosom. Med.* 52: 182–198, 1990.
19. Anderson, N. B., et al. Hypertension in blacks: Psychological and biological perspectives. *J. Hypertens.* 7: 161–172, 1989.
20. Gentry, W. D. Relationship of anger-coping styles and blood pressure among black Americans. In *Anger and Hostility in Cardiovascular and Behavioral Disorders*, edited by M. A. Chesney and R. H. Rosenman, pp. 139–147. Hemisphere, Washington, D.C., 1985.
21. Williams, D. R. Black-white differences in blood pressure: The role of social factors. *Ethnicity Dis.* 2: 12–141, 1992.
22. Krieger, N., et al. Racism, sexism, and social class: Implications for studies of health, disease, and well-being. *Am. J. Prev. Med.* 9(Suppl. 2): 82–122, 1993.
23. Cutter, G. R., et al. Cardiovascular risk factors in young adults: The CARDIA baseline monograph. *Controlled Clin. Trials* 12: 1S–77S, 1991.
24. Friedman, G., et al. Study design, recruitment, and some characteristics of the examined subjects. *J. Clin. Epidemiol.* 41: 1105–1116, 1988.
25. Berrios, D. C., et al. HIV antibody testing in young, urban adults. *Arch. Intern. Med.* 152: 397–402, 1992.
26. Feagin, J., and Sikes, M. P. *Living With Racism: The Black Middle-Class Experience.* Beacon Press, Boston, 1994.
27. Sigelman, L., and Welch, S. *Black Americans' Views of Racial Inequality: The Dream Deferred.* Cambridge University Press, Cambridge, England, 1991.
28. Essed, P. *Understanding Everyday Racism.* Sage, Newbury Park, Calif., 1991.
29. Benokratis, N. V., and Feagin, J. R. *Modern Sexism: Blatant, Subtle, and Covert Discrimination.* Prentice-Hall, Englewood Cliffs, N.J., 1986.
30. Gardner, C. B. Passing by: Street remarks, address rights, and the urban female. *Sociol. Inquiry* 50: 328–356, 1980.
31. Campbell, A., and Schuman, H. *Racial Attitudes in Fifteen American Cities.* Survey Research Center, University of Michigan, Ann Arbor, 1969.
32. Sennett, R., and Cobb, J. *The Hidden Injuries of Class.* Knopf, New York, 1972.
33. Coleman, R. P., and Rainwalter, L. *Social Standing in America: New Dimensions of Class.* Basic Books, New York, 1979.
34. Faderman, L. *Odd Girls and Twilight Lovers: A History of Lesbian Life in Twentieth-Century America.* Penguin, New York, 1991.
35. Katz, J. N. *Gay American History: Lesbians and Gay Men in the U.S.A. A Documentary History*, Rev. Ed. Meridian, New York, 1992 [1976].
36. Galloway, G. (ed.). *Prejudice and Pride: Discrimination against Gay People in Modern Britain.* Routledge & Kegan Paul, London, 1983.
37. U.S. Equal Employment Opportunity Commission. *Facts About Religious Discrimination.* Government Printing Office, Washington, D.C., 1992.
38. U.S. Commission on Civil Rights. *Religious Discrimination: A Neglected Issue.* Government Printing Office, Washington, D.C., 1980.
39. Smith, D. E., et al. Longitudinal changes in adiposity associated with pregnancy: The CARDIA Study. *JAMA* 271: 1747–1751, 1994.
40. Wagenknecht, L. E., et al. Cigarette smoking behavior is strongly related to educational status: The CARDIA Study. *Prev. Med.* 19: 158–69, 1990.

41. Dyer, A. R., et al. Alcohol intake and blood pressure in young adults: The CARDIA study. *J. Clin. Epidemiol.* 43: 1–13, 1990.
42. Krieger, N. Women and social class: A methodological study comparing individual, household, and census measures as predictors of black/white differences in reproductive history. *J. Epidemiol. Community Health* 45: 35–42, 1991.
43. Wright, E. O., et al. The American class structure. *Am. Sociol. Rev.* 47: 709–726, 1982.
44. SAS Institute. *SAS Language Guide for Personal Computers. Release 6.04 Edition.* Cary, N.C., 1990.
45. Laumann, E. O., et al. *The Social Organization of Sexuality: Sexual Practices in the United States.* University of Chicago Press, Chicago, 1994.
46. Diamond, M. Homosexuality and bisexuality in different populations. *Arch. Sex. Behav.* 22: 291–310, 1993.
47. Sell, R. L., Wells, J. A., and Wypij, D. The prevalence of homosexual behavior and attraction in the United States, the United Kingdom, and France: Results of national population-based samples. *Arch. Sex. Behav.* 24: 235–248, 1995.
48. Weeks, J. *Sexuality and Its Discontents: Meaning, Myths, and Modern Sexualities.* Routledge & Kegan Paul, London, 1985.
49. Billy, J. O., et al. The sexual behavior of men in the United States. *Fam. Plann. Perspect.* 25: 52–60, 1993.
50. Stevens, P. E. HIV prevention for lesbians and bisexual women: A cultural analysis of community intervention. *Soc. Sci. Med.* 39: 1565–1578, 1994.
51. Zierler, S. A Comparison of Women's Sexuality According to HIV Status. Paper presented at HIV in Women Conference, Washington, D.C., February 1995.
52. Gomez, J. L., and Smith, B. Taking the home out of homophobia: Black lesbian health. In *Black Women's Health Book: Speaking for Ourselves*, edited by E. C. White, pp. 198–213. Seal Press, Seattle, 1990.
53. Collins, P. H. *Black Feminist Thought: Knowledge, Consciousness, and the Politics of Empowerment.* HarperCollins Academic Press, London, 1990.
54. Mays, V. M., Cochran, S. D., and Rhue, S. The impact of perceived discrimination on the intimate relationships of black lesbians. *J. Homosex.* 25: 1–14, 1993.
55. Parker, H., Botha, J. L., and Haslam, C. "Racism" as a Variable in Health Research— Can It Be Measured? Poster presented at the 38th annual scientific meeting of the U.K. Society for Social Medicine, Leeds, September 14–16, 1994.
56. Neisen, J. H. Heterosexism: Redefining homophobia for the 1990s. *J. Gay Lesbian Psychother.* 1: 21–35, 1990.
57. D'Augelli, A. R. Lesbians' and gay men's experience of discrimination and harassment in a university community. *Am. J. Community Psychol.* 17: 317–321, 1989.
58. Kass, N. E., et al. Homosexual and bisexual men's perceptions of discrimination in health services. *Am. J. Public Health* 82: 1277–1279, 1992.
59. Alexander, F. Emotional factors in hypertension. *Psychosom. Med.* 1: 173–179, 1939.
60. Folkow, B. Sympathetic nervous control of blood pressure: Role in primary hypertension. *Am. J. Hypertens.* 2(3, Pt. 2): 103S–111S, 1989.
61. Kelsey, J. L., Thompson, W. D., and Evans, A. S. *Methods in Observational Epidemiology*, pp. 188–189. Oxford University Press, New York, 1986.

Conclusion

The chapters in this book, not surprisingly, focus on the toll of social inequalities as manifested in social disparities in health. Evidence, while not sufficient to bring about change on its own, is nevertheless necessary—both to galvanize concern and to provide insight into potentially beneficial versus harmful remedies to societal ills, including inequitable distributions of disease. Yet, as has been explicitly argued since at least the time of Engels (and before), raising a critique is not the same as proposing solutions. It is for this reason that new initiatives in public health, building once again on earlier insights, are turning attention to analyzing how policies and interventions promoting social justice and human rights can usefully improve population health and decrease social inequities in disease, disability, and death (1–11). To this new work, social epidemiology can bring a helpful array of conceptual and methodologic tools, including an appreciation for the importance of monitoring trends over time; etiologic period; confounding; and due caution about whether health impacts of specified policies can meaningfully be analyzed (or not) using epidemiologic approaches.

Fittingly, by being true to the historical nature of our work, ideas, and population patterns of health, disease, and well-being, the conclusion of this book thus ends with a beginning, regarding the next set of tasks at hand. Even though the basic concerns of social epidemiology with relationships between social injustice and social inequalities in health are not new, causes of disease, disability, and death have changed over time, as have etiologic explanations. These critical shifts reflect—and at times affect—changes in global and regional economies, policies, physical infrastructures, and ecosystems. For this reason, while a concern about "fundamental causes" of social inequalities is necessary (12), to be concretely relevant, each generation must confront anew the specific exposures, problems, and potential solutions of its time (1, 13–17).

A focus on social disparities in health, from an epidemiologic perspective, is thus at once essential, liberating, and humbling. In challenging us to be as creative and rigorous as we can be in our frameworks, questions, and methods, we can draw on the insights and precedents of our predecessors who forged the field of public health precisely by focusing on social disparities in health and advocating just solutions while continuing to expand the repertoire of conceptual and methodologic tools to conduct our work. By conducting theoretically informed empirical investigations illuminating the determinants, processes, and consequences of the embodiment of inequality, social epidemiologists can make their particular contribution to global coalitions and networks by working for social justice, human rights, and social equity in health as part of improving the well-being of people and this planet.

REFERENCES

1. Krieger, N. Theories for social epidemiology in the 21st century: An ecosocial perspective. *Int. J. Epidemiol.* 30: 668–677, 2001.
2. Krieger, N., et al. and the HIA "promise and pitfalls" conference group. Assessing health impact assessment: Multidisciplinary and international perspectives. *J. Epidemiol. Community Health,* 57: 659-662, 2003.
3. Gruskin, S., and Tarantola, D. Health and human rights. In *The Oxford Textbook of Public Health* (4th ed., pp. 311-335), edited by R. Detels, J. McEwen, R. Beaglehole, K. Tanaka. Oxford University Press, New York, 2001.
4. Mann, J., et al. Health and human rights. In *Health and Human Rights: A Reader,* edited by J. M. Mann, S. Gruskin, M. A. Grodin, and G. J. Annas. Routledge, New York, 1999.
5. Krieger, N., and Gruskin, S. Frameworks matter: Ecosocial and health and human rights perspectives on women and health—The case of tuberculosis. *J. Am. Women's Med. Assoc.* 56: 137–142, 2001.
6. Braverman, P., and Gruskin S. Defining equity in health. *J. Epidemiol. Community Health* 57: 254–258, 2003.
7. Navarro, V. The economic and political determinants of human (including health) rights. *Int. J. Health Serv.* 8: 145–168, 1978.
8. Navarro, V. (ed.). *The Political Economy of Social Inequalities: Consequences for Health and Quality of Life.* Baywood Publishing Co., Amityville, NY, 2002.
9. Graham, N. Building an inter-disciplinary science of health inequalities: The example of lifecourse research. *Soc. Sci. Med.* 55: 2005–2016, 2002.
10. Macintyre, S., et al. Using evidence to inform health policy: Case study. *Br. Med. J.* 322: 222–225, 2001.
11. Davey Smith, G., Ebrahim, S., and Frankel, S. How policy informs the evidence: "Evidence based" thinking can lead to debased policy making. *Br. Med. J.* 322: 184–185, 2001.
12. Link, B. G., and Phelan, J. C. Editorial: Understanding sociodemographic differences in health—The role of fundamental social causes. *Am. J. Public Health* 86: 471–473, 1996.
13. Krieger, N. Epidemiology and social sciences: Towards a critical reengagement in the 21st century. *Epidemiol. Rev.* 11: 155–163, 2001.
14. Davey Smith, G., Dorling, D., and Shaw M. (eds.), *Poverty, Inequality and Health in Britain 1800–2000: A Reader.* Policy Press, Bristol, 2001.
15. Rosen, G. *A History of Public Health (1958).* Introduction by Elizabeth Fee; Bibliographical essay and new bibliography by Edward T. Morman. Expanded ed. Johns Hopkins University Press, Baltimore, MD, 1993.
16. Porter, D. *Health, Civilization and the State: A History of Public Health from Ancient to Modern Times.* Routledge, London, 1990.
17. Hamlin, C. *Public Health and Social Justice in the Age of Chadwick. Britain: 1800–1854.* Cambridge University Press, Cambridge, UK, 1998.

Index

525

Massachusetts, standardizing vital
statistics in, 52
Maternal mortality, 39
Measuring social inequalities, 14–15
See also individual subject headings
Medicaid/Medicare, 87, 281, 282, 312,
476
Medical Nemesis (Illich), 80
Medical Reform, 29, 30
Medical Services of Sonora (SEMESON),
397
Mendel, Gregor, 243
Mental health
homelessness among women, 485,
489–490
lesbian/gay suicide, 261, 267
unemployment, 225–226, 228
See also Psychological stress
Mexican American women and childbirth
mortality rates, 455
Mexico-U.S. border region. *See*
Maquiladora workers
Monitoring, 3
Moral/economic dimensions to public
definition of disability, 280
Morgan, T. H., 243
Motor vehicle *vs.* other unintentional
injury, 429, 430
Multicenter AIDS Study, 517
Multifactorial etiology, 29
Multiracial status and racial data,
164–165

National Center for Health Statistics, 5,
164
National Committee on Vital and Health
Statistics, 5
National Health and Nutrition
Examination Survey
(NHANES-1), 318, 320
National Health and Nutrition
Examination Survey
(NHANES-II), 448, 456, 468
National Health Interview Survey (1979),
227

National Health Survey (1935-1936), 7,
67, 70
National Institutes of Health (NIH), 93,
478
National Longitudinal Survey of Youth,
207–208
National Mortality Followback Survey
(1986), 463
National Opinion Research Surveys
(1996), 183
National Tuberculosis Association,
61–65, 68, 69
Native Americans, 160–161, 247, 249,
266–267
See also data, quality of racial *and*
socioeconomic position *under*
Race/ethnicity and
socioeconomic position;
Discrimination, studying health
consequences of; Whites, racial
ideology/ explanations for health
inequalities among middle-class
Navarro, Vicente, 1
Nazi racial science, 140
New Deal, 68–71
NHANES-1 Epidemiologic Follow-up
Study (NHEFS), 318–323,
326–329
1900-1950: measuring social inequalities
in health in U.S.
Chapin, Charles V., 61
Children's Bureau, 60–61
Cold War, 69–71
conclusions/summary, 72–73
Depression, the Great, 66–69
National Tuberculosis Association,
61–65
retrenchment of socioeconomic
analyses, 66–71
socioeconomic data an vital statistics,
linking, 59–66
studies on income and health, early,
54–59
vital statistics, standardizing U.S.,
52–54

ABOUT THE EDITOR

Nancy Krieger is Associate Professor, Department of Society, Human Development and Health, Harvard School of Public Health; Associate Director, Harvard Center for Society and Health; and co-founder and chair of the Spirit of 1848 Caucus of APHA. A social epidemiologist, she received her PhD in Epidemiology from University of California at Berkeley in 1989; her background includes biochemistry, philosophy of science, and the history of public health, plus 20 years of engagement in issues involving social justice, science, and health. Her work focuses on etiology of, monitoring, and theories to explain population distributions of disease and social disparities in health.

CPSIA information can be obtained
at www.ICGtesting.com
Printed in the USA
FFHW011026261119
56469592-62264FF